Interventional Nephrology

Alexander S. Yevzlin • Arif Asif • Loay Salman

Editors

Interventional Nephrology

Principles and Practice

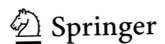 Springer

Editors
Alexander S. Yevzlin, MD
Division of Nephrology
Department of Medicine (CHS)
University of Wisconsin
Madison, WI
USA

Loay Salman, MD
Interventional Nephrology
University of Miami Miller School of Medicine
Miami, FL
USA

Arif Asif, MD, FASN, FNKF
Division of Nephrology and Hypertension
Albany Medical College
Albany, NY
USA

ISBN 978-1-4614-8802-6   ISBN 978-1-4614-8803-3   (eBook)
DOI 10.1007/978-1-4614-8803-3
Springer New York Heidelberg Dordrecht London

Library of Congress Control Number: 2013956233

Printed on acid-free paper

Springer is part of Springer Science+Business Media (www.springer.com)

This textbook is dedicated to my children, Alana, Margarita, and Shayna, whose light shines even on these pages.

– Alexander S. Yevzlin

Dedicated to my sister, Azra Asif, for her love, kindness, devotion and endless support.

– Arif Asif

"To my dear parents, my wonderful wife Rama, and my beautiful children, Zane and Jude, for their endless inspiration."

– Loay Salman

Contents

Contributors

Kenneth Abreo, MD Nephrology Section, Department of Medicine, Louisiana State University Health Sciences Center, Shreveport, LA, USA

Zulqarnain Abro Nephrology Section, Department of Medicine, Louisiana State University Health Sciences Center, Shreveport, LA, USA

Anil K. Agarwal, MD, FACP, FASN, FNKF Division of Nephrology, The Ohio State University, Columbus, OH, USA

Stephen R. Ash, MD, FACP Indiana University Health Arnett, Lafayette, Indiana, USA

HemoCleanse, Inc. and Ash Access Technology, Inc., Lafayette, Indiana, USA

Arif Asif, MD, FASN, FNKF Division of Nephrology and Hypertension, Albany Medical College, Albany, NY, USA

Gerald A. Beathard, MD, PhD, FASN Department of Internal Medicine, University of Texas Medical Branch, Galveston, TX, USA

Mary Buffington, MD, JD Nephrology Section, Department of Medicine, Louisiana State University Health Sciences Center, Shreveport, LA, USA

Micah R. Chan Division of Nephrology, Department of Medicine, University of Wisconsin College of Medicine and Public Health, Madison, WI, USA

Diego A. Covarrubias, MD Vascular Interventional Radiology, Massachusetts General Hospital, Harvard Medical School, Boston, MA, USA

Department of Radiology, Massachusetts General Hospital, Harvard Medical School, Boston, MA, USA

John H. Crabtree Department of Surgery, Kaiser Permanente, Bellflower, CA, USA

Rajiv Dhamija, MD Division of Nephrology, Rancho Los Amigos National Rehabilitation Center, Downey, CA, USA

Internal Medicine, Western University of Health Sciences, Pomona, CA, USA

Ramanath Dukkipati, MD Division of Nephrology, University of California, Torrance, Los Angeles, CA, USA

Talia Eisen, MD Division of Nephrology, Department of Internal Medicine, University of California Davis Medical Center, Sacramento, CA, USA

Marius C. Florescu, MD Division of Nephrology, Department of Internal Medicine, University of Nebraska Medical Center, Omaha, NE, USA

Peter J. Mason Division of Cardiovascular Medicine, Department of Medicine, University of Wisconsin College of Medicine and Public Health, Madison, WI, USA

Laura Maursetter, DO Division of Nephrology, Department of Medicine, University of Wisconsin School of Medicine and Public Health, Madison, WI, USA

K.M.L.S.T. Moorthi, MD Nephrology Associates of Northern Indiana, Merrillville, IN, USA

Rajeev Narayan, MD Clinical and Interventional Nephrology, San Antonio Kidney Disease Center, San Antonio, TX, USA

Vandana Dua Niyyar, MD, FASN Division of Nephrology, Emory University, Atlanta, GA, USA

Jason W. Pinchot Department of Radiology, Vascular and Interventional Radiology Section, University of Wisconsin School of Medicine and Public Health, Madison, WI, USA

Troy J. Plumb, MD Division of Nephrology, Department of Internal Medicine, University of Nebraska Medical Center, Omaha, NE, USA

Karthik Ramani, MD Division of Nephrology and Hypertension, University of Cincinnati, Cincinnati, OH, USA

Jamie Ross, MD Division of Nephrology, Department of Internal Medicine, University of California Davis Medical Center, Sacramento, CA, USA

Bharat Sachdeva, MD Nephrology Section, Department of Medicine, LSU Health Sciences Center, Shreveport, LA, USA

Loay Salman, MD Interventional Nephrology, University of Miami Miller School of Medicine, Miami, FL, USA

Adrian Sequeira Nephrology Section, Department of Medicine, LSU Health Sciences Center, Shreveport, LA, USA

Ravish Shah, MD Division of Nephrology, The Ohio State University, Columbus, OH, USA

Roman Shingarev, MD Division of Nephrology, Department of Medicine, University of Alabama, Birmingham, AL, USA

Chieh Suai Tan, MBBS Vascular Interventional Radiology, Massachusetts General Hospital, Harvard Medical School, Boston, MA, USA

Department of Radiology, Massachusetts General Hospital, Harvard Medical School, Boston, MA, USA

Aris Q. Urbanes, MD Lifeline Vascular Access, Vernon Hills, IL, USA

Tushar J. Vachharajani, MD, FACP, FASN Nephrology Section, W. G. (Bill) Hefner Veterans Affairs Medical Center, Salisbury, NC, USA

Davinder Wadehra, MD, MBBS LMC Diabetes and Endocrinology, Brampton, ON, Canada

Steven Wu, MD Vascular Interventional Radiology, Massachusetts General Hospital, Harvard Medical School, Boston, MA, USA

Department of Medicine, Massachusetts General Hospital, Harvard Medical School, Boston, MA, USA

Department of Radiology, Massachusetts General Hospital, Harvard Medical School, Boston, MA, USA

Alexander S. Yevzlin, MD Division of Nephrology, Department of Medicine (CHS), University of Wisconsin, Madison, WI, USA

Preoperative Evaluation: History

Marius C. Florescu and Troy J. Plumb

1.1 Introduction

An accurate and thorough preoperative history is a key component of any procedure. The preoperative history allows the interventionalist to appropriately plan the procedure. This includes devising the optimal approach, anticipating potential complications, providing safe and effective conscious sedation, ordering the appropriate supplies, and ultimately performing a successful intervention.

It is very important that the history is taken personally by the physician who will perform the procedure. A pertinent history can be obtained relatively quickly, but the extra effort expended taking a thorough history is time well spent. The interaction with the patient while taking a history allows the physician the opportunity to develop an overall evaluation of the patient, establish a good rapport, and often helps to decrease the patient's anxiety before starting the procedure.

Unlike most surgical procedures in which the clinician meets the patient in clinic to evaluate them prior to scheduling a procedure, the interventionalist is often meeting a patient for the first time immediately prior to the procedure. In that short period of time, the interventionalist must determine if the requested procedure is indicated and/or appropriate, and whether it can be safely performed on each individual patient. Despite the fact that it is often colleagues and practice partners requesting a procedure, the well-being of the patient is ultimately the responsibility of the person performing the procedure. The history is a key factor in making these determinations and ensuring the patients safety.

This chapter is intended to highlight the aspects of history the interventional nephrologist needs to focus in order to perform a successful and safe procedure. We strived to explain the clinical use of the information obtained through the preprocedure history. Some of the information may overlap for different procedures. Each subchapter has a table that summarizes the pertinent information needed for each procedure.

1.2 Conscious Sedation

The patient's comfort is paramount to the success of the intervention. A combination of narcotics (usually fentanyl) and benzodiazepines (usually midazolam) is typically used to induce conscious sedation. There is a fine balance between optimal, too much, and not enough sedation. The presence of comorbid conditions which may complicate the procedure or place the patient at increased risk for conscious sedation must be sought [1].

Is the patient at an increased risk of an adverse reaction to conscious sedation? Has the patient had prior difficulties with anesthesia or conscious sedation? Most dialysis patients have had multiple vascular access interventions and are aware of prior problems. Additional questions that may be helpful include inquiry as to the need for reversal of the sedation, unintended intubation, or paradoxical reactions to medications during prior procedures. Has the patient required an extended stay in recovery or did they have to stay overnight?

Patient allergies or adverse reactions to benzodiazepines or narcotics must be identified. What was the nature of the reaction and how severe was it? Many times the patients are not allergic to the whole class of medications and related medications can be safely used. Which narcotic or benzodiazepine was tolerated during previous procedures in order to use it again?

Patients with severe abnormalities of the major organ systems such as diseases of the airways, heart, or liver may be at particular risk for adverse events. A detailed history with regard to these organs/systems should be performed so that conscious sedation and the procedure may be adapted for each particular condition. Patients with severe chronic obstructive pulmonary disease tend to be more sensitive to the respiratory depression induced by conscious sedation so lower doses of both benzodiazepines as well as narcotics should be used. Likewise, patients with severe sleep apnea need to be identified and over sedation avoided.

M.C. Florescu, MD (✉) • T.J. Plumb, MD
Division of Nephrology, Department of Internal Medicine, University of Nebraska Medical Center, Omaha, NE, USA
e-mail: mflorescu@unmc.edu

A.S. Yevzlin et al. (eds.), *Interventional Nephrology*,
DOI 10.1007/978-1-4614-8803-3_1, © Springer Science+Business Media New York 2014

Box 1.1. Conscious Sedation History
1. Severe abnormalities of major organ systems
2. Presence of hepatic insufficiency
3. Presence of severe COPD, sleep apnea
4. Allergic reactions to benzodiazepines and/or narcotics. Type of allergic reaction. What narcotics or benzodiazepines were tolerated during previous procedures?
5. Panic attacks or claustrophobia during previous procedures
6. Previous adverse experiences with sedation
7. Chronic use of narcotic pain medications or benzodiazepines
8. History of drug abuse

Box 1.2. History Information Important for Any Procedure
1. Conditions that are increasing the risk of bleeding: coagulopathies, thrombocytopenia, anticoagulant, or antiplatelet medications
2. What is the medical condition that requires anticoagulant therapy?
3. Allergies to narcotics, benzodiazepines, local anesthetic, radiocontrast dye, latex, heparin
4. Recent myocardial infarction
5. Presence of pacemakers, cardiac prosthetic valves, inferior vena cava filters
6. Previous deficits in mentation or inability to ambulate or move extremities. The baseline needs to be known before starting the procedure
7. Pregnancy test

Patients with severe congestive heart failure or chronic hypotension may have further lowering of their blood pressure with sedation. Patients with orthopnea from congestive heart failure or volume overload cannot lie flat on the procedure table and often benefit from a wedge placed under their chest. Patients with advanced liver disease may have delayed drug metabolism and thus require lower doses of medications and a prolonged period of observation post-procedure.

At the other extreme, patients may require additional sedation or even general anesthesia. It is important to know if the patient has extreme anxiety, a history of panic attacks, or claustrophobia. It is relatively common for patients to be intolerant of having their face covered during the procedure. Oftentimes premedicating the patient or "tenting" the drape will be enough to make the procedure manageable for them. In other cases, deeper sedation or general anesthesia may be required. Likewise, those with chronic pain may require special accommodations, padding, or deeper sedation.

Patient with ongoing drug abuse or chronic narcotic and/or benzodiazepine use may require higher doses than usual to induce effective analgesia and sedation.

Box 1.1 summarizes the pertinent history needed for conscious sedation.

1.3   Medications, Allergies, Preexisting Conditions, and Contraindications

All hemodialysis access procedures target large blood vessels and therefore bleeding is a potentially serious complication. It is of utmost importance to identify those patients at increased risk of bleeding in order to minimize this risk. Interventionalists should inquire regarding the presence of coagulopathies, thrombocytopenia, history of prolonged bleeding, anticoagulant medication, and antiplatelet therapies. One must be aware of the newer classes of medications such as oral direct thrombin inhibitors which are now commonly used to treat atrial fibrillation. Severe coagulation problems should be corrected before the procedure.

In addition to knowing whether an anticoagulant is being used, the interventionalist needs to know the indication for anticoagulation. In some instances, anticoagulation can be safely stopped for a few days (for instance, atrial fibrillation), but in others, like prosthetic cardiac valves, the anticoagulation cannot be stopped and the patient needs bridging anticoagulation.

Careful attention should be paid to the review of the patient's allergies. In the previous section we discussed inquiring about reactions to narcotics and benzodiazepines. Other clinically important allergies include radiocontrast dye, latex, local anesthetic, and heparin. Patients with radiocontrast dye allergy often respond well to preventive treatment. Depending on the protocol, corticosteroid and antihistamine medications administered beginning the day prior to or the day of the procedure can drastically reduce the risk of reactions. Latex allergy can be extremely severe. Latex-free gloves and instruments need to be used in allergic patients. Patients may have allergies to local anesthetics. Heparin is used in many of our procedures and in locking solutions for hemodialysis catheters. Heparin-induced thrombocytopenia needs to be identified and heparin completely avoided in these patients.

It is imperative to be aware of a patient's preexisting conditions such as chronic hypotension, dementia, neurologic deficits, severe congestive heart failure, and chronic pain in order to differentiate these preexisting conditions from possible new changes that may occur during the procedure or conscious sedation. Likewise, the presence of cardiac prosthetic valves, pacemakers, and inferior vena cava filters needs to be known to exercise caution to prevent dislodging these implants.

Although women with end-stage renal disease (ESRD) have a low likelihood of becoming pregnant, this is not something to be overlooked. All women with child-bearing potential should be asked about a possible pregnancy. A pregnancy test should be performed if there is any possibility that the patient could be pregnant. Additionally, elective procedures should be avoided immediately after an acute myocardial infarction.

Box 1.2 summarizes the important aspects of history that need to be taken before any procedure.

1.4 Hemodialysis Catheter Procedures

Tunneled hemodialysis catheter procedures are an important part of the daily activity of any interventional nephrologist and consist of:

- New tunneled hemodialysis catheter placement
- Exchange of a catheter through the same vascular access and tunnel
- Exchange of a catheter through the same vascular access with creation of new tunnel
- Removal of the catheter and placement of another catheter through a different access
- Converting a non-tunneled "temporary" hemodialysis catheter into a tunneled catheter
- Removal of a tunneled catheter
- Obliteration of a fibrous sheath that caused catheter malfunction

Each procedure has a unique indication and addresses specific problems. Before any procedure we must know the precise indication for the procedure to be able to determine which procedure should be performed.

1.4.1 New HD Catheter

In addition to knowing that the patient has committed to HD, we must exclude the presence of an ongoing severe infection which is a contraindication to the procedure. We should inquire about fever, chills, and positive blood cultures.

Most hemodialysis patients have had one or more HD catheters since initiating hemodialysis. The presence of catheters can induce the formation of a stenosis in the veins used for vascular access as well as the superior vena cava. In order to place a new catheter, we need to know the following: how many catheters has the patient had? What was the location and how long ago were the catheters placed and removed? Were there any previous unsuccessful attempts to place HD catheters because of stenosed central veins? The use of external jugular veins for the catheter placement suggests the lack of a suitable internal jugular vein for access.

The presence of superior vena cava stenosis might impede catheter placement. Asking the patient if they have/had upper chest collateral veins, arm, face, or breast swelling can identify the presence of a central vein stenosis. Identifying these abnormalities can be very helpful and may prompt the interventionalist to consider performing a venous angiogram with possible angioplasty through the venous access site before attempting to place the catheter.

Some patients may have malformations of the central veins such as persistent left-sided superior vena cava. Malformations are rare, but can make catheter placement more challenging. Other patients may have had neck surgeries, neck radiation, or trauma which can also alter the anatomy and the availability of central veins. Each of these possibilities should be considered and inquiry made.

Equally important is the presence of cardiac pacemakers or other intravascular devices such as inferior vena cava filters [2, 3]. The location of current or previously placed pacemakers as well as the timing of their placement should be known. The presence of pacemaker leads can often lead to central vein stenosis at the site of the venous access. The presence of pacemaker wires in the SVC should make us cautious during vein dilatation and catheter placement to avoid dislodging these leads. The presence of an inferior vena cava filter can interfere with a femoral vein tunneled catheter placement or an inferior vena cava catheter placement.

During our discussion with the patient, we need to discuss where the catheter exit site will be. Some patients may ask to change the position of the exit site. In the authors' practice, we try to accommodate patient preferences when medically possible.

We need to know the patient's height as this closely correlates with the length of the catheter will use.

1.4.2 Hemodialysis Catheter Removal

The reason for catheter removal should be well understood by both the patient and interventionalist. The most common indications for this procedure are catheter infection and catheter malfunction, or the catheter is no longer needed because of functional arteriovenous access, transition to peritoneal dialysis, or recovery of renal function. It is important to know the precise indication, as to avoid removing a catheter that is still needed.

1.4.3 Hemodialysis Catheter Exchange

What is the reason for exchange? Infection? Malfunction? If the reason is infection, is there a tunnel infection that will require the creation of a new tunnel? Is the patient stable enough to have the catheter safely exchanged over a wire? Has the patient's fever resolved? Are there recent blood cultures to assess for an ongoing infection? Has the infection been appropriately treated [4, 5] ?

Purulent tunnel exit site discharges, pain, redness, and warmth over the tunnel suggest a tunnel infection. If the tunnel is infected, it is sometime possible to exchange the catheter through the same venous access, but a new tunnel needs to be created.

If the reason for exchange is catheter malfunction, we need to know the nature of the malfunction and if thrombolytic medications have been used to lock the catheter [6]. How successful was the thrombolytic in improving catheter blow flow? If the blood flow did not improve following thrombolytics, it suggests the presence of a fibrous sheath, catheter malposition, migration, or the presence of a kink. Catheters that allow fluid to be infused but from which blood cannot be removed or "pulled" often have a fibrous sheath.

In such cases, a pullback angiogram is needed to assess for the presence of a fibrous sheath and to obliterate it if present.

1.4.4 Conversion From a Non-Tunneled to a Tunneled Catheter

This procedure is mainly performed in hospitalized patients. Prior to this procedure it is paramount to exclude the presence of an ongoing generalized or local infection and confirm that the patient requires ongoing dialysis.

Box 1.3 summarizes the main questions for the hemodialysis catheter procedures.

1.5 Angiogram and Angioplasty Procedures

Before starting the procedure, it is important to know the reason the patient was referred for angiogram. The reason can suggest the abnormality that will be found and help in planning the procedure. Prolonged bleeding after hemodialysis needle removal suggests the presence of high pressure in the vascular access and the presence of a tight outflow stenosis. Outflow stenosis is also suggested by increased venous pressures signaled by the hemodialysis machine. Poor blood flow or decreased urea reduction ratio suggests an inflow or outflow stenosis.

The date of access creation and any previous procedures (type and timing) performed must be known. The need for frequent angioplasties (every 2–3 months) suggests a poor prognosis, and referral for surgical revision may be indicated. It is very helpful to know the location of the lesions (stenoses) identified and treated on previous procedures. How severe were the lesions? What size balloons were used for angioplasty and with what results? What pressure was used for angioplasty? Were stents placed, and if so, what size

and types of stents were used? What was the indication and location of the stents? If stents were placed, are the stents being stuck for hemodialysis? Were there any complications such as vessel rupture or hematomas after previous procedures? The patient is unlikely to be able to answer many of these questions, but these can usually be found by looking at the medical record or contacting the dialysis unit [7].

If the access is a graft, it is useful to review the operative note to know the diameter and the type of the graft used in order to use the appropriate balloon size for angioplasty.

It is also important to ask the patient if there have been any changes in the access. Pain, erythema, and increased warmth of the access site can suggest infection. Skin ulceration or skin thinning over the access site mainly when it is associated with the presence of a dilated access (aneurysm or pseudoaneurysm) can suggest impending rupture, and this constitutes an emergency that needs to be recognized and treated promptly.

Box 1.4 summarizes the pertinent history prior to angiogram and angioplasty procedures.

1.6 Thrombectomy

In addition to the history discussed in Sect. 4.4, there is additional information that must be obtained prior to a thrombectomy procedure. When did the access thrombose? When was the last time the access was successfully used for hemodialysis [8]? How many thrombectomy procedures has the patient had on the current vascular access and what was their timing? A vascular access that has required numerous recent thrombectomies may not benefit from another one.

Prior to starting a thrombectomy procedure, the interventionalist must differentiate the arterial from the venous

---

Box 1.5. Thrombectomy
1. Approximate time of thrombosis
2. Last time the access had been used
3. Number and timing of the recent thrombectomy procedures

Box 1.6. Pertinent History Prior to Thrombectomy Procedure
1. Timing of angioplasty
2. Location of the lesions
3. Close attention to lesions that recur in less than 3 months, especially if located in the central veins or venous anastomosis of the AVG

Box 1.7. Fistula Salvage
1. How long since the access was created?
2. Type and access location
3. Were there any complications after AVF creation surgery?
4. Use history: Has the fistula been used? Have there been problems with its use?
5. What other procedures were performed to attempt the salvage of the current access and what were the findings and interventions?
6. Timing of the previous salvage attempts
7. CHF, severe cardiac valve abnormalities, arterial stenoses, central veins stenoses
8. The location and timing of the previous failed vascular accesses

---

portion of the graft. Many times the patient is able to tell us by the color of the needles used for HD. The red needle is placed in the arterial side and the blue needle in the venous side. In the author's experience, this is not always reliable. If available, the orientation of the graft can be found from the operative note. Otherwise, the orientation of the graft may be determined based on the position of the wire when advanced into the vessels of the chest.

It is also a good idea to know the hemodialysis catheter placement history in case the thrombectomy procedure is unsuccessful and a tunneled HD catheter needs to be placed.

Box 1.5 summarizes the pertinent history prior to thrombectomy procedure.

1.7 Stent Placement

The role of the endoluminal stents in the management of hemodialysis (HD) vascular access stenosis is unclear. With the exception of Flair stent graft for AVG venous anastomotic stenosis, there is no FDA indication for the use of stents in HD vascular access [9–11]. In most circumstances, stents add significant cost and the potential for complications with unclear benefit. The possible indications to use stents for the management of hemodialysis vascular access are:
1. Angioplasty failure. Not anymore with the introduction of new, high pressure balloons
2. Venous anastomosis stenosis of the AVG (Flair stent graft).
3. Recurrent stenosis (mainly in the central veins) less than 3 months after angioplasty
4. Vascular access rupture after angioplasty to stop the bleeding

If the use of a stent is contemplated, the preprocedure history should focus on information that would support their use, such as the number and timing of procedures performed on the current access. Frequent, recurrent, and clinically

significant stenosis following successful angioplasty might support the use of a stent. Central lesions may benefit from stent placement more than peripheral lesions

Box 1.6 summarizes the pertinent information needed prior to stent placement.

1.8 Fistula Salvage Procedure for Lack of Maturation

Approximately 50 % of new AVF fail to mature. Endovascular interventions to assist AVF maturation are effective in increasing the rate of AVF maturation. The timing of the procedure is important. Six-week post-AVF creation seems to be the ideal time to intervene if the AVF fails to mature. The preoperative history should focus on location of the AVF, the timing of placement, and intraoperative or postoperative complications of AVF surgery. Was the access ever used for hemodialysis? If so, what problems were encountered? Were other procedures performed to assist in this AVF maturation? If yes, what was the timing, findings, or interventions [12–14]?

Are there any factors that may prevent an increase in AVF blood flow? We should inquire about severe congestive heart failure (CHF) and severe cardiac valvular abnormalities (stenoses or regurgitation) which may decrease cardiac output. Could the patient have arterial stenoses and central veins stenoses, or do they have a pacemaker?

The location and timing of previous failed vascular accesses is important. If the patient still has vascular access sites available, a new AVF might be a better option than repeated attempts to salvage an access that is not maturing despite numerous interventions. If there are no other vascular access sites available, we can consider being more aggressive in hopes that the access will mature.

Box 1.7 summarizes the important data needed prior to fistula salvage procedures.

2. Asif A, Salman L, Lopera G, Haqqie SS, Carrillo R. Transvenous cardiac implantable electronic devices and hemodialysis catheters: recommendations to curtail a potentially lethal combination. Semin Dial. 2012;25(5):582–6.
3. Tourret J, Cluzel P, Tostivint I, Barrou B, Deray G, Bagnis CI. Central venous stenosis as a complication of ipsilateral haemodialysis fistula and pacemaker. Nephrol Dial Transplant. 2005;20(5): 997–1001.
4. Beathard GA, Urbanes A. Infection associated with tunneled hemodialysis catheters. Semin Dial. 2008;21(6):528–38.
5. Krishnasami Z, Carlton D, Bimbo L, et al. Management of hemodialysis catheter-related bacteremia with an adjunctive antibiotic lock solution. Kidney Int. 2002;61(3):1136–42.
6. Beathard GA. Catheter thrombosis. Semin Dial. 2001;14(6):441–5.
7. Beathard GA. Angioplasty for arteriovenous grafts and fistulae. Semin Nephrol. 2002;22(3):202–10.
8. Jain G, Maya ID, Allon M. Outcomes of percutaneous mechanical thrombectomy of arteriovenous fistulas in hemodialysis patients. Semin Dial. 2008;21(6):581–3.
9. Salman L, Asif A. Stent graft for nephrologists: concerns and consensus. Clin J Am Soc Nephrol. 2010;5(7):1347–52.
10. Yevzlin AS, Maya ID, Asif A. Endovascular stents for dialysis access: under what circumstances do the data support their use? Adv Chronic Kidney Dis. 2009;16(5):352–9.
11. Yevzlin A, Asif A. Stent placement in hemodialysis access: historical lessons, the state of the art and future directions. Clin J Am Soc Nephrol. 2009;4(5):996–1008.
12. Mercado C, Salman L, Krishnamurthy G, et al. Early and late fistula failure. Clin Nephrol. 2008;69(2):77–83.
13. Beathard GA. Fistula salvage by endovascular therapy. Adv Chronic Kidney Dis. 2009;16(5):339–51.
14. Asif A, Roy-Chaudhury P, Beathard GA. Early arteriovenous fistula failure: a logical proposal for when and how to intervene. Clin J Am Soc Nephrol. 2006;1(2):332–9.
15. Alvarez AC, Salman L. Peritoneal dialysis catheter insertion by interventional nephrologists. Adv Chronic Kidney Dis. 2009;16(5): 378–85.

Box 1.8. Pertinent Information History Prior to PD Catheter Placement

1. Abdominal surgeries
2. Previous PD catheters placed
3. Peritonitis, diverticulitis, ectopic abdominal pregnancies, ascites

---

1.9 Peritoneal Dialysis (PD) Catheter Placement

Fluoroscopic- or peritoneoscopic-guided peritoneal dialysis catheter placement by interventional nephrologists is gaining popularity. Before the insertion of a new peritoneal dialysis catheter, special attention should be directed towards the condition of the peritoneal cavity. The number, types, and dates of all previous abdominal procedures need to be known [15]. Does the patient have any hernias that may make this procedure contraindicated? A history of abdominal surgeries is not a contraindication to PD tube placement, but it is important to know this prior to the procedure in order to evaluate the chances of a successful and safe procedure as well as the success of peritoneal dialysis as a technique. A history of peritonitis, diverticulitis, ectopic abdominal pregnancies, and severe abdominal trauma should also be elicited.

Any concurrent infection needs to be treated before the catheter insertion. Presence and nature of ascites is important to know before the PD catheter insertion.

Box 1.8 summarizes the pertinent information history prior to PD catheter placement.

References

1. Beathard GA, Urbanes A, Litchfield T, Weinstein A. The risk of sedation/analgesia in hemodialysis patients undergoing interventional procedures. Semin Dial. 2011;24(1):97–103.

Preoperative Evaluation: Physical Examination

Vandana Dua Niyyar

2.1 Introduction

He who studies medicine without books sails an uncharted sea, but he who studies medicine without patients does not go to sea at all.

— William Osler

Physical examination is an invaluable tool that assists in diagnosis and evaluation of the patient and has been used since the advent of medicine. As nephrologists and interventionists, we are well aware that hemodialysis vascular access problems represent an exceedingly important part of the management of the end-stage renal disease patient. A thorough and detailed physical examination is an excellent, non-invasive, and accurate method for initial evaluation and helps guide our interventional procedures – not only those that we do but also those that we do not do.

2.2 General Examination

An abbreviated history and physical should be performed on every patient that presents for an interventional procedure, focusing not only on the presenting symptoms but also on allergies, comorbidities, and a review of systems. A medication history focusing on chronic systemic anticoagulation and pain medication should also be obtained, as adjustments may need to be made to the doses used in conscious sedation and the use of heparin or thrombolytics. A detailed history of previous accesses, including evidence of central venous catheters like scars on the chest wall, swollen extremities and face, and the presence of collaterals, the presence of PICC lines and cardiac rhythm devices, as well as presence and location of previous surgical scars, should be performed and documented.

A thorough physical examination of the access itself is essential prior to performing an interventional procedure. Not only does it provide information with regard to the source of the problem but also aids in planning the interventional procedure and the direction of cannulation. Numerous studies have shown excellent correlation of the accuracy of physical examination as compared to the gold standard (angiography) in both AVF and AVG [1–3]. Indeed, physical examination has shown to be equivalent to, if not superior to, normalized pressure ratios [4], ultrasound [5], or intra-access pressures [6] in detecting access dysfunction. In a comparison of the accuracy of physical examination performed by a trained nephrology fellow as compared to an experienced interventionist, the authors reported a strong correlation between their findings, concluding that physical examination of the dialysis vascular access is an important and easily taught skill that should be incorporated in a formal training curriculum [7].

This chapter details the general physical examination as well as intervention-specific scenarios for particular interventions.

2.3 Physical Examination Prior to Access Placement

The majority of patients in the USA still initiate hemodialysis with a central venous catheter (CVC) as their access [8, 9]. Frequent phlebotomies, peripherally inserted central catheters (PICC) lines [10], and a high prevalence of comorbid conditions including diabetes, obesity, and vascular disease [11] in this high-risk population may negatively impact the vasculature and contribute to early AVF dysfunction. In order to mitigate this complication, preoperative evaluation for arteriovenous fistula (AVF) placement can, and must, be done. The initial physical examination may be done by a simple bedside assessment to determine the patency of the

V.D. Niyyar, MD, FASN
Division of Nephrology, Emory University,
Woodruff Memorial Research Building Rm. 338,
1639 Pierce Drive, Atlanta, GA 30322, USA
e-mail: vniyyar@emory.edu

A.S. Yevzlin et al. (eds.), *Interventional Nephrology*,
DOI 10.1007/978-1-4614-8803-3_2, © Springer Science+Business Media New York 2014

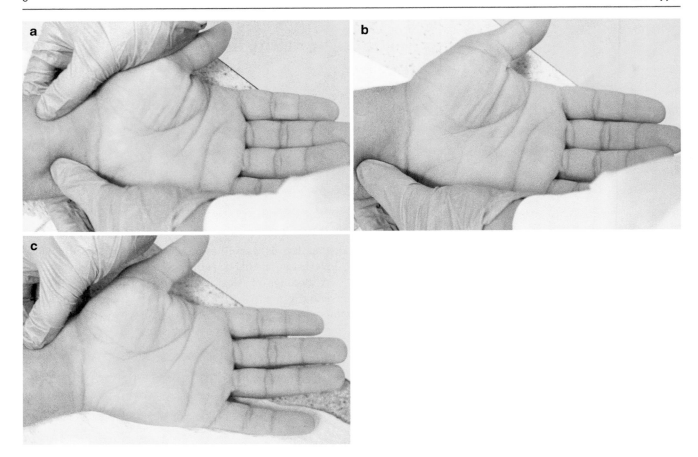

Fig. 2.1 The Allen test. The patient is asked to make a fist and pressure is applied over both the ulnar and the radial arteries to occlude them (**a**). Once the fist is opened, the hand should appear blanched or pale. Then, pressure is alternately released from both the arteries and the hand monitored for return to color. If the color returns rapidly on release of the individual artery, it suggests that the blood supply to the hand is sufficient (**b**, **c**)

arterial and the venous systems. Arterial evaluation is essential as the artery not only provides adequate inflow for access development but also the blood supply of the forearm and hand. It includes documentation of bilaterally equal strong pulses, differential blood pressure measurements in both extremities, and the Allen test. The brachial, radial, and ulnar pulses should be examined in both upper extremities, and their quality should be recorded, whether normal or diminished. Blood pressure measurements should be taken in both arms; a difference of 20 mmHg or greater in systolic blood pressure between the two arms is abnormal and should be recorded. The Allen test helps to confirm the patency of the palmar arch and thereby the collateral circulation to the hand. It should be performed prior to creation of any AVF, but particularly a forearm AVF. The patient is asked to make a fist and pressure is applied over both the ulnar and the radial arteries to occlude them. Once the fist is opened, the hand should appear blanched or pale. Then, pressure is alternately released from both the arteries and the hand monitored for return to color. If the color returns rapidly on release of the individual artery, it suggests that the blood supply to the hand is sufficient (Fig. 2.1).

For the venous examination, a tourniquet is placed sequentially at the upper extremity and the veins are visually inspected to determine the diameter, the distance of the vein from the skin surface, and the length of a straight venous segment suitable for cannulation [12]. An upper extremity physical examination, though valuable, is often inadequate when used alone – particularly in obese patients or those with a history of prior vascular access. In such cases, it may need to be supplemented with additional techniques, such as ultrasonography or venography [13]. In a cohort of 116 patients, the authors classified vein quality as good in patients in whom the cephalic vein was easily visualized, poor with hardly visible veins, and absent when no veins could be seen on physical examination. In patients with poor or absent veins, Duplex sonography was performed, and venography was reserved for those patients who did not have adequate veins on both physical examination and ultrasound. Preoperatively, clinically visualized veins could be found in only 54 of 116 patients (46.5 %), and poor or clinically absent veins were found in 62 patients (53.5 %). Further, of these 62 patients, duplex sonography found adequate veins in 48 patients (77 %), and only 14 patients (23 %) required venography [13].

2.4 Physical Examination Prior to Interventional Procedures on Arteriovenous Fistulae and Early Fistula Failure

Even with an increasing use of preoperative vessel mapping as described above, AVF has a high rate (20–50 %) of primary or early fistula failure (AVF that either does not adequately develop or fail within the first 3 months) that precludes their successful use for dialysis [14].

Though there may be multiple reasons for early fistula failure, they are primarily due to "inflow" problems – arterial or juxta-anastomotic stenosis or due to accessory veins that divert blood away from the main channel and prevent it from developing adequately.

2.4.1 Inflow Problems

Arterial lesions are secondary to diseased, calcified arteries and, ideally, should have been evaluated preoperatively by vascular mapping. Juxta-anastomotic stenosis (a narrowing of the venous segment within 2 cm of the arterial anastomosis) is usually related to surgical trauma as this is the part of the vein that is manipulated to create the anastomosis. Inflow problems are easily diagnosed on physical examination by assessing the AVF for augmentation [15]. On palpation of a normal AVF, there is a pulse at the arterial anastomosis and a soft compressible thrill throughout the AVF. On downstream occlusion (with a tourniquet or just manual pressure), the AVF augments or increases in size. However, in the presence of a juxta-anastomotic stenosis, the AVF itself is pulsatile with a decreased thrill. As the inflow into the access is limited by the stenosis, the augmentation is minimal. Furthermore, the site of the stenosis can be detected by gradually moving proximally along the fistula, as the thrill weakens at the site of stenosis. Auscultation at the stenotic area reveals an auditory whistle suggestive of an obstruction.

2.4.2 Accessory Veins

In an ideal forearm AVF, there is one main channel (cephalic vein) which ultimately develops into a mature, usable AVF. However, the cephalic vein may have additional side branches (Fig. 2.2). Though this may be advantageous in that it allows several channels for the outflow and may even lead to the development of alternative sites for cannulation, in certain cases these accessory veins divert blood flow away from the main channel and may result in inadequate development of the AVF, resulting in early fistula failure.

Accessory veins are readily diagnosed by physical examination, as they are easily visible. Their significance can

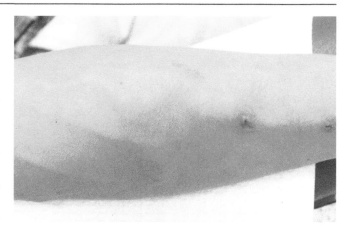

Fig. 2.2 Accessory veins in a forearm radiocephalic AVF. The main channel is well developed and used for hemodialysis

be ascertained by the effect of their occlusion on the main channel; if the AVF augments once the accessory vein is occluded, the accessory vein is significant and ligation may be considered.

2.5 Late Fistula Failure

AVF that fails after 3 months of use is classified under late fistula failure and is commonly due to "outflow" problems as a result of venous stenosis. Other problems that AVF may present with include aneurysm formation, infection, high-output heart failure, and thrombosis. Each of these is individually discussed in detail below.

2.5.1 Venous Stenosis

Venous stenosis in the outflow tract can be detected by a simple bedside test to evaluate for collapse of the AVF [15]. If there is no stenosis, elevation of the arm above the level of the heart will result in collapse of the AVF and a soft thrill. In the presence of a downstream stenosis, the AVF distal to the stenosis does not collapse and becomes hyper-pulsatile. Auscultation reveals an audible high-pitched sound (whistle) with a change in the character of the thrill at the site of stenosis.

2.5.2 Aneurysm Formation

In patients with proximal stenosis, as a result of the increased pressure within the circuit, the AVF wall may weaken over time, leading to dilatation and the development of an aneurysm (Fig. 2.3). A true aneurysm is defined

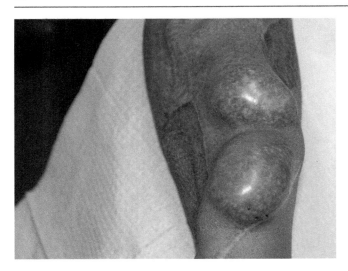

Fig. 2.3 Aneurysmal AVF with associated skin changes

as dilatation of the outflow vein to more than three times the normal vessel diameter with a minimum aneurysm diameter of 2 cm [16]. Aneurysms are more likely to develop distal to the stenosis, especially where the vessel wall has already been weakened by repetitive cannulations (one-site-itis). Aneurysms are not only cosmetically disfiguring, but their size and any associated skin changes should be progressively followed to determine if and when surgical intervention is needed. Aneurysm repair is indicated for symptomatic complications when aneurysms become large enough to impact the patient's quality of life or AVF use including skin changes such as thinning or erosion, pain, thrombosis, venous hypertension, or a shortened area for cannulation [16]. Impending rupture of the AVF is a relative emergency, and signs on physical examination include marked thinning, hypopigmentation, or ulceration of the skin overlying the fistula. The patient should be sent for emergent surgical repair with instructions on occluding the arterial inflow in the event of AVF rupture.

2.5.3 High-Output Heart Failure

The creation of an AVF leads to changes in hemodynamics and cardiac remodeling. In some upper arm AVF, especially brachiocephalic AVF, increased blood flow through the AVF (typically >2 l/min) predisposes patients with preexisting cardiac dysfunction to cardiac decompensation and the development of high-output heart failure [17].

These patients present with symptoms suggestive of worsening heart failure and shortness of breath and have a resting tachycardia on examination. Occlusion of the AVF results in a decrease in the pulse rate (Nicoladoni-Branham sign) and may add important clinical information regarding the hemodynamic significance of the AVF [18]. The management of these patients usually requires reduction or obliteration of the flow through the AVF, which results in symptomatic improvement [19–21].

2.5.4 Distal Ischemia

Hand ischemia in patients with an arteriovenous access is a serious complication, and a detailed history and physical examination helps to delineate the underlying etiology [22]. The key factors in examination are distal arterial pulses, skin temperature, gross sensation, and movement and should be compared to the contralateral side. Patients with preexisting peripheral vascular disease and those with brachial artery AVF (as compared to radial artery AVF) are more predisposed to the development of ischemia [23]. In the classic "steal syndrome" or distal hypoperfusion ischemic syndrome (DHIS) [22], the patient presents with hand pain that worsens on dialysis, a cool hand with cyanotic discoloration, and decreased pulses. In more severe cases, evidence of ischemic changes in the skin, especially at the fingertips, may be present. A distal pulse that is weak on initial examination and strengthens on AVF occlusion is suggestive, though not pathognomonic, of arterial steal, as it suggests that the access is stealing too much blood away from the distal extremity. Differential diagnoses include (a) ischemic monomelic neuropathy that presents acutely with weakness of the muscles with prominent sensory loss from nerve damage due to vascular insufficiency and (b) carpal tunnel syndrome that presents with chronic hand weakness, numbness, and pain unrelated to dialysis. It is essential to identify the pathophysiology of the hand pain prior to the interventional procedure, particularly if the patient presents with a concomitant outflow stenosis, as an angioplasty to improve the blood flow through the access may inadvertently worsen the ischemic symptoms.

2.5.5 Thrombosed Access

When a patient presents with a thrombosed access, there is no palpable thrill or bruit on auscultation throughout the access, though a pulse may still be palpable at the arterial anastomosis. The number of days since the last full hemodialysis session should be noted and the patient placed on a monitor preoperatively to monitor for cardiac effects of hyperkalemia including bradycardia and EKG monitoring suggestive of prolonged P-R or Q-R-S intervals. Additionally, if the patient has a thrombosed "mega-fistula" (Fig. 2.4), it is likely that there is a large thrombus burden leading to a higher risk of symptomatic pulmonary embolism.

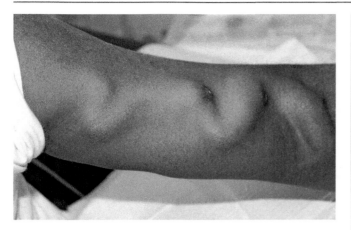

Fig. 2.4 Enlarged brachiocephalic AVF (mega-AVF)

2.6 Physical Examination Prior to Interventional Procedures on Arteriovenous Grafts

2.6.1 Determining the Direction of the Flow

The access circuit begins and ends in the heart; and the direction of flow is from the feeding artery to the draining vein. However, in instances with unusual configurations and loop arteriovenous grafts, it is essential to determine the configuration prior to cannulation to avoid recirculation. At the bedside, the AVG is occluded at the apex of the loop and both sides are palpated (Fig. 2.5). The arterial (inflow) limb of the graft will have an augmented pulse as the blood tries to force past the occlusion, while the venous (outflow) limb of the graft will have a diminished or absent pulse.

2.6.2 Venous Stenosis

Though venous stenosis in an AVG, similar to an AVF, is secondary to outflow stenosis, the underlying pathophysiology differs in that it is a result of the development of neointimal hyperplasia at the vein-graft anastomosis [24]. The graft and draining veins are examined to determine the character of the pulse, the location and intensity of thrills, and the duration and pitch of the bruit. The physical examination reflects the increase in pressure within the access circuit consequent to the downstream stenosis and the AVG is pulsatile throughout, not just at the arterial anastomosis. The normal character of the soft bruit changes, and there is a high-pitched, harsh bruit at the site of maximum turbulence.

2.6.3 Pseudoaneurysms

AVG-associated pseudoaneurysms differ from AVF-associated true aneurysms, as they are composed of skin and

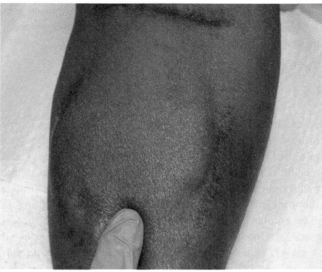

Fig. 2.5 To determine direction of flow, the AVG is occluded at the apex of the loop and both sides are palpated. The arterial (inflow) limb of the graft will have an augmented pulse as the blood tries to force past the occlusion, while the venous (outflow) limb of the graft will have a diminished or absent pulse

fibrous connective tissue and are secondary to a combination of outflow stenosis causing an increase in pressure within the access, with repetitive cannulation at the same sites leading to dilatation at the site of the resultant graft defect. The presence of a pseudoaneurysm necessitates an evaluation for venous stenosis. The overlying skin should be closely monitored for thinning, hypopigmentation, scarring, ulceration, or spontaneous bleeding, as it may rupture leading to massive hemorrhage.

If the diameter of the pseudoaneurysm is greater than twice the diameter of the graft, the patient should be referred for surgical revision [25]. Placement of a stent graft should be avoided in the cannulation area due to concerns for infection and the risk of protrusion of the stent through the skin [26].

2.6.4 Infections

Infection of an AVG is a serious complication, and it is essential to differentiate a reactive inflammation (secondary to thrombosis or postoperative) from a true graft infection. Immediately postoperatively, an inflammatory dermal reaction localized to the graft may be seen; pain and the associated swelling may make it seem similar to a superficial or deep graft infection. Superficial graft infections are generally related to a cannulation site and present as a localized area of cellulitis. On physical examination, there is minimal or no inflammation, swelling, or pain. Deep graft infections are usually at the site of graft surgery or cannulation sites and characterized by the classic signs of inflammation including erythema, warmth, and a fluctuant swelling extending into the surrounding tissues. It is often painful and management involves partial or total graft excision [27].

2.6.5 Thrombosed Access

On examination of a thrombosed AVG, there is no palpable thrill or bruit on auscultation throughout the graft, though a pulse may still be palpable at the arterial anastomosis. There may be a reactive superficial cellulitis in response to the underlying thrombus, which must be differentiated from a true graft infection as detailed above, prior to attempting an endovascular procedure. The mean clot volume in a thrombosed graft has been shown to be much lower than expected (3 cm^3) [28] and by inference, the risk of symptomatic pulmonary emboli may be less than that with mega-fistulas unless there are associated pseudoaneurysms.

2.7 Physical Examination Prior to Interventional Procedures on Central Venous Catheters

2.7.1 Central Venous Stenosis

Central venous stenosis may present with swelling of the arm, neck, and/or face based on the site of stenosis. If the stenosis is in the subclavian vein, the patient presents with unilateral arm swelling, while a stenosis of the superior vena cava presents with swelling of the face and neck as well (SVC syndrome). A detailed history of previous central venous catheters including scars on the chest wall, PICC lines, and cardiac rhythm devices and the presence of collaterals (Fig. 2.6) should be performed and documented. Other risk factors for central venous stenosis include the caliber, site (subclavian > internal jugular), and duration of the catheter [29]. It is important to realize that central venous lesions may be asymptomatic and not all cases are associated with a previous history of a central venous catheter.

2.7.2 Infections

Management of tunneled dialysis catheter infections differs based on their site of involvement. These infections can be classified as exit site infections, tunnel infections, and catheter-related bacteremia (CRB). An exit site infection is restricted to the exit site and is easily recognized on physical examination by redness, crusting, and exudate. An exit site infection is a localized infection and should be treated with topical antibiotics [25]. A tunnel infection is defined as infection within the catheter tunnel – the part of the catheter

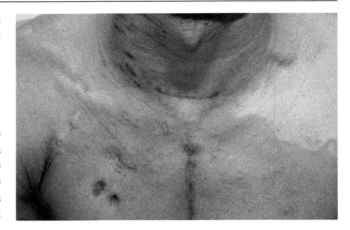

Fig. 2.6 Previous central venous catheter scars on the chest wall and the presence of collaterals

from the cuff to the exit site. The patient presents with warmth, redness, swelling, and exquisite tenderness over the catheter tunnel, and occasionally an exudate may be expressed from the tunnel. Appropriate treatment consists of removal of the catheter and systemic antibiotics based on culture results. If the patient needs dialysis prior to resolution of the infection, a catheter should be placed at an alternative site. Catheter-related bacteremia reflects bloodstream infection, and these patients present with systemic symptoms including fever, chills, and a positive blood culture. There are no other clearly visible signs on physical examination, though a CRB may present with a concomitant exit site or tunnel infection. The management is based on the infecting organism, the need for dialysis, and the hemodynamic stability of the patient [30].

Conclusions

Even with the advent of elaborate and expensive technology, physical examination is far from obsolete. An inexpensive, quick, and thorough physical examination performed at the bedside provides essential clues to the management of vascular access in hemodialysis patients. It is an invaluable, easily teachable skill in the nephrologists and interventionists armamentarium and should be utilized more widely and frequently.

References

1. Asif A, Leon C, Orozco-Vargas LC, Krishnamurthy G, Choi KL, Mercado C, et al. Accuracy of physical examination in the detection of arteriovenous fistula stenosis. Clin J Am Soc Nephrol. 2007;2(6):1191–4.
2. Leon C, Orozco-Vargas LC, Krishnamurthy G, Choi KL, Mercado C, Merrill D, et al. Accuracy of physical examination in the detection of arteriovenous graft stenosis. Semin Dial. 2008;21(1):85–8.

3. Agarwal R, McDougal G. Buzz in the axilla: a new physical sign in hemodialysis forearm graft evaluation. Am J Kidney Dis. 2001; 38(4):853–7.

4. Trerotola SO, Ponce P, Stavropoulos SW, Clark TW, Tuite CM, Mondschein JI, et al. Physical examination versus normalized pressure ratio for predicting outcomes of hemodialysis access interventions. J Vasc Interv Radiol. 2003;14(11):1387–94.

5. Trerotola SO, Scheel Jr PJ, Powe NR, Prescott C, Feeley N, He J, et al. Screening for dialysis access graft malfunction: comparison of physical examination with US. J Vasc Interv Radiol. 1996;7(1):15–20.

6. Campos RP, Chula DC, Perreto S, Riella MC, do Nascimento MM. Accuracy of physical examination and intra-access pressure in the detection of stenosis in hemodialysis arteriovenous fistula. Semin Dial. 2008;21(3):269–73.

7. Leon C, Asif A. Physical examination of arteriovenous fistulae by a renal fellow: does it compare favorably to an experienced interventionalist? Semin Dial. 2008;21(6):557–60.

8. Asif A, Cherla G, Merrill D, Cipleu CD, Briones P, Pennell P. Conversion of tunneled hemodialysis catheter-consigned patients to arteriovenous fistula. Kidney Int. 2005;67(6):2399–406.

9. Wasse H, Speckman RA, Frankenfield DL, Rocco MV, McClellan WM. Predictors of central venous catheter use at the initiation of hemodialysis. Semin Dial. 2008;21(4):346–51.

10. Allen AW, Megargell JL, Brown DB, Lynch FC, Singh H, Singh Y, et al. Venous thrombosis associated with the placement of peripherally inserted central catheters. J Vasc Interv Radiol. 2000;11(10):1309–14.

11. Ethier J, Mendelssohn DC, Elder SJ, Hasegawa T, Akizawa T, Akiba T, et al. Vascular access use and outcomes: an international perspective from the dialysis outcomes and practice patterns study. Nephrol Dial Transplant. 2008;23(10):3219–26.

12. Asif A, Ravani P, Roy-Chaudhury P, Spergel LM, Besarab A. Vascular mapping techniques: advantages and disadvantages. J Nephrol. 2007;20(3):299–303.

13. Malovrh M. Native arteriovenous fistula: preoperative evaluation. Am J Kidney Dis. 2002;39(6):1218–25.

14. Allon M, Robbin ML. Increasing arteriovenous fistulas in hemodialysis patients: problems and solutions. Kidney Int. 2002;62(4):1109–24.

15. Beathard GA. An algorithm for the physical examination of early fistula failure. Semin Dial. 2005;18(4):331–5.

16. Pasklinsky G, Meisner RJ, Labropoulos N, Leon L, Gasparis AP, Landau D, et al. Management of true aneurysms of hemodialysis access fistulas. J Vasc Surg. 2011;53(5):1291–7.

17. MacRae JM, Levin A, Belenkie I. The cardiovascular effects of arteriovenous fistulas in chronic kidney disease: a cause for concern? Semin Dial. 2006;19(5):349–52.

18. Velez-Roa S, Neubauer J, Wissing M, Porta A, Somers VK, Unger P, et al. Acute arterio-venous fistula occlusion decreases sympathetic activity and improves baroreflex control in kidney transplanted patients. Nephrol Dial Transplant. 2004;19(6): 1606–12.

19. Anderson CB, Codd JR, Graff RA, Groce MA, Harter HR, Newton WT. Cardiac failure and upper extremity arteriovenous dialysis fistulas. Case reports and a review of the literature. Arch Intern Med. 1976;136(3):292–7.

20. Bailey WB, Talley JD. High-output cardiac failure related to hemodialysis arteriovenous fistula. J Ark Med Soc. 2000;96(9): 340–1.

21. Murray BM, Rajczak S, Herman A, Leary D. Effect of surgical banding of a high-flow fistula on access flow and cardiac output: intraoperative and long-term measurements. Am J Kidney Dis. 2004;44(6):1090–6.

22. Leon C, Asif A. Arteriovenous access and hand pain: the distal hypoperfusion ischemic syndrome. Clin J Am Soc Nephrol. 2007; 2(1):175–83.

23. Tordoir JH, Dammers R, van der Sande FM. Upper extremity ischemia and hemodialysis vascular access. Eur J Vasc Endovasc Surg. 2004;27(1):1–5.

24. Lee T, Roy-Chaudhury P. Advances and new frontiers in the pathophysiology of venous neointimal hyperplasia and dialysis access stenosis. Adv Chronic Kidney Dis. 2009;16(5):329–38.

25. Schwab S, Besarab A, Beathard G, Brouwer D, Levine M, McCann R et al. Vascular Access 2006 Work Group. Clinical practice guidelines for vascular access. Am J Kidney Dis. 2006;48 Suppl 1:S248–73.

26. Asif A, Gadalean F, Eid N, Merrill D, Salman L. Stent graft infection and protrusion through the skin: clinical considerations and potential medico-legal ramifications. Semin Dial. 2010;23(5): 540–2.

27. Ryan SV, Calligaro KD, Scharff J, Dougherty MJ. Management of infected prosthetic dialysis arteriovenous grafts. J Vasc Surg. 2004;39(1):73–8.

28. Winkler TA, Trerotola SO, Davidson DD, Milgrom ML. Study of thrombus from thrombosed hemodialysis access grafts. Radiology. 1995;197(2):461–5.

29. Agarwal AK, Patel BM, Haddad NJ. Central vein stenosis: a nephrologist's perspective. Semin Dial. 2007;20(1):53–62.

30. Schwab SJ, Beathard G. The hemodialysis catheter conundrum: hate living with them, but can't live without them. Kidney Int. 1999;56(1):1–17.

Admission After Intervention: When and Why

Bharat Sachdeva

Dialysis access care is integral to wholesome management of an ESRD patient. Access care contributes to major mortality and morbidity in ESRD and is also associated with tremendous cost to the system [1]. Over the last 15 years, there has been approximately 50 % drop in the rate of hospitalizations for access-related complications in ESRD [1]. Untimely, improper and low priority care of access resulted in nephrologists stepping up to take care of problems affecting their patients. Nephrologists traditionally had performed kidney biopsies and inserted temporary dialysis catheters. Interventional nephrologists have shown excellent outcomes when performing endovascular procedures with minimal complications [2, 3]. Over the years, growth in interventional nephrology (IN) has occurred primarily as freestanding access centers bringing financial value to the practice. Timely care, convenience, comfort, and improved outcomes are all benefits delivered to patients by IN, but safety during the intervention should remain the prime goal and responsibility of the operator. Decision of admission to hospital is taken after careful assessment of risk to a patient before, during, and after a procedure.

3.1 Are There Patients That Will Require Hospitalization Prior to a Procedure?

The ability to deliver safe and effective moderate sedation is crucial to the ability to perform invasive procedures [4]. Intraoperative procedure experience should be as smooth for the patient as can be and should start with preemptive assessment of patient's comorbid conditions, physical examination, history of allergies, or prior experiences with medications

used in procedure sedation analgesia (PSA). Sedative drugs used for PSA should have a quick onset of action, maintain moderate sedation during surgical treatment, provide rapid and clear-headed recovery, and be easy to administer and monitor. Sedation and analgesia comprise a continuum of states ranging from minimal sedation (anxiolysis) through general anesthesia. Decision to apply level of sedation/analgesia has to be individualized to a given patient taking into account factors including but not limited to nature of the procedure, comorbid medical conditions, patient's level of anxiety, history of complications in prior procedures with use of anesthetic drugs, and operator experience with sedating procedure.

Preoperative work-up should incorporate a focused physical examination, including vital signs, auscultation of the heart and lungs, and evaluation of the airway. Laboratory testing should be guided by the patient's underlying medical condition and the likelihood that the results will affect the management of sedation/analgesia. Most commonly used agents for PSA include a combination of benzodiazepines, opioids providing amnesia, and analgesia, respectively.

Ability to maintain airway and ventilation is directly affected by sedation/analgesia. The effect of sedative medications on patient's ability to maintain and protect airway is exacerbated in CKD patients, and PSA may be relatively contraindicated in patients who may have a difficult airway. Key to minimizing risk is to identify and monitor patients at higher risk. Uncooperative patients, morbid obesity, potentially difficult airway, and sleep apnea are all associated with an increased risk of ventilation/oxygenation complication and may benefit from preprocedure consultation to anesthesia. There is no specific age above which PSA may not be performed, though the risk is higher for elderly patients [5, 6]. Comorbid conditions including heart failure, dehydration, chronic obstructive pulmonary disease (COPD), and neuromuscular disease should be assessed prior to the procedure and corrective measures be taken to optimize hemodynamics [7]. Several recent studies have supported the use of PSA across a broad patient population with careful clinical

B. Sachdeva, MD
Nephrology Section, Department of Medicine,
LSU Health Sciences Center, Shreveport, LA 71106, USA
e-mail: bsachd@lsuhsc.edu

A.S. Yevzlin et al. (eds.), *Interventional Nephrology*,
DOI 10.1007/978-1-4614-8803-3_3, © Springer Science+Business Media New York 2014

supervision. When careful attention is paid to examine subject and modus operandi individualized, most procedures can be completed with minimal complications and no hospitalization [8–10].

The risk to patient for complications may persist after their procedure is completed. Decreased procedural stimulation and slow drug elimination in chronic kidney disease (CKD) patients may contribute to residual sedation and cardiorespiratory depression during the recovery period.

Continued monitoring will be required if patient is not fully alert and oriented; infants and patients whose mental status was initially abnormal should have returned to their baseline status [5, 7]. Abnormal vital signs should be watched till they return to acceptable limits. If the patient required a reversal agent during the procedure, practicing physician needs to be aware of the short half-life of these agents (naloxone, flumazenil) and up to 2 h should have elapsed after the last administration of reversal agent [7]. This would ensure that patients do not become resedated after reversal effects have worn off.

In summary, comprehensive assessment prior to a procedure will identify patients at high risk for complication. PSA can be safely administered in all patients with adequate planning and preparation [7].

3.2 Does the Nature of Procedure Require Inpatient Care?

The last decade has seen tremendous growth in vascular access centers and the role of nephrologists has been redefined, from being passive facilitator of patient care to an interventionist rendering solutions to complex dialysis access demands. List of procedures performed by nephrologists continues to grow, with more complex procedure being added to the roll [2, 11–14]. So as more complex cases are performed at freestanding access centers without any backup, are there any interventions that will warrant inpatient care? Reviewed below are common procedures and recommendations for the place of service.

3.2.1 Percutaneous Needle Biopsy of Kidney

Native kidney biopsy is frequently performed for diagnostic purposes. Minor complications are defined as gross hematuria and perinephric hematoma that resolve without the need for transfusion or intervention. Major complications are defined as those requiring a blood transfusion, invasive radiological procedure (angiogram/coil), nephrectomy, and bowel perforation [15–17]. Automated spring-loaded biopsy gun is widely accepted to be standard approach and biopsies

are done under real-time ultrasonography [18]. The standard of care has been to observe patient post-biopsy for 24 h as suggested by most studies [15–17]. There was correlation with the 6-h post-hematocrit drop with rate of complication in one study [15], yet another study suggested that >20 % of complications may be missed if patient is discharged within 8-h post-renal biopsy [17]. The only randomized control study comparing manual to automated kidney biopsy noted 11 % incidence of perirenal hematoma post-kidney biopsy. All patients were required to have 12 h of strict bed rest after the biopsy [18]. Based on above data it is safe practice that patient be observed for 24-h post-biopsy.

3.2.2 Interventions Directed at Vascular Access

Wide spectrum of services are now offered at access centers with an objective to create, maintain, and salvage hemodialysis access. Data over the last decade, from several operators, supports safe application of these techniques in freestanding access centers with minimal complications [2, 19–21]. Ability of nephrologist to provide wholesome care has helped improve overall access health [1], and we strive to attain goals set by CMS and fistula first for hemodialysis patients [22].

Angiogram, Angioplasty, and Stent Placements
Success of angiography/angioplasty procedures has been upwards of 98 % [21] and the complications associated with the procedures are low [21]. Complications graded as high-grade complications are noted to be less than 0.05 % [2], and though the data is not available as to what percentage of these may require admission for management of the complication, the overall numbers may be lower than 1 out of 2,000 patients at risk [2]. 99.9 % of procedures performed in access center have no complication (>98 %) or minor complications noted during the procedure managed with nominal interventions [2].

Central Vein Catheter Placement/Tunneled/Port
About a quarter of all dialysis patients require a central venous catheter for long-term dialysis causing considerable morbidity and mortality. Infections continue to be a major cause of admissions into hospitals and contribute to a high mortality [1]. Since 1993 infection-related hospitalizations have increased a whopping 43 % [1], and a majority of these are associated with tunneled dialysis catheter (TDC).

TDC patients on hemodialysis have 0.9–2.0 episodes of bacteremia per year of catheter use. If we account for the total dialysis population inUSA, this would account for 100,000 incidents of bacteremia and with roughly 10 % of these developing infection-related complications, over 10,000 admissions for catheter infection [23–25]. Complications from catheter infection include sepsis, metastatic infection to the cardiac valves or the spine most commonly, septic arthritis, skin abscess, and thrombosis of the insertion vein.

Port-a-catheters are similar to TDC with subcutaneous port reservoir and are primarily used for central vein access for chemotherapy. Successful placement and management of port-a-catheters will involve the nephrologists to be aware of indications for catheter removal and management of infections at times requiring hospitalization and intravenous antibiotics [13].

Indications for hospitalization and management of infection from a TDC or a port-a-catheter will be severe sepsis with hemodynamic instability, diagnosis and management of a suspected metastatic infection after bacteremia, treatment of deep vein thrombosis associated with catheter insertion/infection, amongst other clinical indications.

If catheter-related bacteremia is suspected clinically, empiric antibiotic therapy should be started quickly, without waiting for the culture report. Bacteriological data from several studies show a mixture of gram-negative/gram-positive rods, thus mandating broad-spectrum antibiotic coverage for both gram-positive and gram-negative organisms pending culture results. Many staphylococcal infections in hemodialysis patients are caused by methicillin-resistant species, requiring empiric therapy with vancomycin pending sensitivity reports.

Treatment of catheter-related bacteremia with systemic antibiotics without catheter removal has a high failure rate. Hospitalized patients should get a catheter-free period with a temporary dialysis catheter used in the interval for dialysis. TDC can be replaced on clinical improvement [23].

Peritoneal Dialysis [PD] Catheter Placement Using Fluoroscopy/Peritoneoscopy

Growing interest amongst nephrologists and dialysis chains for peritoneal dialysis has sparked tremendous interest for placement and management of PD catheters by nephrologists themselves. Several studies have shown risk of complication to be very low when catheters are placed under PSA using either fluoroscopy [26, 27] or peritoneoscopy [28]. Complications associated with PD catheter placement can be classified into intraoperative and postoperative. Intraoperative complication that may require hospital admission will include bowel perforation, bladder perforation, intraperitoneal bleeding, and laceration of the inferior epigastric artery [14, 26]. The risk of above complications is extremely low, and most patients can be safely discharged after the PD catheter placement within the same day [26].

PD catheter infections are associated with major morbidity and require dedicated personnel geared towards rapid identification/classification of infection. As more interventionists are performing PD catheter placement procedures, it is required a wholesome care approach be used when a catheter does get infected. Exit site infections are treated with oral/topical antibiotics alone, but a tunnel infection or peritonitis may require PD catheter removal/replacement [29].

Removal of PD catheter poses challenge to continue renal replacement therapy (RRT), occasionally requiring admission for acute hemodialysis.

Peripheral Arterial Interventions

Arterial stenosis accounts for significant number of immature fistulae and plays a major role in late access complications including distal ischemia hypoperfusion syndrome [DHIS], commonly identified as "steal" [30]. Arterial interventions involve at times arterial approach where femoral or radial artery puncture is used to place a sheath for access. Removal of sheath may be done once the anticoagulation given during the course of the procedure has dissipated. Observation will be required until homeostasis can be secured using a closure device for femoral access or band for radial access [31].

Rare and mostly unforeseen, significant complications will require admission and inpatient care of the asymptomatic patient prior to the intervention. An arterial embolus to the brain with ischemic cerebral vascular accident (CVA) after percutaneous fistula thrombectomy [32], suppurative thrombophlebitis (Lemierre's syndrome) of the internal jugular vein after a central venous catheter placement [33], phlegmasia cerulea dolens (PCD) characterized by massive venous thrombosis leading to arterial compromise and tissue ischemia [34], severe acute pancreatitis after percutaneous mechanical thrombectomy of arterial thrombus occlusion [35], rapidly progressing superior vena cava syndrome with a thrombus around a central venous catheter in superior vena cava [36, 37], breakage and migration of hemodialysis catheter on removal [38], and catheter tip embedded into the wall of the superior vena cava on attempted removal of catheter [38] are all examples of what makes interventional field unpredictable. These and other unpredicted complications underline importance of being ready for every case and to take into account that even a trivial case of TDC removal can turn into a major cardiac bypass surgical event for a patient [38].

3.3 Recording Procedure-Related Complications [PRC]

A procedural-related complication is defined as an unanticipated adverse event that requires therapy. In general, unanticipated events that do not require therapy are not considered procedure complications [19, 39, 40]. Complications which occur during or immediate postoperative period should, in most instances, be attributed to the procedure. Uniform classification and reporting of these events has been supported by all interventional societies including Society of Interventional Radiology (SIR) [40], Society of Vascular Surgery (SVS) [39], and American Society of Diagnostic and Interventional Nephrology [19]. Hospitalization of a patient for a procedure-related event should be noted as a major complication and is graded as a grade 3 or grade 4 complication based on the severity and number of days spent in the hospital.

Patients may experience an adverse reaction to intravascular radiographic contrast media or medications administered for PSA. Adverse reactions to medications typically occur soon after administration of the drug, although significant reactions may occur several hours after completion of the procedure [5]. Hospital admission may be required and major complication will be recorded when prolonged (>30 s) decrease in O_2 saturation (<90 %) is recognized and it fails to improve with minor therapy [19, 39, 40]. Hemodynamic instability with profound and persistent hypotension, cardiac arrhythmias refractory to reversal of sedation and requiring antiarrhythmic medications, or a persistent mental status change that fails to return to baseline during recovery ought to be charted as major complication and infrequently may require hospitalization [5, 19, 39, 40].

Conclusion

There is no absolute indication for admission to hospital for a given procedure. All procedures can be done safely as outpatient visits, saving disruptions in patient's schedule and providing batter value to the insurers. Decision of admission to hospital should be taken after careful assessment of risk associated with procedure itself and the PSA.

References

1. USRDS: U S Renal Data System, USRDS 2011 Annual Data Report: atlas of chronic kidney disease and end-stage renal disease in the United States. National Institutes of Health, National Institute of Diabetes and Digestive and Kidney Diseases, Bethesda; 2011.
2. Beathard GA, Litchfield T, Physician Operators Forum of RMS Lifeline, Inc. Effectiveness and safety of dialysis vascular access procedures performed by interventional nephrologists. Kidney Int. 2004;66(4):1622–32.
3. Vachharajani TJ, Moossavi S, Salman L, et al. Dialysis vascular access management by Interventional Nephrology Programs at University Medical Centers in the United States. Semin Dial. 2011;24(5):564–9.
4. Gan TJ. Pharmacokinetic and pharmacodynamic characteristics of medications used for moderate sedation. Clin Pharmacokinet. 2006;45(9):855–69.
5. Beathard GA, Urbanes A, Litchfield T, Weinstein A. The risk of sedation/analgesia in hemodialysis patients undergoing interventional procedures. Semin Dial. 2011;24(1):97–103.
6. Mace SE. 190: Adverse events of emergency department procedural sedation. Ann Emerg Med. 2006;48(4):59.
7. American Society of Anesthesiologists Task Force on Sedation and Analgesia by Non-Anesthesiologists. Practice guidelines for sedation and analgesia by non-anesthesiologists. Anesthesiology. 2002;96(4):1004–17.
8. Holdgate A, Taylor DM, Bell A, et al. Factors associated with failure to successfully complete a procedure during emergency department sedation. Emerg Med Australas. 2011;23(4):474–8.
9. Sacchetti A, Senula G, Strickland J, Dubin R. Procedural sedation in the community emergency department: initial results of the ProSCED registry. Acad Emerg Med. 2007;14(1):41–6.
10. Weaver CS, Terrell KM, Bassett R, et al. ED procedural sedation of elderly patients: is it safe? Am J Emerg Med. 2011;29(5):541–4.
11. Asif A, Yevzlin AS. Arterial stent placement in arteriovenous dialysis access by interventional nephrologists. Semin Dial. 2009;22(5):557–60.
12. Carrillo RG, Garisto JD, Salman L, Merrill D, Asif A. A novel technique for tethered dialysis catheter removal using the laser sheath. Semin Dial. 2009;22(6):688–91.
13. Pervez A, Zaman F, Aslam A, et al. Port catheter placement by nephrologists in an interventional nephrology training program. Semin Dial. 2004;17(1):61–4.
14. Zaman F, Pervez A, Atray NK, Murphy S, Work J, Abreo KD. Fluoroscopy-assisted placement of peritoneal dialysis catheters by nephrologists. Semin Dial. 2005;18(3):247–51.
15. Khajehdehi P, Junaid SMA, Salinas-Madrigal L, Schmitz PG, Bastani B. Percutaneous renal biopsy in the 1990s: safety, value, and implications for early hospital discharge. Am J Kidney Dis. 1999;34(1):92–7.
16. Manno C, Strippoli GF, Arnesano L, et al. Predictors of bleeding complications in percutaneous ultrasound-guided renal biopsy. Kidney Int. 2004;66(4):1570–7.
17. Marwah DS, Korbet SM. Timing of complications in percutaneous renal biopsy: what is the optimal period of observation? Am J Kidney Dis. 1996;28(1):47–52.
18. Kim D, Kim H, Shin G, et al. A randomized, prospective, comparative study of manual and automated renal biopsies. Am J Kidney Dis. 1998;32(3):426–31.
19. Vesely TM, Beathard G, Ash S, Hoggard J, Schon D, ACPC: Classification of complications associated with hemodialysis vascular access procedures. A position statement from the American Society of Diagnostic and Interventional Nephrology. Semin Dial. 2007;20(4):359–64.
20. Asif A, Salman L, Carrillo RG, et al. Patency rates for angioplasty in the treatment of pacemaker-induced central venous stenosis in hemodialysis patients: results of a multi-center study. Semin Dial. 2009;22(6):671–6.
21. Lifeline Access 2011 Outcomes Report, LifelineAcess.com, Three Hawthorn Parkway, Suite 410; Vernon Hills 60061.
22. Schinstock CA, Albright RC, Williams AW, et al. Outcomes of arteriovenous fistula creation after the fistula first initiative. Clin J Am Soc Nephrol. 2011;6(8):1996–2002.
23. Allon M. Dialysis catheter-related bacteremia: treatment and prophylaxis. Am J Kidney Dis. 2004;44(5):779–91.
24. Lee T, Barker J, Allon M. Tunneled catheters in hemodialysis patients: reasons and subsequent outcomes. Am J Kidney Dis. 2005;46(3):501–8.
25. Beathard GA, Urbanes A. Infection associated with tunneled hemodialysis catheters. Semin Dial. 2008;21(6):528–38.
26. Sharma M, Sachdeva B. Percutaneous peritoneal dialysis catheter insertion: making a case for an outpatient procedure. J Invest Med. 2012;60(1):1.
27. Maya ID. Ambulatory setting for peritoneal dialysis catheter placement. Semin Dial. 2008;21(5):457–8.
28. Alvarez AC, Salman L. Peritoneal dialysis catheter insertion by interventional nephrologists. Adv Chronic Kidney Dis. 2009;16(5):378–85.

29. Li PK, Szeto CC, Piraino B, et al. Peritoneal dialysis-related infections recommendations: 2010 update. Perit Dial Int. 2010;30(4):393–423.
30. Leon C, Asif A. Arteriovenous access and hand pain: the distal hypoperfusion ischemic syndrome. Clin J Am Soc Nephrol. 2007;2(1):175–83.
31. Yevzlin AS, Schoenkerman AB, Gimelli G, Asif A. Arterial interventions in arteriovenous access and chronic kidney disease: a role for interventional nephrologists. Semin Dial. 2009;22(5):545–56.
32. Pinard EA, Fazal S, Schussler JM. Catastrophic paradoxical embolus after hemodialysis access thrombectomy in a patient with a patent foramen ovale. Int Urol Nephrol. 2012;45(4):1215–7.
33. Kar S, Webel R. Septic thrombophlebitis: percutaneous mechanical thrombectomy and thrombolytic therapies. Am J Ther. 2011.
34. Mufarrij AJ, Hitti E. A case of phlegmesia cerulea dolens after dialysis catheter insertion. Emerg Med Australas. 2011;23(5):644–6.
35. Hershberger R, Bornak A, Aulivola B, Mannava K. Acute pancreatitis after percutaneous mechanical thrombectomy: case report and review of the literature. Cardiovasc Intervent Radiol. 2011;34 Suppl 2:S25–30.
36. Rabinstein A, Wijdicks E. Fatal brain swelling due to superior vena cava syndrome. Neurocrit Care. 2009;10(1):91–2.
37. Küçükarslan N, Yilmaz M, Us M, Arslan Y, Güler A, Yilmaz A. Superior vena cava syndrome caused by dialysis catheter. Ulus Travma Acil Cerrahi Derg. 2007;13(1):63–6.
38. Sequeira A, Sachdeva B, Abreo K. Uncommon complications of long-term hemodialysis catheters: adhesion, migration, and perforation by the catheter tip. Semin Dial. 2010;23(1):100–4.
39. Sidawy AN, Gray R, Besarab A, et al. Recommended standards for reports dealing with arteriovenous hemodialysis accesses. J Vasc Surg. 2002;35(3):603–10.
40. Sacks D, McClenny T, Cardella J, Lewis C. Society of interventional radiology clinical practice guidelines. J Vasc Interv Radiol. 2003;14(9 Pt 2):S199–202.

Communicating Effectively for Interventional Nephrologists

Jamie Ross and Talia Eisen

4.1 Introduction: Why a Chapter on Communication in an Interventional Text?

The finest work in medicine will go unnoticed by patients, referring physicians, colleagues, payers, and other large organizations if the information regarding the procedure, the outcome, future plans, and implications for care are not effectively communicated. This chapter will discuss the most current thinking regarding individual and organizational communication to assist the physician in creating and sustaining a robust practice.

Improved communications between physicians and their patients have been clearly shown to lead to both improved patient and physician satisfaction but also to better outcomes [1–4]. An extensive review of this literature is beyond the scope of this chapter. What is becoming clearer, however, is that not only is direct communication with the patient important but good communication with other colleagues and the entire system of care clearly improves patient safety and outcomes [5, 6]. In addition, good treatment or mistreatment of the medical staff will be reflected in the physician's ability to deliver care [7]. Therefore, developing effective communication becomes an important skill to deliver effective care.

One of the cornerstones of the success of an interventional practice has been communication with referral sources. Communication between the interventional physician and the referral source can take multiple forms: verbal, written, and imaging. The use of as many avenues as possible to transmit information can improve the results and satisfaction of the patients, dialysis clinics, nephrologists, surgeons, and primary care practitioners. Each of the recipient's will have unique pieces of information that they need to achieve a satisfactory interaction.

Satisfaction of a referral source with the results of your work has been shown to be proportional to the communications received from the consultant [8]. The information stated as most valued by referral sources was direct feedback, both written and verbal, with acknowledgement of the patient's history, suggestions or need for future care, scheduled follow-up if needed, and plans for comanaging care in the future. Of all of these, the inclusion of the plans for comanaging the patient's care in the future was directly proportional to the referring physician's overall satisfaction [9–11]. For interventional nephrology, one can substitute the dialysis facility, the general nephrologists, and access surgeon for the above entities.

4.2 What Is Good Communication and How Does It Impact Care?

The essence of good communication is the effective transfer of information. Communication is effective when these transfers occur in such a way as to build relationship, trust, confidence, and synchronicity. Much has been written on the art and science of good communication. Many organizations will cite the issue of communication as a central one in their quest for effectiveness and efficiency [12, 13]. It is a common theme. In spite of this, it is possible for good communication can happen without great effort. There are often small but important changes that can make a big difference.

What elements are the markers of excellence in communication? Although information can be transferred without attention to relationship, the result is not as effective. The reason is simple: Communication must occur between human parties. It is of vital importance that a level of trust is established and maintained to ensure the best results from all parties. People must feel they can trust one another to do their best work, to be reliable and dependable. Communication

J. Ross, MD (✉) • T. Eisen, MD
Division of Nephrology, Department of Internal Medicine,
University of California Davis Medical Center,
Sacramento, CA, USA
e-mail: jamie.ross@ucdmc.ucdavis.edu

can inspire confidence in the abilities of the individuals involved. It brings a more profound level of commitment from people when they have confidence in those with whom they work [14, 15].

Any complex system will function most efficiently when its members function with a high level of synchronicity. If parties are functioning in isolation, not informing one another of their efforts or updating needed information, then a murkiness and confusion develop. None of the participants has all the needed tools to be truly successful. Muddled and ad hoc processes result, leaving many people feeling entirely incapable of addressing simple, let alone complex, problems. It is important for a physician to realize that any health care is delivered in a complex system that starts with a patient-physician interaction and then involves multiple caregivers and systems.

Physicians work in concert with many. Although it may seem not to be the case, there is a high level of interdependence that exists in the world of the interventional physician. At the core is the partnership with the patient. Without getting all necessary information from the patient, the physician cannot do his/her best work as all issues are not taken into consideration. In turn, the physician must transfer information to the patient in such a way as to encourage the patient to follow the plan of care with confidence. In other words, the patient has a large part in the maintenance of their own health, and if they do not have a sufficient understanding of their role, they are not as likely to do their part [4].

An interventional needs referrals to maintain their practice. These are ongoing relationships that require good communication. However, in the course of busy days and under much pressure, a strained dynamic may develop. Staff and doctors may find it hard to get information they need from each other, and tempers may flare as both parties face the pressure of long days and high levels of stress. Good communication skills help decrease the stress of these situations. Finally, most doctors work within some sort of institution and are dependent upon that institution for patients, contracts, funding, and support. Likewise, the institution depends on the doctor to complete their part in a cost-effective and quality manner to keep the business viable. So it is clear that doctors function not in isolation but as part of a complex web of human activity. This interdependence requires constant continued effective communication and relationship building for all parties to function with excellence.

4.3 Strategies for Excellent Communication

It is important to note that delivering information is not the same as communicating. Communication is not a one-way delivery but a multitrack exchange. Information must travel back and forth between parties (two or more) to be considered communication. To begin with, different people have very different learning styles. This has been analyzed in many ways. For our purpose, we will look at the following element: Some learn best visually, some by auditory means, and some kinetically [16]. Therefore it is very important to deliver information in at least two of these three ways, at all times.

This means that the delivery of a pamphlet alone is not a communication. The individual receiving the pamphlet must then read it and understand it and be able to interact with the material. If they do not, the pamphlet may as well be blank. So handing someone a pamphlet must not be construed as a communication. However, checking with someone about the material contained therein and answering questions as needed, or discussing the material, constitute successful communication. In this example, two modes of communication have been employed: both visual and auditory. The visual is the pamphlet which is a reading material, and the auditory exchange is the conversation. In the same way, sending a memo, writing a report, or leaving a message is not a complete communication cycle. The information must be confirmed and shared in some other way via vocal or pictorial means.

Several strategies may help physicians improve their communication skills. We will look at three: active listening, use of questions, and the feedback model. Although there are numerous methods to improve communication, these three are excellent core skill-building strategies that will empower physicians to become great communicators without setting up complex new systems or changing organizational structures. These are skills that can be learned, practiced, and employed right away and do not take up excessive time or energies in already busy, stressful work days.

4.4 Active Listening

Listening is a key skill in the pursuit of good communication. For many, "listening" means waiting for the other person to stop speaking so we can make our point. For some who think quickly and grasp concepts easily, hearing someone out at length may be tiresome. For those who are under tremendous time constraints and have crucial information to impart, both of these reactions can hinder the ability to communicate effectively. In order to communicate well, one must cultivate real empathy. Empathy is an understanding of the situation from the other person's point of view. Without this shared understanding, there is no real or effective communication that will happen [17, 18].

The solution is a technique called active listening. It comes from psychologist Carl Rogers, PhD, who also pioneered the ideas of congruence and unconditional positive regard [19]. Congruence means being aware of our own reactions and emotions so we can convey those in a clear and honest way. The misconception is that when we are feeling irritated, for example, we can plaster on a smile and no one will know. That is rarely the case. Usually those around us are aware on some level that something is not right, though they may only be able to guess at the reason. It is simply a better, cleaner approach to become very aware of our reactions and deal with them directly. For instance, that same irritation, once recognized, can be examined to understand its cause. It may come from a time crunch, a poor diagnosis, or a bad breakfast. Being aware helps us deal with the issue and not project it upon those around us or try to hide and come across as "false."

Unconditional positive regard is an attitude taken by a practitioner in which one holds the client or patient in a positive regard. This means understanding them as human beings doing their best with what they have, as worthy and acceptable, despite any possible perceived shortcomings. This level of regard engenders tremendous trust as it allows the person to feel accepted on a deep level.

Both these practices support the technique of active listening. The technique is done by first finding a baseline level of regard for the person speaking, then actually listening to what they say, without working on our response or preparing our thoughts. When the person is done speaking, the listener checks for understanding. This is important. The listener reflects or returns the information back as they have understood it, checking to see if they have captured the meaning. "I hear you say you need more lead time to get those reports complete." The speaker is thereby given the opportunity to clarify as needed. This clarity results in a much greater level of shared understanding. This is really a very simple technique and can become a valuable tool. It can be used in any situation in which the exchange of information is very important, be that between physician and patient, physician and staff, or physician and referring doctor. It is especially useful when there has been some misunderstanding or shortcoming in communication in the past. This may seem more time consuming, but the clarity of information, lack of misunderstandings, and absence of a need for repeated communications will actually result in a more efficient exchange (Fig. 4.1).

4.5 Use of Questions

Much conflict arises in any workplace as a result of "jumping to conclusions." Of course it is the most natural thing to draw conclusions from what we see around us and the assumptions we make about what we see. The problem is when we confuse our assumptions with fact. However, facts cannot be determined without checking those assumptions. This is illustrated by the "ladder of inference" [20] (Fig. 4.2).

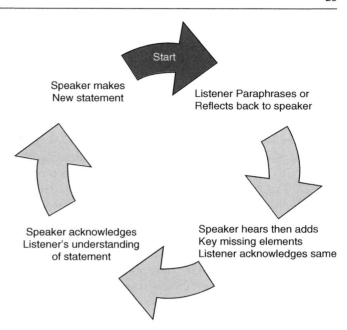

Fig. 4.1 Active listening cycle

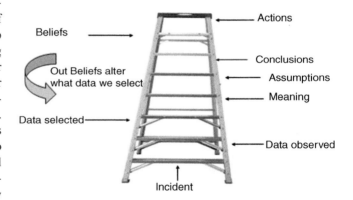

Fig. 4.2 Ladder of inference

The ladder shows how we take observations and begin to climb the ladder forming beliefs that inform our actions. However, the data we draw from our observations, the meaning we give that data, the assumptions, and conclusions we draw are all subjective. Without taking time to check things through, to question our own impressions, we may end up building belief systems that are structurally flawed.

The solution is in exploring perceptions through use of questions. The first place to intervene on the ladder is at the lowest level, checking with others about the information available and its possible meaning, before we make assumptions and draw conclusions. We all tend to work, unconsciously, in a network of assumptions and preconceptions. It is a very effective technique to begin asking question on a regular basis. Recognizing where we have assumed information is the hardest part. It might be helpful to start with a few generic questions to use regularly, such as "What have I missed?" or "What more would you like to hear about?"

Physicians use questions as a tool routinely to collect data. The types of questions normally used are closed-ended questions that allow only specific responses. "On a scale of 1–10, what is your pain?" or "Did you eat breakfast today?" To explore our assumptions, we must use open-ended questions, allowing the responder to choose what information to share. "Can you help me understand the choice you made there?" "I see a strong reaction from you; can you tell me what is going on?" "Is there something more you need from me to make this work better?"

Each type of question has its place. One of the things to learn is that "yes" or "no" questions will limit the communication rather than expand it. Those closed-ended questions make it far too easy to evade real communication for both parties. While closed-ended questions can be useful, they rarely enhance a relationship. Ask questions that inspire some thought, and require some explanation. Those thoughtful answers may actually produce needed information. Most importantly, they make the person feel appreciated and relationship building occurs. There is great power in recognizing an individual by offering them the opportunity to reflect and be heard.

4.6 Feedback Model

Some situations in the workplace can be contentious. Conflict is not easy to handle for many people. Some avoid it by closing their office doors, some by barking or snapping after letting things build up, and some by exhausting themselves by pretending to be "fine" at all times. The problem with allowing conflict to submerge in these unhealthy ways is that true solutions to problems are never addressed. Conflict is most often the result not of individual relational issues but of more complex sets of circumstances or misunderstandings. Something small can sometimes grow out of proportion, or the original cause may even get lost over time with only the conflict and avoidance remaining. The cost is tremendous exertion of energy that could better be used in more productive ways. Unresolved conflict can be very taxing indeed to the individuals and systems involved.

One solution to deal with conflict is to handle it right away and not let it fester. This involves a simple way of phrasing issues that makes it possible for both parties to view the situation in a new light without blame or hostility. We require tools to handle conflict, however, and many are never taught any of those tools. One tool is the feedback model. The essence of this approach is that we choose to address the conflict by talking about specific behavior, and our reactions to that behavior, rather than speak in generalities.

The first principle of this model is to understand that when we are upset or irritated by something, it is our own issue. The irritation is our own. The upset is because of our perception, history, viewpoint, and values. The other person may or may not have meant the insult or offense.

Remember the ladder of inference. What may seem like a fact, "She obviously disdains my work," may come from a series of assumptions based on misunderstood data. What makes this conclusion seem real? "I saw the look on her face." As above, the use of questions can be very helpful. "What was that look on your face about?" The answer may be, "I have indigestion." Or even something surprising like, "I was impressed with your work and suddenly felt inadequate. Did I make a face?" If the answer in fact is "I wasn't impressed with your work," then the good news is that issue is out in the open and can be discussed. Use questions such as "Can you tell me what your judgment is based on?" Maybe there is more hidden misunderstanding that now has an opportunity to come to light. If the objective is one of data collection, the mining effort can be very helpful. As painful as certain answers may be, carrying around worry and distress as we imagine things, and make up stories about reasons, is usually far worse.

The feedback model is a way of reflecting our experience to bring deeper understanding. The first step is to figure out what is the behavior in the other person that is upsetting. The second step is to identify that behavior to the person and let them know the effect it has on you and the conclusions you draw. The reason this works is because it takes both parties into account in the behavior and reaction cycle. The conflict is not just due to the initiator of a certain behavior but also the reactions and conclusions of the other person. This way of giving feedback is collaborative, because it takes ownership of reactions, rather than blaming the other for our reactions [21] (Table 4.1).

Compare this to the usual approach, "You're such a jerk! You are always nasty to me and treat me like dirt." Sadly, this more common approach undermines resolution by using vague and broad, even insulting descriptions that cannot be addressed in any concrete way. What is a "jerk?" The accused must respond to the insults in a defensive manner, rather than gain understanding about the behavior which is something that can be addressed.

The above technique does not guarantee a change in behavior, but it will successfully let the person know the effect they have with their chosen behavior. At that point,

Table 4.1 Three steps for productive feedback

	What is said	What is the process
1.	"When you snap at me in front of patients…"	This is the behavior
2.	"It causes me embarrassment…"	This is the effect
3.	"And I assume you have no respect for me."	This is the conclusion

both parties must "own" their individual part. The answer may be, "I do respect you… I just get frustrated, but it is not personal." Now both people know where they stand. If this is not comfortable, then it would be important to seek additional support within your company or an outside consultant if needed.

4.7 Communicating with Referral Sources

The principles discussed above will assist you in communicating with your referral sources. Each of the referral sources will want a different part of the information you have as a result of your care. In this section the specifics needed from each party are discussed. However, it is still important that the information be effectively communicated using the techniques described above.

4.7.1 The Patient

The patient may want an understanding of the importance of the dialysis access in their lives, the risks of the procedure, the probability that they will need future procedures, and the expected outcome for them in the future. They may also want a sense of confidence and safety with the procedure that does not necessarily come from verbal communication alone but nonverbal as well. While general information describing the procedure and the known risks may be communicated in handouts or pamphlets, nothing can take the place of the availability and willingness of the physician to directly speak with the patient. Pictures printed or drawn or copies of the actual images will clarify an enormous amount of technical information,

and using techniques like active listening and asking questions will help build that confidence and safety (Table 4.2).

4.7.2 Nephrologists

Nephrologists need to know different information. Most nephrologists are "on the road" a lot and might not be able to immediately take the time to receive oral communication. Some physicians may even prefer written to oral communication and it easy to ask them when the opportunity presents itself. This may be very individual, but written information will reliably be available via email, fax, or ideally the same electronic medical records as long as HIPAA standards are met. As to the type of information needed, it is important to estimate the degree of the procedural success and the ability of the patient to dialyze immediately. Images, if you are able to provide them, will help the physician to understand your communications better. Use questions to check for mutual understanding, and use more than one type of communication to insure complete clarity.

4.7.3 Surgeons

Surgeons are very individual in the specifics they want. The communication with your surgeon may need to be oral until you understand what they individually need and then it can be predominately written. This would be primarily in the form of your dictation. Complete imaging of the venous and sometimes arterial anatomy will assist in surgical planning. There is no substitute for actual images and a detailed description of the anatomy in surgical care. Clearly, several

Table 4.2 Communicating to referral sources

Entity	Mode	Required data	Future needs	Making it better
Patient	1. Oral	1. Risks/benefits	1. When?	Pre-tx pamphlets
	2. Pictures	2. Why?	2. What?	Post-tx images
	3. Written	3. Results	3. How?	
Nephrologists	1. Written	1. Success?	1. How long?	Know which doctors like phone calls
	2. Oral	2. Dialysis now	2. Tx options	Send images with reports
	3. Pictures		3. Next site?	
			4. Referral?	
Surgeons	1. Oral	1. Anatomy	1. Tx options	Send images
	2. Pictures	2.Tx response	2. How long	Specifics in report and images
	3. Written	3. Alter surgery	3. New sites	
Dialysis units	1. Pictures	1. Use today?	1. Is more tx needed? When?	Images of access –especially "stick zone"
	2. Written	2. Where to stick?	2. Needed f/u?	
	3. Oral	3. New orders	3. Orders?	
Payers	Written	Justify tx	Practice trends?	Know requirements

Evidence for the table is based on research from studies of radiological literature [22–25]

modes of information delivery are required. Be aware of your ladder of inference, and check facts and understanding with surgeons as you establish a working relationship.

4.7.4 Dialysis Units

Dialysis units are very specific and immediate in their needs. Can they dialyze now? Do they need to be rescheduled? Dialysis staff often does not have time to come to the phone. Unless it is urgent with regard to the care of the patient today, it may not be really useful. If verbal communications are needed, of course they are readily appreciated. However, for routine information, a written report and ideally a picture of where the problems are and where to "stick" will be appreciated. Remember to conclude by checking for understanding. Repeat back information to confirm you have it right. Ask an open-ended question like "is there anything else you need to know?" The ability to successful communicate with the dialysis staff may be most important in terms of your ability to grow your practice.

4.7.5 Payers

For now the primary source of communication with payers is your dictation. It should include the diagnosis, name of procedure, and indication for the procedure. It should also document the degree of abnormality that made the intervention necessary and the immediate response to treatment. The K/ DOQI standards are the most pertinent [26]. For instance, the minimum degree of stenosis that will qualify for angioplasty is 50 %, and a successful angioplasty is judged by the response of the lesion to be decreased to less than 30 % residual stenosis. The ASDIN coding manual may be very useful in this regard [27].

Legal issues may arise from performing procedures. While no pre-procedure plans to communicate with attorneys in advance should exist, it is important that elements of your written documentation satisfy the standards of care in your community and in this field of medicine. Documentation of your consent and explanation of the procedure are needed. Some documentation of pre-sedation assessment will be needed for cases where sedation is used. Documenting the "time-out" or a procedural "pause" in the procedure room is now standard of care at most facilities. The procedural dictation itself should be as detailed as needed for payers and for the above physician referral sources. Again all your communications, oral, written, or imaging, will be viewed by different people in different contexts. It is important to be aware of this as you perform each procedure and discuss the outcome with the interested parties.

Taking these last two areas of communication into account may seem tedious, but the fact remains that the physician must interact, again, with the larger web of human and organizational structures that make up the whole. They do not function in isolation and cannot simply do their "job" without understanding their dependence upon the larger structure and the dependence that structure has upon them.

4.7.6 Organizational Communication

Corporations can be seen as living entities. They have their own needs, such as maintaining a reputation and increasing revenue year to year. At the same time, the corporation is made up of networks of individuals with their own needs. They wish to be respected, appreciated, and understood. This is why the skill of communicating with individuals and relationship building with those individuals with whom you have contact within the corporation is so important. They make up the pieces of the whole.

Just like people, organizations adopt cultures and personalities. Organizational communication is far more difficult to understand and more difficult to change than individual interactions. Whether it is the government, professional societies, hospitals, health maintenance organizations, large dialysis groups, or the newly developing accountable care organizations, physicians will have to interact with large organizations in some way. It is important to realize that some of the strategies for communication are the same for this sort of communication and some are different [28–31].

Companies like to align themselves with others who share their view of the "world." Companies will not participate in enterprises that have too large an investment without a guaranteed return or enterprises they do not believe will make money in the long run or might be negative for public relations. Understanding this will influence what you say and how you say it when discussing your practice with potential partners and contractors. If you do not understand the wants and needs of the organization you are working with, then questioning techniques as described above are helpful to understand what the issues are. "What is the company looking for? What is your role in the company? Is there specific information you need to assist you in making this decision?" Empathy or the ability to understand the information you have from the view of the organization is extremely advantageous.

Do not forget that each conversation you have with an employee of an organization is with a person. So active listening will assist in building trust and better understanding between people. The specifics of the information exchanged will be different, but the people and techniques are the same. Your ability to present the data needed in an effective manner may become important in the survival of your practice. As the evolution of health care continues, you may need to present data ranging from the ability of your staff to communicate to your complication rate and the cost efficiency of your practice. All this data is highly valued by many organizations.

It is therefore upon the presenter to have the data to back up their statements. It will not be enough to say "I practice good medicine." Information will be needed regarding the delivery of quality service, cost efficiency, and rate of complications compared to the rest of those in your field. Thus it may be important in the future to participate in national databases which collect patient safety information. In the corporate world, such by data can be obtained using continuous quality improvement techniques [32]. Many of the lessons from manufacturing have been applied with some success to health care [33, 34]. Quality improvement in the manufacturing business is a large field that is beyond the scope of this chapter, but the techniques can be useful in maintaining and improving your practice. Even when there is a large amount of data available, it is still essential to communicate the information well to your corporate colleagues in order to be successful. The techniques described for improving individual communication can apply to corporations.

Conclusion

Much depends on continued individual, institutional, and corporate communications to survive in a changing health-care landscape. While practicing medicine can be done without good communications, practicing excellent medicine cannot.

References

1. Auerbach AD, Sehgal NL, Biegen MA, et al. Effects of a multicentre teamwork and communication programme on patient outcomes: results from the Triad for Optimal Patient Safety (TOPS) project. BMJ Qual Saf. 2012;21(2):118–26.
2. Davenport DL, Henderson WG, Mosca CL, Khuri SH, Mentzer Jr RM. Risk-adjusted morbidity in teaching hospitals correlates with reported levels of communication and collaboration on surgical teams but not with scale measures of teamwork climate, safety climate, or working conditions. J Am Coll Surg. 2007;205(6):778–84.
3. Shaw JR. Four core communication skills of highly effective practitioners. Vet Clin North Am Small Anim Pract. 2006;36(2):385–96.
4. Teutsch C. Patient-doctor communication. Med Clin North Am. 2003;87(5):1115–45.
5. Solomon P, Salfi J. Evaluation of an interprofessional education communication skills initiative. Educ Heatlh (Abingdon). 2011;24(2):616.
6. Tamuz M, Giardina TD, Thomas EJ, Menon S, Singh H. Rethinking resident supervision to improve safety: from hierarchical to interprofessional models. J Hosp Med. 2011;6(8):445–52.
7. Dupree E, Anderson R, McEvoy MD, Brodman M. Professionalism: a necessary ingredient in a culture of safety. Jt Comm J Qual Patient Saf. 2011;37(10):447–55.
8. Forrest CB, Glade GB, Baker AE, Bocian A, von Schrader S, Starfield B. Coordination of specialty referrals and physician satisfaction with referral care. Arch Pediatr Adolesc Med. 2000;154(5):499–506.
9. Williams PT, Peet G. Differences in the value of clinical information: referring physicians versus consulting specialists. J Am Board Fam Pract. 1994;7(4):292–302.
10. Piterman L, Koritsas S. Part II. General practitioner-specialist referral process. Intern Med J. 2005;35(8):491–6.
11. Barnett ML, Keating NL, Christakis NA, O'Malley AJ, Landon BE. Reasons for choice of referral physician among primary care and specialist physicians. J Gen Intern Med. 2012;27(5):506–12.
12. Harolds JA. Communicating in organizations, part I: general principles of high-stakes discussions. Clin Nucl Med. 2012;37(3):274–6.
13. Roberts C, Roper C. The four C's of leadership development. Adv Health Care Manag. 2011;10:125–49.
14. Tsai Y, Wu SW. Using internal marketing to improve organizational commitment and service quality. J Adv Nurs. 2011;67(12):2593–604.
15. MacDavitt K, Chou SS, Stone PW. Organizational climate and health care outcomes. Jt Comm J Qual Patient Saf. 2007;33 (11 Suppl):45–56.
16. Shams L, Seitz AR. Benefits of multisensory learning. Trends Cogn Sci. 2008;12(11):411–7.
17. Tavakol S, Dennick R, Tavakol M. Empathy in UK medical students: differences by gender, medical year and specialty interest. Educ Prim Care. 2011;22(5):297–303.
18. Brown T, Boyle M, Williams B, et al. Predictors of empathy in health science students. J Allied Health. 2011;40(3):143–9.
19. Rogers CR. Client-centered therapy: its current practice, implications and theory. London: Constable; 1951.
20. Senge PM, Kleiner A, Roberts C, Ross RB, Smith BJ. The fifth discipline fieldbook: strategies and tools for building a learning organization". New York: Doubleday; 1994.
21. Seashore CN, Seashore EW, Weinberg GM. What did you say?: the art of giving and receiving feedback. North Attenbough: Douglas Charles Press; 1992.
22. Plumb AA, Grieve FM, Khan SH. Survey of hospital clinicians' preferences regarding the format of radiology reports. Clin Radiol. 2009;64(4):386–96.
23. Grieve FM, Plumb AA, Khan SH. Radiology reporting: a general practitioner's perspective. Br J Radiol. 2010;83(985):17–22.
24. Cinger NJ, Hunter TB, Hillman BJ. Radiology reporting: attitudes of referring physicians. Radiology. 1988;169(3):825–6.
25. Siskin G. Outpatient care of the interventional radiology patient. Semin Intervent Radiol. 2006;23(4):337–45.
26. Hayashi R, Huang E, Nissenson AR. Vascular access for hemodialysis. Nat Clin Pract Nephrol. 2006;2(9):504–13.
27. ASDIN coding manual. www.asdin.org.
28. Lok P, Rhodes J, Westwood B. Mediating the role of organizational subcultures in health care organizations. J Health Organ Manag. 2011;25(5):506–25.
29. Zhou P, Bundorf K, Le Chang J, Huang JX, Xue D. Organizational culture and its relationship with hospital performance in public hospitals in China. Health Serv Res. 2011;46(6 pt 12):2139–60.
30. Morrison EE, Burke 3rd GC, Greene L. Meaning in motivation: does your organization need an inner life? J Health Hum Serv Adm. 2007;30(1):98–115.
31. Kirschbaum K. Physician communication in the operating room: expanding application of face-negotiation theory to the health communication context. Health Commun. 2012;27(3):292–301.
32. Stapleton FB, Hendricks J, Hagan P, DelBeccaro M. Modifying the Toyota production system for continuous performance improvement in an academic children's hospital. Pediatr Clin North Am. 2009;56(4):799–813.
33. Chung KC, Shauver MJ. Measuring quality in health care and its implications for pay-for-performance initiatives. Hand Clin. 2009;25(1):71–81.
34. Caplan JP, Querques J, Epstein LA, Stern TA. Consultation, communication, and conflict management by out-of-operating room anesthesiologists: strangers in a strange land. Anesthesiol Clin. 2009;27(1):111–20.

Anticoagulants and Thrombolytics

5

K.M.L.S.T. Moorthi

5.1 Introduction

Anticoagulants and thrombolytics are used during several procedures that the interventionalist performs. In this chapter we will review patient safety issues with the use of these agents.

5.2 Heparin

Heparin is used in several access interventions. Two formulations of heparin exist – unfractionated heparin (UFH) and low molecular weight heparin (LMWH). UFH has a molecular weight of 15,000 Da, and LMWH, which is prepared by depolymerization of UFH, has a molecular weight of approximately 5,000 Da. Since LMWH is typically not used in the interventional nephrology setting, discussions in this chapter will be limited to UFH.

Heparin is an indirect thrombin inhibitor (Fig. 5.1). It forms a complex with the heparin binding site of antithrombin. Antithrombin is a circulating cofactor and at baseline is a slow inactivator of thrombin, factor Xa, and to a lesser extent, factors XIIa, XIa, and IXa. The binding of heparin accelerates the inactivating function of antithrombin 1,000–4,000-fold [1, 2].

With IV dosing, the onset of action is immediate. The half-life of elimination is dose dependent. With the usual doses used in interventional nephrology procedures (3,000–5,000 units), the half-life is 30 min.

The limitations of heparin include a narrow therapeutic window of anticoagulation (without bleeding) and a highly variable dose–response relation. In addition, heparin has a reduced ability to inactivate thrombin bound to fibrin as well

as factor Xa bound to activated platelets within a thrombus. As a result, a thrombus may continue to grow during heparin therapy [3].

The most dreaded adverse reaction to heparin is bleeding. Although there is a strong clinical correlation between subtherapeutic activated partial thromboplastin time (aPTT) and recurrent thromboembolism, the relation between supratherapeutic aPTT and bleeding is less clear. Patients who have had recent surgery or trauma, or who have other clinical factors which predispose to bleeding, such as occult malignancy, liver disease, hemostatic defects, age >65 years, female gender, and a reduced baseline hemoglobin concentration, seem to be at a higher risk for bleeding with heparin.

5.3 Bleeding During Interventional Procedures

The incidence of bleeding complications during and after thrombectomy (Fig. 5.2) is about 2–3 %, with the incidence increasing to 10–15 % with the use of pharmacologic thrombolysis. Bleeding, when it occurs, is usually seen at the sites of cannulation. Bleeding from the sites of attempted cannulation by dialysis staff is unfortunately common. Education of dialysis staff to examine the AV access for patency before attempting to cannulate can help reduce the incidence of such bleeding. Placement of percutaneous sutures at the sites of cannulation is usually adequate to prevent/treat such bleeding.

Peri-access hematomas are also possible. Most are small hematomas that do not impede flow in the access. Rarely expanding hematomas may occur, and these may impede flow. Such hematomas can be treated by prolonged angioplasty of the affected site (the angioplasty balloon catheter is held dilated at the affected site for 1–2 min) (Fig. 5.3: plates d–f) and/or placing a stent across the site of bleeding. In extreme cases the hematoma may not stabilize and may lead to arterial insufficiency of the upper extremity by compression of the brachial artery. In such instances, external

K.M.L.S.T. Moorthi, MD
Nephrology Associates of Northern Indiana,
8668 Broadway, Merrillville, IN 46410, USA
e-mail: kmlstmoorthi@yahoo.com

A.S. Yevzlin et al. (eds.), *Interventional Nephrology*,
DOI 10.1007/978-1-4614-8803-3_5, © Springer Science+Business Media New York 2014

Fig. 5.1 Coagulation cascade

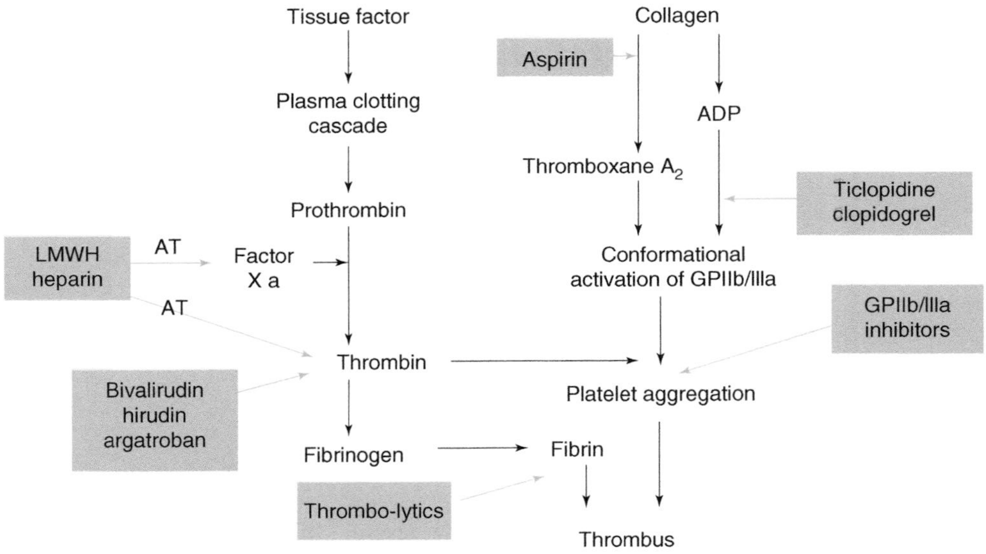

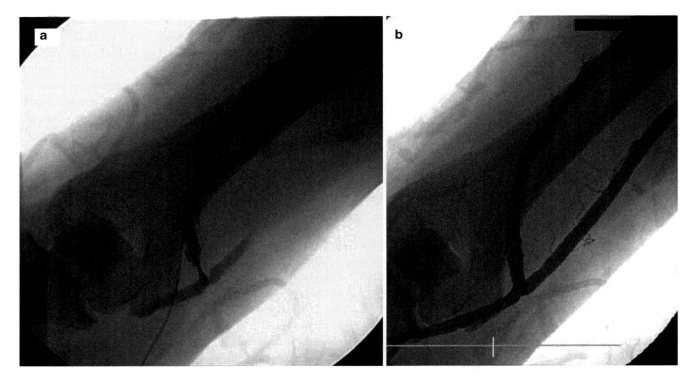

Fig. 5.2 Lesion leading to thrombosis (**a**) and eventual thrombectomy (**b**)

compression and occlusion of inflow with an inflated angio-plasty balloon catheter while the patient is transported to the hospital may be limb and life saving.

Hematomas can also occur at the site of angioplasty of juxta-anastomotic stenoses. After angioplasty of the juxta-anastomotic stenoses, the inflow artery is usually selectively catheterized, and an arteriogram is performed to evaluate for complications of the angioplasty and to avoid vein rupture

associated with retrograde injection. While withdrawing the catheter, it could inadvertently "flip" and injure the vessel wall and result in a hematoma (Fig. 5.3). To avoid this, it is advisable to introduce a guidewire into the catheter and remove the catheter over the guidewire.

Delayed bleeding is possible, when patients are sent back to their dialysis centers after thrombectomy and they receive additional doses of heparin. It is standard practice at our center,

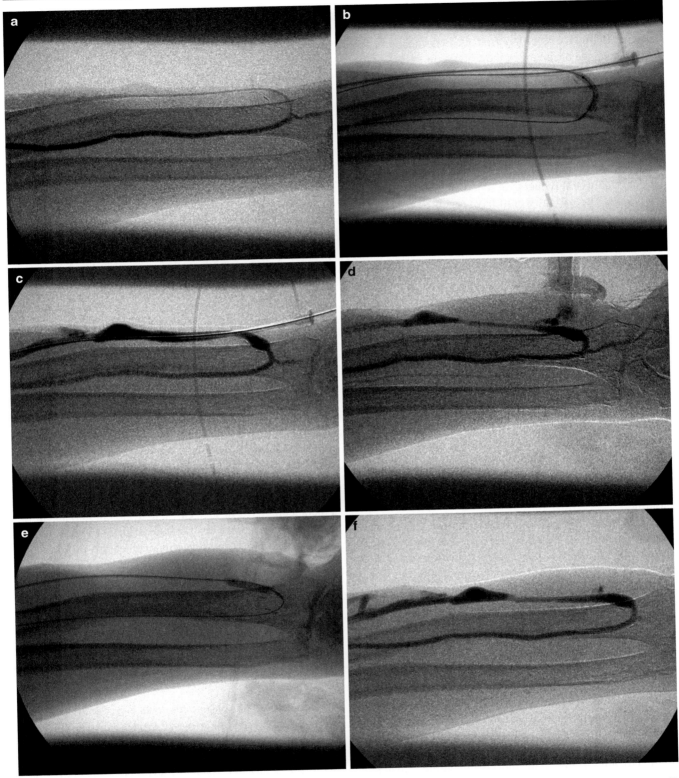

Fig. 5.3 Extravasation at the site of juxta-anastomotic stenosis. (**a**) Severe juxta-anastomotic stenosis with minimal flow into the fistula. (**b**) Angioplasty of the stenosis. (**c**) Post-angioplasty angiogram with improved flow. (**d**) Extravasation/hematoma after withdrawal of the vascular catheter – the catheter "flipped" and injured the vessel wall. There is sluggish flow in the fistula. (**e**) Prolonged angioplasty. (**f**) Resolution of extravasation and improved flow

where a call is placed to the dialysis center and instructions are given to the dialysis staff to deduct the dose of heparin that was given during the procedure from the bolus dose scheduled to be given at the beginning of the dialysis run.

5.4 Dialysis Catheter Procedures

During tunneled dialysis catheter insertion, heparin is used to pack the catheter ports at the end of the procedure. However, after failed thrombectomy procedures, the patient would likely need a tunneled dialysis catheter placement. The patient would have received heparin during the thrombectomy procedure. As described above, the half-life of heparin in the usual doses used for outpatient interventions is 30 min. It is safe to place a tunneled dialysis catheter after a failed thrombectomy. Central venous patency should be evaluated with an angiogram, as central venous stenoses could increase the pressure the jugular vein and if untreated could lead to bleeding from the venotomy or from the exit site.

5.5 Heparin-Induced Thrombocytopenia

Heparin is used routinely as an anticoagulant during hemodialysis and in dialysis access interventions. HIT is a well-recognized complication of heparin therapy. As many as 10–20 % of patients receiving unfractionated heparin will experience a decrease in platelet count to less than the normal range or a 50 % decrease in platelet count from the baseline.

There are two major mechanisms causing thrombocytopenia. In majority of the cases, the thrombocytopenia occurs within the first 48–72 h after heparin initiation. The platelet counts return to normal with continued heparin use. This is Type 1 HIT and is of no clinical consequence. The mechanism is nonimmune and appears to be due to a direct effect of heparin on platelet activation.

Type 2 occurs in 0.5–3 % of patients receiving heparin. These patients develop an immune thrombocytopenia, mediated by antibodies to a heparin-platelet factor 4 complex [4].

In contrast to other autoimmune thrombocytopenias, the platelet count usually does not drop below 50,000, and spontaneous bleeding is unusual. However, in patients who have been diagnosed with HIT, the subsequent 30-day risk of a thrombotic event (arterial and/or venous) is 53 % [5]. Pulmonary embolism was the most common life-threatening thrombotic event.

HD patients are continually exposed to heparin and are at risk of developing heparin-platelet factor 4 complex antibodies. Reports have described the prevalence of these antibodies in HD with frequencies ranging from 0 to 12 % [6, 7].

It is important to note that the mere presence of heparin-platelet factor 4 complex antibodies does not suggest a diagnosis of HIT in the absence of other clinical events.

In addition, several case reports have reported a dramatic improvement in access patency after discontinuing heparin with HD and beginning treatment with Coumadin. This suggests that heparin antibodies have a role in recurrent vascular access occlusion in some patients [8].

5.6 Interventions in Patients on Warfarin

Dialysis patients who present to the interventionalist may be on warfarin therapy for various reasons. For instance, the prevalence of atrial fibrillation is about 10 % in US dialysis patients. [9]. A large proportion of these patients can be expected to be treated with warfarin. The question arises as to the safety of performing vascular access interventions in these patients. There is a paucity of data regarding this.

The placement of tunneled dialysis catheters in patients on warfarin is safe [10].

We routinely evaluate patients on warfarin for central venous stenosis and perform angioplasty on any such lesions before placing a tunneled dialysis catheter. As described before in this chapter, this decreases the pressure in the jugular vein and the chances of postoperative bleeding.

During thrombectomy procedures, it is unknown whether the dose of heparin given systemically should be reduced. In the absence of specific data, we reduce the dose of heparin to 3,000 units (instead of the 5,000 units that we usually use in thrombectomy procedures) in patients who have a therapeutic INR. In such cases, to avoid embolizing all the thrombus material, we also aspirate as much of the thrombus with the aid of a 6 French vascular catheter. A 6 Fr vascular catheter is passed over a guidewire and several passes are made, while applying negative pressure and thrombus material is aspirated and discarded. This reduces the volume of the thrombus centrally embolized.

5.7 Warfarin to Prevent Thrombosis of Dialysis Accesses

Warfarin does not prevent thrombosis/failure of an AV graft, and its use is associated with increased incidence of bleeding. In a multicenter randomized control study, 107 patients with new grafts were randomly assigned to receive warfarin (target INR of 1.4–1.9) or placebo. There was no difference in graft thrombosis between the two groups. The incidence of major hemorrhage was 10 % despite close monitoring of the INR [11].

A subset of dialysis patients in whom thrombosis of the AV graft occurs within the first 48 h of surgery, and those who have recurrent graft thrombosis may have a hypercoagulable state that contributes to the thrombosis. In such patients evaluation for a hypercoagulable state could be performed, and if such a condition is present, warfarin therapy could be considered [12–14]. However, there is paucity of strong data supporting this recommendation. A case could be made for performing a hypercoagulable state evaluation in select patients as follows:

1. Patients in whom the graft thrombosis is in the first 48 h of surgery
2. Patients in whom the graft thromboses are without an anatomical lesion AND in whom the blood pressure is normal
3. Patients who have had more than three episodes of thrombosis in a calendar year

Antiphospholipid antibodies, activated protein C resistance, protein C and S levels, and evaluation for antithrombin deficiency could be obtained. If the work-up above is positive, then low-dose warfarin therapy (target INR of 1.5–2.0) could be considered.

5.8 Newer Anticoagulant Medications

We avoid the use of the new orally active anticoagulants (dabigatran, rivaroxaban, and apixaban) in our dialysis patients as there are no long-term data on the safety of these medications in this subset of patients and there is a lack of effective antidotes. Interventions in patients who are on these agents cannot be advocated at this time.

5.9 Thrombolytics

Thrombolytic therapy is used in management of thrombosed AV accesses. The most commonly used agent is Alteplase (recombinant tissue plasminogen activator – rtPA). When given intravenously, the onset is almost instantaneous. The drug binds to fibrin in a thrombus and converts entrapped plasminogen into plasmin, thus initiating local fibrinolysis. It is a short-acting drug with about half the drug present in the plasma cleared by 5 min after termination of the infusion and more than 80 % cleared within 10 min.

Reteplase (onset of thrombolysis in 30–90 min and half-life of elimination of 13–15 min) and urokinase have been used as well. Due to the delayed onset of reteplase and the predominantly extravascular activation of fibrinolysis by urokinase (in contrast to tPA which is largely responsible for initiating intravascular fibrinolysis), neither is used commonly by the interventionalist.

Doses of 0.5–2 mg of tPA are usually used. With such doses the incidence of complications is about 10–15 % [15]. Most are minor complications and include bleeding from dialysis cannulation sites and peri-access hematomas. Major complications are uncommon and include vein rupture. These can be treated with prolonged angioplasty and/or stenting. Rarely arterial rupture can be a complication (Fig. 5.4). If this happens, the first and only priority is to save the limb. A stent could be placed across the rupture. More often than not, ligation of the access and arterial bypass may be needed. It is of paramount importance to evaluate the artery with an arteriogram after arterial angioplasty to recognize this complication.

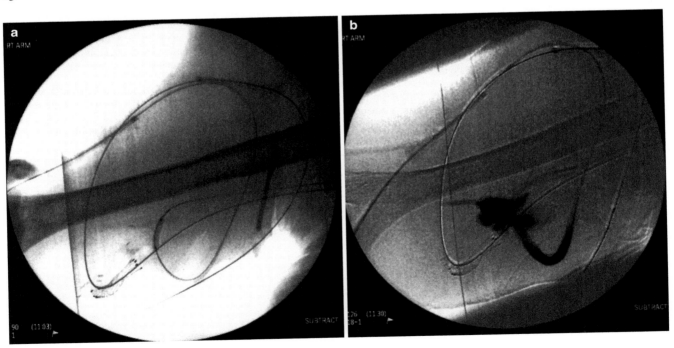

Fig. 5.4 Arterial anastomotic angioplasty complicated by arterial rupture. The patient underwent brachial artery bypass

Given the rapid clearance of rtPA, it is safe to place tunneled dialysis catheters should a thrombectomy be unsuccessful.

In the in-patient setting, continuous rtPA infusion has been used to achieve thrombolysis. While there exists little data on the incidence of complications, we have encountered two instances of cerebral bleeding in our dialysis patients who underwent rtPA infusion (out of a total of 12 patients whom we referred for in-patient thrombolysis due to large thrombus load).

5.10 Summary and Recommendations

1. The use of anticoagulants and thrombolytics in percutaneous interventions of dialysis accesses is safe.
2. The most common complication of the use of anticoagulants and thrombolytics is bleeding.
3. Bleeding from access cannulation sites can be controlled with percutaneous sutures.
4. Bleeding from sites of angioplasty can be treated with prolonged angioplasty and/or stenting.
5. After selective catheterization of an artery, removal of the catheter over a guidewire should be considered.
6. If a tunneled dialysis catheter is needed after the patient has received anticoagulants and/or thrombolytics, central venous patency should be evaluated with an angiogram. If central venous stenoses are noted, then these should be treated before placement of a catheter.

References

1. Hirsh J, Bauer KA, Donati MB, Gould M, Samama MM, Weitz JI, American College of Chest Physicians SO Chest. Parenteral anticoagulants: American College of Chest Physicians Evidence-Based Clinical Practice Guidelines (8th Edition). Chest. 2008;133(6 Suppl):141S.
2. Hirsh J, Anand SS, Halperin JL, Fuster V, American Heart Association. Guide to anticoagulant therapy: heparin: a statement for healthcare professionals from the American Heart Association. Circulation. 2001;103(24):2994.
3. Weitz JI, Hudoba M, Massel D, Maraganore J, Hirsh J. Clot-bound thrombin is protected from inhibition by heparin-antithrombin III but is susceptible to inactivation by antithrombin III-independent inhibitors. J Clin Invest. 1990;86(2):385.
4. Visentin GP, Ford SE, Scott JP, Aster RH. Antibodies from patients with heparin-induced thrombocytopenia/thrombosis are specific for platelet factor 4 complexed with heparin or bound to endothelial cells. J Clin Invest. 1994;93(1):81–8.
5. Warkentin TE, Kelton JG. A 14-year study of heparin-induced thrombocytopenia. Am J Med. 1996;101(5):502.
6. Yamamoto S, Koide M, Matsuo M, Suzuki S, Ohtaka M, Saika S, Matsuo T. Heparin-induced thrombocytopenia in hemodialysis patients. Am J Kidney Dis. 1996;28(1):82–5.
7. de Sancho M, Lema MG, Amiral J, Rand J. Frequency of antibodies directed against heparin-platelet factor 4 in patients exposed to heparin through chronic hemodialysis. Thromb Haemost. 1996;175(4):695–6.
8. O'shea SI, Lawson JH, Reddan D, Murphy M, Ortel TL. Hypercoagulable states and antithrombotic strategies in recurrent vascular access site thrombosis. J Vasc Surg. 2003;38(3):541–8.
9. United States renal data system: cardiovascular special studies. The National Institutes of Health, National Institute of Diabetes and Digestive and Kidney Diseases, Bethesda. 2005.
10. Lee O, Raque JD, Lee LJ, Wivell W, Block CA, Bettmann MA. Retrospective assessment of risk factors to predict tunneled hemodialysis catheter outcome. J Vasc Interv Radiol. 2004;15(5):1457–61.
11. Crowther MA, Clase CM, Margetts PJ, Julian J, Lambert K, Sneath D, Nagai R, Wilson S, Ingram AJ. Low-intensity warfarin is ineffective for the prevention of PTFE graft failure in patients on hemodialysis: a randomized controlled trial. J Am Soc Nephrol. 2002;13(9):2331.
12. Brunet P, Aillaud MF, San Marco M, Philip-Joet C, Dussol B, Bernard D, Juhan-Vague I, Berland Y. Antiphospholipids in hemodialysis patients: relationship between lupus anticoagulant and thrombosis. Kidney Int. 1995;48(3):794.
13. Prakash R, Miller 3rd CC, Suki WN. Anticardiolipin antibody in patients on maintenance hemodialysis and its association with recurrent arteriovenous graft thrombosis. Am J Kidney Dis. 1995;26(2):347.
14. Molino D, De Lucia D, Marotta R, Perna A, Lombardi C, Cirillo M, De Santo NG. In uremia, plasma levels of anti-protein C and anti-protein S antibodies are associated with Thrombosis. Kidney Int. 2005;68(3):1223.
15. Abigail Falk MD, Harold Mitty MD, Jeffrey Guller MD, Victoria Teodorescu MD, Jaime Uribarri MD, Joseph Vassalotti MD. Thrombolysis of clotted hemodialysis grafts with tissue-type plasminogen activator. J Vasc Interv Radiol. 2001;12(3):305–11.

Noninvasive Screening and Testing for PAD in CKD Patients

Alexander S. Yevzlin and Peter J. Mason

6.1 Introduction

Cardiovascular disease (CVD) is the cause of death in nearly half of end-stage renal disease (ESRD) patients [1]. An individual with ESRD has a CVD mortality rate 15 times that found in the general population. Moreover, CVD is the leading cause of death in patients with chronic kidney disease (CKD), and a patient even with early-stage CKD is five to ten times more likely to die from a cardiovascular event than progress to ESRD [2]. As nephrologists we are aware of the importance of CVD risk factor detection and modification. We are instructed by a multitude of guidelines to evaluate our ESRD and CKD patients for atherosclerotic coronary artery disease (CAD) with cardiologic referral, lipid management, and stress testing.

The prevalence of PAD increases significantly with age and is high regardless of age in patients with diabetes or tobacco abuse [14]. Previous studies have shown that peripheral arterial disease (PAD) is associated with a significantly elevated risk of cardiovascular disease morbidity and mortality and is generally regarded as a CVD equivalent in terms of mortality risk [3–5]. Despite these facts, PAD remains underdiagnosed and undertreated [14]. Patients with PAD are often asymptomatic or present with atypical symptoms, and although the severe complications of PAD are devastating and should be aggressively prevented, the benefits of detection and treatment of PAD beyond the recommended guidelines for its associated comorbid conditions remain somewhat uncertain. This may be especially true for the subset of CKD patients with PAD. The purpose of this chapter is to describe an approach to PAD screening in CKD patients.

6.2 Pathophysiology of PAD in CKD Patients

The pathophysiology of vascular disease in the CKD population differs from the nonrenal disease population. Vascular disease associated with traditional atherosclerotic disease risk factors such as diabetes, dyslipidemia, hypertension, tobacco abuse, and aging is characterized by intimal disease with lipid-rich plaques producing focal stenoses and the potential for plaque rupture and subsequent thrombosis. In CKD, on the other hand, plaques are characterized by intense medial calcification, which tends toward chronic stenotic disease rather than acute plaque rupture [6]. Although medial calcification does occur in the aging population, the form seen in the CKD population occurs at a much earlier age and with much greater severity [7–9].

The most evident factors in the development of medial arterial calcification are serum levels of calcium and phosphate. Relatively early in the progression of CKD, the kidneys retain phosphate. The tissue most exposed to the serum is the vascular endothelium. Recent epidemiologic data suggest that there is a direct correlation between serum phosphate levels and all-cause and cardiovascular mortality in CKD and ESRD [10]. Vascular smooth muscle cells (VSMC) also appear central to the process of medial calcification. Vascular smooth muscle cells may undergo trans-differentiation into phenotypically distinct cells that are capable of generating calcification in the presence of inflammation [11].

A.S. Yevzlin, MD (✉)
Division of Nephrology,
Department of Medicine (CHS),
University of Wisconsin, Madison, WI 53705, USA
e-mail: asy@medicine.wisc.edu

P.J. Mason
Division of Cardiovascular Medicine,
Department of Medicine,
University of Wisconsin College of Medicine
and Public Health, Madison, WI, USA

6.3 Epidemiology of PAD in CKD Population

Prior estimates of PAD prevalence in the USA have ranged from 3 to 30 % in US adult populations [12–15]. A study by Selvin et al. analyzed data from 2,174 participants aged 40 years and older from the 1999–2000 National Health and Nutrition Examination Survey [16]. PAD was defined as an ankle-brachial index less than 0.90 in either leg. The prevalence of PAD among adults aged 40 years and over in the USA was 4.3 %, which corresponds to approximately five million individuals. Among those aged 70 years or over, the prevalence was 14.5 %. Among the risk factors identified, CKD (OR 2.00, 95 % CI 1.08–3.70) conferred a twofold increased risk of PAD. Interestingly, fibrinogen and C-reactive protein levels, which are known to be disproportionately elevated in CKD patients, are also associated with PAD [16]. In an updated analysis of NHANES including data from 1999 to 2004, the estimated prevalence of PAD among US adults over 40 years of age was 5.9 %, or approximately 7.1 million individuals.

Our understanding of PAD prevalence is further enhanced by two epidemiological studies in at-risk individuals followed in community-based primary care practices. The peripheral arterial disease detection, awareness, and treatment in primary care (PARTNERS) trial assessed the prevalence of PAD in 6,979 American adults aged 70 years and older and 50 years of age or older with diabetes or tobacco abuse [14]. PAD was defined by questionnaire and ankle-brachial index testing. The study found that 29 % of all patients had PAD based on an abnormal ABI (<0.9) but that only 9 % of these patients reported typical claudication symptoms [14]. The German epidemiological trial on ankle brachial index (GETABI) determined the prevalence of PAD in 6,821 German adults by practitioner history and ankle-brachial index testing. Unlike in PARTNERS, the only inclusion criterion in the GETABI trial was that patients were aged 65 years and older. The study found that 21 % of patients had either symptomatic or asymptomatic PAD (ABI <0.9).

Most studies of cardiovascular disease in patients with CKD have not examined lower-extremity PAD per se [17–19], despite exceedingly high amputation rates in this patient population [20]. A study by O'Hare et al. examined the cross-sectional association of PAD, defined as an ankle-brachial index (ABI) <0.9, and CKD stage 3–5, defined as an estimated creatinine clearance (CRCL) <60 mL per min, among 2,229 eligible participants in the National Health and Nutrition Examination Survey (NHANES) 1999–2000 [22]. Univariate logistic regression analysis showed that compared with their counterparts with CKD stage 2 or higher kidney function, patients with moderate to severe CKD were at ninefold increased risk to have an ABI <0.9 (versus an ABI of 1–1.3). The authors developed two multivariable models to adjust sequentially for demographic characteristics and comorbid conditions that might confound the association between renal insufficiency and ABI. After adjustment for age, gender, and race, moderate to severe CKD remained strongly associated with an ABI <0.9 (OR 3.0, 95 % CI 1.7–5.3, $P < 0.001$). This association persisted after further adjustment for comorbid conditions including diabetes, coronary artery disease, and history of stroke; measures of diabetes severity (glycosylated hemoglobin, self-reported retinopathy, and insulin use); history of diagnosed hypertension; and measured blood pressure, total cholesterol, BMI, and smoking history. The authors concluded that clinicians should be aware of the remarkably high prevalence of PAD among patients with CKD. Moreover, they argued that accurate identification of patients with CKD combined with routine ABI measurement in this group would greatly enhance efforts to detect subclinical PAD.

Given the increased incidence of PAD in CKD, the K/DOQI guidelines recommend screening all patients upon initiation of dialysis [21]. The K/DOQI guidelines, however, in this particular area, must be taken with caution given the weakness in evidence supporting them. In addition, the guidelines address only dialysis patients and do not make specific recommendations for those with CKD. The issue is further complicated by the fact that there is no consensus regarding optimal treatment strategies. The issues regarding cardiovascular mortality, lower limb mortality, patient's functional status, and candidacy for available medical and interventional therapies must be weighed when making the decision to screen for PAD in CKD. Put simply, patients with CKD and ESRD may not be candidates for revascularization, which would be an argument against screening in these situations in the first place.

Therefore, before screening methods are discussed, it is important to determine risk factors for the presence of PAD. Data from waves 1, 3, and 4 of the US Renal Data System Dialysis Morbidity and Mortality Study were used to examine cross-sectional associations of a range of conventional cardiovascular risk factors and uremia- or dialysis-related variables with PAD in a recent study [22]. PAD was positively associated with the duration of dialysis (vintage) and malnourished status and was negatively associated with serum albumin and parathyroid hormone levels and predialysis diastolic BP. Kt/V was negatively associated with PVD in waves 3 and 4 but not in wave 1. PAD was associated with increasing age, white (versus nonwhite) race, male gender, diabetes mellitus, coronary artery disease, cerebrovascular disease, smoking, and left ventricular hypertrophy, as for the general population, but not with hypertension or hyperlipidemia [23].

6.4   Noninvasive Screening Methods

6.4.1   Physical Exam and History

Diagnosis begins with a detailed medical history and exam in patients who are at risk for PAD, which in our patient population includes all CKD stage 3–5 patients. The medical history should focus on symptoms of claudication, rest pain, impaired ability to walk, and nonhealing lower-extremity ulcerations. Claudication, the symptom classically associated with PAD, usually presents as reproducible muscle pain that occurs with activity and improves with rest. It results from a mismatch between oxygen supply to and demand of muscle group during exercise. Conditions other than lower-extremity atherosclerosis can result in claudication-like symptoms, such as compartment syndromes, deep venous thrombosis, and spinal stenosis. Therefore, an astute clinician should distinguish between these various diagnoses, looking for signs of trauma, edema, or back problems in addition to PAD. Although claudication is classically associated with PAD, most patients (up to 90 %) are asymptomatic or present with atypical leg symptoms [14, 24]. At more advanced stages, PAD may manifest as rest pain, nonhealing leg ulcers, or gangrene. Physical examination should focus on skin integrity (e.g., hair loss, presence of wounds or ulcers) and assessment of peripheral pulses with accurate documentation of all pulses at each visit. Diminished bilateral peripheral pulses, femoral bruits, and prolonged capillary refill are very specific for PAD [25, 26].

6.4.2   Noninvasive Testing

The ankle-brachial BP index is a simple, noninvasive, and reliable test for the detection of PAD and assessment of its severity. Clinical guidelines for PAD recommend ABI as a screening test for asymptomatic PAD of the lower extremities [27, 28]. ABI has also been reported to correlate well with PAD severity and angiographic findings [29]. One method of measurement uses a 10–12 cm sphygmomanometer cuff placed just above the ankle and a Doppler instrument used to measure the systolic pressure of the posterior tibial and dorsalis pedis arteries of each leg (Fig. 6.1). These pressures are then divided by the higher brachial pressure of either arm to form the ankle-brachial ratio or "index." A reduced ABI in symptomatic patients confirms the existence of hemodynamically significant occlusive disease between the heart and the ankle, with a lower ABI (<0.9) indicating a greater degree of hemodynamic significance of the occlusive disease. The reproducibility of the ABI varies in the literature, but it is significant enough that reporting standards require a change of 0.15 in an isolated measurement for it to be considered clinically relevant or >0.10 if associated with a change in clinical status. The typical cutoff point for diagnosing PAD is

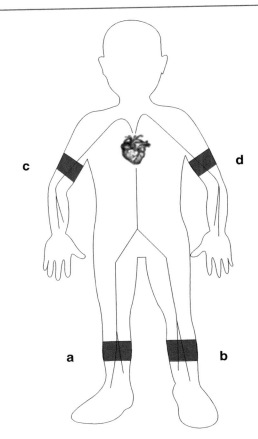

Fig. 6.1 ABI methodology. *Right ABI* right ankle systolic BP (*a*)/higher upper extremity systolic BP (left (*c*) or right (*d*)). *Left ABI* left ankle systolic BP (*b*)/higher upper extremity systolic BP (left (*c*) or right (*d*))

≤0.90 at rest. However, patients with borderline reduced values (0.9–1.0) are also at increased risk of adverse cardiovascular events and mortality and should be considered for further testing and/or treatment.

In patients with PAD who do not have classic claudication (asymptomatic patients), a reduced ABI is highly associated with cardiovascular events [30]. This risk is related to the degree of reduction of the ABI (lower ABI predicts higher risk) and is independent of other standard risk factors. The purpose of screening asymptomatic patients in the general population is to attempt to modify their CVD risk by prescribing aspirin, lipid medications, diet, etc., if they are discovered to have PAD. For this reason, ABI testing is recommended in a variety of "at-risk" patient subgroups frequent to primary care practices (Table 6.1) [31]. In CKD patients, the presence of CKD alone is an independent risk factor for CVD. Thus, by virtue of CKD alone, independent of PAD diagnosis, patients should be treated with an aggressive CVD risk reduction regimen. For this reason, screening of asymptomatic CKD patients for PAD is not recommended (Tables 6.1 and 6.2). For a detailed algorithmic approach to PAD screening in the CKD population, see Fig. 6.2.

Table 6.1 Recommendations for ankle-brachial index (ABI) screening to detect PAD in the general population and in CKD population

An ABI should be measured in a non-CKD patient:	An ABI should be measured in a CKD patient:
All patients who have exertional leg symptoms	All patients who have exertional leg symptoms
All patients between the age of 50 and 69 and who have a cardiovascular risk factor (particularly diabetes or smoking)	
All patients age ≥70 years regardless of risk factor status	
All patients with a Framingham risk score 10–20 %	

Table 6.2 The value of a reduced ABI in the general population differs from that in CKD population

General population	CKD
Confirms the diagnosis of PAD	Confirms the diagnosis of PAD
Detects significant PAD in (sedentary) asymptomatic patients	Used in the differential diagnosis of leg symptoms to identify a vascular etiology
Used in the differential diagnosis of leg symptoms to identify a vascular etiology	Identifies patients with reduced limb function (inability to walk defined distances or at usual walking speed)
Identifies patients with reduced limb function (inability to walk defined distances or at usual walking speed)	
Provides key information on long-term prognosis, with an ABI ≤0.90 associated with a three- to sixfold increased risk of cardiovascular mortality	
Provides further risk stratification, with a lower ABI indicating worse prognosis	
Highly associated with coronary and cerebral artery disease	
Can be used for further risk stratification in patients with a Framingham risk score between 10 and 20 %	

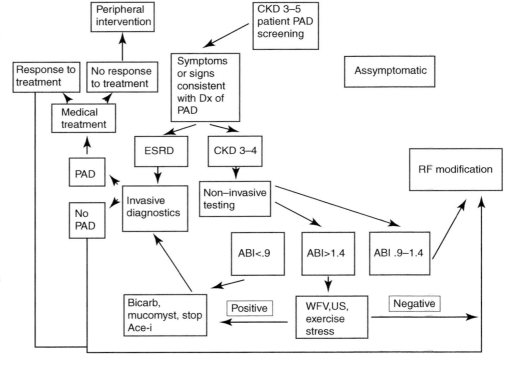

Fig. 6.2 Diagnostic approach to the CKD patient with suspected PAD. Patients with symptoms and borderline reduced ABI (0.9–1.0) values should be considered for additional testing (e.g., exercise ABI/PVR, CTA/MRA, or arterial duplex). Hemodynamically significant inflow (e.g., aortoiliac) disease may not cause a significant resting pressure gradient but will cause symptoms and can be detected with a postexercise ABI or vascular imaging study. Patients with borderline reduced ABI (0.9–1.0) regardless of symptoms are known to be at increased risk of all-cause mortality and CVD morbidity and mortality and should also be targeted for aggressive risk factor modification

However, ABI has been suggested to be unsuitable for assessing PAD in patients with diabetes, older age, history of intervention for PAD, or advanced chronic kidney disease (CKD) [18, 32, 33]. In particular, increased arterial stiffness might interfere with ABI measurements and affect the sensitivity of ABI for detecting PAD among dialysis patients. These patients typically have an ABI >1.40.

In some of these patients, the Doppler signal at the ankle cannot be obliterated even at cuff pressures above 300 mmHg [31]. In these patients additional noninvasive diagnostic testing should be performed to evaluate the patient for PAD (Fig. 6.2).

In an attempt to establish a screening test for PAD that has sufficient diagnostic value and is safe and inexpensive, Ogata et al. attempted to use duplex ultrasound [34]. Of the 315 patients evaluated in their study, 23.8 % had PAD. The receiver operating characteristic analysis (area under the receiver operating characteristic curve = 0.846) showed that sensitivity and specificity of ABI values for PAD were 49.0 and 94.8 %, respectively. As a result of the limitations of ABI and ultrasonographic studies in PAD screening, alternative diagnostic strategies have been employed, including magnetic resonance (MR) angiography and computed tomographic (CT) angiography. While both of these modalities have been shown to be reliably accurate in providing information regarding the presence and extent of vascular disease, they are not without limitations. Alternative tests include toe systolic pressures, pulse volume recordings, transcutaneous oxygen measurements, or vascular imaging (most commonly with duplex ultrasound).

6.4.3 Invasive Testing

Unfortunately, CT and MR, once thought to be noninvasive in nature due to their safety profile, are fraught with potential problems for the CKD population. CT uses ionizing radiation and requires the use of iodinated contrast, which is nephrotoxic and could potentially exacerbate CKD. Contrast MR angiography of the lower extremities is a highly accurate modality, which does not utilize ionizing radiation or iodinated contrast. The emergence of nephrogenic systemic fibrosis (NSF) as a complication of gadolinium use in patients with compromised renal failure has limited the continued use of MRA in the CKD population [35].

As a result, conventional angiography remains the gold standard for diagnosis of PAD in CKD patients with multiple risk factors. Angiography is a highly accurate method for evaluation of PAD. Although invasive, it offers the distinct advantage of allowing for treatment with percutaneous transluminal angioplasty (PTA) or stenting of significant lesions discovered at the time of assessment. The disadvantages of angiography include the use of iodinated contrast and ionizing radiation, relative cost, need for patient sedation and monitoring, and the potential occurrence of associated complications. The potential complications of arterial angiography include bleeding, infection, and vascular injury. Patients with CKD not yet on dialysis, and even those on dialysis in whom residual renal function is an issue, may not be able to safely undergo conventional angiography. However, the use of various preparatory methods prior to angiography seems to diminish the risk of acute kidney injury in the setting of CKD [36]. Furthermore, contrast dose can be very strictly managed in these patients by a careful and deliberate approach to diagnostic evaluation in the CKD population (Fig. 6.2).

Conclusion

PAD is a problem that affects CKD patients out of proportion to the general population and mirrors CVD outcomes very closely. Unlike the general population, PAD in CKD occurs in association with traditional atherosclerotic disease risk factors and in combination with the process of medial calcification. Screening for PAD should be performed in symptomatic patients, and CVD risk factor modification should occur in all CKD patients, regardless of the presence of PAD.

References

1. USRDS: United States Renal Data System Annual Data Report, Bethesda, National Institutes of Health, National Institute of Diabetes and Digestive and Kidney Diseases, Division of Kidney Urologic and Hematologic Diseases. 2000. p. 339–48.
2. Foley RN, Murray AM, Li S, et al. Chronic kidney disease and the risk for cardiovascular disease, renal replacement, and death in the United States medicare population, 1998 to 1999. J Am Soc Nephrol. 2005;16(2):489–95.
3. Murabito JM, Evans JC, Larson MG, et al. The ankle-brachial index in the elderly and risk of stroke, coronary disease, and death: the Framingham study. Arch Intern Med. 2003;163(16):1939–42.
4. Newman AB, Shemanski L, Manolio TA, et al. Ankle-arm index as a predictor of cardiovascular disease and mortality in the cardiovascular health study: the cardiovascular health study group. Arterioscler Thromb Vasc Biol. 1999;19(3):538–45.
5. Criqui MH, Langer RD, Fronek A, et al. Mortality over a period of 10 years in patients with peripheral arterial disease. N Engl J Med. 1992;326(6):381–6.
6. Kerr PG, Guérin AP. Arterial calcification and stiffness in chronic kidney disease. Clin Exp Pharmacol Physiol. 2007;34(7):683–7.
7. Robinson RF, Nahata MC, Sparks E, et al. Abnormal left ventricular mass and aortic distensibility in pediatric dialysis patients. Pediatr Nephrol. 2005;20(1):64–8.
8. Goodman WG, Goldin J, Kuizon BD, et al. Coronary artery calcification in young adults with end-stage renal disease who are undergoing hemodialysis. N Engl J Med. 2000;342(20):1478–83.
9. Block GA, Klassen PS, Lazarus JM, Ofsthun N, Lowrie EG, Chertow GM. Mineral metabolism, mortality, and morbidity in maintenance hemodialysis. J Am Soc Nephrol. 2004;15:2208–18.
10. Young EW, Akiba T, Albert JM, et al. Magnitude and impact of abnormal mineral metabolism in hemodialysis patients in the dialysis outcomes and practice patterns study (DOPPS). Am J Kidney Dis. 2004;44(5 Suppl 2):34–8.
11. Cooper BA, Penne EL, Bartlett LH, Pollack CA. Protein malnutrition and hypoalbuminemia as predictors of vascular events and mortality in ESRD. Am J Kidney Dis. 2004;43(1):61–6.
12. Hiatt WR. Medical treatment of peripheral arterial disease and claudication. N Engl J Med. 2001;344(21):1608–21.
13. Braunwald E, Zipes DP, Libby P. Heart disease: a textbook of cardiovascular medicine. Philadelphia: Saunders; 2001.
14. Hirsch AT, Criqui MH, Treat-Jacobson D, et al. Peripheral arterial disease detection, awareness, and treatment in primary care. JAMA. 2001;286(11):1317–24.
15. Hirsch AT, Hiatt WR, PARTNERS Steering Committee. PAD awareness, risk, and treatment: new resources for survival–the USA PARTNERS program. Vasc Med. 2001;6(3 Suppl):9–12.

16. Selvin E, Erlinger TP. Prevalence of and risk factors for peripheral arterial disease in the United States: results from the National Health and Nutrition Examination Survey, 1999–2000. Circulation. 2004;110(6):738–43.

17. Lamar Welch VL, Casper M, Greenlund K, Zheng ZJ, Giles W, Rith-Najarian S. Prevalence of lower extremity arterial disease defined by the ankle-brachial index among American Indians: the Inter-Tribal Heart Project. Ethn Dis. 2002;12:S1-63-S7.

18. Leskinen Y, Salenius JP, Lehtimäki T, Huhtala H, Saha H. The prevalence of peripheral arterial disease and medial arterial calcification in patients with chronic renal failure: requirements for diagnostics. Am J Kidney Dis. 2002;40(3):472–9.

19. Newman AB, Siscovick DS, Manolio TA, et al. Ankle-arm index as a marker of atherosclerosis in the cardiovascular health study: cardiovascular heart study (CHS) collaborative research group. Circulation. 1993;88(3):837–45.

20. Eggers PW, Gohdes D, Pugh J. Nontraumatic lower extremity amputations in the Medicare end-stage renal disease population. Kidney Int. 1999;56:1524–33.

21. DeLoach SS, Mohler 3rd ER. Peripheral arterial disease: a guide for nephrologists. Clin J Am Soc Nephrol. 2007;2(4):839–46.

22. O'Hare AM, Glidden DV, Fox CS, Hsu CY. High prevalence of peripheral arterial disease in persons with renal insufficiency. Circulation. 2004;109(3):320–3.

23. O'Hare AM, Hsu CY, Bacchetti P, Johansen KL. Peripheral vascular disease risk factors among patients undergoing hemodialysis. J Am Soc Nephrol. 2002;13(2):497–503.

24. Mcdermott MM, Greenland P, Liu K, et al. Leg symptoms in peripheral arterial disease: associated clinical characteristics and functional impairment. JAMA. 2001;286(13):1599–606.

25. McGee SR, Boyko EJ. Physical examination and chronic lower-extremity ischemia: a critical review. Arch Intern Med. 1998;158(12):1357–64.

26. McDermott MM, Criqui MH, Liu K, et al. Lower ankle/brachial index, as calculated by averaging the dorsalis pedis and posterior tibial arterial pressures, and association with leg functioning in peripheral arterial disease. J Vasc Surg. 2000;32(6):1164–71.

27. Norgren L, Hiatt WR, Dormandy JA, et al. Inter-society consensus for the management of peripheral arterial disease (TASC II). Eur J Vasc Endovasc Surg. 2007;33 Suppl 1:S1–75.

28. K/DOQI Workgroup. K/DOQI clinical practice guidelines for cardiovascular disease in dialysis patients. Am J Kidney Dis. 2005;45 (4 Supple 3):S1–153.

29. Rutherford RB, Baker JD, Ernst C, et al. Recommended standards for reports dealing with lower extremity ischemia: revised version. J Vasc Surg. 1997;26(3):517–38.

30. Heald CL, Fowkes FG, Murray GD, Price JF. Ankle brachial index collaboration: risk of mortality and cardiovascular disease associated with the ankle-brachial index: systematic review. Atherosclerosis. 2006;189(1):61–9.

31. Steffen LM, Duprez DA, Boucher JL, Ershow AG, Hirsch AT. Management of peripheral arterial disease. Diabetes Spectrum. 2008;21(3):171.

32. McLafferty RB, Moneta GL, Taylor Jr LM, Porter JM. Ability of ankle-brachial index to detect lower-extremity atherosclerotic disease progression. Arch Surg. 1997;132(8):836–40.

33. Okamoto K, Oka M, Maesato K, et al. Peripheral arterial occlusive disease is more prevalent in patients with hemodialysis: comparison with the findings of multidetector-row computed tomography. Am J Kidney Dis. 2006;48(2):269–76.

34. Ogata H, Kumata-Maeta C, Shishido K, et al. Detection of peripheral artery disease by duplex ultrasonography among hemodialysis patients. Clin J Am Soc Nephrol. 2010;5(12):2199–206.

35. Haemel AK, Sadowski EA, Shafer MM, Djamali A. Update on nephrogenic systemic fibrosis: are we making progress? Int J Dermatol. 2011;50(6):659–66.

36. Li JH, He NS. Prevention of iodinated contrast-induced nephropathy. Chin Med J (Engl). 2011;124(23):4079–82.

Overview of PAD Treatment in the CKD Population: Indications, Medical Strategies, and Endovascular Techniques

Alexander S. Yevzlin and Micah R. Chan

7.1 Introduction

Cardiovascular disease (CVD) is the cause of death in nearly half of end-stage renal disease (ESRD) patients [1, 2]. An individual with ESRD has a CVD mortality rate 15 times that found in the general population. Previous studies have shown that peripheral arterial disease (PAD) is associated with a significantly elevated risk of cardiovascular disease morbidity and mortality and is generally regarded as a CVD equivalent in terms of mortality risk [3–5]. The purpose of this chapter is to describe an approach to PAD treatment in CKD patients with a discussion of indications, outcomes, techniques, and precautions.

7.2 Indications

The pathophysiology of vascular disease in the CKD population differs from the nonrenal disease population. Traditional vascular disease comprises intimal disease with lipid-rich plaques producing focal stenoses and the potential for plaque rupture and subsequent thrombosis. In CKD, on the other hand, plaques are characterized by intense medial calcification, which tends toward chronic stenotic disease rather than acute plaque rupture [6, 7]. What is more, PAD appears to be more common in the CKD population than in the general population [8], with some studies suggesting that patients with moderate to severe CKD were at ninefold increased risk to have an ABI <0.9 [9]. In addition, lower extremity amputations resulting from PAD are more prevalent in the ESRD population than in the general population with PAD [10].

Given the prevalence of PAD in CKD, the K/DOQI guidelines recommend screening all patients upon initiation of dialysis [9]. However, the recommendation to screen CKD/ESRD patients for PAD who are asymptomatic is not supported by clinical data. In patients with PAD who do not have classic claudication (asymptomatic patients), a reduced ABI is highly associated with cardiovascular events [11]. The purpose of screening asymptomatic patients in the general population is to attempt to modify their CVD risk by prescribing aspirin, lipid medications, diet, etc., if they are discovered to have PAD. For this reason, the ABI has become a routine measurement in the primary care practice of medicine [12]. In CKD and ESRD patients, however, the presence of CKD alone is an independent risk factor for CVD. Thus, by virtue of CKD alone, independent of PAD diagnosis, patients should be treated with an aggressive CVD risk reduction regimen. For this reason, screening of asymptomatic CKD patients for PAD is not recommended.

Likewise, treatment of PAD is only indicated if the CKD/ESRD patient exhibits symptoms and signs of claudication, rest pain, impaired ability to walk, or nonhealing lower extremity ulcerations. Claudication, the symptom classically associated with PAD, usually presents as reproducible muscle pain that occurs with activity and improves with rest. It results from a mismatch between oxygen supply to and demand of muscle group during exercise. Physical examination should focus on skin integrity (e.g., hair loss, presence of wounds or ulcers) and assessment of peripheral pulses with accurate documentation of all pulses at each visit. Diminished bilateral peripheral pulses, femoral bruits, and prolonged capillary refill are very specific for PAD [13]. If a CKD patient complains of the symptoms outlined above and if the suspected diagnosis is corroborated with noninvasive screening tests (ABI < .9), then treatment should be strongly considered.

A.S. Yevzlin, MD (✉)
Division of Nephrology,
Department of Medicine (CHS),
University of Wisconsin, Madison, WI 53705, USA
e-mail: asy@medicine.wisc.edu

M.R. Chan
Division of Nephrology, Department of Medicine,
University of Wisconsin College of Medicine and Public Health,
Madison, WI, USA

A.S. Yevzlin et al. (eds.), *Interventional Nephrology*,
DOI 10.1007/978-1-4614-8803-3_7, © Springer Science+Business Media New York 2014

7.3   Medical Treatment of PAD

The evidence for medical therapies that reduce symptoms and attenuate disease progression is strongest for antiplatelet therapies. There may be a modest benefit with clopidogrel over aspirin, as suggested by Clopidogrel versus Aspirin in Patients at Risk of Ischemic Events (CAPRIE) trial found a reduced cardiovascular risk in the clopidogrel-treated group [14]. Although the ACC/AHA guidelines recommend clopidogrel as an aspirin alternative, severe CKD was an exclusion criterion for enrollment in the CAPRIE trial, so the potential benefits of clopidogrel versus aspirin in our patients are unclear [15]. However, the TransAtlantic Inter-Society Consensus (TASC) guidelines recommend either aspirin or clopidogrel [16]. A recent meta-analysis which evaluated the effects of antiplatelet agents on maximal walking distance (MWD), one of the key parameters of symptom relief in the general PAD population [17], found that the overall pooled estimate was in favor of treatment but with a modest increase in MWD of 59 m.

Cilostazol and pentoxifylline are phosphodiesterase inhibitors that reduce platelet aggregation and act as mild vasodilator. Several studies have suggested that cilostazol can reduce claudication and increase walking times [18–20]. Studies with cilostazol showed a significant effect on walking distance at doses of 50 and 100 mg. MWD increased 36 m (95 % CI: 30e41 m) with 50 mg, but almost twice that, 70 m (95 % CI: 47e93) with the 100-mg dose [17]. It is

important to note that the use of cilostazol is contraindicated in patients with congestive heart failure, although there are no studies in this population. In addition, information in the package insert indicates that cilostazol has reduced clearance in severe renal impairment. Since this drug has not been studied in dialysis patients, caution is advised for use in individuals with a creatinine clearance <25 ml/min [9]. Pentoxifylline was similarly found to be of modest benefit on MWD [17], clearance is reduced in renal failure, so dosages must be adjusted appropriately in those settings.

A comprehensive medical therapy algorithm based on the above observations is offered in Fig. 7.1.

7.4   Invasive Diagnostics of PAD

Severe forms of PAD often manifest as the clinical entity known as critical limb ischemia, which is defined by rest pain and ischemic skin lesions such as ulcers and gangrene. In the general population, revascularization is the optimal therapy for critical limb ischemia [15, 21]. Revascularization via percutaneous transluminal angioplasty (PTA) procedures is preferred to surgical revision in most cases. There are no randomized, controlled trial data regarding revascularization techniques in patients with CKD and dialysis patients, however. Not surprisingly, a retrospective analysis of patients who had CKD and underwent lower limb revascularization found lower rates of limb loss and mortality compared with

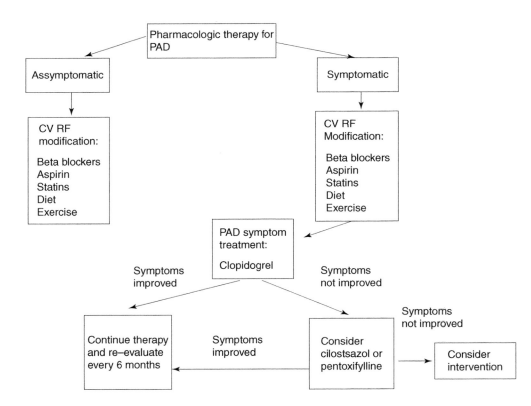

Fig. 7.1 Medical treatment algorithm for PAD in CKD patients

ESRD [22]. What is more, mortality rates were found to be inversely correlated with kidney function [23]. Patients with ESRD often are not good candidates for PTA because of distal disease and vascular calcifications. Nevertheless, a retrospective analysis of hemodialysis patients saw lower mortality and higher limb salvage rates in those who underwent percutaneous revascularization compared with a surgical approach [24].

Once a patient is judged to be a likely candidate to benefit from intervention, an angiogram is scheduled. Contrast angiography remains the gold standard for diagnosis and the assessment of the severity of atherosclerotic PAD. The value of this diagnostic modality has been buoyed by the recently described association of nephrogenic systemic fibrosis (NSF) with magnetic resonance contrast agents, as such are required for MR angiography [25]. Angiography, further, allows evaluation of the abdominal aorta, renal arteries and branch vessels, the presence of accessory renal arteries, as well as cortical blood flow and renal dimensions [26]. Moreover, pressure gradients across arterial lesions can be obtained to evaluate its hemodynamic significance of the said lesions if the angiographic or noninvasive testing data is equivocal. Digital subtraction angiography (DSA) has become available in many institutions and, although its resolution is inferior to film, it permits the use of lower concentrations of iodinated contrast, as well as of alternative contrast agents such as CO_2 [27].

The disadvantages of angiography include the use of iodinated contrast and ionizing radiation, relative cost, need for patient sedation and monitoring, and the potential occurrence of associated complications. The potential complications of arterial angiography include bleeding, infection, cholesterol embolization, and vascular injury. Patients with CKD not yet on dialysis, and even those on dialysis in whom residual renal function is an issue, may not be able to safely undergo conventional angiography. However, the use of various preparatory methods prior to angiography seems to diminish the risk of acute kidney injury in the setting of CKD [28]. Furthermore, contrast dose can be very strictly managed in these patients by a careful and deliberate approach to diagnostic evaluation in the CKD population.

Typically, an abdominal aortogram is performed with distal runoff, usually positioning a pigtail catheter at the lower edge of the first lumbar vertebra and power-injecting 40 ml of dye at 20 ml/s. The abdominal aortogram will provide information regarding the aorta itself, the position of the renal arteries, and the presence of iliac calcification. Runoff into the lower extremities must be done properly by moving the image intensifier or table such that the flow of contrast can be followed. This takes a certain degree of experience and can lead to repeated aortograms if not performed properly. In most instances, the aortogram provides adequate visualization of the peripheral arterial tree, but if optimal imaging or pressure gradient measurement are needed, selective catheterization becomes necessary. This can be achieved with a variety of different 4–6 F diagnostic catheters. Whatever catheter shape is used, the goal is to achieve selective cannulation of the artery in question without excessive catheter manipulation, as atheromas are often adjacent to areas of disease and distal embolization can occur [26].

7.5 Interventional Approach

Percutaneous intervention on PAD in CKD patients should be considered only if one of the following conditions is met:
1. Symptomatic and refractory to medical therapy.
2. Critical limb ischemia is present.

Medical therapy of the CKD patient with claudication is described above. If the CKD patient has been treated with medical therapy with no improvement in symptoms, then percutaneous revascularization may be considered (Fig. 7.1). Critical limb ischemia (CLI) is different from claudication per se and can be defined as limb pain that occurs at rest or impending limb loss that is caused by severe compromise of blood flow to the affected extremity. All CKD patients with rest pain, ulcers, or gangrene attributable to objectively proven arterial occlusive disease should be categorized as CLI. Unlike individuals with claudication, patients with CLI have resting perfusion that is inadequate to sustain viability in the tissue bed and which frequently leads to amputation (Fig. 7.2). Therefore, CLI should be considered for percutaneous revascularization at the same time that medical therapy is initiated [15].

Claudication and CLI exist on a continuum, which makes it challenging to simplify this complex disease state into two distinct categories. For this reason, guidelines have been developed to subcategorize PAD into several distinct subtypes based on characteristics of lesion morphology [21]. These classifications are summarized in Tables 7.1 and 7.2 for supra- and infrainguinal disease, respectively. The symptoms that a given lesion is causing can also be divided into stages (Table 7.3) [29]. Based on classification of symptoms and lesion morphology, the interventional plan can then be determined based on the algorithms described in Figs. 7.3 and 7.4.

7.6 Precautions

Careful attention to contrast dye load is required, especially in patients at high risk for contrast nephropathy. As mentioned above, CO_2 can be used as alternative contrast agents at least during some parts of the intervention.

Adjuvant pharmacology before and after peripheral percutaneous intervention has not been systemati-

Fig. 7.2 Natural history of PAD in non-CKD patients

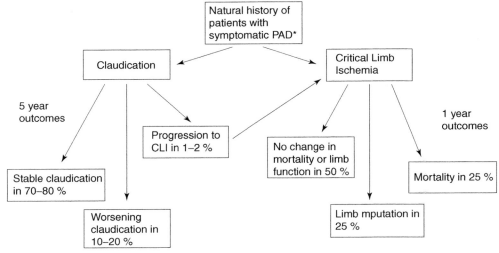

* outcomes in non-CKD patients

Table 7.1 TASC stratification of suprainguinal lesions

Type A lesions

Single stenosis less than 3 cm of the CIA or EIA (unilateral/bilateral)

Type B lesions

Single stenosis 3–10 cm in length, not extending into the CFA

Total of 2 stenoses less than 5 cm long in the CIA and/or EIA and not extending into the CFA

Unilateral CIA occlusion

Type C lesions

Bilateral 5- to 10-cm-long stenosis of the CIA and/or EIA, not extending into the CFA

Unilateral EIA occlusion not extending into the CFA

Unilateral EIA stenosis extending into the CFA

Bilateral CIA occlusion

Type D lesions

Diffuse, multiple unilateral stenoses involving the CIA, EIA, and CFA (usually more than 10 cm long)

Unilateral occlusion involving both the CIA and EIA

Bilateral EIA occlusions

Diffuse disease involving the aorta and both iliac arteries

Iliac stenoses in a patient with an abdominal aortic aneurysm or other lesion requiring aortic or iliac surgery

Table 7.2 TASC stratification of infrainguinal lesions

Type A lesions

Single stenosis less than 3 cm of the superficial femoral artery or popliteal artery

Type B lesions

Single stenosis 3–10 cm in length, not involving the distal popliteal artery

Heavily calcified stenoses up to 3 cm in length

Multiple lesions, each less than 3 cm (stenoses or occlusions)

Single or multiple lesions in the absence of continuous tibial runoff to improve inflow for distal surgical bypass

Type C lesions

Single stenosis or occlusion longer than 5 cm

Multiple stenoses or occlusions, each 3–5 cm in length, with or without heavy calcification

Type D lesions

Complete common femoral artery or superficial femoral artery occlusions or complete popliteal and proximal trifurcation occlusions

Table 7.3 Rutherford classification of PAD symptoms

Category	Clinical description
0	Asymptomatic
1	Mild claudication
2	Moderate claudication
3	Severe claudication
4	Ischemic rest pain
5	Minor tissue loss
6	Ulceration or gangrene

cally studied. Heparin to maintain an ACT of 250–300 s is frequently used as the anticoagulant of choice during interventional procedures; most interventionalists are quite familiar with its use, and it can be easily reversed with protamine. Patients are usually pretreated with aspirin which is continued indefinitely. The use of clopidogrel seems theoretically necessary following percutaneous intervention; however, there are no controlled studies exploring its use on CKD patients with PAD. However, if

the CKD patient has symptoms of PAD justifying intervention, they should be treated with clopidogrel by virtue of that alone. Other possible intra-procedural anticoagulants,

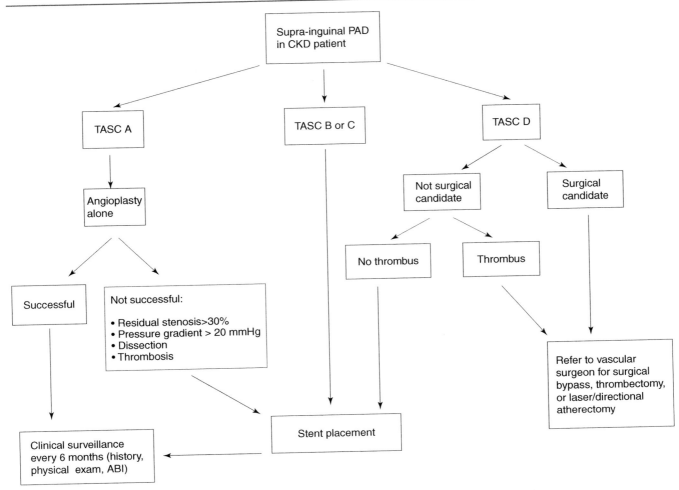

Fig. 7.3 Suprainguinal lesion treatment algorithm

such as glycoprotein 2B3A receptor antagonists, and direct thrombin inhibitors, such as bivalirudin, have not been formally studied in peripheral interventions in CKD.

PAD intervention requires close attention to several important details that are typically not a major concern in the venous system. When performing arterial intervention, one must not oversize the balloon or undersize the stent [30]. In addition, there is no reason to use a longer balloon than you need, and one should aim for 5-mm extension beyond the length of the lesion when selecting balloon length. The guidewire should be kept across the lesion at all times, even when retracting the balloon in what one feels is a successful intervention. One should seldom intervene before giving anticoagulation. One should not inflate an angioplasty balloon over nominal pressure in the arterial system, since balloon rupture can lead to acute limb ischemia in the arterial system. A partially inflated balloon should not be retracted, and it is best to intervene in the

arterial system with a sheath that engages the lesion in question [26]. Most importantly, one must not allow air into the arterial system, especially when operating on the great vessels of the thoracic aorta. In most cases a manifold can be used to minimize the probability of air embolization.

Given the above precautions, PAD intervention should be performed only by skilled interventionalists who are specifically trained for PAD intervention. These practitioners should have a thorough knowledge of the medical/cognitive components of the decision making process as described above. To date, there is no entity that trains, certifies, or accredits nephrologists in this discipline. Furthermore, the procedures described above should only be performed if there is adequate monitoring and surgical backup to allow detection and treatment of the potential complications of PAD intervention, including but not limited to acute limb ischemia, arterial thrombosis, and arterial dissection.

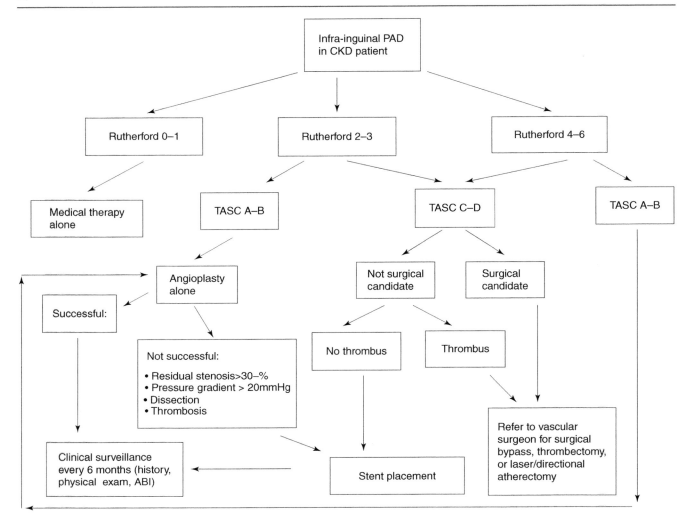

Fig. 7.4 Infrainguinal lesion treatment algorithm

Conclusion

PAD is a problem that affects CKD patients out of proportion to the general population and mirrors CVD outcomes very closely. Unlike the general population, PAD in CKD occurs due to medial calcification; as opposed to an intimal atherosclerotic process, PAD intervention should be performed in select symptomatic patients, as described by the guidelines, and CVD risk factor modification should occur in all CKD patients, regardless of the presence of PAD.

As a discipline, interventional nephrology has emerged out of a desire to create better outcomes for our patients and to "fix a problem." The core values of our discipline have evolved out of this fundamental desire to meet an unmet clinical need, provide insight into a disease state specific to our patients, and offer clinical/academic excellence in doing so. We must endeavor to follow a similar path in our approach to PAD.

References

1. USRDS: United States renal data system annual data report, Bethesda, National Institutes of Health, National Institute of Diabetes and Digestive and Kidney Diseases, Division of Kidney Urologic and Hematologic Diseases. 2000. p. 339–48.
2. Murabito JM, Evans JC, Larson MG, et al. The ankle-brachial index in the elderly and risk of stroke, coronary disease, and death: the Framingham study. Arch Intern Med. 2003;163(16):1939–42.
3. Newman AB, Shemanski L, Manolio TA, et al. Ankle-arm index as a predictor of cardiovascular disease and mortality in the cardiovascular health study: the cardiovascular health study group. Arterioscler Thromb Vasc Biol. 1999;19(3):538–45.
4. Criqui MH, Langer RD, Fronek A, et al. Mortality over a period of 10 years in patients with peripheral arterial disease. N Engl J Med. 1992;326(6):381–6.
5. Kerr PG, Guérin AP. Arterial calcification and stiffness in chronic kidney disease. Clin Exp Pharmacol Physiol. 2007;34(7):683–7.
6. Guérin AP, Pannier B, Marchais SJ, London GM. Cardiovascular disease in the dialysis population: prognostic significance of arterial disorders. Curr Opin Nephrol Hypertens. 2006;15(2):105–10.

7. Leskinen Y, Salenius JP, Lehtimäki T, Huhtala H, Saha H. The prevalence of peripheral arterial disease and medial arterial calcification in patients with chronic renal failure: requirements for diagnostics. Am J Kidney Dis. 2002;40(3):472–9.

8. Selvin E, Erlinger TP. Prevalence of and risk factors for peripheral arterial disease in the United States: results from the National Health and Nutrition Examination Survey, 1999–2000. Circulation. 2004;110(6):738–43.

9. DeLoach SS, Mohler 3rd ER. Peripheral arterial disease: a guide for nephrologists. Clin J Am Soc Nephrol. 2007;2(4):839–46.

10. Eggers PW, Gohdes D, Pugh J. Nontraumatic lower extremity amputations in the Medicare end-stage renal disease population. Kidney Int. 1999;56(4):1524–33.

11. Heald CL, Fowkes FG, Murray GD, Price JF, Ankle Brachial Index Collaboration. Risk of mortality and cardiovascular disease associated with the ankle-brachial index: systematic review. Atherosclerosis. 2006;189(1):61–9.

12. Steffen LM, Duprez DA, Boucher JL, Ershow AG, Hirsch AT. Management of peripheral arterial disease. Diabet Spectr. 2008;21(3).

13. McDermott MM, Criqui MH, Liu K, et al. Lower ankle/brachial index, as calculated by averaging the dorsalis pedis and posterior tibial arterial pressures, and association with leg functioning in peripheral arterial disease. J Vasc Surg. 2000;32(6):1164–71.

14. Clagett GP, Sobel M, Jackson MR, Lip GY, Tangelder M, Verhaeghe R. Antithrombotic therapy in peripheral arterial occlusive disease. The seventh ACCP conference on antithrombotic and thrombolytic therapy. Chest. 2004;126(3 Suppl):609S–26.

15. Hirsch AT, Haskal ZJ, Hertzer NR, et al. ACC/AHA 2005 practice guidelines for the management of patients with peripheral arterial disease (lower extremity, renal, mesenteric, and abdominal aortic): a collaborative report from the American Association for Vascular Surgery/Society for Vascular Surgery, Society for Cardiovascular Angiography and Interventions, Society for Vascular Medicine and Biology, Society of Interventional Radiology, and the ACC/AHA Task Force on Practice Guidelines. Circulation. 2006;113(11):e463–654.

16. Norgren L, Hiatt WR, Dormandy JA, et al. Inter-society consensus for the management of peripheral arterial disease (TASC II). J Vasc Surg. 2007;45(Suppl S):S5–67.

17. Momsen AH, Jensen MB, Norager CB, Madsen MR, Vestersgaard-Andersen T, Lindholt JS. Drug therapy for improving walking distance in intermittent claudication: a systematic review and meta-analysis of robust randomised controlled studies. Eur J Vasc Endovasc Surg. 2009;38(4):463–74.

18. Beebe HG, Dawson DL, Cutler BS, et al. A new pharmacological treatment for intermittent claudication: results of a randomized, multicenter trial. Arch Intern Med. 1999;159(17):2041–50.

19. Mohler 3rd ER, Beebe HG, Salles-Cuhna S, et al. Effects of cilostazol on resting ankle pressures and exercise-induced ischemia in patients with intermittent claudication. Vasc Med. 2001;6(3): 151–6.

20. Reilly MP, Mohler 3rd ER. Cilostazol: treatment of intermittent claudication. Ann Pharmacother. 2001;35(1):48–56.

21. Dormandy JA, Rutherford RB. Management of peripheral arterial disease (PAD). TASC working group. TransAtlantic Inter-Society Consensus. J Vasc Surg. 2000;31(1 Pt 2):S1–296.

22. O'Hare AM, Sidawy AN, Feinglass J, et al. Influence of renal insufficiency on limb loss and mortality after initial lower extremity surgical revascularization. J Vasc Surg. 2004;39(4):709–16.

23. O'Hare AM, Feinglass J, Sidawy AN, et al. Impact of renal insufficiency on short-term morbidity and mortality after lower extremity revascularization: data from the Department of Veterans Affairs' National Surgical Quality Improvement Program. J Am Soc Nephrol. 2003;14(5):1287–95.

24. Jaar BG, Astor BC, Berns JS, Powe NR. Predictors of amputation and survival following lower extremity revascularization in hemodialysis patients. Kidney Int. 2004;65(2):613–20.

25. Sadowski EA, Bennett LK, Chan MR, et al. Nephrogenic systemic fibrosis: risk factors and incidence estimation. Radiology. 2007; 243(1):148–57.

26. Yevzlin AS, Schoenkerman AB, Gimelli G, Asif A. Arterial interventions in arteriovenous access and chronic kidney disease: a role for interventional nephrologists. Semin Dial. 2009;22(5):545–56.

27. Hawkins Jr IF, Wilcox CS, Kerns SR, Sabatelli FW. CO_2 digital angiography: a safer contrast agent for renal vascular imaging? Am J Kidney Dis. 1994;24(4):685–94.

28. Li JH, He NS. Prevention of iodinated contrast-induced nephropathy. Chin Med J (Engl). 2011;124(23):4079–82.

29. Rutherford RB, Baker JD, Ernst C, et al. Recommended standards for reports dealing with lower extremity ischemia: revised version. J Vasc Surg. 1997;26(3):517–38.

30. Asif A, Yevzlin AS. Arterial stent placement in arteriovenous dialysis access by interventional nephrologists. Semin Dial. 2009;22(5): 557–60.

Unconventional Venous Access: Percutaneous Translumbar and Transhepatic Venous Access for Hemodialysis

8

Jason W. Pinchot

8.1 Introduction

The National Kidney Foundation Kidney Disease Outcomes Quality Initiative™ (NKF KDOQI™) Clinical Practice Guidelines on chronic kidney disease (CKD) estimate that CKD affects more than 50 million people worldwide and more than one million of these patients are receiving hemodialysis [1]. In the USA alone, more than 382,000 patients were receiving hemodialysis for ESRD through 2008 [2]. Maintenance of functional venous access for hemodialysis often determines the survival of patients with end-stage renal disease [3]. Despite ongoing initiatives to reduce central venous catheter use for hemodialysis such as KDOQI and the CMS Fistula First program, the use of catheters has remained 17–18 % in prevalent hemodialysis patients since 2003 [2]. Published data support the use of the internal jugular veins as the initial vascular access site for placement of central venous catheters for hemodialysis [4, 5]. Prolonged central venous catheterization commonly results in endoluminal thrombosis, stenosis, or occlusion. Eventual exhaustion of venous access options often occurs prior to the availability of a surgical vascular access or suitable renal transplant donor. In patients with chronic total occlusion of the jugular, subclavian, and femoral veins, alternative unconventional access sites must be explored. This includes use of the inferior vena cava (IVC) via the translumbar and transhepatic approaches. There are only a small number of studies to date reporting on translumbar and transhepatic catheters for hemodialysis [3, 6–13]. Nonetheless, familiarity with the patient selection and technical considerations of percutaneous translumbar and transhepatic venous access for hemodialysis and the management of related complications is requisite for any practitioner who cares for the catheter-dependent hemodialysis patient.

8.2 Catheter-Based Hemodialysis

Catheter hemodialysis presents a conundrum—catheters provide access that is immediately available, but complications of catheter use remain quite high [14]. As per recommendations of the KDOQI, the ideal hemodialysis access permits a flow rate to the dialyzer adequate for the dialysis prescription, has a long-use life, and has a low rate of complications (e.g., infection, thrombosis, stenosis, aneurysm, and distal limb ischemia) [15]. Undoubtedly, a surgically created arteriovenous fistula provides the most optimal and durable fulfillment of these criteria. Although fistulae have been shown to have the lowest rate of thrombosis and require the fewest interventions [16], an arteriovenous graft is often requisite for patients in whom a fistula cannot be created because of anatomic or technical limitations. Catheter hemodialysis remains the least desirable and often the last option for patients with end-stage renal disease. In an effort to reduce morbidity in the hemodialysis population, KDOQI has proposed a limitation of less than 10 % of patients using catheters as a primary mode of access [15].

Hemodialysis catheters can be defined based on design, intent, and duration of use. Acute or short-term catheters (three to five dialysis sessions within 1 week) are typically non-cuffed and placed such that the catheter tips reside in the superior vena cava. On the contrary, long-term catheter systems—those intended for vascular access for hemodialysis over weeks to months—are cuffed catheters and are frequently tunneled in the subcutaneous tissues to permit catheter retention and minimize infectious complications. Such catheters should have their tips in the right atrium to permit optimal flow. Contemporary hemodialysis catheters are usually dual lumen with a tip design that is either stepped (i.e., the arterial and venous tips are staggered by 1–2 cm) or split

J.W. Pinchot
Department of Radiology,
Vascular and Interventional Radiology Section,
University of Wisconsin School of Medicine and Public Health,
Madison, WI, USA
e-mail: jpinchot@uwhealth.org

so that the tips are not next to each other [15]. Newer designs such as the Tal Palindrome catheter (Covidien, Mansfield, Massachusetts) have a symmetric tip design that incorporates a spiral separator that allows reversal of the arterial and venous lines during hemodialysis with reduced risk of recirculation.

Tunneled cuffed hemodialysis catheters should be placed in a vein that is easily accessible using sonographic and fluoroscopic guidance. The internal jugular veins are generally favored as the initial choice for central venous access [5]. The right internal jugular vein is preferable to the left because this site offers a more direct route to the right atrium. If both of the internal jugular veins become occluded, alternative access sites must be explored. Choices include the external jugular, subclavian, and femoral veins. Unfortunately, the high-rate of venous thrombosis and occlusion associated with prolonged central venous catheter use results in the exhaustion of even these unconventional access sites. Elaborate vascular surgical procedures have evolved to bypass stenoses with the interposition of prosthetic graft material to create a patent arteriovenous circuit that supports hemodialysis, but such surgical intervention may not always be acceptable or feasible [17]. Unconventional approaches to central venous access may be entertained only when all other surgical and endovascular options have been exhausted. Translumbar and transhepatic cannulation of the inferior vena cava, the former first described over 20 years ago, reflect two such unconventional approaches into a central vein that have been described in the literature [6–13]. To be sure, these sites require considerable technical expertise for catheter placement, and maintenance of catheters at these sites may be somewhat more problematic. Transhepatic guidance of translumbar hemodialysis catheter placement has been described in the setting of chronic infrarenal inferior vena cava occlusion [3], but this technique is technically challenging and remains an infrequent method of central venous access. Percutaneous puncture of the renal vein via the transrenal approach was first described by Murthy et al. [18], but widespread use of this technique remains limited due to a potentially high risk of bleeding and limited precedent in the literature.

8.3 Patient Selection

8.3.1 Indications

For those patients in whom translumbar or transhepatic cannulation of the inferior vena cava is contemplated, most options for surgical vascular access have been exhausted or have become impractical due to thrombosis or chronic total occlusion of the central veins. Translumbar or transhepatic placement of inferior vena cava catheters has been accepted as the last useful and reliable alternative in patients who require long-term hemodialysis but have exhausted all other conventional access sites.

8.3.2 Contraindications

Similar to more conventional sites of central venous access, there are no absolute contraindications to placement of a tunneled cuffed hemodialysis catheter into the central veins via the translumbar or transhepatic routes. When more permanent surgical access options exist (e.g., AV fistulae and grafts), the use of catheters as a primary mode of hemodialysis should be discouraged. Most interventionalists avoid placement in patients with uncorrectable coagulopathy, active infection, or proven bacteremia. In our institution, blood cultures must be negative for at least 24 h prior to considering placement of a tunneled hemodialysis catheter. Coagulopathy is a relative contraindication to placement of a translumbar or transhepatic catheter, and in those patients with a bleeding diathesis or those taking systemic anticoagulants should ideally be corrected prior to catheter insertion. Platelet replacement or the administration of fresh frozen plasma can be performed if necessary. Available data suggest an international normalized ratio (INR) of less than 1.5, and a platelet count greater than 50,000/mm^3 carries less risk of bleeding during and after tunneled central venous catheter placement [19].

Morbid obesity may be considered a relative contraindication to translumbar placement of tunneled hemodialysis catheters. Several studies have suggested an increased risk of catheter migration out of the inferior vena cava and into the subcutaneous soft tissues or retroperitoneum in these patients [6, 8, 9]. Patient selection criteria based on obesity are very subjective, although truncal obesity is considered a more definite risk factor for translumbar catheter migration [8]. If a translumbar catheter is placed in a child, the performing physician must be aware that interval growth may lead to displacement of the catheter tip to an extravascular location [20]. Plain radiographs may be used to monitor for appropriate positioning of the catheter tip over time.

Infrarenal caval occlusion may result in technical failure of the translumbar approach and should be considered a relative contraindication to translumbar cannulation of the inferior vena cava. In these patients, a transhepatic route may provide their final percutaneous access site, although it may be complicated by a high rate of catheter thrombosis (0.18–0.24 per 100 catheter days) [11, 13] and migration (14–37.4 %) [11–13]. Ascites is considered a relative contraindication to transhepatic catheter placement. Pre-procedure paracentesis may lessen the bleeding risk of the transhepatic route, however.

8.4 Technique

8.4.1 Translumbar IVC Catheter Placement

Easily accessed by direct percutaneous puncture, the inferior vena cava provides a durable conduit for central venous access. Percutaneous puncture of the inferior vena cava with subcutaneous tunneling of a catheter was first described by Kenney et al. [21] in 1985 as an alternative means of access to the central venous circulation for long-term parenteral nutrition. The safety and efficacy of larger, long-term translumbar hemodialysis catheters (14 French) was first demonstrated by Lund et al. [6] several years later. This group detailed insertion of 17 double-lumen hemodialysis catheters in 12 adult patients. Cumulative patency was 52 % at 6 months and 17 % at 12 months [6]. Despite this early data, there remain only a small number of studies to date reporting on translumbar placement of hemodialysis catheters.

Placement of translumbar hemodialysis catheters has been described in both the pediatric and adult patient populations [6–10, 22]. The technique for translumbar hemodialysis catheter placement is identical for pediatric and adult patients, although general anesthesia is used in the pediatric population at our institution. At present, there is no support in the literature for prophylactic antibiotic administration prior to placement of tunneled hemodialysis catheters. This is supported by the Centers for Disease Control in a type I-A recommendation published in 2002 [23]. Nonetheless, at many health-care centers patients still receive intravenous antibiotic prophylaxis, usually with a first-generation cephalosporin such as cefazolin.

Insertion technique may vary depending on the presence of preexisting iliofemoral thrombosis or obstruction. When the iliofemoral veins are patent but conditions such as a local cutaneous infection or systemic neutropenia necessitate an alternative approach to tunneled femoral venous access, transfemoral placement of a pigtail catheter or guidewire into the inferior vena cava has significant utility. The presence of an intra-caval catheter or guidewire facilitates subsequent direct inferior vena cava puncture, while minimizing potential morbidity from errant needle passes. In such instances, the patient is brought to the angiography suite and initially placed in the supine position. Ultrasonography is used to confirm patency of one or both common femoral veins. A suitable groin site is then prepped and draped in the usual sterile fashion. Buffered 1 % lidocaine is infiltrated to provide local analgesia prior to percutaneous puncture of the common femoral vein. Using sonographic guidance, the right or left common femoral vein is punctured with a 21-gauge needle. A 0.018-in. guidewire is passed through the access needle into the common femoral vein. Over the guidewire, the needle is exchanged for a coaxial microintroducer sheath, which facilitates exchange of the 0.018-in. guidewire

for a larger 0.035-in. working wire. A 4- or 5-French vascular sheath is then advanced over the guidewire into the accessed common femoral vein. A guidewire or pigtail flush catheter is advanced through the transfemoral access into the inferior vena cava to act as the fluoroscopic marker for direct percutaneous puncture of the inferior vena cava. A cavogram should be performed if the patency of the inferior vena cava has not been pre-procedurally evaluated with cross-sectional imaging. [20] Once the guidewire or catheter is secured in place, the patient is placed in the prone position for puncture of the inferior vena cava.

Percutaneous cannulation of the inferior vena cava is performed from a right paramedian approach, irrespective of the presence or absence of a transfemoral inferior vena cava catheter or guidewire. The right flank and anterolateral abdomen are prepped and draped in the usual sterile fashion. Local anesthesia is administered immediately superior to the right iliac crest, approximately 8–10 cm lateral to the midline. Using fluoroscopic guidance, a 21-gauge, 15-cm-long needle is used to puncture the inferior vena cava by targeting the previously placed guidewire or pigtail catheter. If there is known obstruction of both iliofemoral veins and a transfemoral fluoroscopic marker cannot be placed, the inferior vena cava is directly punctured using bony fluoroscopic landmarks for guidance. In this setting, the needle is advanced craniomedially, targeting the anterolateral margin of the L2–L3 vertebral bodies so as to puncture the inferior vena cava just below the renal veins. Intraluminal position is confirmed by free aspiration of blood through the needle. If the needle appears to be in the location of the inferior vena cava but blood cannot be aspirated, gentle administration of contrast media can help confirm intravascular needle position. Contrast administration also excludes unintended entry into the renal vein and thereby avoids the potential complications of renal vein thrombosis and catheter dysfunction [8]. A 0.018-in. platinum-tipped mandril guidewire is then introduced through the access needle and advanced to the inferior cavoatrial junction or right atrium. The needle is exchanged for a coaxial transitional sheath (Accustick system, Boston Scientific, Natick, Massachusetts), which permits replacement of the 0.018-in. guidewire with a 0.035-in. guidewire. Intravascular catheter length is measured and selected in standard fashion. The selected dual-lumen, cuffed hemodialysis catheter is then tunneled through the subcutaneous tissues of the right flank and brought out at the initial access site, keeping the retention cuff approximately 2 cm from the catheter exit site. The tunnel should form a gentle angle with respect to the venotomy site, and the catheter exit site should be located as far laterally as possible to facilitate improved catheter care and patient comfort [20]. Creating a tunnel that is too long can make future catheter manipulations through the same tunnel difficult, if not impossible. Attention is once again directed toward the initial percutaneous access into the inferior vena cava. The transitional dilator is exchanged over the guidewire for an appropriately sized peel-away sheath. Longer introducer sheaths may be necessary for larger patients. Great care should be taken to avoid kinking the guidewire as it can hinder intravascular placement of the introducer sheath and increase the risk of retroperitoneal bleeding. Once the peel-away sheath is placed, the inner dilator and guidewire are removed, and the catheter is inserted through the sheath in standard fashion. Completion radiographs centered on the right hemidiaphragm should demonstrate the catheter tip in the right atrium. The catheter is sutured in place, and the initial puncture site is closed using interrupted sutures or Steri-Strips (3 M, St. Paul, Minnesota). Both lumens of the catheter should be heparinized to minimize the risk of catheter thrombosis.

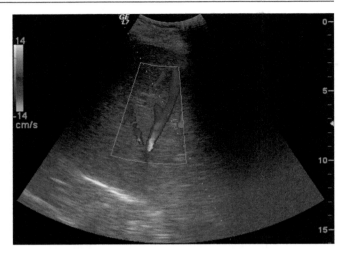

Fig. 8.1 Pre-procedure transverse color Doppler image shows planned route of transhepatic puncture into the middle hepatic vein

8.4.2 Transhepatic Catheter Placement

In some instances, occlusion of the infrarenal inferior vena cava may result in technical failure of the translumbar approach for hemodialysis catheter placement. Percutaneous transhepatic puncture of a hepatic vein for hemodialysis access was first described by Po et al. [24] in a case report in 1994. Since this time, several retrospective studies have sought to verify long-term safety and effectiveness of the transhepatic route for central venous access [11–13]. As with the translumbar route, placement of transhepatic hemodialysis catheters has become commonplace in both the pediatric and adult patient populations. General anesthesia is used at our institution when transhepatic access to the inferior vena cava is requisite in a child.

The technique for transhepatic cannulation of the inferior vena cava is rather straightforward and requires fewer steps than the translumbar route. As with translumbar placement of hemodialysis catheters, antibiotic prophylaxis is controversial and not universally practiced [23]. Pre-procedure ultrasonography of the right upper quadrant is performed to identify a patent middle or right hepatic vein (Fig. 8.1). The right upper quadrant is prepped and draped in the usual sterile fashion. Buffered 1 % lidocaine is administered for local analgesia taking special care to anesthetize the superficial and deep soft tissues including the liver capsule. Using ultrasound guidance, a 21-gauge, 15-cm-long needle is advanced into the middle or right hepatic vein from an anterior subcostal or midaxillary intercostal approach (Fig. 8.2a). The subcostal approach may help to limit future catheter migration [12]. Transhepatic cannulation of a hepatic vein is preferred over direct inferior vena cava puncture because it permits a longer intravascular tract and decreases the chance of migration out of the vessel [11]. A 0.018-in. platinum-tipped mandril guidewire is then advanced through the needle and into the right atrium. Intravascular catheter length is measured

and selected in standard fashion. The initial access needle is exchanged over the guidewire for a coaxial transitional sheath (Accustick system, Boston Scientific, Natick, Massachusetts), which permits replacement of the 0.018-in. guidewire with a 0.035-in. guidewire (Fig. 8.2b). In obese patients or in those with cirrhosis, a stiff guidewire may be necessary to facilitate transhepatic passage of the peel-away sheath.

Additional local anesthesia is administered inferior and lateral to the venous entry site, and a subcutaneous tunnel is fashioned. The hemodialysis catheter is pulled through the tunnel and brought out at the initial venous entry site. Over the guidewire, the transitional dilator is exchanged for an appropriately sized peel-away sheath, which is advanced into the hepatic vein. Once the sheath is in place, the inner dilator and guidewire are removed, and the catheter is introduced through the sheath and into the central venous circulation (Fig. 8.2c). Some interventionalists opt to keep a stiff hydrophilic guidewire in place and then advance the catheter through the sheath and over the guidewire into the hepatic vein until the tip lies within the right atrium [20]. Both catheter ports are flushed, heparinized,

Fig. 8.2 Images of a 45-year-old female with end-stage renal disease in whom transhepatic dialysis catheter placement was pursued because she had no remaining peripheral access sites. (**a**) Frontal view of the abdomen. A 21-gauge needle (*open arrow*) has been used to puncture the appropriate hepatic vein. Of note, the venous outflow component of a failed HeRO vascular access device (Hemosphere, Inc., Eden Prairie, Minnesota) is seen within the inferior vena cava (*arrowhead*). (**b**) A coaxial transitional sheath (*arrow*) has been placed over a guidewire into the central hepatic vein near the confluence with the inferior vena cava. (**c**) Dual-lumen hemodialysis catheter has been placed with the tip in the right atrium just beyond the inferior cavoatrial junction (*arrowhead*)

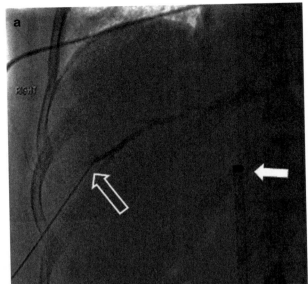

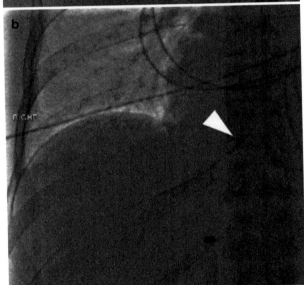

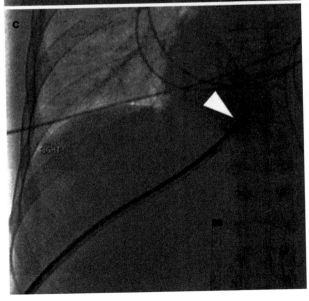

and secured. The initial venous access site is closed using interrupted sutures or Steri-Strips (3 M, St. Paul, Minnesota).

8.5 Complications

Complications of translumbar and transhepatic placement of hemodialysis catheters can be divided into two groups: early (periprocedural) and late. Early complications occur at the time of or immediately following catheter placement and include failure to gain access, guidewire- or catheter-induced atrial or ventricular dysrhythmia, bleeding, air embolism, and catheter malposition or kinking. Acute bleeding following translumbar puncture of the inferior vena cava is quite rare in the setting of acceptable coagulation parameters (INR < 1.5, platelet count > 50,000/mm^3). Rates of air embolism have decreased dramatically with the introduction of valved introducer sheaths several years ago. Most of the other aforementioned immediate complications are avoided with meticulous technique and imaging guidance.

Late complications of translumbar and transhepatic hemodialysis catheters may occur days to months following placement (Table 8.1). One such late complication unique to translumbar hemodialysis catheter placement is spontaneous migration and dislodgement resulting in bleeding. Translumbar catheter migration has been noted to be most common in obese patients, particularly in those with excess adipose tissue concentrated in the truncal area [8, 9]. In such patients, catheter migration or dislodgement out of the inferior vena cava can result in retroperitoneal hemorrhage. According to Biswal et al. [8], bleeding in the form of retroperitoneal hemorrhage has been demonstrated as a common occurrence in several studies. If a translumbar dialysis catheter appears to have migrated on routine or surveillance radiographs, it should be exchanged for a new catheter over a guidewire to facilitate proper placement.

Catheter thrombosis and fibrin sheath formation are late complications common to both translumbar and transhepatic hemodialysis catheter placements. Catheter thrombosis may be treated with outpatient thrombolysis performed through the catheter over 30 min to 1 h. If pharmacologic thrombolysis is unsuccessful, catheter exchange may be performed over a guidewire, thereby maintaining the original access site. Catheter thrombosis rates may be lowered by consistent use of heparin after each hemodialysis session and at the conclusion of placement and exchanges to reduce the risk of intra-catheter thrombosis. Fibrin sheath formation is quite common with chronic indwelling catheters and commonly manifests as catheter dysfunction with impaired ability to aspirate blood despite appropriate catheter tip position on a radiograph. Pharmacologic fibrinolysis and catheter exchange over a guidewire are often the only ways to

Table 8.1 Study comparison – translumbar dialysis catheter placement

	Power et al. [10]	Bennett et al. [7]	Biswal et al. [9]	Lund et al. [6]
No. patients	26 (11 M, 15 F)	22 (10 M, 12 F)	10 (6 M, 4 F)	12
Age (years)	61.9±12.1	37.0±11.9	59±14.2	–
Total catheters	39	29	10	17
Total follow-up	15,864 days	3,510 days	2,252 days	–
Mean catheter duration in situ	–	121 days (14–536)	250 days (30–530)	–
Patients with retroperitoneal hemorrhage	2	1	1	–
Infection rate	2.84 per 1,000 catheter-days	2.80 per 1,000 catheter days	–	2.80 per 1,000 catheter days
Catheter-related bacteremia	0.82 per 1,000 catheter-days	–	–	1.40 per 1,000 catheter days
Exit-site infection	2.01 per 1,000 catheter-days	–	–	–
Catheter thrombosis requiring lysis	0.63 per 1,000 catheter days			330 per 1,000 catheter days

rid a translumbar or transhepatic catheter of a fibrin sheath, as transjugular access for fibrin sheath stripping with a loop snare is often not feasible due to supracardiac central venous occlusion.

Additional late complications of translumbar and transhepatic cannulation of the central veins include infection (Table 8.1) and nonocclusive or occlusive thrombosis of the central veins. Infection can involve the exit site, the subcutaneous tunnel, or the bloodstream. Exit site and subcutaneous tunnel infections are typically caused by skin flora with direct extension from the adjacent skin. *Staphylococcus epidermidis* is the most common organism. In three large retrospective studies detailing experience with transhepatic dialysis catheter placement [11–13], authors noted an infection rate of 0.22–0.24 per 100 catheter days. Unfortunately, infection necessitated catheter removal in nearly all patients because the catheter was presumed to be the nidus of infection

Hepatic tract embolization after elective removal of transhepatic catheters is controversial and to date is a subject that has not achieved consensus on an appropriate course of action [13]. Stavropoulos et al. [11] routinely performed tract embolization with Gelfoam pledgets (Upjohn Pharmacia, Kalamazoo, Michigan). On the contrary, Smith et al. [12] and Younes et al. [13] did not perform hepatic tract embolization after removal of transhepatic catheters, and neither study noted any associated bleeding complications.

Conclusion

Despite ongoing initiatives to reduce catheter use for hemodialysis, a large number of end-stage renal disease patients continue to utilize catheters as a primary mode of access for treatment. Prolonged catheter use eventually leads to the exhaustion of conventional modes of central venous access. The translumbar and transhepatic routes of access require expert technical skill and close surveillance to maintain patency, but each remains an invaluable tool in the armamentarium for interventionalists treating patients that require chronic central venous access for

hemodialysis. Translumbar and transhepatic hemodialysis catheters each have proven long-term functionality and provide remarkably durable access in patients who have otherwise exhausted all access options.

References

1. Dirks JH, de Zeeuw D, Agarwal SK, et al. Prevention of chronic kidney and vascular disease: toward global health equity—the Bellagio 2004 declaration. Kidney Int Suppl. 2005;98:S1–6.
2. U.S. Renal Data System. USRDS 2010 annual data report: atlas of end-stage renal disease in the United States. Bethesda: National Institutes of Health, National Institute of Diabetes and Digestive and Kidney Diseases; 2010.
3. Lorenz J, Regalado S, Navuluri R, Zangan S, Vanha T, Funaki B. Transhepatic guidance of translumbar hemodialysis catheter placement in the setting of chronic infrarenal IVC occlusion. Cardiovasc Intervent Radiol. 2010;33(3):635–8.
4. Schillinger F, Schillinger D, Montagnac R, Milicent T. Post catheterization vein stenosis in haemodialysis: comparative angiographic study of 50 subclavian and 50 internal jugular accesses. Nephrol Dial Transplant. 1991;6(10):722–4.
5. Cimochowski GE, Worley E, Rutherford WE, Sartain J, Blondin J, Harter H. Superiority of the internal jugular over the subclavian access for temporary dialysis. Nephron. 1990;54(2):154–61.
6. Lund GB, Trerotola SO, Scheel Jr PJ. Percutaneous translumbar inferior vena cava cannulation for hemodialysis. Am J Kidney Dis. 1995;25(5):732–7.
7. Bennett J, Papadouris D, Rankin R, et al. Percutaneous inferior vena caval approach for long-term central venous access. J Vasc Interv Radiol. 1997;8(5):851–5.
8. Rajan D, Croteau DL, Sturza SG, Harvill ML, Mehall CJ. Translumbar placement of inferior vena caval catheters: a solution for challenging hemodialysis access. Radiographics. 1998;18(5):1155–67.
9. Biswal R, Nosher J, Siegel R, Bodner LJ. Translumbar placement of paired hemodialysis catheters (Tesio catheters) and follow-up in 10 patients. Cardiovasc Intervent Radiol. 2000;23(1):75–8.
10. Power A, Singh S, Ashby D, et al. Translumbar central venous catheters for long-term haemodialysis. Nephrol Dial Transplant. 2010;25(5):1588–95.
11. Stavropoulos SW, Pan JJ, Clark TW, et al. Percutaneous transhepatic venous access for hemodialysis. J Vasc Interv Radiol. 2003;14(9 Pt 1):1187–90.

12. Smith TP, Ryan JM, Reddan DN. Transhepatic catheter access for hemodialysis. Radiology. 2004;232(1):246–51.

13. Younes HK, Pettigrew CD, Anaya-Ayala JE, et al. Transhepatic hemodialysis catheters: functional outcome and comparison between early and late failure. J Vasc Interv Radiol. 2011;22(2): 183–91.

14. Hakim R, Himmelfarb J. Hemodialysis access failure: a call to action. Kidney Int. 1998;54(4):1029–40.

15. Vascular Access 2006 Work Group. NKF-DOQI clinical practice guidelines for vascular access. National kidney foundation—dialysis outcomes quality initiative. Am J Kidney Dis. 2006;48 Suppl 1:S176–247.

16. Perera GB, Mueller MP, Kubaska SM, Wilson SE, Lawrence PF, Fujitani RM. Superiority of autogenous arteriovenous hemodialysis access: maintenance of function with fewer secondary interventions. Ann Vasc Surg. 2004;18(1):66–73.

17. Chemla E, Korrakuti L, Makanjuola D, et al. Vascular access in haemodialysis patients with central venous obstruction or stenosis: one center's experience. Ann Vasc Surg. 2005;19:692–8.

18. Murthy R, Arbabzadeh M, Lund G, Richard 3rd H, Levitin A, Stainken B. Percutaneous transrenal hemodialysis catheter insertion. J Vasc Interv Radiol. 2002;13(10):1043–6.

19. Waybill P, Brown D, editors. SIR syllabus series, patient care in vascular and interventional radiology. Fairfax: SIR Press; 2010.

20. Weeks SM. Unconventional venous access. Tech Vasc Interv Radiol. 2002;5(2):114–20.

21. Kenney P, Dorfman G, Denny Jr DF. Percutaneous inferior vena cava cannulation for long-term parenteral nutrition. Surgery. 1985;97(5):602–5.

22. Robertson LJ, Jaques PF, Mauro MA, Azizkhan RG, Robards J. Percutaneous inferior vena cava placement of tunneled silastic catheters for prolonged vascular access in infants. J Pediatr Surg. 1990;25(6):596–8.

23. O'Grady A, Dellinger E, et al. Guidelines for the prevention of intravascular catheter-related infections. MMWR. 2002;51:1–26.

24. Po CL, Koolpe HA, Allen S, Alvez LD, Raja RM. Transhepatic PermCath for hemodialysis. Am J Kidney Dis. 1994;24(4): 590–1.

Approach to a Nonfunctioning Catheter

Roman Shingarev and Alexander S. Yevzlin

9.1 Introduction

Despite substantial efforts by nephrology community to reduce utilization of dialysis catheters, majority of end-stage renal disease (ESRD) patients in the USA initiate hemodialysis (HD) with a tunneled dialysis catheter (TDC) with approximately one-quarter of them remaining catheter-dependent thereafter [1]. TDCs are associated with decreased patient survival [2], as well as multiple complications, such as central venous stenosis [3, 4], infection [5, 6], and thrombosis [7]. In many cases, these lead to catheter dysfunction defined by KDOQI as "failure to attain and maintain an extracorporeal blood flow of 300 mL/min or greater at a prepump arterial pressure more negative than −250 mmHg" [8]. Besides increases in arterial and venous pressures registered by dialyzer that necessitate decrease in blood flow, catheter dysfunction can result in significant recirculation leading to lower Kt/V. Left untreated, such catheters require premature removal when they become nonfunctional (i.e., with one or both lumens that cannot be aspirated) [9]. To detect catheter dysfunction early, KDOQI recommends monitoring the ratio of dialyzer blood flow rate divided by the prepump arterial limb pressure (normal is greater than 1.2) and the trends in changes of catheter blood flow rates.

TDC dysfunction is usually viewed as presenting early or late, which helps determining etiology of the problem and guides subsequent management. Dysfunction noted immediately after the catheter placement is likely due to the positioning of the catheter, preexisting vascular abnormalities (e.g., central venous stenosis) (Fig. 9.1), or mechanical damage to the catheter (e.g., tight suture or perforation). Dysfunction developing after successful initial use is usually due to thrombosis, fibrin sheath formation around the catheter, mural thrombus adhering to the catheter tip, or new central venous stenosis.

9.2 Initial Evaluation and Treatment

Catheter dysfunction is usually detected at a dialysis unit where several steps can be taken to evaluate and resolve the problem. Improvement of blood flows after patient repositioning is indicative of catheter tip malposition. Reversal of inlet and outlet lumens may overcome the ball valve effect of the fibrin sheath or a vessel wall in direct contact with one of the catheter tips. Dialysis equipment should be assessed

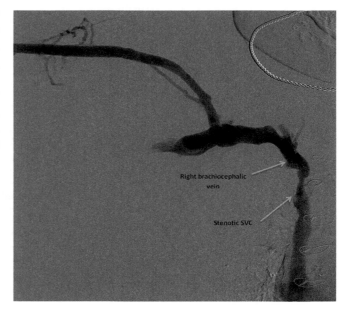

Fig. 9.1 Central vein stenosis

R. Shingarev, MD (✉)
Division of Nephrology, Department of Medicine,
University of Alabama, Birmingham, AL, USA
e-mail: roman@uab.edu

A.S. Yevzlin, MD
Division of Nephrology,
Department of Medicine (CHS),
University of Wisconsin, Madison, WI 53705, USA

A.S. Yevzlin et al. (eds.), *Interventional Nephrology*,
DOI 10.1007/978-1-4614-8803-3_9, © Springer Science+Business Media New York 2014

for malfunction leading to activation of pressure alarms. Examples of equipment problems include line kinking, dialyzer pump failure, and dialyzer clotting. Instillation of a thrombolytic agent in TDC lumens for 1 h to up to 24 h is usually performed when intraluminal stenosis is suspected. Endoluminal fibrin analysis system (FAS) brush has been employed in attempt to improve catheter flows by few dialysis centers; however, only one small study sought to evaluate its effectiveness reporting positive results [10]. Figure 9.2 suggests a diagnostic and therapeutic algorithm for general nephrologists and dialysis unit staff to follow when catheter dysfunction is present.

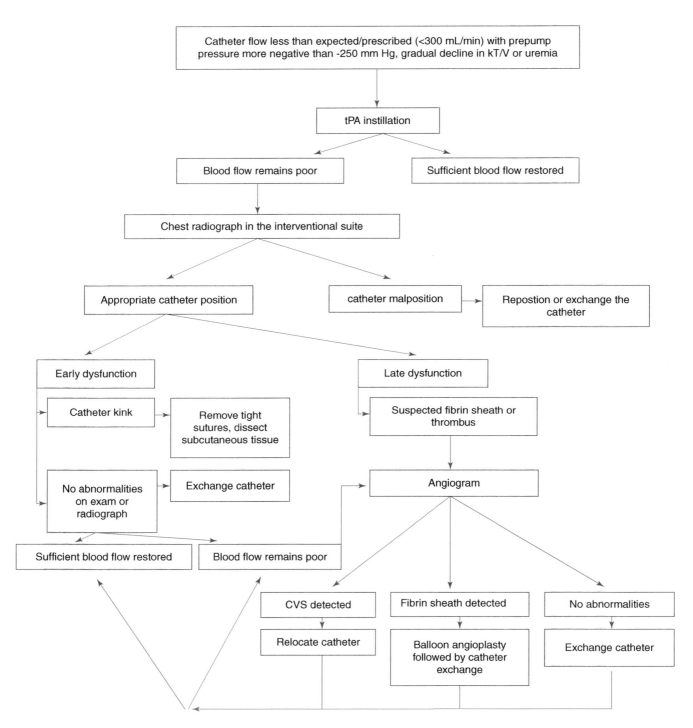

Fig. 9.2 Diagnostic and therapeutic algorithm for catheter dysfunction

9.3 Diagnostic Evaluation in an Interventional Suite

If adequate blood flows cannot be reestablished at the dialysis unit, referral to the interventional suite is indicated. There, a physical examination of the malfunctioning catheter should be performed as the first step in evaluation and should include aspiration of luminal contents, assessment for kinks, integrity, and tunnel infection of the TDC. Next, a radiograph should be obtained to evaluate the catheter positioning. This may reveal a kink in the catheter, a catheter tip that migrated into the superior vena cava (SVC) or even into either of the brachiocephalic veins. The latter may happen in obese patients, whose cuff-to-vein catheter length may increase considerably with movement, thereby shortening the intravascular catheter length due to immovable subcutaneous cuff position. A curved caudal portion of the catheter or a doughnut ("down the barrel") appearance of the edge of the catheter's tip is indicative of azygos vein cannulation. Location of the distal portion of the catheter in the midsternal or left parasternal region should raise a suspicion of intra-aortic placement of the catheter. A lateral radiograph showing the catheter projecting toward anterior mediastinum may further strengthen this suspicion [11, 12].

If there is a suspicion for a pericatheter thrombus or fibrin sheath, angiogram can be performed by slowly injecting 10–15 ml of contrast by hand through each catheter port. In presence of a fibrin sheath, the contrast will outline the sheath flowing retrograde from the catheter tip (Fig. 9.3). Antegrade contrast flow may also demonstrate a pericatheter

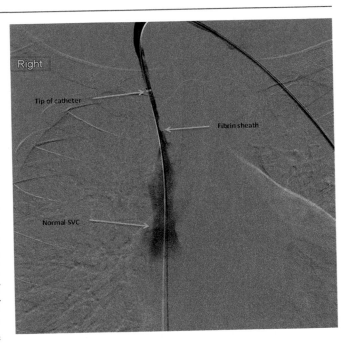

Fig. 9.4 Fibrin sheath

filling defect consistent with a mural thrombus [13]. Alternatively, the catheter may be retracted over an Amplatz wire to position its tip in the internal jugular vein. In this case, the contrast flows antegrade clearly outlining the lumen of the fibrin sheath (Fig. 9.4) [14].

9.4 Interventions Directed at Specific Causes of Catheter Dysfunction

9.4.1 Catheter Damage

If a catheter wall integrity is compromised anywhere along its extravascular portion, either as a result of a manufacturing defect or an operator's mistake, the patient may present with either persistent bleeding from the tunnel or symptoms of air embolism [15, 16]. Diagnostic test of choice in this case is a catheterogram that can be performed by hand-injecting 10 cc of contrast into each catheter lumen. Extravasation of contrast confirms the diagnosis necessitating exchange of the malfunctioning catheter for a new one.

9.4.2 Catheter Kinking

The initial radiograph taken in the IR suite may immediately expose a problem such as a catheter kink. Kinking occurs either as a result of a "high stick," when the entry in the internal jugular vein was made high above the clavicle in the neck forcing the catheter to take a sharp turn from the tunnel and

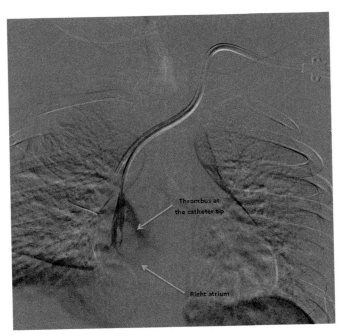

Fig. 9.3 Thrombus at the catheter tip

into the vein or when the catheter gets caught in the insufficiently dissected subcutaneous tissue at the neck incision site after it has been inserted in the vein through the split sheath or over the wire. In the first scenario, the existing TDC has to be removed and a new one has to be placed lower in the internal jugular vein after sufficient hemostasis has been achieved. In the second scenario, an Amplatz wire placed in the IVC through one of the lumens may be used to stabilize the catheter. Next, an incision in the skin overlying the kink is made with care taken not to nick the catheter, and a blunt-tip hemostat is used to dissect the tissue underneath the kink. Moving the catheter back and forth over the wire while applying pressure to the catheter bend usually allows the operator to eliminate the kink.

9.4.3 Tip Malposition

Due to complex anatomy of the thoracic veins, catheter malposition is common [17]. In the settings of SVC stenosis (itself common in HD patients) and venous aberrations that follow, such as dilatation of the azygos vein, the likelihood of incorrect catheter positioning is even higher [18]. Even if initially appropriately positioned, catheters have been described to migrate spontaneously, most commonly in the contralateral innominate vein generating an array of complications [11, 19]. TDC dysfunction in these cases is due to direct contact of the catheter tip or its side holes with the vessel wall causing obstruction of blood flow. A TDC placed through the left internal jugular vein may induce thrombus formation even if its tip only moves up into the upper portion of the SVC [20], because of the 90° turn the catheter has to take from the left brachiocephalic vein into the SVC. If the catheter length is too short, its tip will be sticking against the right lateral wall of the SVC irritating endothelium.

If the TDC is found to be malpositioned within the first week of its placement, attempts can be made to advance it into the lower portion of the SVC over an Amplatz wire placed through one or both catheter lumens. Older TDCs will have fibrous tissue formed around the cuff necessitating subcutaneous dissection and subsequent exchange for a new TDC. An operator may choose to advance the new TDC further into the SVC to minimize the future catheter migration; however, observations from a small patient series reported by Haygood et al. [11] suggest this strategy does not necessarily change the outcomes. Nevertheless, this option may still be appropriate for TDCs with split-tip design, as its tips are preformed to separate at an angle making it more likely for the shorter tip to end up in an inappropriate position. Because of that, some experts recommend placing the tips of a split-tip catheter in the right atrium [21]. This recommendation is somewhat controversial, as there are reports of higher incidence of atrial thrombi, vessel wall perforation leading to cardiac tamponade, and cardiac arrhythmias [22, 23], associated with atrial positioning of a catheter. Supporting evidence, however, is rather insufficient to advice against such practice. If the TDC is to be exchanged, an operator may also consider changing a split-tip catheter for a step-tipped one, which should theoretically lower the chances of tip migration.

9.4.4 Catheter Thrombosis

Intraluminal thrombosis remains the most common cause of TDC dysfunction despite routine use of anticoagulant locking solutions [24, 25]. After the initial evaluation ruling out a positional or mechanical problem, instillation of a thrombolytic agent is recommended. Several drugs, such as urokinase and streptokinase, have been used in the past, but of drugs currently available on the market only two – alteplase and reteplase – have been used for TDC thrombosis. Reteplase has been purported to have superior clot penetration [26]; it is rather cumbersome to use requiring frozen storage and aliquoting individual doses [27]. Therefore, use of alteplase or tPA is more common in clinical practice. The dose of 2 mg per lumen is usually instilled for about an hour; however, if blood flow is not restored, the alteplase is aspirated from the lumens and another dose may be instilled for longer duration (usually 10–24 h), although evidence exists that prolonged dwell time may not influence subsequent rates of TDC patency [28]. In general, treatment of intraluminal thrombosis with thrombolytics is associated with 70–88 % immediate success rate of restoring adequate blood flow [28–32]. At 2 weeks following instillation of thrombolytics only half of the TDCs remain patent [28]. These unsatisfactory patency rates are likely explained by the fact that catheter dysfunction in many patients included in these studies was due to thrombi extending outside of the catheter lumen or fibrin sheath that require a more intensive therapy than described above.

As described above, a FAS brush can be employed in the interventional suite in attempt to mechanically remove an intraluminal thrombus; however, the outcome and complication data are limited to a small trial reported by Tranter et al. [10]. The immediate success rate of 73 % and 6-week patency of 50 % are comparable to those of thrombolytic use, and it is unclear if this novel strategy can improve outcomes if used in combination with thrombolytic therapy.

9.4.5 Fibrin Sheath

Recurring use of thrombolytics should in itself raise suspicion for the presence of fibrin sheath around the catheter (Fig. 9.4) [33] – a problem affecting 40–100 % of central venous catheters [34–36]. While thrombolytic therapy was demonstrated to have immediate success rate of 91 %, 2-month patency was, expectedly, quite low at around 36 % [37]. Subsequently, four other strategies for restoration of catheter patency have been evaluated. Those included TDC exchange, percutaneous fibrin sheath stripping (PFSS), angioplasty disruption, and internal snare maneuver. In one study, patency rates were shown to be superior with catheter exchange compared to PFSS at 4 months [14] and in another one, PFSS did not improve catheter patency rates when compared to urokinase over 45 days following the procedure [13]. Yet another study showed no differences in immediate or long-term (6 months) outcomes following TDC exchange, PFSS, and angioplasty disruption [38]. Most recently, Oliver et al. [34] demonstrated significantly improved median times to recurrent TDC dysfunction associated with angioplasty disruption followed by TDC exchange compared to TD exchange alone (373 days versus 97.5 days, $p = 0.22$). Based on these findings and procedure cost analysis, current KDOQI guidelines currently recommend the latter strategy for treatment of TDC-associated fibrin sheaths. A novel technique of fibrin sheath removal by an "internal snare" has been described in 2007 and has not been compared head-to-head with other fibrin sheath disruption procedures. Authors, however, report 100 % immediate success and 100 % patency rate at a mean follow-up of 17 weeks [39]. Below is the brief description of these procedures.

TDC Exchange

One or two Amplatz wires are placed in the IVC under fluoroscopic guidance. Subcutaneous tissue around the cuff is dissected under local anesthesia with a hemostat and the indwelling TDC is retracted over the wires that are then sterilized. A new TDC is then inserted through the existing tunnel over the wires into the appropriate position.

Percutaneous Fibrin Sheath Stripping

A standard 6-French sheath is placed in the femoral (usually right) vein and a diagnostic angiographic catheter is advanced into the SVC over a guide wire. Next, the guide wire is exchanged for a 25 or 35-mm diameter nitinol loop snare, which is then engaged and advanced cranially to encircle the catheter. An Amplatz wire placed in the IVC through one of the TDC lumens may facilitate this maneuver. After the snare device reaches the catheter insertion site in the internal jugular vein, it should be tightened and retracted all the way out to manually clean it thereby minimizing the risk of distal embolization of fibrin. Contrast can be injected through the catheter to evaluate the outcome of this procedure.

Angioplasty Disruption

The indwelling TDC needs to be retracted over two Amplatz wires as described in the "TDC Exchange" section above. A long (20 cm) 7-French sheath is then advanced over one of

the Amplatz wires into the SVC and a 12-mm balloon is inserted through the sheath and inflated several times along the fibrin sheath tract. To maximize the fibrin sheath disruption, the balloon may be moved back and forth in the SVC while inflated. Post-procedure angiography should be performed to ascertain success of the procedure.

Internal Snare

A 0.089 mm nitinol Terumo wire is folded in the middle to form a U-shaped loop and advanced through each TDC lumen under fluoroscopic guidance until the loop emerges from the catheter tip. Moving the loop back and forth around the tip of the catheter disrupts the fibrin sheath overlying the distal and proximal ports and restores the catheter flow.

9.4.6 Central Vein Stenosis

Stenosis of the brachiocephalic vein or SVC does not affect the TDC function as long as its tip remains outside the stenotic segment, not in direct contact with the vessel wall (Fig. 9.5). If patient develops SVC syndrome, however, the catheter has to be relocated. In the settings of SVC stenosis, the usual choice is either femoral vein. In many patients with long history of vascular access problems, internal jugular and femoral veins may become inaccessible, either due to stenosis (Fig. 9.6) or venous stents placed in arteriovenous thigh grafts. Uncommon approaches to cannulation of these patients have been described, including translumbar

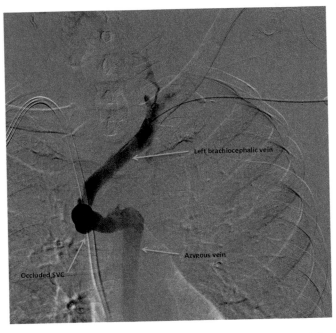

Fig. 9.5 SVC stenosis in the presence of catheter with blood draining via the azygos vein

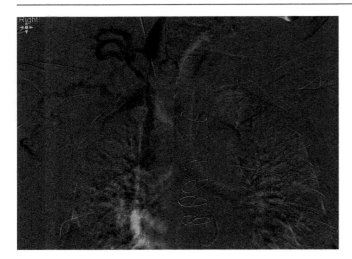

Fig. 9.6 Right internal jugular vein stenosis

approach [40, 41] or transhepatic approach [42, 43]. Decision to undertake one approach or the other should be based on an individual patient's anatomy and an operator experience with these procedures.

References

1. Collins AJ, Foley RN, Gilbertson DT, Chen SC. The state of chronic kidney disease, ESRD, and morbidity and mortality in the first year of dialysis. Clin J Am Soc Nephrol. 2009;4 Suppl 1:S5–11.
2. Xue JL, Dahl D, Ebben JP, Collins AJ. The association of initial hemodialysis access type with mortality outcomes in elderly Medicare ESRD patients. Am J Kidney Dis. 2003;42(5): 1013–9.
3. Agarwal AK, Patel BM, Haddad NJ. Central vein stenosis: a nephrologist's perspective. Semin Dial. 2007;20(1):53–62.
4. Wilkin TD, Kraus MA, Lane KA, Trerotola SO. Internal jugular vein thrombosis associated with hemodialysis catheters. Radiology. 2003;228(3):697–700.
5. Lee T, Barker J, Allon M. Tunneled catheters in hemodialysis patients: reasons and subsequent outcomes. Am J Kidney Dis. 2005;46(3):501–8.
6. Stevenson KB, Hannah EL, Lowder CA, et al. Epidemiology of hemodialysis vascular access infections from longitudinal infection surveillance data: predicting the impact of NKF-DOQI clinical practice guidelines for vascular access. Am J Kidney Dis. 2002; 39(3):549–55.
7. Schwab SJ, Buller GL, McCann RL, Bollinger RR, Stickel DL. Prospective evaluation of a Dacron cuffed hemodialysis catheter for prolonged use. Am J Kidney Dis. 1988;11(2):166–9.
8. National Kidney Foundation. KDOQI clinical practice guidelines and clinical practice recommendations for vascular access. Am J Kidney Dis. 2006;48 Suppl 1:S176–322.
9. Ponikvar R, Buturović-Ponikvar J. Temporary hemodialysis catheters as a long-term vascular access in chronic hemodialysis patients. Ther Apher Dial. 2005;9(3):250–3.
10. Tranter SA, Donoghue J. Brushing has made a sweeping change: use of the endoluminal FAS brush in haemodialysis central venous catheter management. Aust Crit Care. 2000;13(1):10–3.
11. Haygood TM, Malhotra K, Ng C, Chasen B, McEnery KW, Chasen M. Migration of central lines from the superior vena cava to the azygous vein. Clin Radiol. 2012;67(1):49–54.
12. Parry W, Dhillon R, Salahudeen A. Carotid pseudoaneurysm from inadvertent carotid artery catheterization for haemodialysis. Nephrol Dial Transplant. 1996;11(9):1853–5.
13. Gray RJ, Levitin A, Buck D, et al. Percutaneous fibrin sheath stripping versus transcatheter urokinase infusion for malfunctioning well-positioned tunneled central venous dialysis catheters: a prospective, randomized trial. J Vasc Interv Radiol. 2000;11(9): 1121–9.
14. Merport M, Murphy TP, Egglin TK, Dubel GJ. Fibrin sheath stripping versus catheter exchange for the treatment of failed tunneled hemodialysis catheters: randomized clinical trial. J Vasc Interv Radiol. 2000;11(9):1115–20.
15. Huang EY, Cohen S, Lee J, et al. Diagnosis of unexplained bleeding from tunneled dialysis catheter. Am J Nephrol. 2001;21(5):397–9.
16. Yu AS, Levy E. Paradoxical cerebral air embolism from a hemodialysis catheter. Am J Kidney Dis. 1997;29(3):453–5.
17. Godwin JD, Chen JT. Thoracic venous anatomy. AJR Am J Roentgenol. 1986;147(4):674–84.
18. Chasen MH, Charnsangavej C. Venous chest anatomy: clinical implications. Eur J Radiol. 1998;27(1):2–14.
19. Skandalos I, Hatzibaloglou A, Evagelou I, et al. Deviations of placement/function of permanent central vein catheters for hemodialysis. Int J Artif Organs. 2005;28(6):583–90.
20. Puel V, Caudry M, Le Métayer P, et al. Superior vena cava thrombosis related to catheter malposition in cancer chemotherapy given through implanted ports. Cancer. 1993;72(7):2248–52.
21. Ash SR. Fluid mechanics and clinical success of central venous catheters for dialysis–answers to simple but persisting problems. Semin Dial. 2007;20(3):237–56.
22. Gilon D, Schechter D, Rein AJ, et al. Right atrial thrombi are related to indwelling central venous catheter position: insights into time course and possible mechanism of formation. Am Heart J. 1998;135(3):457–62.
23. Kalen V, Medige TA, Rinsky LA. Pericardial tamponade secondary to perforation by central venous catheters in orthopaedic patients. J Bone Joint Surg Am. 1991;73(10):1503–6.
24. Moss AH, Vasilakis C, Holley JL, Foulks CJ, Pillai K, McDowell DE. Use of a silicone dual-lumen catheter with a Dacron cuff as a long-term vascular access for hemodialysis patients. Am J Kidney Dis. 1990;16(3):211–5.
25. Shaffer D, Madras PN, Williams ME, D'Elia JA, Kaldany A, Monaco AP. Use of Dacron cuffed silicone catheters as long-term hemodialysis access. ASAIO J. 1992;38(1):55–8.
26. Fischer S, Kahnert U. Major mechanistic differences explain the higher clot lysis potency of reteplase over alteplase: lack of fibrin binding is an advantage for bolus application of fibrin specific thrombolytics. Fibrinolysis Proteolysis. 1997;11(3):129–35.
27. Hyman G, England M, Kibede S, Lee P, Willets G. The efficacy and safety of reteplase for thrombolysis of hemodialysis catheters at a community and academic regional medical center. Nephron Clin Pract. 2004;96(2):39–42.
28. Macrae JM, Loh G, Djurdjev O, et al. Short and long alteplase dwells in dysfunctional hemodialysis catheters. Hemodial Int. 2005;9(2):189–95.
29. Davies J, Casey J, Li C, Crowe AV, McClelland P. Restoration of flow following haemodialysis catheter thrombus. Analysis of rt-PA infusion in tunnelled dialysis catheters. J Clin Pharm Ther. 2004; 29(6):517–20.
30. Zacharias JM, Weatherston CP, Spewak CR, Vercaigne LM. Alteplase versus urokinase for occluded hemodialysis catheters. Ann Pharmacother. 2003;37(1):27–33.
31. Eyrich H, Walton T, Macon EJ, Howe A. Alteplase versus urokinase in restoring blood flow in hemodialysis-catheter thrombosis. Am J Health Syst Pharm. 2002;59(15):1437–40.
32. Daeihagh P, Jordan J, Chen J, Rocco M. Efficacy of tissue plasminogen activator administration on patency of hemodialysis access catheters. Am J Kidney Dis. 2000;36(1):75–9.

33. Cassidy FP, Zajko AB, Bron KM, Reilly JJ, Peitzman AB, Steed DL. Noninfectious complications of long-term central venous catheters: radiologic evaluation and management. AJR Am J Roentgenol. 1987;149(4):671–5.

34. Oliver MJ, Mendelssohn DC, Quinn RR, et al. Catheter patency and function after catheter sheath disruption: a pilot study. Clin J Am Soc Nephrol. 2007;2(6):1201–6.

35. Xiang DZ, Verbeken EK, Van Lommel AT, Stas M, De Wever I. Composition and formation of the sleeve enveloping a central venous catheter. J Vasc Surg. 1998;28(2):260–71.

36. Brismar B, Hårdstedt C, Jacobson S. Diagnosis of thrombosis by catheter phlebography after prolonged central venous catheterization. Ann Surg. 1981;194(6):779–83.

37. Savader SJ, Ehrman KO, Porter DJ, Haikal LC, Oteham AC. Treatment of hemodialysis catheter-associated fibrin sheaths by rt-PA infusion: critical analysis of 124 procedures. J Vasc Interv Radiol. 2001;12(6):711–5.

38. Janne d'Othée B, Tham JC, Sheiman RG. Restoration of patency in failing tunneled hemodialysis catheters: a comparison of catheter exchange, exchange and balloon disruption of the fibrin sheath, and femoral stripping. J Vasc Interv Radiol. 2006;17(6): 1011–5.

39. Reddy AS, Lang EV, Cutts J, Loh S, Rosen MP. Fibrin sheath removal from central venous catheters: an internal snare manoeuvre. Nephrol Dial Transplant. 2007;22(6):1762–5.

40. Lund GB, Lieberman RP, Haire WD, Martin VA, Kessinger A, Armitage JO. Translumbar inferior vena cava catheters for long-term venous access. Radiology. 1990;174(1): 31–5.

41. Gupta A, Karak PK, Saddekni S. Translumbar inferior vena cava catheter for long-term hemodialysis. J Am Soc Nephrol. 1995;5(12):2094–7.

42. Po CL, Koolpe HA, Allen S, Alvez LD, Raja RM. Transhepatic PermCath for hemodialysis. Am J Kidney Dis. 1994;24(4): 590–1.

43. Stavropoulos SW, Pan JJ, Clark TW, et al. Percutaneous transhepatic venous access for hemodialysis. J Vasc Interv Radiol. 2003;14(9 Pt 1):1187–90.

Approach to the Infected Catheter

10

Laura Maursetter

10.1 Introduction

Vascular access is a continuous challenge for any patient receiving either acute or chronic hemodialysis (HD). The type of access used and its maintenance can impact the outcome of the patient. It is imperative that the practicing nephrologist knows how to deal with complications of vascular access including infections. This chapter will focus on the approach to a patient with an infected catheter.

10.2 Background

Use of central venous catheters (CVC) is essential to the practice of critical care medicine with more than seven million sold annually in the USA [1]. A life-threatening complication of CVC is a bloodstream infection. Approximately 80,000 episodes of catheter-related bloodstream infections (CRBSI) occur in the USA annually at a cost of approximately $25,000–$45,000 per episode [1, 2]. Serious complications of this illness can occur in as many as 44 % of bacteremic episodes making optimal treatment imperative. Serious complications include endocarditis, osteomyelitis, thrombophlebitis, septic arthritis, epidural abscess, and death [3]. These data are not specific to the HD population, but CVC are essential to many patients who require dialysis making management of the infected catheters an important topic for nephrologists.

Over the last decade there has been a push to place fistulas earlier in chronic kidney disease patients. This was started because the United States Renal Data System (USRDS) showed that patients using a catheter were four times more likely to get an infection than those using a graft and eight times more likely than those using a fistula [4]. The Fistula First initiative has decreased the number of chronic kidney disease patients who initiate HD with a catheter, but more than 65 % of US patients will still have their first HD session using a catheter. This is compared to 14 % who use arterial-venous fistulas [5]. With 116,395 incident cases of end-stage renal disease in 2009, this means more than 75,000 patients experienced catheter use at the start of their dialysis careers [5].

Many HD patients are rapidly transitioned to other means of venous access, but the increased risk associated with catheters is imposed on the majority of end-stage renal disease (ESRD) patients at dialysis initiation. The use of CVC as an option for permanent hemodialysis access began in the mid-1980s. Current first-year infection-related mortality is 2.4 times higher than it was in 1981, much of which has been attributed to CVC use [3, 5]. In addition, when comparing total cost of a patient receiving dialysis through an arterial-venous fistula, those with a catheter have a 25 % higher cost, mostly attributed to catheter-related infection costs [5]. The increased mortality from catheter use heightens the already elevated mortality rate for this high-risk population [6]. It is imperative that the dialysis care team works to prevent, suspect, manage, and treat infections related to catheters appropriately as patient outcomes depend on this practice.

10.3 Risk Factors for Infection

Before an infection can be diagnosed, it needs to be suspected. Risk factors have been identified that increase the possibility of an infection. These include recent or prolonged hospitalization, poor patient hygiene, prior catheter-related infection, inadequate dialysis, low albumin levels, diabetes, hypertension, and longer duration of catheter use [1, 3, 7–9]. A review of 96 studies was conducted to highlight common risk factors present for all CVC-related infections. The leading events that increased risk for catheter-related infections include insertion without maximal sterile barriers (relative risk 2.1), placement of a catheter via guidewire exchange

L. Maursetter, DO
Division of Nephrology, Department of Medicine,
University of Wisconsin School of Medicine and Public Health,
Madison, WI, USA
e-mail: lmaursetter@uwhealth.org

A.S. Yevzlin et al. (eds.), *Interventional Nephrology*,
DOI 10.1007/978-1-4614-8803-3_10, © Springer Science+Business Media New York 2014

into an old site (relative risk 2), heavy cutaneous colonization of the insertions site (relative risk 5.5), contamination of the catheter hub, and duration of the catheter for more than 7 days (relative risk 2) [1]. Guidelines to decrease or eliminate these risk factors have been published and are available for review [10].

10.3.1 Mechanisms of Infection

Catheter-related bloodstream infections (CRBSI) can occur by three main mechanisms. Organisms that are present on the skin can gain entry through the exit site of a newly placed catheter. This can occur at the time of initial placement or, in the case of tunneled line placement, before the subcutaneous tunnel has had time to endothelialize. The organism can enter at the catheter exit site and migrate down the path of the catheter on its external surface where it can either colonize the tissue, device, or eventually make it to the bloodstream to be hematogenously spread during hemodialysis [1, 11, 12]. The second mechanism of infection occurs when there is contamination of the catheter hub, usually by contact with patient's skin or clothing or from health-care workers' hands when accessing the catheter. This leads to intraluminal colonization of the catheter and is spread during high blood flows during hemodialysis [12]. Lastly, infections elsewhere in the body can hematogenously seed the catheter as it sits in its venous environment [2].

As quickly as 24 h after insertion, a fibrin sheath can form around the catheter as it occupies its position in the vein [13]. Fibrin can cause difficulty with catheter blood flow but can also promote biofilm formation and be a nidus for infection [14]. The layer of glycomatrix that makes up the fibrin sheath can protect against the effects of antibiotics on the organisms hiding in its layers making clearance with antimicrobial therapy difficult [3]. The biofilm that adheres to the catheter does not universally have colonization of bacteria as was previously believed. This was confirmed by scanning electron microscopy, therefore prevention of colonization may be useful [13].

10.3.2 Suspecting an Infection

Due to an immunocompromised state, patients requiring dialysis may not present with common signs and symptoms of bacteremia, and surveillance cultures are an ineffective way of monitoring for infection [7]. Al-Solaiman et al. investigated the rate of infection and associated symptoms in catheter-dependent HD patients. The study followed 172 catheter-dependent patients over a 1.5-year period of time and found the rate of infection was 4.6 infections per 1,000

catheter days [15]. This was similar to published data that cited rates from 0.6 to 6.5 episodes per 1,000 catheter days [3]. The most common symptoms leading to assessment for infection were fever, rigors, altered mentation, change in exit-site appearance, and unexplained hypotension. Only 47 % of catheter-related bacterial infections presented with fever. In fact, symptoms were evenly distributed between fevers alone, fever and rigors, and rigors alone but as many as 20 % had none of these findings [15]. Therefore, a wide array of symptoms should raise suspicion for catheter-related infection and fever is not a defining criterion (Fig. 10.1).

As the exit site is one of the portals of entry that can lead to catheter-related bacteremia, it is important to do a careful examination whenever there is a change appearance or symptoms are noted. Manipulation of the catheter through daily wear and tear can cause increased erythema, but any drainage, tenderness, or associated fevers should be carefully monitored.

10.3.3 Diagnosis of Suspected Catheter-Related Bloodstream Infection (CRBSI)

Once symptoms suggest that infection is present, blood cultures should be drawn from the catheter and a peripheral site simultaneously. It is important that diligent skin and catheter hub antiseptic practices are followed prior to taking the culture and that the same volume of blood is obtained per culture bottle to have an accurate and comparable measure. If the catheter happens to be immediately removed, the tip should be sent for culture as well [7] (Fig. 10.1).

Two different cultures are done to help differentiate between the infection coming from the catheter and an alternative source. A definitive diagnosis of CRBSI can be made if the same organism is identified from a peripheral culture and the catheter tip. Alternative means of diagnosis includes a quantitative blood culture from the catheter hub that shows a colony count three-fold greater than a culture from the peripheral vein. The same criteria can be used for cultures taken from two different catheter lumens. Lastly, differential time to positivity can assist in diagnosis if the catheter lumen turning positive a minimum of 2 h before the alternative culture [7]. If physical examination reveals drainage at the exit site of the catheter during examination, it should be cultured. The diagnosis of catheter-related infection is strengthened if the same organism is found at both sites [3, 7, 16] (Fig. 10.1).

Given the unique venous access challenges posed by HD patients, attempts to obtain peripheral cultures from veins that may be used for future vascular access should be avoided. The Infectious Disease Society of America (ISDA),

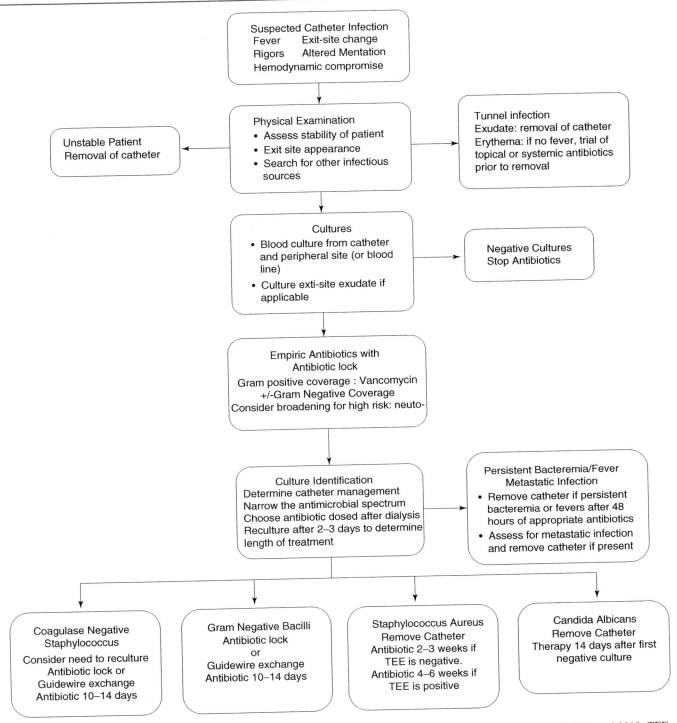

Fig. 10.1 Approach to tunneled catheter-related infection (Information adapted from ISDA Guidelines 2009 and ERA-EDTA of 2010. TEE: Transesophageal echocardiography)

the European Renal Association-European Dialysis and Transplantation Association (ERA-EDTA) have accepted an alternative approach to diagnosis of CRBSI in these patients. If peripheral cultures are not available, cultures can be taken from the CVC and a second set from the bloodline connected to the catheter after HD is started [3, 7, 16]. The high blood flows necessary for HD makes this sample similar to a peripheral assessment.

10.4 Management of Confirmed Infections

10.4.1 Catheter Management

Catheter lock, removal, or guidewire exchange needs to be a part of the treatment plan for CRBSI as there is a high incidence of treatment failure with systemic antibiotics alone [17–19]. Prompt removal of the catheter in any patient with severe sepsis is necessary. In patients who have persistent bacteremia after 48–72 h of appropriate antibiotic therapy, thrombophlebitis, endocarditis, or the presence of any metastatic infection also require catheter removal [17, 20]. Some organisms have been shown to have a high incidence of relapse when these devices are retained. Therefore removal is recommended if *Staphylococcus aureus, Pseudomonas aeruginosa*, fungi, or mycobacteria are identified [7]. The timing of reinsertion of permanent or temporary access for hemodialysis after removal is important to management of infections. Insertion can be considered after the patient has been afebrile for 48–72 h, has normalization of C-reactive protein, and has negative blood cultures [7, 16]. If these parameters are not met and hemodialysis is necessary, a single-use catheter may be placed, but the risk and benefits must be balanced prior to removal [16]. Short-term catheters should be removed if CRBSI is found to be due to gram-negative bacilli, *S. aureus*, enterococci, fungi, and mycobacteria [7].

At times, there are HD patients who have absolutely no alternative sites for vascular access placement. In these situations, it is reasonable to consider either guidewire exchange with an antimicrobial catheter and/or systemic antibiotics with antibiotic lock when any infection occurs [7]. Many studies have been conducted concerning techniques to preserve the current location of the catheter. These evaluated removal of the catheter with delayed replacement, exchanging the catheter over a wire or preservation of the present catheter with use of antibiotic locks in addition to systemic antibiotic administration. The studies are difficult to compare because different end points were used, but it was clearly evident that removal of the catheter was the best way to eradicate the organism. The small success seen with salvage techniques is overshadowed by a failure rate of at least 65 %, and a cost was at least twice as high as other management methods [17].

Current recommendations by the ISDA suggest catheter salvage can be tried using antibiotic lock and systemic antibiotics for uncomplicated infections by organisms other than *S. aureus, P. aeruginosa*, Bacillus species, Micrococcus species, propionibacteria, fungi, or mycobacteria. Surveillance cultures should be obtained 1 week after completion of antibiotic course. If blood cultures are persistently positive despite appropriate antibiotics, catheter removal is necessary [7]. Alternatively, if the symptoms prompting suspicion of

CRBSI resolve in 2–3 days and none of the aforementioned organisms are present, guidewire exchange can be done without continued antibiotic lock or negative cultures [21– 23]. Risks of this technique include increased sclerosis and stenosis of the venous access; therefore the new catheter may have functional compromise [16].

Exit-site infections leading to bacteremia are more likely to occur in recently placed tunneled line due to skin trauma and decreased time for endothelialization and fibrosis of the catheter tunnel [12]. Both the natural creation of the biofilm, which can harbor organisms, and abscess formation in the tunnel can lead to less antibiotic penetration [24]. Often tunneled line infections are unable to be treated solely with systemic antibiotics and removal of catheters is necessary, especially when fever is present. Topical antibiotics can be attempted for exit-site infections without fevers. If the infection is not quickly cleared, systemic antibiotics should be initiated and catheter removal if this therapy fails [16].

10.4.2 Identifying the Organism

Empiric Therapy

In addition to catheter management, defining the organism that is causing the infection is necessary to determine treatment. Often there are no culture results available at the time when antibiotics are initiated. Guidance to the appropriate antibiotic should be based on local infection trends where available [16]. Fifty to eighty percent of catheter-related infections are due to gram-positive organisms: the most common being *Staphylococcus aureus* or *coagulase-negative staphylococcus* [7, 18]. Given the high incidence of *S. aureus* infections being methicillin resistant, vancomycin or teicoplanin should be the first-line agent for all patients when empiric therapy is started [3, 7, 16]. If the patient is immunocompromised or neutropenic and if the local culture trend in the HD unit has a high incidence of gram-negative organisms, then empiric coverage with third-generation cephalosporin, carbapenem, or b-lactam/b-lactamase combination should be added [11]. Also, if the catheter is in the femoral vein, empiric fungal and gram-negative coverage is recommended [7] (Table 10.1).

Antibiotic locks are included in the 2009 ISDA guidelines as part of empiric therapy when the catheter is retained and cultures are being processed [7]. This therapy should be used in conjunction with systemic antibiotics and not as a monotherapy. A reasonable approach would be to start with a vancomycin antibiotic locks until organism identification is available. Gram-negative organisms respond well to treatment with antibiotic locks as the success rate has been shown to be 87–100 %. This is not true with *S. aureus* with only 40–55 % success rate and is one reason why catheter removal is part of management of infection by this organism [25, 26].

Table 10.1 Recommended duration of antibiotic therapy

Type of infection	Length of antimicrobial treatment
Uncomplicated with line removed	
Coagulase-negative staphylococci	5–7 days
Staphylococcus Aureus	14 days
Enterococcus	7–14 days
Gram-negative bacilli	7–14 days
Candida	14 days
Tunneled infection	
No fungemia or bacteremia, lineremoved	7–10 days
Complicated infection, line removed	
Bacteremia fungemia persists >48 h	4–6 weeks
Endocarditis	
Intravascular infection	6–8 weeks
Osteomyelitis	
Uncomplicated with line retained (not *S. aureus, P. aeruginosa*, Bacillus species, Mia-ococcus species, propionibacteria, fungi or mycobacteria)	2 weeks of systemic antibiotics with antibiotic lock
Coagulase-negative staphylococci	or
Gram negative organism	Guidewire exchange with 2 weeks of systemic antibiotics
Enterococcus	

Note that day 1 of therapy is the first day of negative blood cultures after appropriate antibiotics were started

Tailoring Antibiotics

Empiric antibiotics should be adjusted as soon as culture results are available. For example, if *S. aureus* is found to be resistant to vancomycin, a change to daptomycin is indicated [7]. Alternatively, if *S. aureus* is found to be methicillin sensitive, it is worthwhile to change to cefazolin as continuation with vancomycin increases the risk of treatment failure [7, 27]. Blood cultures should be done after 48 h of antibiotic treatment to ensure that the infection is cleared. The day of the first negative culture can be considered day 1 of therapy. Also, tailoring antibiotics to better suit administration with dialysis is preferred. Vancomycin, ceftazidime, or cefazolin can be given after each dialysis session (Fig. 10.1).

Gram-negative species are seen in approximately one-third of the isolates [7, 18]. Most of these organisms are susceptible to aminoglycosides, but the risk of ototoxicity and diminishing any residual renal function makes their use less preferred [7]. Cephalosporins, namely, ceftazidime, are suggested for ease of dosing and low side effect profile. These organisms are rather responsive to treatment and can be managed with systemic antibiotics and antibiotic lock without catheter removal [7]. Guidewire exchange in conjunction with systemic antibiotics is an alternative therapy (Fig. 10.1).

Fungi make up the remaining <10 % of CRBSI. Catheter removal is necessary to treat these infections as prospective studies have shown worse outcomes with catheter salvage management [28–30]. Antibiotic locks are experimental and have not shown good salvage results.

10.4.3 Duration of Antibiotics

When determining the duration of antibiotic therapy, it is important to obtain daily blood cultures after starting antibiotics. The first day when blood cultures are negative is noted to be day 1 of therapy. The treatment timeline varies depending on catheter management strategies and if systemic complications are present. Many infections can be treated with a 7–14-days course, but if severe complications occur, the duration can be extended. For example, if endocarditis is present, treatment will be extended to 4–6 weeks and osteomyelitis will prompt continuation of antibiotics to 8 weeks of therapy [7, 11] (Table 10.2).

10.5 Prevention

The best means to reducing catheter-related infections would be to eliminate catheters. This is not possible in a large number of patients in whom vasculature is not amenable to AV fistula or graft placement. There are a variety of ideas that have been explored as means to reduce the risk of infection.

10.5.1 Sterile Technique in Placement of Catheter

The use of sterile technique including maximal barrier precautions including mask, cap, sterile gown, sterile gloves, and large sterile drape can decrease bloodstream infections

Table 10.2 Antimicrobial therapy for hemodialysis catheter-related bloodstream infections

	Antimicrobial	Dose	Alternative	Notes
Empiric choice				
Gram-positive—use in all suspected cases when cultures pending	Vancomycin	20 mg/kg loading dose then 500 mg during the last 30 min of each HD session	Teicoplanin	No linezolid
Gram-negative—per local susceptibilities/culture pattern usually third or fourth generation cephalosporin	Ceftazidime	1 g IV after each HD	Gentamicin 1 mg/kg after each HD session (max 100 mg)	
If femoral catheter—add gram-negative and yeast coverage	Caspofungin	70 mg IV loading dose then 50 mg IV daily	Micafungin 100 mg IV daily	
If neutropenic—add gram-negative coverage	Ceftazidime	1 g IV after each HD		
Antibiotic lock if catheter retained	Vancomycin	5 mg/mL in heparin or saline	Ceftazidime 0.5 mg/mL	
After culture identified gram-positive				
Staphylococcus aureus				Catheter should be removed
Methicillin sensitive	Cefazolin	20 mg/kg to nearest 500 mg after HD	Vancomycin	Vancomycin shown to have higher failure rate
Methicillin resistant	Vancomycin	20 mg/kg loading dose then 500 mg during the last 30 min of each HD session	Daptomycin 6 mg/kg after dialysis	
Vancomycin resistant	Daptomycin	6 mg/kg after HD	Linezolid 600 mg oral twice daily	
Coagulase-negative staphylococci				If single culture then repeat with peripheral culture; colonization can occur and antibiotic lock may be acceptable
Methicillin sensitive	Cefazolin	20 mg/kg to nearest 500 mg after HD	Vancomycin or Bactrim	
Methicillin resistant	Vancomycin	20 mg/kg loading dose then 500 mg during the last 30 min of each HD session	Daptomycin 6 mg/kg after dialysis	Linezolid also acceptable
Enterococcus faecalis/faecium				Catheter can be retained
Ampicillin sensitive	Ampicillin	500 mg oral after dialysis		
Ampicillin resistant	Vancomycin	20 mg/kg loading dose then 500 mg during the last 30 min of each HD session	Daptomycin 6 mg/kg after dialysis	
Amp/vancomycin resistant	Daptomycin	6 mg/kg after dialysis	Linezolid 600 mg oral twice daily	
Gram-negative				
Pseudomonas aeruginosa	Cefepime	1 g IV once then 500 mg IV daily after HD	Piperacillin/tazobactam 2.25 mg q 8 h	Catheter should be removed
Escherichia coli and Klebsiella				Catheter can be retained with antibiotic lock or guidewire exchange
ESBL negative	Ceftriaxone	1 g IV daily	Ciprofloxacin 250–500 mg po daily after dialysis or 200 mg IV q 12 h after dialysis	
ESBL positive	Ertapenem	1 g daily	Ciprofloxacin 250–500 mg po daily after dialysis or 200 mg IV q 12 h after dialysis	
Enterobacter	Ertapenem	1 g daily	Cefepime or cipro	Catheter can be retained with antibiotic lock or guidewire exchange
Acinetobacter	Ampicillin/ sulbactam	1–2 g IV daily	Imipenem	Catheter can be retained with antibiotic lock or guidewire exchange
Stenotrophomonas	Bactrim		Ticarcillin	Catheter can be retained with antibiotic lock or guidewire exchange
Fungus				Removal of catheter
Candida	Caspofungin	70 mg IV loading dose then 50 mg IV daily	Micafungin 100 mg IV daily	Fluconazole (if C. Krusei or glabrata is low) 200 mg daily

and save approximately $167 per CVC inserted [31, 32]. Also, the use of chlorhexidine can reduce the risk of catheter colonization when compared to other skin-cleaning techniques [33, 34]. No data has shown prophylactic antibiotics at the time of insertion is helpful in preventing catheter-related infections [11].

10.5.2 Vascular Access Team

Often CRBSI occurs in patients in the outpatient dialysis unit who do not need admission to the hospital. Rarely is consideration given to catheter removal as part of their treatment plan as the outpatients are not as ill as those seen in the hospital setting. Implementation of an access-care team for the outpatient hemodialysis setting has been shown to decrease treatment failure and reduce death from sepsis. Much of this success was based on decreased catheter salvage practices [3, 17, 35].

10.5.3 Antibiotic Impregnated Catheters

In the general population requiring CVC, it has been shown that the use of CVC impregnated with chlorhexidine and silver sulfadiazine or minocycline and rifampin has lowered the rate of infection from 7.6 infections per 1,000 catheter days to 1.6 infections per 1,000 catheter days ($P = 0.03$ with CI 0.0–30.95). This was estimated to decrease medical costs by approximately $196 per catheter inserted [36]. This data has not been consistent in the dialysis population; therefore, Kidney Disease Outcomes Quality Initiative (KDOQI) and the IDSA do not have specific recommendations for routine use.

10.5.4 Daily Handling

As per guidelines established from studies on general CVC access placement, all staff accessing catheters should wear masks and gloves as well as perform good hand hygiene regimens [37]. Chlorhexidine and alcohol solutions should be used as antiseptics for exit-site cleanings. This solution has been shown to be superior to povidone-iodine solution when they were directly compared [38].

10.5.5 Exit-Site Care

Studies have shown more than 75 % decreased rate of infection with topical ointment application around exit sites. A Cochrane review was done on topical ointment

and found that mupirocin ointment reduced the risk of catheter-related bacteremia, including the infections caused by *S. aureus*, but did not have any effect on infection-related mortality. There was insufficient evidence to show if topical honey or other types of ointments are beneficial [39]. There is no consensus on the optimal frequency of dressing changes or the type of exit-site dressing that is used [3, 33, 39].

10.5.6 Catheter Lock

Many clinical trials have been performed to assess the efficacy of catheter locks containing antibiotics for infection prophylaxis. Of the published trials, it seems that using these locks can reduce the rate of catheter-related infections by as much as 51–99 % [3, 40]. In a systematic review, it was found that the number needed to treat was three patients to prevent 1 CRSBI [41]. The drawback to this practice may be increased antibiotic resistance [3]. Another locking technique has been an attempt to eradicate the biofilm with solutions such as ethylenediaminetetraacetic acid (EDTA) or high-concentration citrate. Successful reduction in biofilm was noted, but data has varied on reducing the time to catheter-related bacteremia [40, 42]. There will be more data on the horizon to establish the optimal use of these solutions to improve patient care.

10.5.7 Scheduled Catheter Exchange

For patients that need prolonged catheterization, no benefit has been seen with routine exchange of the catheter over a wire or schedule replacement of the catheter at a new site. More risk of mechanical complications are present with these protocols [11].

10.6 Summary

Catheters are associated with an increased risk of mortality in the hemodialysis population largely due to their heightened threat of infection. The best means to prevent associated complications is to avoid their use by having arterial-venous fistulas or arterial-venous grafts in place. At times, acute illness or poor vascular access can limit the ability of these alternative forms of vascular access which leaves catheters as the only option for treatment. In these situations, meticulous care for the catheter and prompt recognition and management of infections are important. Continued research on prevention of infections is necessary to decrease the mortality related to catheter use.

References

1. Safdar N, Maki DG. Inflammation at the insertion site is not predictive of catheter-related bloodstream infection with short-term, noncuffed central venous catheters. Crit Care Med. 2002;30(12):2632–5.

2. Pronovost P, Needham D, Berenholtz S, et al. An intervention to decrease catheter-related bloodstream infections in the ICU. N Engl J Med. 2006;355(26):2725–32.

3. Lok CE, Mokrzycki MH. Prevention and management of catheter-related infection in hemodialysis patients. Kidney Int. 2011;79(6):587–98.

4. Quarello F, Forneris G. Prevention of hemodialysis catheter-related bloodstream infection using an antimicrobial lock. Blood Purif. 2002;20(1):87–92.

5. Collins AJ, Foley RN, Herzog C, et al. US renal data system 2010 annual data report. Am J Kidney Dis. 2011;57(1 Suppl 1):A8. e1-526.

6. Dhingra RK, Young EW, Hulbert-Shearon TE, Leavey SF, Port FK. Type of vascular access and mortality in U.S. hemodialysis patients. Kidney Int. 2001;60(4):1443–51.

7. Mermel LA, Allon M, Bouza E, et al. Clinical practice guidelines for the diagnosis and management of intravascular catheter-related infection: 2009 update by the Infectious Diseases Society of America. Clin Infect Dis. 2009;49(1):1–45.

8. Mermel LA. Prevention of intravascular catheter-related infections. Ann Intern Med. 2000;132(5):391–402.

9. Oliver MJ, Callery SM, Thorpe KE, Schwab SJ, Churchill DN. Risk of bacteremia from temporary hemodialysis catheters by site of insertion and duration of use: a prospective study. Kidney Int. 2000;58(6):2543–5.

10. O'Grady NP, et al. Guidelines for the prevention of intravascular catheter-related infections. Am J Infect Control. 2002;30(8):476–89.

11. McGee DC, Gould MK. Preventing complications of central venous catheterization. N Engl J Med. 2003;348(12):1123–33.

12. Cheesbrough JS, Finch RG, Burden RP. A prospective study of the mechanisms of infection associated with hemodialysis catheters. J Infect Dis. 1986;154(4):579–89.

13. Kanaa M, Wright MJ, Sandoe JA. Examination of tunnelled haemodialysis catheters using scanning electron microscopy. Clin Microbiol Infect. 2010;16(6):780–6.

14. Saxena AK, Panhotra BR, Sundaram DS, et al. Tunneled catheters' outcome optimization among diabetics on dialysis through antibiotic-lock placement. Kidney Int. 2006;70(9):1629–35.

15. Al-Solaiman Y, Estrada YE, Allon M. The spectrum of infections in catheter-dependent hemodialysis patients. Clin J Am Soc Nephrol. 2011;6(9):2247–52.

16. Vanholder R, Canaud B, Fluck R, et al. Catheter-related blood stream infections (CRBSI): a European view. Nephrol Dial Transplant. 2010;25(6):1753–6.

17. Mokrzycki MH, Zhang M, Cohen H, Golestaneh L, Laut JM, Rosenberg SO. Tunnelled haemodialysis catheter bacteraemia: risk factors for bacteraemia recurrence, infectious complications and mortality. Nephrol Dial Transplant. 2006;21(4):1024–31.

18. Saad TF. Bacteremia associated with tunneled, cuffed hemodialysis catheters. Am J Kidney Dis. 1999;34(6):1114–24.

19. Marr KA, Sexton DJ, Conlon PJ, Corey GR, Schwab SJ, Kirkland KB. Catheter-related bacteremia and outcome of attempted catheter salvage in patients undergoing hemodialysis. Ann Intern Med. 1997;127(4):275–80.

20. Kovalik EC, Raymond JR, Albers FJ, et al. A clustering of epidural abscesses in chronic hemodialysis patients: risks of salvaging access catheters in cases of infection. J Am Soc Nephrol. 1996;7(10):2264–7.

21. Carlisle EJ, Blake P, McCarthy F, Vas S, Uldall R. Septicemia in long-term jugular hemodialysis catheters; eradicating infection by changing the catheter over a guidewire. Int J Artif Organs. 1991;14(3):150–3.

22. Shaffer D. Catheter-related sepsis complicating long-term, tunnelled central venous dialysis catheters: management by guidewire exchange. Am J Kidney Dis. 1995;25(4):593–6.

23. Robinson D, Suhocki P, Schwab SJ. Treatment of infected tunneled venous access hemodialysis catheters with guidewire exchange. Kidney Int. 1998;53(6):1792–4.

24. Stewart PS. New ways to stop biofilm infections. Lancet. 2003;361(9352):97.

25. Krishnasami Z, Carlton D, Bimbo L, et al. Management of hemodialysis catheter-related bacteremia with an adjunctive antibiotic lock solution. Kidney Int. 2002;61(3):1136–42.

26. Maya ID, Carlton D, Estrada E, Allon M. Treatment of dialysis catheter-related Staphylococcus aureus bacteremia with an antibiotic lock: a quality improvement report. Am J Kidney Dis. 2007;50(2):289–95.

27. Stryjewski ME, Szczech LA, Benjamin Jr DK, et al. Use of vancomycin or first-generation cephalosporins for the treatment of hemodialysis-dependent patients with methicillin-susceptible Staphylococcus aureus bacteremia. Clin Infect Dis. 2007;44(2):190–6.

28. Nguyen MH, Peacock Jr JE, Tanner DC, et al. Therapeutic approaches in patients with candidemia. Evaluation in a multi-center, prospective, observational study. Arch Intern Med. 1995;155(22):2429–35.

29. Rex JH, Bennett JE, Sugar AM, et al. Intravascular catheter exchange and duration of candidemia. NIAID mycoses study group and the candidemia study group. Clin Infect Dis. 1995;21(4):994–6.

30. Nucci M, Colombo AL, Silveira F, et al. Risk factors for death in patients with candidemia. Infect Control Hosp Epidemiol. 1998;19(11):846–50.

31. Raad II. The pathogenesis and prevention of central venous catheter-related infections. Middle East J Anesthesiol. 1994;12(4):381–403.

32. Raad II, Hohn DC, Gilbreath BJ, et al. Prevention of central venous catheter-related infections by using maximal sterile barrier precautions during insertion. Infect Control Hosp Epidemiol. 1994;15(4 Pt 1):231–8.

33. Maki DG, Ringer M. Evaluation of dressing regimens for prevention of infection with peripheral intravenous catheters. Gauze, a transparent polyurethane dressing, and an iodophor-transparent dressing. JAMA. 1987;258(17):2396–403.

34. Mimoz O, Pieroni L, Lawrence C, et al. Prospective, randomized trial of two antiseptic solutions for prevention of central venous or arterial catheter colonization and infection in intensive care unit patients. Crit Care Med. 1996;24(11):1818–23.

35. Mokrzycki MH, Singhal A. Cost-effectiveness of three strategies of managing tunnelled, cuffed haemodialysis catheters in clinically mild or asymptomatic bacteraemias. Nephrol Dial Transplant. 2002;17(12):2196–203.

36. Veenstra DL, Saint S, Sullivan SD. Cost-effectiveness of antiseptic-impregnated central venous catheters for the prevention of catheter-related bloodstream infection. JAMA. 1999;282(6):554–60.

37. III. NKF-K/DOQI clinical practice guidelines for vascular access: update 2000. Am J Kidney Dis. 2001;37(1 Suppl 1):S137–81.

38. Maki DG, Ringer M, Alvarado CJ. Prospective randomised trial of povidone-iodine, alcohol, and chlorhexidine for prevention of infection associated with central venous and arterial catheters. Lancet. 1991;338(8763):339–43.

39. McCann M, Moore ZE. Interventions for preventing infectious complications in haemodialysis patients with central venous catheters. Cochrane Database Syst Rev. 2010;1, CD006894.

40. Moran J, Sun S, Khababa I, Pedan A, Doss S, Schiller B. A randomized trial comparing gentamicin/citrate and heparin locks for central venous catheters in maintenance hemodialysis patients. Am J Kidney Dis. 2012;59(1):102–7.

41. Snaterse M, Rüger W, Scholte Op Reimer WJ, Lucas C. Antibiotic-based catheter lock solutions for prevention of catheter-related bloodstream infection: a systematic review of randomised controlled trials. J Hosp Infect. 2010;75(1):1–11.

42. Solomon LR, Cheesbrough JS, Ebah L, et al. A randomized double-blind controlled trial of taurolidine-citrate catheter locks for the prevention of bacteremia in patients treated with hemodialysis. Am J Kidney Dis. 2010;55(6):1060–8.

Approach to Patient Referred for Vascular Mapping

Vandana Dua Niyyar

11.1 Introduction

The population of patients with end-stage renal disease (ESRD) in the USA is progressively increasing, with hemodialysis (HD) as the major mode of renal replacement therapy [1]. Arteriovenous fistulae (AVF), though not perfect, are the most preferred of the three types of hemodialysis vascular access. They have higher patency rates [2], lower infection rates [3], and lower overall costs [1] than either grafts or catheters. As a result, the National Kidney Foundation's Dialysis Outcomes and Quality Initiative recommends that AVF be placed in 50 % of all incident patients and 40 % of all prevalent dialysis patients use an AVF [4]. The Fistula First Initiative, jointly formed by CMS and the ESRD networks, with the help of specific change concepts to promote AVF placement and maintenance, has further expanded this goal to have 66 % of prevalent hemodialysis patients dialyzing with an AVF [5].

Unfortunately, despite these efforts, the majority of patients still initiate hemodialysis with a central venous catheter (CVC) as their primary access [6, 7]. Frequent phlebotomies, peripherally inserted central catheters (PICC) [8], and a high prevalence of comorbid conditions including diabetes, obesity, and vascular disease [9] in this high-risk population negatively impact the vasculature. These, in turn, may contribute to early AVF dysfunction and the high rate (20–50 %) of primary failure that prevents their successful use for dialysis [7]. Thus, preoperative vascular mapping is recommended prior to AVF creation for both pre-dialysis chronic kidney disease (CKD) and ESRD patients on hemodialysis. This chapter aims to review the approach to the patient who has presented for vascular mapping, the various techniques (physical examination, ultrasonography, and angiography)

currently available for venous mapping, as well as their effect on AVF creation and use.

11.2 The Techniques

Vascular mapping includes assessment of both arterial and venous systems prior to access placement. One of three techniques may be used: physical examination, ultrasonography, and angiography.

11.3 Physical Examination

A simple bedside assessment may be done to evaluate the patency of the arterial and the venous systems. Arterial evaluation includes documentation of bilaterally equal strong pulses and differential blood pressure measurements in both extremities. The Allen's test assesses the collateral circulation to the hand by confirming the patency of the palmar arch and should be performed prior to creation of any forearm AVF. The patient is asked to make a fist and pressure is applied over both the ulnar and the radial arteries to occlude them. Once the fist is opened, the hand should appear blanched or pale. Then, pressure is alternately released from both the arteries and the hand monitored for return to color. If the color returns rapidly on release of the individual artery, it suggests that the blood supply to the hand is sufficient.

For the venous examination, a tourniquet is placed sequentially at the upper extremity and the veins are visually inspected to determine the diameter, the distance of the vein from the skin surface, and the length of a straight venous segment suitable for cannulation [10].

An upper extremity physical examination, though valuable, is often inadequate when used alone – particularly in obese patients or those with a history of prior vascular access. In such cases, it may need to be supplemented with additional techniques, such as ultrasonography or venography [11]. In a cohort of 116 patients, the authors classified vein

V.D. Niyyar, MD, FASN
Division of Nephrology, Emory University,
Woodruff Memorial Research Building, Rm 338,
1639 Pierce Drive, Atlanta, GA 30322, USA
e-mail: vniyyar@emory.edu

A.S. Yevzlin et al. (eds.), *Interventional Nephrology*,
DOI 10.1007/978-1-4614-8803-3_11, © Springer Science+Business Media New York 2014

quality as good in patients in whom the cephalic vein was easily visualized, poor with hardly visible veins, and absent when no veins could be seen on physical examination. In patients with poor or absent veins, duplex sonography was performed and venography was reserved for those patients who did not have adequate veins on both physical examination and ultrasound. Preoperatively, clinically visualized veins could be found in only 54 of 116 patients (46.5 %), and poor or clinically absent veins were found in 62 patients (53.5 %). Further, of these 62 patients, duplex sonography found adequate veins in 48 patients (77 %), and only 14 patients (23 %) required venography [11].

11.4 Ultrasound Examination

Ultrasonography is an excellent tool that provides an objective and noninvasive assessment of the venous and arterial systems prior to fistula creation. Real-time imaging using a linear transducer with a frequency of 10–12 MHz should be performed and images recorded. The preoperative criteria currently used to support successful AVF maturation include a minimal venous diameter of 2.5 mm and a minimal arterial diameter of 2.0 mm in the upper extremities at the site of the anastomosis [12]. The technique for vessel imaging by ultrasonography is thoroughly detailed in prior publications, and the salient points are as follows [7, 13–15].

11.4.1 Arterial Examination

The patient's arm is positioned comfortably, at approximately 45° from the body and the nondominant arm is examined first. The artery is evaluated with grayscale and spectral Doppler imaging. The internal luminal diameter of the artery is measured at the site of the expected anastomosis. Any arterial calcification should be recorded, as the surgery can be technically difficult if significant calcification is present.

Evaluation of the upper extremity arteries includes measurement of arterial wall thickness, the internal diameter, arterial flow with peak-systolic/end-diastolic velocities, and the presence of calcifications and/or other abnormalities. The radial and ulnar arteries are measured at the wrist, and the brachial artery at the antecubital fossa (Figs. 11.1, 11.2, and 11.3).

11.4.2 Venous Examination

The primary goal of the venous examination is to find veins appropriate for AVF formation and, if they are unsuitable, to identify alternate veins for an AVG. In order to visualize the venous system, the nondominant arm is examined first. The

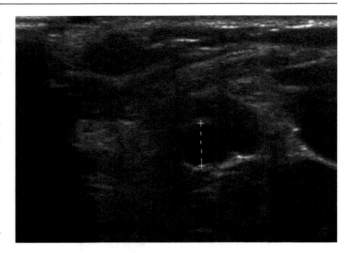

Fig. 11.1 US vascular mapping: brachial artery at elbow, diameter 0.54 cm

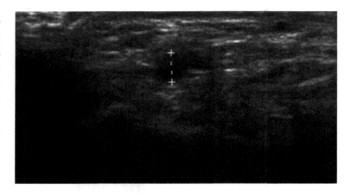

Fig. 11.2 US vascular mapping: radial artery at wrist, diameter 0.32 cm

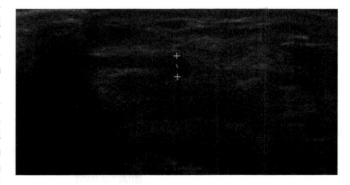

Fig. 11.3 US vascular mapping: ulnar artery at wrist, diameter 0.32 cm

entire upper extremity is evaluated, and the cephalic, basilic, and axillary vein diameters are measured throughout their course (Figs. 11.4, 11.5, and 11.6). A tourniquet is then sequentially placed at the mid-forearm, antecubital area, and at the upper arm; the diameters are again measured and recorded.

The veins are also evaluated for compressibility throughout the course as well as the depth from the skin

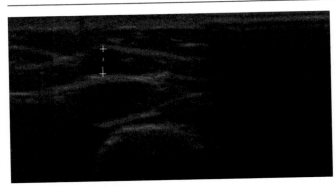

Fig. 11.4 US vascular mapping: cephalic vein at wrist, diameter 0.30 cm

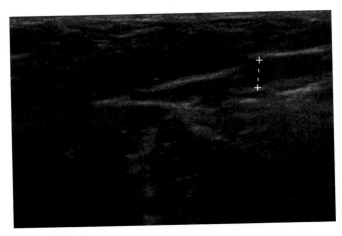

Fig. 11.5 US vascular mapping: cephalic vein above elbow, diameter 0.39 cm

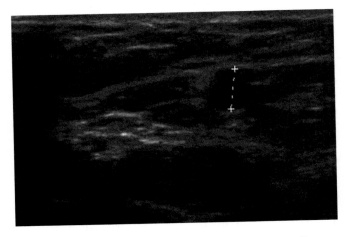

Fig. 11.6 US vascular mapping: basilic vein above elbow, diameter 0.60 cm

surface. If the veins are deeper than 6 mm, the distance from the skin surface should be recorded to assist in planning for superficialization. All abnormalities should be noted including venous stenosis, branches of veins near the future AVF site, or sclerotic, thick-walled veins.

If no suitable upper arm vein for AVF creation is found, the basilic and axillary veins should be measured for potential graft placement as previously described. A vein with a proximal diameter (at the site of the venous anastomosis) of at least 4 cm is needed for graft placement.

The routine use of preoperative venous mapping led to a significant increase in the use of autogenous AVF (5–68 %) in a study designed to evaluate the impact of DOQI (Kidney Dialysis Outcome and Quality Initiative) guidelines [16]. Preoperative mapping resulted in a change in the planned procedure in 31 % of the patients in another prospective evaluation to assess the effect of preoperative vessel mapping by ultrasonography. Unsuccessful surgical explorations decreased from 11 to 0 %, and the AVF placement rate increased from 32 to 58 % [13]. Encouraged by these promising initial data, the authors expanded their intervention over a 17-month period. The proportion of fistulas placed increased to 64 % with preoperative vascular mapping as compared to 34 % in the historical controls. Further, their intervention resulted in essentially doubling the proportion of patients dialyzing with a fistula (from 16 to 34 %) [17].

A limitation of ultrasonography is that it provides only indirect evaluation of central venous vasculature. The central veins are assessed for stenosis or thrombosis by analysis of the waveform for changes in respiratory phasicity and transmitted cardiac pulsatility. Thus, especially among patients with a history of central venous catheter use, additional techniques may be needed to fully delineate the central venous system.

11.5 Angiography

Venous mapping can also be performed with iodinated contrast [10, 18] or carbon dioxide (CO_2) [19]. The arm is then placed in the anatomic position, and a peripheral vein on the dorsum of the hand is cannulated. To visualize the veins using iodinated contrast, sequential tourniquets are then applied – one at the elbow and the other at the axilla. Low iso-osmolar contrast diluted with normal saline is injected through the cannula, and images are obtained throughout the course of the veins using calibrated fluoroscopy. Once the forearm is examined, the distal tourniquet is removed, to allow contrast to pass into the upper arm. The criteria used to determine suitability of veins for AVF placement are the same as those for ultrasonography [12]: vein diameters of at least 2.5 mm, a 6 cm long straight cannulation segment, and patent draining and central veins.

Angiography offers the advantage of direct imaging of the central veins and is often utilized in patients with a history of long-term central venous catheter use. On the other hand, administration of radiocontrast material may expose the patient to the risk of potential nephrotoxicity.

Encouragingly, recent data have shown that small doses of low iso-osmolar contrast agent for venous mapping may be safe in patients with stages 4 and 5 CKD [20, 21]. In a prospective study, 25 consecutive patients who underwent angiograms with 10–20 ml of contrast were evaluated for contrast nephropathy. Of those 21 patients who had pre- and post-procedure GFR measurements, there were no significant differences in the two measurements [21]. In another dataset, a total of 65 procedures for endovascular salvage were performed on 34 patients over 2 years, and the safety of low-dose contrast was evaluated. The incidence of contrast-induced nephropathy was reported as 4 % at 2 days and 4.7 % at 1 week. All patients returned to baseline renal function at 2 weeks, and none required dialysis. The authors concluded that even in advanced CKD, fistulas could be salvaged with low-dose contrast [20]. In yet another subset of 28 patients, with CKD stage 4 and 5, upper arm venography was done preoperatively with 10–15 ml of dilute radiocontrast. There were no significant differences in GFR pre- and post-intervention; one patient developed a decrease in the GFR, but it returned to baseline within 7 days [22]. Nonetheless, larger studies with long-term follow-up are needed prior to establishing the safety of contrast in this high-risk population.

In order to minimize the risk of contrast-induced nephropathy, some authors have proposed the use of CO_2 angiography as compared to iodinated media. CO_2 venography has been shown to have a sensitivity of 97 % and a specificity of 85 % in the assessment of upper limb and central vein patency and stenosis, with conventional iodinated venography used as the reference standard [23]. The procedure is described in detail in the publication, and the salient features are as follows [23]. A superficial vein in the dorsum of the hand is cannulated, and a CO_2 injector is used to inject 10 ml of CO_2 initially to accustom the patient to the sensation of a CO_2 injection. Thereafter, the volume varies between 10 and 30 ml for upper extremities and 30–50 ml for central veins. Using this technique, in a retrospective evaluation of 209 CO_2 venograms in 116 patients, surgical findings correlated with angiographic findings in 90 % of the patients. The overall maturation rate was 84 % with 1-year primary patency rates of 63 %, which is comparable to those with conventional venography [19]. The authors noted that the CO_2 was less useful in delineating the forearm veins, secondary to the lower viscosity of CO_2 as compared to iodine. On the other hand, it has also been noted that CO_2 may inadvertently overestimate the degree of stenosis in certain cases [24]; a proposed mechanism is that CO_2 dissolves in the blood immediately after the injection. Thus, CO_2 angiography could be an acceptable alternative for those patients with either an allergic reaction to iodinated contrast or with residual renal function.

11.6 Which Technique Should Be Used?

Thus far, no randomized studies have compared the various techniques for AVF vascular mapping. Nonetheless, each technique has advantages in certain clinical settings. A detailed and focused physical examination alone may be sufficient if clearly defined criteria and careful clinical examination are used. In a European analysis of 145 consecutive patients, 106 patients (73 %) were referred for vascular access surgery on the basis of clinical examination alone, with favorable (77 %) subsequent patency results [25]. However, as there is a high prevalence of central venous catheter use and because an increasing proportion of the HD population in the USA has multiple comorbidities which may affect the vasculature, physical examination alone may be inadequate in the vast majority of these patients.

A large number of studies support the use of ultrasonography to increase AVF creation, as detailed in Table 11.1. It has the advantage of providing noninvasive assessment of both arterial and venous diameters and depth from the surface without exposure to radiation or potentially nephrotoxic contrast. A limitation is that it only provides indirect assessment of central venous patency. Interestingly, in a retrospective comparison of two surgical practices, preoperative duplex ultrasonography resulted in a decrease in AVF creation when compared to physical examination [27]. This was attributed to be secondary to underestimation of cephalic vein size by ultrasonography.

Angiography offers the advantage of direct imaging of the central veins and is often employed in patients with a history of long-term central venous catheter use. It also allows for measurement of the venous diameter as well as any stenosis or accessory veins. Nevertheless, administration of radiocontrast material is contraindicated in patients with contrast allergy and does expose the patient to the risk of potential nephrotoxicity. Though recent data have shown that small doses of low iso-osmolar contrast agent for venous mapping or fistula salvage may be safe in patients with stages 4 and 5 CKD [20, 21], larger studies with long-term follow-up are needed prior to establishing the safety of contrast in this high-risk population. This can be mitigated by the use of CO_2 angiography, but it is currently not widely available.

Currently, there is no evidence to support one vessel mapping technique over another; the procedure used should be individualized to each patient, with careful consideration of the advantages and disadvantages of each method. The use of ultrasonography in patients with poorly visualized vessels on physical examination may expedite placement of fistulae by early referral for surgery [25]. Though minimal vessel diameter criteria have been established for ultrasonography [12], these clearly have limitations, as shown by the poor AVF maturation rates reported in the DAC study. Thus, perhaps additional variables including resistive indices, internal vessel diameter, and blood flow before and after reactive

Table 11.1 Effect of preoperative vascular mapping on AVF creation

Author and technique used (%)	AVF creation rate – prior to intervention (%)	AVF creation rate – post-intervention (%)
Silva et al. (1998) – US [12]	14	63
Robbin et al. (2000) – US [13]	32	58
Ascher et al. (2000) – US + DOQI [16]	5	68
Allon et al. (2001) – US [17]	34	64
Gibson – US	11	95
Dalman et al. (2002) – US [26]	35	85
Fullerton et al. (2002) – US + DOQI [27]	23	39
Huber et al. (2002) – US + angiography [28]	0	90
Patel et al. (2003) – physical examination + US + angiography [29]	61	73
Wells et al. (2005) [25]	Physical examination (73); US (27)	100 (physical examination) to 76.5 (US)
Asif et al. (2005) – US [21, 30]	0	77
Elsharawy and Moghazy (2006) – physical examination (26); angiography (74) [31]	0	95

US ultrasonography, *DOQI* Dialysis Outcomes and Quality Initiative

hyperemia might be considered in order to maximize AVF placement and maturation [14, 32, 33].

Indeed, a combination of techniques, as detailed in a prospective algorithm, was successful in creating a native AVF in an overwhelming majority of patients presenting for a new hemodialysis access [28]. In another recent cohort of 422 patients, the authors first identified preoperative clinical characteristics that are predictive of failure to mature AVF and then devised and validated a scoring system to stratify the patient's risk for failure to mature (FTM) [34]. The clinical characteristics associated with a failure to mature included age >65 years, coronary artery disease, peripheral vascular disease, and race (white race being protective). Using a prediction model and the odds ratio, the scores were categorized into probability risks for failure to mature as follows: scores <2, low risk; 2–3, moderate risk; 3.1–7.9, high risk; and >8.0, very high risk. The authors suggested the following clinical application for preoperative evaluation using the scoring system. If the patient is low risk for FTM, a physical examination and/or duplex US should suffice. In high-risk patients, a venogram and arteriogram may be necessary with appropriate preoperative interventions as needed and close postoperative follow-up after AVF creation. In extremely high-risk patients, the authors recommended abandoning AVF and considering an AVG [28, 34]. This is yet to be validated in the clinical setting, and prospective studies are needed to further delineate the impact of these measures on the creation of mature, functional AVF.

11.7 Summary and Future Directions

Though preoperative vessel mapping increases AVF creation [12, 13, 16, 26, 28, 31, 35], there is limited and conflicting evidence regarding the effect of vessel mapping on AVF

maturation [17, 29]. It is essential to differentiate an increase in the number of AVF created from an increase in mature fistulae that are successfully used for dialysis. In a landmark historical cohort study, the authors compared primary failure rates and patency rates of AVF before and after implementation of ultrasonographic assessment of the upper extremity vasculature [12]. The outcomes included not only a significant increase in the creation and use of AVF but also a reduction in early AVF failure rates and an increase in cumulative AVF patency. Other investigators had comparable results after using various techniques for preoperative evaluation, including physical examination, ultrasonography, angiography, or a combination thereof, as well as establishment of a comprehensive multipronged approach to maximize AVF placement [13, 16, 17, 26, 28, 31, 35]. A prospective analysis using angiography involved an organized program by an interventional nephrology team (including vascular access education and vascular mapping) for tunneled catheter-assigned patients [30]. The patients were divided into two groups – those with no prior AV access and those with at least one previous AV access. After angiographic mapping, 97 % of patients in the first group and 90 % of the patients in the second group had adequate veins for AVF creation. Overall, they had a notable success rate with 77 % of the tunneled catheter-consigned patients achieving functional AVF and 5 % receiving AVG.

Though it could be reasonably concluded that a preoperative strategy to identify suitable vessels for AVF creation would translate into decreased early failure rates and an increased proportion of prevalent patients dialyzing with an AVF, it may not always be the case. In one such review, routine preoperative vascular mapping resulted in a marked increase in AVF creation and an increased maturation rate for forearm AVF, but it did not improve the maturation of upper arm AVF [17]. In another protocol, despite the fact that the implementation of preoperative ultrasonography and angiography increased AVF creation, the maturation rate decreased from 73 to 57 % [29]. This decline was ascribed to a change in practice patterns, with more complicated surgeries being performed in the study group as compared to the historical controls. Furthermore, they only performed ultrasonography in those patients in whom physical examination was inadequate to identify suitable vessels for AVF placement.

A synopsis of the evidence in this field is summarized in Table 11.1, keeping in mind that most of the studies demonstrating a benefit of preoperative mapping are not randomized. In the vast majority, the primary outcome has been AVF creation, rather than AVF maturation, or usability, and only 3 of the 12 previous studies report favorable outcomes related to venous mapping and AVF maturation. Incidentally, it must also be noted that a majority of these studies were published alongside promotion of AVF creation by major national initiatives [7]. Future research should focus on prospective, randomized controlled trials to evaluate the efficacy of preoperative mapping techniques on the creation, maturation, and patency of AVF.

References

1. U.S. Renal Data System, USRDS. Annual data report: atlas of chronic kidney disease and end-stage renal disease in the United States. Bethesda: National Institutes of Health, National Institute of Diabetes and Digestive and Kidney Diseases; 2010.
2. Pisoni RL, Young EW, Dykstra DM, et al. Vascular access use in Europe and the United States: results from the DOPPS. Kidney Int. 2002;61(1):305–16.
3. Kalman PG, Pope M, Bhola C, Richardson R, Sniderman KW. A practical approach to vascular access for hemodialysis and predictors of success. J Vasc Surg. 1999;30(4):727–33.
4. Vascular Access Work Group. Clinical practice guidelines for vascular access. Am J Kidney Dis. 2006;48 Suppl 1:S248–73.
5. Peters VJ, Clemons G, Augustine B. "Fistula First" as a CMS breakthrough initiative: Improving vascular access through collaboration. Nephrol Nurs J. 2005;32:686–87.
6. Wasse H, Speckman RA, Frankenfield DL, Rocco MV, McClellan WM. Predictors of central venous catheter use at the initiation of hemodialysis. Semin Dial. 2008;21(4):346–51.
7. Allon M, Robbin ML. Increasing arteriovenous fistulas in hemodialysis patients: problems and solutions. Kidney Int. 2002;62(4):1109–24.
8. Allen AW, Megargell JL, Brown DB, et al. Venous thrombosis associated with the placement of peripherally inserted central catheters. J Vasc Interv Radiol. 2000;11(10):1309–14.
9. Ethier J, Mendelssohn DC, Elder SJ, et al. Vascular access use and outcomes: an international perspective from the Dialysis Outcomes and Practice Patterns Study. Nephrol Dial Transplant. 2008;23(10):3219–26.
10. Asif A, Ravani P, Roy-Chaudhury P, Spergel LM, Besarab A. Vascular mapping techniques: advantages and disadvantages. J Nephrol. 2007;20(3):299–303.
11. Malovrh M. Native arteriovenous fistula: preoperative evaluation. Am J Kidney Dis. 2002;39(6):1218–25.
12. Silva Jr MB, Hobson 2nd RW, Pappas PJ, et al. A strategy for increasing use of autogenous hemodialysis access procedures: impact of preoperative noninvasive evaluation. J Vasc Surg. 1998;27(2):302–7; discussion 307–8.
13. Robbin ML, Gallichio MH, Deierhoi MH, Young CJ, Weber TM, Allon M. US vascular mapping before hemodialysis access placement. Radiology. 2000;217(1):83–8.
14. Malovrh M. The role of sonography in the planning of arteriovenous fistulas for hemodialysis. Semin Dial. 2003;16(4):299–303.
15. American Institute of Ultrasound in Medicine, American College of Radiology, Society of Radiologists in Ultrasound. AIUM practice guideline for the performance of ultrasound vascular mapping for pre-operative planning for dialysis access. J Ultrasound Med. 2012;31(1):173–81.
16. Ascher E, Gade P, Hingorani A, et al. Changes in the practice of angioaccess surgery: impact of dialysis outcome and quality initiative recommendations. J Vasc Surg. 2000;31(1 Pt 1):84–92.
17. Allon M, Lockhart ME, Lilly RZ, et al. Effect of preoperative sonographic mapping on vascular access outcomes in hemodialysis patients. Kidney Int. 2001;60(5):2013–20.
18. Beathard GA. Manual of endovascular skills and procedures for the interventional nephrologist. 2002.
19. Heye S, Fourneau I, Maleux G, Claes K, Kuypers D, Oyen R. Preoperative mapping for haemodialysis access surgery with CO_2 venography of the upper limb. Eur J Vasc Endovasc Surg. 2010;39(3):340–5.
20. Kian K, Wyatt C, Schon D, Packer J, Vassalotti J, Mishler R. Safety of low-dose radiocontrast for interventional AV fistula salvage in stage 4 chronic kidney disease patients. Kidney Int. 2006;69(8):1444–9.
21. Asif A, Cherla G, Merrill D, et al. Venous mapping using venography and the risk of radiocontrast-induced nephropathy. Semin Dial. 2005;18(3):239–42.
22. Won YD, Lee JY, Shin YS, et al. Small dose contrast venography as venous mapping in predialysis patients. J Vasc Access. 2010;11(2):122–7.
23. Heye S, Maleux G, Marchal GJ. Upper-extremity venography: CO_2 versus iodinated contrast material. Radiology. 2006;241(1):291–7.
24. Ehrman KO, Taber TE, Gaylord GM, Brown PB, Hage JP. Comparison of diagnostic accuracy with carbon dioxide versus iodinated contrast material in the imaging of hemodialysis access fistulas. J Vasc Interv Radiol. 1994;5(5):771–5.
25. Wells AC, Fernando B, Butler A, Huguet E, Bradley JA, Pettigrew GJ. Selective use of ultrasonographic vascular mapping in the assessment of patients before haemodialysis access surgery. Br J Surg. 2005;92(11):1439–43.
26. Dalman RL, Harris Jr EJ, Victor BJ, Coogan SM. Transition to all-autogenous hemodialysis access: the role of preoperative vein mapping. Ann Vasc Surg. 2002;16(5):624–30.
27. Fullerton JK, McLafferty RB, Ramsey DE, Solis MS, Gruneiro LA, Hodgson KJ. Pitfalls in achieving the Dialysis Outcome Quality Initiative (DOQI) guidelines for hemodialysis access? Ann Vasc Surg. 2002;16(5):613–7.
28. Huber TS, Ozaki CK, Flynn TC, et al. Prospective validation of an algorithm to maximize native arteriovenous fistulae for chronic hemodialysis access. J Vasc Surg. 2002;36(3):452–9.
29. Patel ST, Hughes J, Mills Sr JL. Failure of arteriovenous fistula maturation: an unintended consequence of exceeding dialysis outcome quality initiative guidelines for hemodialysis access. J Vasc Surg. 2003;38(3):439–45; discussion 45.
30. Asif A, Cherla G, Merrill D, Cipleu CD, Briones P, Pennell P. Conversion of tunneled hemodialysis catheter-consigned patients to arteriovenous fistula. Kidney Int. 2005;67(6):2399–406.
31. Elsharawy MA, Moghazy KM. Impact of pre-operative venography on the planning and outcome of vascular access for hemodialysis patients. J Vasc Access. 2006;7(3):123–8.
32. Yerdel MA, Kesenci M, Yazicioglu KM, Döşeyen Z, Türkçapar AG, Anadol E. Effect of haemodynamic variables on surgically created

arteriovenous fistula flow. Nephrol Dial Transplant. 1997;12(8):1684–8.

33. Lockhart ME, Robbin ML, Allon M. Preoperative sonographic radial artery evaluation and correlation with subsequent radiocephalic fistula outcome. J Ultrasound Med. 2004;23(2):161–8; quiz 169–71.

34. Lok CE, Allon M, Moist L, Oliver MJ, Shah H, Zimmerman D. Risk equation determining unsuccessful cannulation events and failure to maturation in arteriovenous fistulas (REDUCE FTM I). J Am Soc Nephrol. 2006;17(11):3204–12.

35. Hafeez M, Asif S, Hanif H. Profile and repair success of vesico-vaginal fistula in Lahore. J Coll Physicians Surg Pak. 2005;15(3):142–4.

Approach to Arteriovenous Access

12

Ravish Shah and Anil K. Agarwal

12.1 Introduction

A well-functioning and reliable vascular access is an absolute requirement to provide life-sustaining dialysis treatment in end-stage renal disease (ESRD) patients and
rightfully referred to as their "lifeline" [1]. Hemodialysis
(HD) vascular access (VA) dysfunction is the single most
important cause of morbidity in ESRD patients [1, 2]. The
rising incidence and prevalence of ESRD have led to an
increased burden on the US health-care system. The social
and economic cost of ESRD care is disproportionately
high. In 2009, the total ESRD cost rose to $29 billion,
amounting to 5.9 % of the entire Medicare budget [2]. Care
of vascular access accounts for over a billion dollars of this
expense annually.

To optimize VA care, procedural aspects of nephrology have steadily evolved over the past decade. Despite
the concerted efforts of the nephrologists, surgeons, and
radiologists to deliver timely care, treatment delays persist [3–5]. Endovascular procedures are increasingly
being performed by the "interventional" nephrologists
[6, 7]. The American Society of Diagnostic and
Interventional Nephrology (ASDIN) was founded in
2000 to fulfill this unmet need, and its published training
guidelines have generated a renewed interest among
nephrologists to master procedural skills in an effort to
reduce morbidity and improve quality of life in the dialysis population [8, 9].

12.2 Types of Vascular Access

The three principal forms of vascular access are native AV
fistulae, synthetic AV grafts, and tunneled cuffed hemodialysis catheters.

12.2.1 AV Fistulae

AV fistulae are typically constructed with an end-to-side
vein-to-artery anastomosis between an artery and vein.
Creation of an AV fistula at the wrist was first described by
Brescia and Cimino [1, 10] (Fig. 12.1). The fistula with the
best outcome is the lower forearm radiocephalic (RCF);
however this access often fails to mature in the elderly
patient with underlying vascular disease, particularly in diabetics [11]. The next recommended site for fistula is the
upper arm brachiocephalic fistula (Fig. 12.2). This type of
fistula is being placed with increased frequency because of
the high failure rate of RCF or as a secondary AVF in patients
with failed forearm AV grafts [12]. Less commonly, native
fistulae are created between the brachial artery and basilic
vein, for which the basilic vein is usually mobilized laterally
and superficially to allow easier cannulation (transposed brachiobasilic fistula) (Fig. 12.3) [13]. Radiocephalic native
vessel fistula is recommended as the first choice followed by
brachiocephalic and brachiobasilic fistula as the second and
third choice, respectively [14, 15].

Fistulae in the lower extremity, such as the superficial
femoral and common femoral thigh transpositions, are rare,
although adequate outcomes have been reported with good
patient selection [16].

AVF is the preferred dialysis access given their superior
longevity, fewer complication rates, cost-effectiveness, and
their salutary impact on patient outcomes have made them
the most "desirable" access for dialysis [12]. However, successful creation of AVF requires patent and good-sized arteries and veins, and despite creation of AVF, there is a high rate
of failure to mature that often requires more than one

R. Shah, MD • A.K. Agarwal, MD, FACP, FASN, FNKF (✉)
Division of Nephrology, The Ohio State University,
395 W 12th Avenue, Ground Floor, Columbus, OH 43210, USA
e-mail: anil.agarwal@osumc.edu

A.S. Yevzlin et al. (eds.), *Interventional Nephrology*,
DOI 10.1007/978-1-4614-8803-3_12, © Springer Science+Business Media New York 2014

Fig. 12.1 Illustration for radiocephalic arteriovenous fistula (Brescia-Cimino) (With permission from Vachharajani [47])

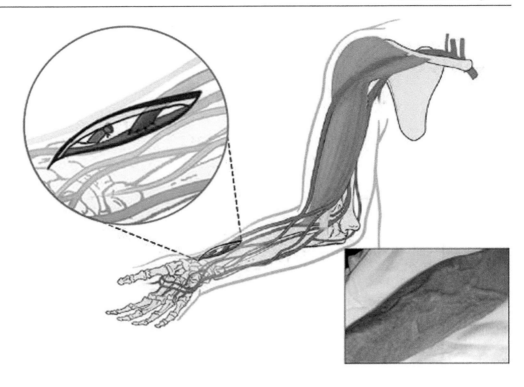

Fig. 12.2 Illustration for brachiocephalic AV fistula (With permission from Vachharajani [47])

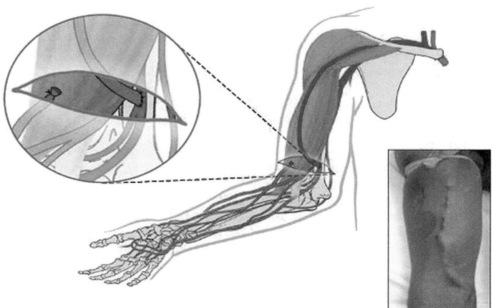

intervention. AVF usually require a maturation period of 4–6 weeks prior to cannulation for dialysis.

12.2.2 Synthetic Grafts

When the location or condition of the native blood vessels is not adequate, a synthetic graft can be substituted. Synthetic grafts are constructed by anastomosing a synthetic conduit,

usually polytetrafluoroethylene (PTFE), between an artery and vein [17, 18]. PTFE grafts are the second most preferred form of permanent dialysis vascular access. They have the advantage of being easier to create surgically, require a maturation time of only 2–3 weeks, and have a relatively large cannulation area [19]. Unfortunately, PTFE dialysis grafts have a poor primary patency rate (50 % at 1 year and 25 % at 2 years) [20]. Aggressive preemptive monitoring and intervention can result in a cumulative patency for PTFE grafts

Fig. 12.3 Illustration for transposed brachiobasilic AV fistula (With permission from Vachharajani [47])

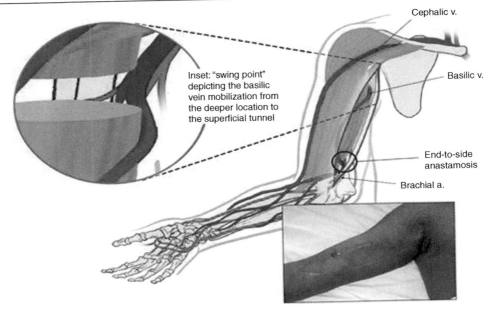

Cephalic v.

Basilic v.

Inset: "swing point" depicting the basilic vein mobilization from the deeper location to the superficial tunnel

End-to-side anastamosis

Brachial a.

Fig. 12.4 Illustration for forearm loop graft (brachiocephalic) (With permission from Vachharajani [47])

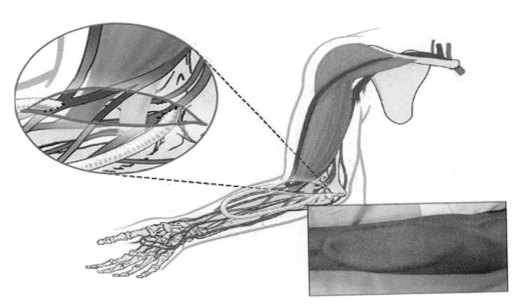

that matches the results for AV fistulae. This increase in cumulative patency, however, requires a sixfold increase in interventions (thrombectomies and angioplasties) [1].

Common graft locations and configurations are straight forearm (radial artery to cephalic vein), looped forearm (brachial artery to cephalic vein) (Fig. 12.4), straight upper arm (brachial artery to axillary vein), or looped upper arm (axillary artery to axillary vein). Thigh grafts (Fig. 12.5), looped chest grafts, axillary-axillary (necklace), and axillary-atrial grafts have also been reported [21, 22]. Many synthetic materials other than PTFE have been used for construction of graft. The use of autologous tissue-engineered vascular grafts and drug-eluting grafts remains a subject of active

research and not widely used in the clinical practice at the current time [23, 24].

12.2.3 Tunneled Cuffed Catheters

Tunneled cuffed catheters are dual-lumen catheters usually composed of silicone or polyurethane composites. Catheters are commonly placed in the internal jugular vein and tunneled superficially to exit on the upper, anterior chest. Patency of central veins should be confirmed with ultrasound prior to insertion. Direct guidance with ultrasound is highly recommended. The catheters are commonly positioned under fluo-

Fig. 12.5 Illustration for thigh AV graft (external iliac artery to femoral vein) (With permission from Vachharajani [47])

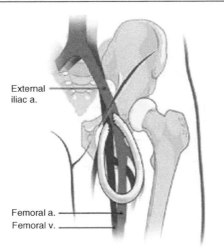

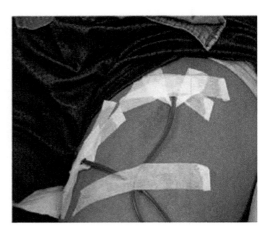

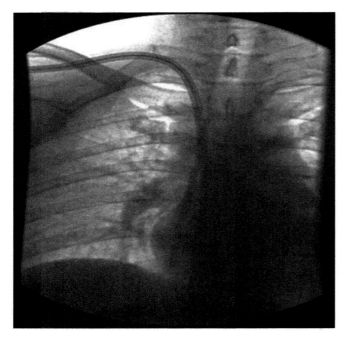

Fig. 12.6 Chest X-ray showing a right internal jugular split-tip tunneled dialysis catheter

roscopy such that the tip rests in the middle of the right atrium when the patient is supine as it tends to move up with erect posture (Fig. 12.6). The use of subclavian catheters should be discouraged given high incidence of subclavian vein stenosis with their use [15, 25]. The main advantage of using tunneled dialysis catheter as dialysis access (>3 weeks) is that they can be used immediately after placement [1]. However, these catheters have many disadvantages including a significant morbidity caused by thrombosis and infection, a substantial risk of permanent central venous stenosis or occlusion, a far shorter life span than with AV fistulae or PTFE grafts [26], and relatively lower blood-flow rates resulting in inadequate

dialysis. There is a significantly negative impact of these catheters on patient outcomes. Ideally, these catheters should be used only as bridge catheters while an AV fistula matures [1]. Every attempt should be made to limit the use of cuffed tunneled dialysis catheters whenever possible [1].

12.3   Pre-dialysis Evaluation

Process of approaching vascular access begins long before the patient is referred for the creation of access. With the increase of comorbid conditions related to age and diabetes, vascular problems are increasingly prevalent as evidenced by progressive peripheral vascular, carotid, and coronary artery disease [27]. Additionally, damage to the venous vasculature occurs from numerous blood samplings, infusions, and intravenous lines during hospitalizations especially in patients with advance chronic kidney disease (CKD). Venous damage may thus occur even before the patient is referred to a nephrologists or access surgeon, emphasizing the need for timely nephrology referral along with the intensive strategies for vein preservation in CKD patients (Fig. 12.7) [27]. The KDOQI and NVAII recommend timely referral of CKD patients to a nephrologist usually at stage 4 so that the education for dialysis options including dialysis access evaluation can begin [28]. Thus, the timing of access placement, preferably an AVF, and the process of patient evaluation are extremely important for the successful use of vascular access.

12.3.1   Timing of AVF Creation

Creating the AVF well before it is required for dialysis allows for this process to take place in an adequate fashion prior to use. NKF-K/DOQI guidelines suggest that the patient be referred for the creation of an AVF when the patient's creati-

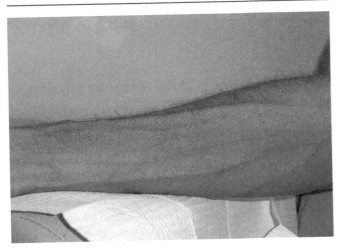

Fig. 12.7 Well-preserved veins in the forearm and upper arm for creating a functional arteriovenous fistula (With permission from Vachharajani [47])

nine clearance is at 25 mL/min or less, their serum creatinine is 4 mg/dL or more, or within 1 year of anticipated need [29]. Early referral allows time for a second AV access attempt at an alternative site in patients with failed first attempt of AVF, without having to depend on tunneled dialysis catheter for dialysis initiation [30].

12.3.2 Patient Evaluation Prior to Access Placement

In order to determine the type of access most suitable for an ESRD patient, a thorough physical examination along with a focused medical history is imperative [30, 31]. Any scars should be noted in the neck or upper chest region, since this might suggest use of a previous central venous catheter (CVC) or previous surgery and ensuing anatomical abnormalities [32]. Patient's chest, breast, and upper arms should be evaluated for the presence of swelling or collateral veins, if present; they are strongly suggestive of central venous stenosis. Both the size and anatomical characteristics of the venous and arterial components of the AVF can affect the success of AVF placement and maturation. Prior to AVF creation, both arterial and venous evaluation must be conducted.

Arterial Evaluation
The feeding artery must be capable of delivering blood flow at a rate adequate to support dialysis while simultaneously not jeopardizing the blood flow to the hand and digits. There are three important clinical features relative to the arterial system for a successful AVF creation [33]. Firstly, the patient should have less than 20 mmHg differential in blood pressure between the two arms; a greater difference suggests the presence of arterial disease that needs to be evaluated further, before access placement. Secondly, the palmar arch should be patent. The palmar arch can be tested for patency using the Allen test [34]. The test has been criticized as being unreliable given considerable inter-operator variation in performance and interpretation, partly because of the subjective nature. Use of either a pulse oximeter, to detect the pulse wave, or a vascular Doppler, to evaluate pulse augmentation, can increase the efficacy of the Allen test [35]. Failure of palmar arch pressures to increase during this maneuver suggests inadequate collateral circulation in the hand and predicts a higher risk for vascular steal if the dominant artery is used for access creation. And lastly, the arterial lumen should be at least 2 mm in diameter at the site proposed for AV anastomosis, which can be determined using color flow Doppler.

Venous Evaluation
The cephalic vein is ideal for an AVF because of its location on the ventral surface of the forearm and the lateral surface of the upper arm, making it easily accessible for cannulation with the patient in a sitting position [30]. Venous mapping should be performed in all patients prior to the placement of an access. Routine preoperative mapping results in a marked increase in placement of AV fistulae, as well as an improvement in the adequacy of forearm fistulae for dialysis [33, 36].

The main goal of venous mapping is to identify a cephalic vein that is suitable for the creation of an AV fistula. In addition to a thorough physical examination, venous mapping can be done by Doppler ultrasound and angiography study as needed. During the physical examination, a blood pressure cuff is inflated to a pressure about 5 mmHg above diastolic pressure for no more than 5 min. Although in many patients venous anatomy can be evaluated by physical examination only, most surgeons prefer to get a detailed venogram performed using either color flow Doppler ultrasound or angiography prior to surgery. Color flow Doppler ultrasound is considered to be the best method for visualizing the venous anatomy primarily because it avoids the use of radiocontrast. Optimum features on venogram for the creation of an AVF are a luminal diameter at the point of anastomosis of 2.5 mm or greater, a straight segment of vein, absence of stenosis, and continuity with the proximal central veins [33].

12.4 Alternative Strategies for Arteriovenous Fistula Creation

Use of nondominant arm is preferred as an initial AV access site; however, if suitable anatomy is not found, the dominant arm should be evaluated. In instances in which the cephalic vein in the lower arm is not large enough to meet the size criteria, consideration should shift to an upper forearm or upper arm region [30]. If the cephalic vein is not deemed suitable for the AV access placement, attention must be directed towards evaluation of basilic venous system. In cases where a straight segment of vein suitable for cannulation is not present, the novel vein transposition techniques should be considered [37]. By this procedure, an otherwise unsuitable forearm vein is identified, exteriorized and, transposed to an optimal position on the volar surface of the forearm. This technique has yielded a primary patency rate of 84 % at 1 year [30, 37]. If mapping reveals the presence of a suitable but a deep vein, superficial transposition can yield a usable fistula.

12.5 Factors Related to Successful Fistula Use

Once a fistula is created, it must develop to the point that it can be cannulated for successful dialysis. This requires an adequate blood flow to support dialysis and physical characteristics to permit for repetitive cannulation. Without adequate inflow, the fistula will simply not develop. The issue of repetitive cannulation involves characteristics that are often referred to as "maturation." For the most part, this relates to its size, position on the arm, configuration, and depth. In addition there are subjective elements including the feel of the AVF by an experienced operator, which cannot be quantified.

Robin et al. have shown that if fistula diameter was 0.4 cm or greater, the likelihood it would be adequate for dialysis was 89 % versus 44 % if it was less than 0.4 cm [38]. In addition, the chances that the fistula would be adequate for dialysis were 84 % if the flow was 500 mL/min or greater but only 43 % if it was less than this level. Combining both the parameters, a minimum fistula diameter of 0.4 cm and a minimum flow volume of 500 mL/min resulted in a 95 % chance that the fistula would be adequate versus 33 % if neither of the minimum criteria were met [38]. Of considerable interest was the fact that experienced dialysis nurses had an 80 % accuracy in predicting the ultimate utility of a fistula for dialysis.

Evaluation at 30 days to detect problems with adequacy has been recommended [39]. This practice is based upon the observation that an AVF that did not appear to be adequate at that time was generally not adequate at a later date. Studies have suggested that there is no significant difference in fistula blood flow in the second, third, or fourth month following creation and that vessel diameter changes very little [40]. Given the fact that there is very little change in the fistula blood flow or diameter after first month along with the finding that that AVF maturation can be judged with high accuracy via physical examination, it is recommended that all newly created AVF should be evaluated by an experienced examiner at 4 weeks [30]. An angiographic study should be performed for non-maturing or poorly mature AVF, so that a

procedure to mature the AVF can be undertaken, if necessary.

12.6 Assessment of AV Access by Physical Examination

Physical examination of the AV access is easily performed, is inexpensive to apply, and provides a high level of accuracy [17, 41]. The examination of AV access – both AVF and AVG – has the following essential components:

Pulse: A normal AVF should not be pulsatile. When a pulse is felt, it is indicative of a downstream obstruction. The severity of this obstruction is reflected in the strength of the pulse.

Thrill: A thrill, or bruit, at the anastomosis is indicative of flow. When feeling for the thrill (or listening to a bruit), it is important to focus on both the diastolic and systolic components [17]. Normally, a very prominent continuous thrill is present at the anastomosis. A thrill at any point other than the anastomosis is indicative of turbulence in the flow, indicating a stenotic lesion at that point. With stenosis, the diastolic portion of the thrill becomes shortened and will eventually disappear, leaving only the systolic component [18]. The thrill generated by a central venous stenosis may be palpable in the axillary or subclavian region, especially in thin-chested individuals.

Arm elevation: When the extremity is elevated to a level above the heart, there should be collapse of the fistula, at least partially. If stenosis is present at some point in the fistula's drainage circuit, then the portion of the fistula distal (peripheral) to the lesion will stay distended while the proximal (central) portion will collapse [17].

Pulse augmentation: If the body of the fistula is manually occluded several centimeters from the anastomosis, the pulse in the fistula distal to that point should become hyperpulsatile. This maneuver is referred to as "checking the pulse augmentation." The degree of pulse augmentation is directly proportional to the arterial inflow pressure. In a hyperpulsatile fistula, the degree of augmentation can be used to gauge the degree of stenosis. Although this is a subjective assessment, very useful information can often be obtained from this evaluation, especially by an experienced examiner.

When an abnormality is detected by physical examination, further diagnostic evaluation of the access should be pursued. The development of an inflow or outflow stenosis perpetually results in access dysfunction which can not only cause inadequate dialysis but also culminate in access thrombosis with the risk of losing the access permanently. Further AV access diagnostic testing can be accomplished by using ultrasound imaging or angiography. If a lesion is detected, it can be treated by percutaneous endovascular intervention with a high success rate [42]. The interventions include angioplasty of a stenosis or ligation of an accessory vein and are out of the scope of this chapter.

12.6.1 Special Considerations Related to AVG Examination

AV graft examination entails the following additional points.

Detection of Direction of Flow

The direction of blood flow in an AVG can vary depending upon the surgeon's choice or due to the location of the suitable vessels. If the orientation of the dialysis needles does not correspond to the direction of blood flow, a gross recirculation is unavoidable. The blood flow can be determined easily by occluding the graft with the tip of the finger and palpating on each side of the occlusion point for a pulse (Fig. 12.8). The side without a pulse is the downstream side of the graft, also referred to as a venous limb. The upstream pulse will increase in intensity during the occlusion, also known as the arterial limb. This should also be communicated to the dialysis staff to ensure proper use of the AVG.

Detecting Recirculation

Recirculation occurs when the blood flow of the graft falls below the rate demanded by the blood pump. This results in varying degrees of reversal of flow between the needles depending upon the severity of the recirculation [17]. Presence of access recirculation can be detected by simple physical examination. To perform this maneuver, simply occlude the graft between the two needles while patient is on dialysis, and observe the venous and arterial pressure gauges (Fig. 12.9). With a normal well-functioning graft, very little or no change is observed in either the venous or arterial pressure readings. If recirculation is secondary to outflow obstruction (venous stenosis), the venous pressure will rise since the lower resistance, recirculation route has been occluded [17]. As pressure limits are exceeded, the alarm

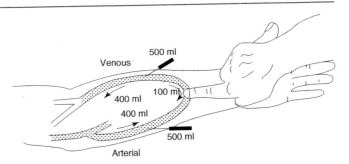

Fig. 12.9 The technique of graft occlusion to detect recirculation (*Source*: Beathard [17])

will sound and the blood pump will stop. The arterial pressure may become slightly more negative as the pressure head generated by the venous side is no longer transmitted given the graft occlusion [17]. If recirculation is due to poor inflow (arterial stenosis or insufficiency), arterial pressures with become more negative as the blood pump demands more blood than is available with the recirculation route cutoff. In this instance, the venous pressure may remain unchanged [17]. If the needles are too close together, this assessment might not be possible.

Diagnosis of Venous Stenosis

Unfortunately, venous stenosis is a very common occurrence. A strong pulse or a vigorous thrill is often mislabeled as a good access with excellent flow rather than an abnormal finding [18]. A well-functioning graft has a soft, easily compressible pulse with a continuous thrill present only at the arterial anastomosis. The normal graft has a low-pitched bruit, which is continuous with both systolic and diastolic components. With the development of significant venous stenosis, downstream resistance is increased and the graft becomes hyperpulsatile. The increase in the force of the pulse within the graft proximal to the stenosis is noted and may have a "water-hammer" character particularly in the presence of severe stenosis [17]. Similar to the AVF exam, as the degree of stenosis increases, the velocity of flow increases, and the pitch of the bruit rises, and with severe stenosis, the bruit is high pitched and only the systolic component is audible.

The diagnosis of intra-graft stenosis is even more perplexing. Abnormal thrills are generally not present. In some instances, it is possible to detect a change in pulsation within the graft as one crosses the stenotic lesion, although this is not a uniform finding and often the area distal to the stenosis becomes pulseless [17]. Normally, if the outflow of the AVG is manually occluded, there is considerable augmentation of the pulse. In cases of diffuse intra-graft stenosis, this augmentation does not occur [18]. The bruit does reflect the hemodynamic changes characteristic of a stenotic lesion – it is high pitched and of short duration.

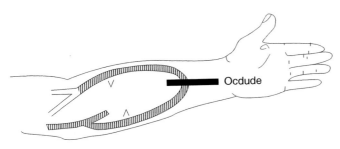

Fig. 12.8 Detection of direction of flow in a graft. When the graft is occluded, the upstream portion (*A*, arterial limb) continues to be pulsatile while the downstream portion (*V*, venous limb) should be non-pulsatile (*Source*: Beathard [17])

12.7 Secondary AV Fistula Creation

A SAVF is defined as an AVF that is created following the failure of a previous access. Type 1 SAVF utilizes the outflow vein of a previous distal failing AV access. Since this vein has been exposed to prolonged pressure and high flow, it has already undergone the process of maturation. This change makes these veins excellent candidate for the creation of an AVF when the primary access fails. In type 2 SAVF, the fistula can be created anywhere other than the outflow vein of previous AV access, including a different extremity. The main advantage of SAVF includes minimum or no exposure to catheter.

A large percentage of patients with dialysis access dysfunction are excellent candidates for an SAVF. In one study, for example, 74 % with a forearm loop graft had one or both of the upper arm veins that appeared to be optimum for the creation of an SAVF, based on the angiographic images [43].

To create an SAVF, the venous anatomy should be evaluated preferably when the lower arm access is still functioning and the veins of the upper arm are under pressure [44]. Although, vascular mapping is usually the first step, angiographic studies are often performed. The 1-year patency rates for SAVF are encouraging, with one study reporting the 1-year patency rate for SAVF (58 %) although lower than that for primary AVF (75 %), and are superior to the reported primary patency of the synthetic grafts at 1 year (25–50 %%) [45, 46].

Conclusions

A functioning vascular access is the key to successful management of a hemodialysis patient and can be cultivated by early nephrology referral, multidisciplinary collaboration among nephrologist, access surgeon, interventional nephrologist/radiologist, and preferably a vascular access coordinator. A nephrologist's knowledge and understanding of ESRD patients and their needs demands them to attain a lead role in creating and maintaining a functional AV access. Once the access is placed, physical examination is the key to monitor access maturation and should be a part of the standard care of dialysis patients. Surveillance with access blood flow and venous pressures should be used as an "adjunct" and should not "substitute" for the monitoring by access examination [17, 18]. Providing conscientious and high-quality access care will lead to early identification and treatment of access-related problems. In addition, it has a great potential to reduce morbidity, improve quality of life, and reduce costs of health care in the dialysis population.

References

1. Roy-Chaudhury P, Kelly BS, Melhem M, et al. Vascular access in hemodialysis: issues, management, and emerging concepts. Cardiol Clin. 2005;23(3):249–73.
2. Shah R, Bhatt UY, Cleef SV, et al. Vascular access thrombosis and interventions in patients missing hemodialysis sessions. Clin Nephrol. 2011;76(6):435–9.
3. Vachharajani TJ, Salman L, Yevzlin AS, et al. Successful models of interventional nephrology at academic medical centers. Clin J Am Soc Nephrol. 2010;5(11):2130–6.
4. Asif A, Besarab A, Roy-Chaudhury P, Spergel LM, Ravani P. Interventional nephrology: from episodic to coordinated vascular access care. J Nephrol. 2007;20(4):399–405.
5. Asif A, Byers P, Gadalean F, Roth D. Peritoneal dialysis underutilization: the impact of an interventional nephrology peritoneal dialysis access program. Semin Dial. 2003;16(3):266–71.
6. Beathard GA. The treatment of vascular access graft dysfunction: a nephrologist's view and experience. Adv Ren Replace Ther. 1994;1(2):131–47.
7. Beathard GA. Percutaneous venous angioplasty in the treatment of stenotic lesions affecting dialysis fistulas. ASAIO Trans. 1991;37(3):M224–5.
8. American Society of Diagnostic and Interventional Nephrology. Guidelines for training, certification, and accreditation in placement of permanent tunneled and cuffed peritoneal dialysis catheters. Semin Dial. 2003;15(6):440–2.
9. American Society of Diagnostic and Interventional Nephrology. Guidelines for training, certification, and accreditation for hemodialysis vascular access and endovascular procedures. Semin Dial. 2003;16(2):173–6.
10. Brescia MJ, Cimino JE, Appel K, Hurwich BJ. Chronic hemodialysis using venipuncture and a surgically created arteriovenous fistula. N Engl J Med. 1966;275(20):1089–92.
11. Miller PE, Tolwani A, Luscy CP, et al. Predictors of adequacy of arteriovenous fistulas in hemodialysis patients. Kidney Int. 1999;57(1):275–80.
12. Hammes M. Hemodialysis access: the fistula. Technical problems in patients on hemodialysis.
13. Rodriguez JA, Armadans L, Ferrer E, et al. The function of permanent vascular access. Nephrol Dial Transplant. 2000;15(3):402–8.
14. Jindal K, Chan CT, Deziel C, et al. Hemodialysis clinical practice guidelines for the Canadian Society of Nephrology. J Am Soc Nephrol. 2006;17 Suppl 1:S1–27.
15. National Kidney Foundation. KDOQI clinical practice guidelines and clinical practice recommendations for 2006 updates: hemodialysis adequacy, peritoneal dialysis adequacy and vascular access. Am J Kidney Dis. 2006;48 Suppl 1:S1–322.
16. Gradman WS, Laub J, Cohen W. Femoral vein transposition for arteriovenous hemodialysis access: improved patient selection and intraoperative measures reduce postoperative ischemia. J Vasc Surg. 2005;41(2):279–84.
17. Beathard GA. Physical examination of the dialysis vascular access. Semin Dial. 1998;11(4):231–6.
18. Beathard GA. Physical examination: the forgotten tool. In: Gray R, Sands J, editors. A multidisciplinary approach for hemodialysis access. New York: Lippincott Williams & Wilkins; 2002. p. 111–8.
19. Schwab SJ, Oliver MJ, Suhocki P, McCann R. Hemodialysis arteriovenous access: detection of stenosis and response to treatment by vascular access blood flow. Kidney Int. 2001;59(1):358–62.
20. Schwab SJ, Harrington JT, Singh A, et al. Vascular access for hemodialysis [clinical conference]. Kidney Int. 1999;55(5):2078–90.
21. Miller CD, Robbin ML, Barker J, Allon M. Comparison of arteriovenous grafts in the thigh and upper extremities in hemodialysis patients. J Am Soc Nephrol. 2003;14(11):2942–7.
22. Ram SJ, Sachdeva BA, Caldito GC, Zibari GB, Abreo KD. Thigh grafts contribute significantly to patients' time on dialysis. Clin J Am Soc Nephrol. 2010;5(7):1229–34.
23. McAllister TN, Maruszewski M, Garrido SA, et al. Effectiveness of haemodialysis access with an autologous tissue-engineered vascular graft: a multicentre cohort study. Lancet. 2009;373(9673):1440–6.
24. Baek I, Bai CZ, Hwang J, Park J, Park JS, Kim DJ. Suppression of neointimal hyperplasia by sirolimus-eluting expanded PTFE hae-

modialysis grafts in comparison with paclitaxel-coated grafts. Nephrol Dial Transplant. 2012;27(5):1997–2004.

25. Agarwal AK, Haddad NJ, Patel BM. Central vein stenosis: a nephrologist's perspective. Semin Dial. 2007;20(1):53–62.

26. Hodges TC, Fillinger MF, Zwolak RM, Walsh DB, Bech F, Cronenwett JL. Longitudinal comparison of dialysis access methods: risk factors for failure. J Vasc Surg. 1997;26(6):1009–19.

27. Konner K, Hulbert-Shearon TE, Roys EC, Port FK. Tailoring the initial vascular access for dialysis patients. Kidney Int. 2002;62(1):329–38.

28. Hoggard J, Saad T, Schon D, et al. Guidelines for venous access in patients with chronic kidney disease. A position statement from the American Society of Diagnostic and Interventional Nephrology, Clinical Practice Committee and the Association for Vascular Access. Semin Dial. 2008;21(2):186–91.

29. National Kidney Foundation. NKF-K/DOQI clinical practice guidelines for vascular access, guideline 8: timing of access placement. Am J Kidney Dis. 2001;37 Suppl 1:S137–81.

30. Beathard, GA. Hemodialysis arteriovenous fistulas. 2003. Retrieved on Mar 2012 from www.esrdnetwork.org

31. National Kidney Foundation. NKF-K/DOQI clinical practice guidelines for vascular access: guideline 1: patient history and physical examination prior to permanent access selections. Am J Kidney Dis. 2001;37 Suppl 1:S141.

32. Beathard GA. Complications of vascular access. In: Lamiere N, Mehta R, editors. Complications of dialysis – recognition and management. New York: Marcel Dekker, Inc; 2000. p. 1–27.

33. Silva MB, Hobson RW, Pappas PJ, et al. A strategy for increasing use of autogenous hemodialysis access procedures: impact of preoperative noninvasive evaluation. J Vasc Surg. 1998;27(2):302–7.

34. Hirai M, Kawai S. False positive and negative results in Allen test. J Cardiovasc Surg (Torino). 1980;21(3):353–60.

35. Ruland O, Borkenhagen N, Prien T. [The Doppler palm test]. Ultraschall Med. 1988;9(2):63–6.

36. Allon M, Lockhart ME, Lilly RZ, et al. Effect of preoperative sonographic mapping on vascular access outcomes in hemodialysis patients. Kidney Int. 2001;60(5):2013–20.

37. Silva MB, Hobson RW, Pappas PJ, et al. Vein transposition in the forearm for autogenous hemodialysis access. J Vasc Surg. 1997;26(6):981–6.

38. Robbin ML, Chamberlain NE, Lockhart ME, et al. Hemodialysis arteriovenous fistula maturity: US evaluation. Radiology. 2002;225(1):59–64.

39. Beathard GA, Settle SM, Shields MW. Salvage of the nonfunctioning arteriovenous fistula. Am J Kidney Dis. 1999;33(5):910–6.

40. Robbin ML, Gallichio MH, Deierhoi MH, Young CJ, Weber TM, Allon M. US vascular mapping before hemodialysis access placement. Radiology. 2000;217(1):83–8.

41. Migliacci R, Selli ML, Falcinelli F, et al. Assessment of occlusion of the vascular access in patients on chronic hemodialysis: comparison of physical examination with continuous-wave Doppler ultrasound. Nephron. 1999;82(1):7–11.

42. Beathard GA, Arnold P, Jackson J, Litchfield T. Physician Operators Forum Of RMS Lifeline. Aggressive treatment of early fistula failure. Kidney Int. 2003;64(4):1487–94.

43. Beathard GA. Interventionalist's role in identifying candidates for secondary fistulas. Semin Dial. 2004;17(3):233–6.

44. Oliver MJ, McCann RL, Indridason OS, Butterly DW, Schwab SJ. Comparison of transposed brachiobasilic fistulas to upper arm grafts and brachiocephalic fistulas. Kidney Int. 2001;60(4):1532–9.

45. Ascher E, Hingorani AP, Yorkovich WR. Techniques and outcome after brachiocephalic and brachiobasilic arteriovenous AVF creation. In: Gray R, Sands J, editors. A multidisciplinary approach for hemodialysis access. New York: Lippincott Williams & Wilkins; 2002. p. 84.

46. Beathard GA. Complications of vascular access. In: Lamiere N, Mehta R, editors. Complications of dialysis – recognition and management. New York: Marcel Dekker, Inc; 2000.

47. Vachharajani T. Atlas of hemodialysis access. 2010.

Approach to a Patient with Non-maturing AV Fistula

13

Ravish Shah and Anil K. Agarwal

13.1 Introduction

The superiority of the native arteriovenous fistula (AVF) over other types of accesses including arteriovenous graft (AVG) and tunneled dialysis catheters (TDC) for chronic hemodialysis is a well-recognized fact. It has been shown to have superior patency rates and lower complication rate including a low risk of infection and a lower intervention rate to maintain its patency [1, 2]. This is the core reason underlying the development of guidelines and the Fistula First project that have led to AVF creation in a majority of patients with end-stage renal disease (ESRD). Unfortunately, a considerable number of fistulas (28–53 %) fail to mature sufficiently to support dialysis therapy [3–6]. Failure to mature (FTM) often commits these patients to a tunneled dialysis catheter for a variable length of time until they have a well-functioning arteriovenous (AV) access [3]. In addition to the risk of infection and central venous stenosis, the catheters also contribute to inadequate dialysis and poor patient outcomes [3]. Therefore, early recognition and timely intervention in cases of an AVF with FTM are critically important [3].

13.1.1 Failure to Mature: Definition

Fistula failure can be classified as early and late. Early failure is a true FTM that refers to the cases in which the AV fistula never develops to the point that it can be used or fails within the first 3 months of usage [1]. Late failure refers to those cases where the AVF fails after 3 months of successful usage [7, 8]. Although there might be considerable overlap in the causes of both early and late failure, early failure has gained significant attention as recent data have demonstrated that a great majority of the failed fistulas can be salvaged using percutaneous interventions [9–12]. While it not infrequent to abandon these AVFs with early failure, aggressive evaluation and treatment have been shown to result in the salvage of vast majority of these accesses [10].

13.1.2 Risk Factors for Failure of Maturation

FTM is a common problem occurring in 28–53 % of native AVF [3–6, 13]. Several studies have looked at factors that might predict fistula maturation. Preoperative vascular mapping has been shown to improve the rate of fistula placement and overall surgical success rate [14–16]. Creation of AVF using very small arteries (e.g., < 1.6 mm in diameter) and veins is likely to fail, although the precise cutoff hinges on the available surgical experience and expertise [14]. Perhaps the most critical determinant of fistula maturation is the functional ability of the artery and vein to dilate and achieve a rapid increase in blood flow after surgery [14]. Several studies have shown that postoperative flow rate measured by Doppler ultrasound in a forearm fistula is a moderately good predictor of fistula maturation [17, 18]. In addition, these studies have reported using a cutoff between 400 and 500 ml/min at 2–8 weeks as a predictor of fistula maturation. Clinical examination of the fistula may be as accurate as Doppler flow measurements [17–19]. Other predictors of AVF failure include age >65 year, diabetes, female gender, and high body mass index (>27), although in the majority of the patients with early FTM, anatomic abnormalities as detected by angiography are present [1].

13.1.3 Causes of Early Fistula Failure

Fistulas can fail to mature for a number of reasons including:
1. Inflow problems: poor arterial inflow and juxta-anastomotic venous stenosis (JAVS).
2. Outflow problems: failure for the vein to "arterialize" and presence of large and/or multiple accessory veins.

R. Shah, MD • A.K. Agarwal, MD, FACP, FASN, FNKF (✉)
Division of Nephrology, The Ohio State University,
395 W 12th Avenue, Ground Floor, Columbus, OH 43210, USA
e-mail: anil.agarwal@osumc.edu

A.S. Yevzlin et al. (eds.), *Interventional Nephrology*,
DOI 10.1007/978-1-4614-8803-3_13, © Springer Science+Business Media New York 2014

3. Other technical factors at the time of surgery: a deep fistula, although mature, might not be easily accessible for cannulation and may require transposition in order to support dialysis adequately. Majority of these causes can and must be identified early in order to salvage the AVF, frequently using percutaneous interventions.

Inflow Problems

A good inflow is critical for fistula maturation and for attaining adequate flow rates to deliver dialysis. After AVF creation, the arterial flow is expected to increase, with increasing arterial diameter and changes in flow pattern [14]. Vascular remodeling and dilation are typically attained by longitudinal shear stress and circumferential deformation, in the milieu of vasoactive factors [14, 20]. This process may continue over a long period of time and contributes to maturation. Rarely, a small-size artery or presence of arterial disease such as atherosclerosis can result in early fistula failure. However, this can be identified and prevented by a comprehensive patient evaluation prior to access placement.

JAVS is one of the most common causes of maturation failure in angiographically evaluated AVF [15] (Fig. 13.1). Although precise etiology is not clear, it is postulated that the JAVS occurs in the swing segment of the vein, where the vein is mobilized to connect with the artery and suffers stretching, torsion, and spasm [21]. It is unclear as to what extent these factors contribute to JAVS; however, the net effect of JVAS is to reduce fistula inflow. JVAS often occurs early in the process and often results in early access failure. In one single-center retrospective study, the authors reported their 12-year experience of radiological management of stenosis and thrombosis in both AVF and AVGs [22]. Of the total 283 patients with AVF, majority of the patients had forearm AVF (74 %) and 74 patients had upper arm AVF. In patients with forearm AVF, JVAS was present in almost half of these patients leading to an inflow problem (Fig. 13.2a). However, of the 74 patients with the upper arm AVF, outflow venous stenosis was predominantly reported in 55 % of cases

($n = 41$) (Fig. 13.2b). The vast majority of the stenoses (86 %) were less than two cm long [22]. Fortunately, JVAS is amenable to treatment. It can generally be successfully treated by percutaneous angioplasty surgically [1, 10, 23]. A retrospective analysis of prospectively collected data compared outcomes and cost of surgery ($n = 21$) and percutaneous transluminal angioplasty (PTA) ($n = 43$) for JAVS in a total of 64 patients [24]. Although the results showed similar cost and success rate, adjusted relative risk was 2.77 for restenosis within the PTA group. The primary 1-year unassisted patency rate for surgery was 91 ± 6 % as compared with 54 ± 8 % with PTA, although adjusted-assisted primary patency rates were similar in the two groups. The surgical approach that had the advantage of less restenosis however was more invasive, involved small but significant risk of loss of venous capital, and was associated with a higher median cost, primarily because of the procedure-related hospitalization. It is important to note that the study was not randomized and only included patients with mature AVF based on the choice made on the basis of available expertise and technical facilities as suggested by the authors. It is worth reemphasizing that JAVS can be easily diagnosed by physical examination [25, 26].

Outflow Problems

Venous dilatation ensues after AVF creation, initially as a result of increased venous pressure and later because of the increase in flow-mediated shear stress [14, 15]. For an AVF to develop and provide satisfactory hemodialysis, there must also be sufficient blood flow through the outflow vein. The absence of good outflow will result in failure of the access. Anomalies that lead to outflow problems include veins that are too small for fistula development, veins that are fibrotic or stenotic, or presence of side branches, referred to as accessory veins. Failure of the dilation of outflow vein has been suggested to be a common cause of maturation failure [27]. Venous stenosis causes failure of the majority of AVF, and endovascular techniques have become popular in the treat-

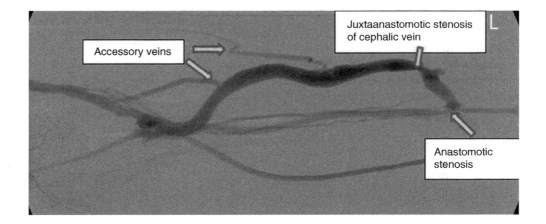

Fig. 13.1 Fistulogram of radiocephalic AVF showing arteriovenous anastomotic stenosis and juxta-anastomotic stenosis of cephalic vein and accessory veins in the forearm

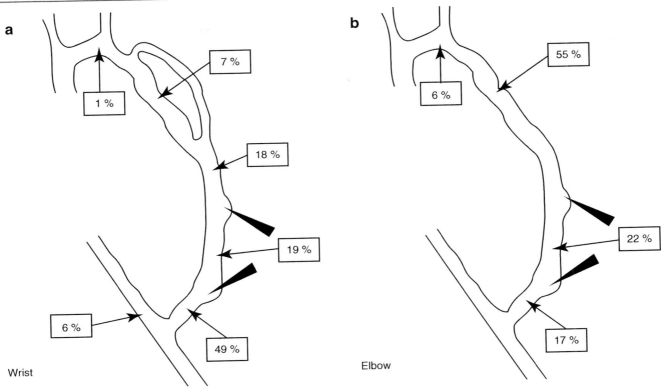

Fig. 13.2 (**a**, **b**) Common sites of stenosis in AVF. (**a**) In wrist AVF. (**b**) In upper arm AVF (Adapted from Turmel-Rodrigues et al. [22])

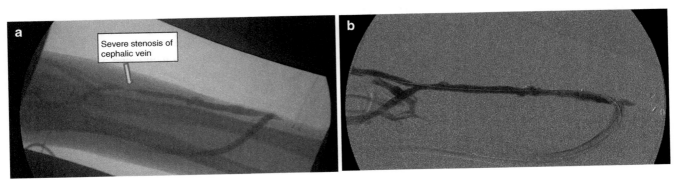

Fig. 13.3 (**a**) Cephalic vein in forearm with severe stenosis that can be angioplastied for maturation of AVF. (**b**) Cephalic vein in forearm after angioplasty leading to maturation of AVF

ment of most venous stenoses (Fig. 13.3a, b). However, recurrent lesions remain problematic, especially with long segment of severely narrow lesions [28]. Close surveillance and repeated interventions are generally required to maintain patency, although the restenosis at 6 month is significantly less with AVF, compared with AVG [29].

Although, a single cephalic vein stretching from the wrist to the antecubital space is preferred, in many cases, it may be accompanied by one or more accessory veins [25]. These accessory veins are normal anatomy. All of the veins receiving the drainage from the newly created anastomosis enlarge after creation of AVF, and a small accessory vein may

become enlarged with time. The accessory veins must be distinguished from the collateral veins which are pathological and are associated with a downstream (antegrade) stenosis. Ideally the presence of an accessory vein may be viewed as an advantage since it might provide an additional venous channel suitable for cannulation. However, when large (>25 % of the diameter of main AVF), these can steal enough blood flow so that the main fistula channel does not dilate, often resulting in early AVF failure [25, 30] (Fig. 13.4). The accessory veins can often be diagnosed by physical examination [31, 32]. Frequently they are visible or can be detected by palpating the fistula. Also, the thrill that is palpable over

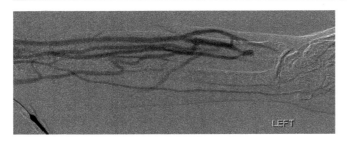

Fig. 13.4 Fistulogram of forearm radiocephalic AVF showing multiple large accessory veins

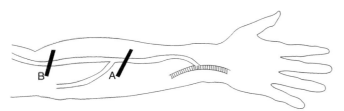

Fig. 13.5 Physical examination of accessory vein. When the fistula is occluded at *point A*, the thrill will disappear at the anastomosis. As the point of occlusion is moved upward past the accessory vein to *point B*, the thrill will continue when the fistula is occluded (Adapted from Beathard [25])

the arterial anastomosis usually disappears when the downstream (antegrade) fistula is manually occluded, but it does not disappear if an outflow channel (accessory vein) is present below the point of occlusion [25] (Fig. 13.5). Ligation of these accessory veins will redirect the flow to the main channel and promote the development of a usable AVF [1, 10]. Accessory veins together with the JAVS represent the two most common causes of early AVF failure [33, 34]. These two lesions are often present simultaneously [22, 35].

13.1.4 Identification and Management of Early AVF Failure

Identification of patients who are at risk of early AVF failure is critical in order to perform timely intervention to salvage the AVF [1, 15]. Physical examination of the AV access is not only easy to perform and inexpensive, it provides a high level of accuracy [25, 36]. Both accessory veins along with JAVS can be easily identified by a thorough physical examination of the AV access [7]. Please refer to the chapter on "Approach to an AV Access" for details regarding access examination. While ultrasonography can identify these lesions successfully, it is not readily available in all centers and is not free of added cost.

Given the fact that there is very little change in the fistula blood flow or diameter after the first month along with the finding that AVF maturation can be judged with high accuracy via physical examination, it is recommended that all

newly created AVFs should be evaluated by an experienced examiner at 4 weeks [1, 10, 37, 38]. An angiographic study must be performed for non-maturing or poorly mature AVF [3]. In patients who have not initiated dialysis, there is often a concern with use of radiocontrast. However, a small amount of contrast use has been shown to be safe in the evaluation of AVF.

An early identification and intervention approach is critical to the successful maturation of AVF for two reasons. First, a majority of fistulas with early failure demonstrate stenotic lesions within the access circuit [1, 10, 11]. In addition, vascular stenosis is a progressive process eventually culminating in access thrombosis, with the risk of permanently losing the access. Failure to act promptly in these AVFs will result in a loss of the opportunity to salvage an AVF. Second, those patients with early fistula failure are often committed to a tunneled dialysis catheter exposing them to all the dreaded complications of catheter use. Hence, early intervention to identify and salvage early AVF failure becomes an important part of preventing AVF loss and minimizing complications related to tunneled dialysis catheters. Such an approach also supports the "catheter last" approach that the experts advocate.

13.1.5 Specific Interventions

Once a patient with early AVF failure has been identified, appropriate action to salvage the AVF should be taken in a timely manner. As previously mentioned, studies have demonstrated that the two most common problems observed in early AVF failure are the presence of stenosis and accessory veins [9–11]. Fortunately, a great majority of these failed fistulas can be salvaged using percutaneous techniques [1, 11, 39].

13.2 Angioplasty

Endovascular intervention to salvage an immature or failing AVF has become routine. Using radiocontrast, an angiogram of the AVF (commonly termed as "fistulogram") is done to diagnose the presence of anatomic abnormalities, which can commonly be treated with percutaneous transluminal angioplasty (PTA). PTA is typically indicated when there is >50 % stenosis of AVF or AVG [15, 32]. In addition, an inflow lesion, if identified, may be amenable to PTA via a retrograde fistula approach. In a prospective observational study, 100 patients with early failure underwent evaluation and treatment at six freestanding outpatient vascular access centers [1]. Vascular stenosis and the presence of a significant accessory vein alone or in combination were found to be the most common offenders. Venous stenosis was present in 78 % of the cases. A majority (48 %) of these lesions were found to be close to the anastomosis (JAVS). A significant accessory vein was present in 46 % of the cases. Percutaneous balloon angioplasty and accessory vein obliteration using one of the three techniques (percutaneous ligation using 3/0 nylon, venous cut down, or coil insertion) were used to salvage the failed AVF. Angioplasty was performed with a 98 % success rate, and there was 100 % success rate for accessory vein ligation. These interventions resulted in dialysis initiation using the AVF in 92 % of the cases [1]. Upon further analysis, 84 % of the AVF were functional at 3 months, 72 % at 6 months, and 68 % at 12 months [1]. The overall complication rate in this series was 4 %, exclusively seen in patient who underwent angioplasty. Of these, only one patient (1 %) had a major complication consisted of a vein rupture with an expanding hematoma resulting in loss of the access. The three minor complications included low-grade hematomas requiring no treatment and no sequelae [1].

13.3   Accessory/Branching Vein Ligation

Ligation of the accessory veins can be performed surgically or percutaneously with suture ligation and/or embolization. Suture ligation is useful in patients with superficial accessory veins given minimal distance for subcutaneous dissection [40]. Coils within superficial veins can be irritating to patients and possibly erode through the skin. However, coil embolization is preferred in those with deep accessory veins as cutdown suture ligation is more difficult with potential risks of nerve/muscle and tendon injury [40]. Using a percutaneous ligation technique, a separate report also described accessory vein ligation of fistulas that failed to achieve adequate blood flow or size for successful cannulation. Authors reported that of the 17 AV fistulas, 15 (88 %) successfully matured at 1.7 months (± 1 month) after the procedure and were functioning at 44.5 (± 12 weeks) after the first use [9]. In another series of 119 patients with AVF complicated by maturation failure, 29.4 % had a significant accessory vein but that was the sole cause of AVF dysfunction in only 3.4 % [39]. The AVF salvage rate for all lesions was 83 % in this series. These reports suggest that early intervention for maturation failure can salvage a majority of AVF using endovascular techniques [1, 11, 15].

13.4   Sequential Dilation

Occasionally early fistula failure is found due to a long segment of the vein which is diffusely small or stenosed. Recent reports have highlighted a newer technique (sequential dilation or balloon-assisted maturation) to salvage an AVF that fails to develop because of diffuse stenosis [5, 41]. In this technique, the AVF is gradually dilated with a progressively increasing size of angioplasty balloon at 2- to 4-weeks intervals until a size that is optimal for dialysis cannulation is achieved. The goal is to progressively dilate the outflow vein to a point that is usable for repetitive cannulation and will also deliver adequate blood flow. Dilation time is typically <20 s mainly to reduce the chance of thrombosis [40]. In addition, shutting down or occluding flow to the AVF by compressing the anastomosis during vein dilation is recommended to prevent venous tears resulting in blood leaking out subsequently causing ecchymosis [40]. In addition, balloon dilation is usually performed starting from the central to the peripheral vein to reduce the likelihood of blood extravasation as it is easier to pull back a balloon than push it forward [40].

13.5   Surgical Techniques

Surgical interventions include patch angioplasty, creation of a combination of fistula and graft ("graftula"), creation of a new anastomosis for a juxta-anastomotic lesion, and superficialization procedures [3, 40]. However, large-scale randomized prospective studies examining the role of surgical approach in the salvage of AVF with early failure are lacking. Inability to navigate the wire across a stenotic lesion during percutaneous approach and deep location of an AVF are some of the indications for surgical intervention [3].

13.6   Stents in AV Access

Stents have a very limited role in salvage of immature AVF. When dealing with the stenosis, patients with >30 % residual stenosis after PTA of venous stenosis or those with recurrence of the stenosis within 3 months and requiring repeated intervention should be considered for a stent placement [15]. Stents can also be useful in the case of vessel rupture during angioplasty that does not respond to conservative measures. However, the latter is generally associated with poor primary patency [42]. Stents can also be used when PTA has failed and surgery is not feasible due to a variety of reasons. Although stents have been used in coronary and peripheral arterial circulation with decent success, dialysis access demonstrates unique pathologies being in a venous circulation. Self-expanding rather than balloon-expanded stents are commonly used for VA [43]. These include bare metal stainless steel stents or nitinol shape memory alloy recoverable technology (SMART) stents that are made of nickel titanium alloy [15]. These have physical characteristics that allow more deformability as compared with bare metal stents. Stent grafts are composed of nitinol skeleton covered by graft material on both sides. Stents available until recently have been used off-label to improve patency in patients with VA stenosis, primarily in AVG, with variable results. Stent placement has several disadvantages including migration, fracture, and in-stent restenosis [15]. Infectious complications are usually not evident until many days after the procedure [44]. In addition, due to the stent placed in the venous segment, loss of vein length may jeopardize future AVF creation [15]. Despite the recent advances in knowledge, both technical and theoretical, the role of stent placement in the management of hemodialysis access dysfunction remains controversial. It will remain so until large, multicenter, prospective, randomized, controlled trials are conducted [44]. Stent placement should be utilized only after considering the type, location, and frequency of recurrence of the lesion. Possibility of a secondary AVF must be considered to avoid the loss of available venous length from stent placement.

13.7 Thrombectomy

If the immature AVF is thrombosed, then one can perform a thrombectomy with simple PTA maceration of the clot in most cases [5]. There is typically a minimal amount of thrombus usually located at the juxta-anastomotic region. Use of heparin is typically indicated. The treatment should also include prompt detection and treatment of the underlying anatomic abnormality and evaluation and management of outflow, including central veins. Percutaneous declotting of AVF is more difficult than declotting of AVG, with success rates that vary between 73 and 96 % in published literature [45]. With the advent of new technology and growing expertise in the field on interventional nephrology, the results of percutaneous techniques have improved significantly and are now comparable to surgical thrombectomy with restoring AVF patency in >90 % of cases [46]. However, the results seem to vary with operator experience and available resources.

13.8 Prevention of Early FTM

Appropriate preoperative evaluation of the patients prior to AVF creation will not only increase chances of AVF creation but also of AVF maturation. Use of physical examination, ultrasonography, and occasional venography are recommended based on individual case. Use of certain pharmacologic agents, especially the antiplatelet agents, has been noted to be associated with improved survival of AVF but has not been proved conclusively to improve the use of AVF in randomized controlled trials despite reduction in AVF thrombosis [47–50]. Many novel therapies are being evaluated to improve maturation of AVF. Local delivery of endothelial cells as a wrap can reduce development of neointimal hyperplasia at the arteriovenous anastomosis [51]. Perivascular wraps of antiproliferative agents (paclitaxel) and gene therapy with adenoviral vectors have been tried [52]. Use of venous and arterial allografts as well as decellularized xenografts has been tried in those with unsuitable veins. Better hemodynamics by way of using a premade arteriovenous anastomosis is also being tried in clinical studies.

Conclusion

It is crucial to evaluate a newly created AVF at 4–6 weeks after placement to identify candidates with early AVF failure. Physical examination is a simple but efficient modality of identifying such candidates. Once identified, these patients then should be referred to an interventionalist for evaluation and appropriate intervention. Delays in such intervention may result in the delivery of dialysis with a tunneled dialysis catheter, rendering the patient susceptible to higher complications as well as to a risk of eventual thrombosis leading to permanent loss of access. By use of the percutaneous endovascular techniques such as balloon angioplasty and vein obliteration, majority of early fistula failures can be rescued.

References

1. Beathard GA, Arnold P, Jackson J, Litchfield T, Physician Operators Forum of RMS Lifeline, Inc. Aggressive treatment of early fistula failure. Kidney Int. 2003;64:1487–94.
2. Allon M, Robbin ML. Increasing arteriovenous fistulas in hemodialysis patients: problems and solutions. Kidney Int. 2002;62: 1109–24.
3. Asif A, Roy-Chaudhury P, Beathard GA. Early arteriovenous fistula failure: a logical proposal for when and how to intervene. Clin J Am Soc Nephrol. 2006;1:332–9.
4. Allon M, Lockhart ME, Lilly RZ, et al. Effect of preoperative sonographic mapping on vascular access outcomes in hemodialysis patients. Kidney Int. 2001;60:2013–20.
5. Asif A, Cherla G, Merrill D, Cipleu CD, Briones P, Pennell P. Conversion of tunneled hemodialysis catheter-consigned patients to arteriovenous fistula. Kidney Int. 2005;67:2399–406.
6. Won T, Jang JW, Lee S, Han JJ, Park YS, Ahn JH. Effects of intraoperative blood flow on the early patency of radiocephalic fistulas. Ann Vasc Surg. 2000;14:468–72.
7. Beathard GA. Strategy for maximizing the use of arteriovenous fistulae. Semin Dial. 2000;13:291–6.
8. Beathard GA. Angioplasty for arteriovenous grafts and fistulae. Semin Nephrol. 2002;22:202–10.
9. Faiyaz R, Abreo K, Zaman F, et al. Salvage of poorly developed arteriovenous fistulae with percutaneous ligation of accessory veins. Am J Kidney Dis. 2002;39:824–7.
10. Beathard GA, Settle SM, Shields MW. Salvage of the nonfunctioning arteriovenous fistula. Am J Kidney Dis. 1999;33:910–6.
11. Turmel-Rodrigues L, Mouton A, Birmele B, et al. Salvage of immature forearm fistulas for hemodialysis by interventional radiology. Nephrol Dial Transplant. 2001;16:2365–71.
12. Corpataux JM, Haesler E, Silacci P, et al. Low-pressure environment and remodelling of the forearm vein in Brescia-Cimino haemodialysis access. Nephrol Dial Transplant. 2002;17:1057–62.

13. Miller PE, Tolwani A, Luscy CP, Deierhoi MH, Bailey R, Redden DT, Allon M. Predictors of adequacy of arteriovenous fistulas in hemodialysis patients. Kidney Int. 1999;56:275–80.

14. Dixon BS. Why don't fistulas mature? Kidney Int. 2006;70:1413–22.

15. Agarwal A, Asif A. Maintenance and salvage of vascular access: current concepts. Intervent Nephrol. 2009;8(5):353–9.

16. Silva Jr MB, Hobson II RW, Pappas PJ, et al. A strategy for increasing use of autogenous hemodialysis access procedures: impact of preoperative noninvasive evaluation. J Vasc Surg. 1998;27:302–7.

17. Lin SL, Chen HS, Huang CH, et al. Predicting the outcome of hemodialysis arteriovenous fistulae using duplex ultrasonography. J Formos Med Assoc. 1997;96:864–8.

18. Robbin ML, Oser RF, Allon M, et al. Hemodialysis access graft stenosis: US detection. Radiology. 1998;208:655–61.

19. Wong V, Ward R, Taylor J, et al. Factors associated with early failure of arteriovenous fistulae for haemodialysis access. Eur J Vasc Endovasc Surg. 1996;12:207–13.

20. Kim YO, Choi YJ, Kim JI, et al. The impact of intima-media thickness of radial artery on early failure of radiocephalic arteriovenous fistula in hemodialysis patients. J Korean Med Sci. 2006;21:284–9.

21. Konner K, Nonnast-Daniel B, Ritz E. The arteriovenous fistula. J Am Soc Nephrol. 2003;14:1669–80.

22. Turmel-Rodrigues L, Pengloan J, Baudin S, et al. Treatment of stenosis and thrombosis in haemodialysis fistulas and grafts by interventional radiology. Nephrol Dial Transplant. 2000;15:2032–6.

23. Romero A, Polo JR, Morato EG, et al. Salvage of angioaccess after late thrombosis of radiocephalic fistulas for hemodialysis. Int Surg. 1999;71:122–4.

24. Tessitore N, Mansueto G, Lipari G, et al. Endovascular versus surgical preemptive repair of forearm arteriovenous fistula juxta-anastomotic stenosis: analysis of data collected prospectively from 1999 to 2004. Clin J Am Soc Nephrol. 2006;1:448–54.

25. Beathard GA. Physical examination of the dialysis vascular access. Semin Dial. 1998;11:231–6.

26. Beathard GA. Physical examination: the forgotten tool. In: Gray R, Sands J, editors. A multidisciplinary approach for hemodialysis access. New York: Lippincott Williams & Wilkins; 2002. p. 111–8.

27. Tordoir JH, Rooyens P, Dammers R, Van der Sande FM, De Haan M, Yo TI. Prospective evaluation of failure modes in autogenous radiocephalic wrist access for hemodialysis. Nephrol Dial Transplant. 2003;18:378–83.

28. Clark TW, Hirsch DA, Jindal KJ, et al. Outcome and prognostic factors of restenosis after percutaneous treatment of native hemodialysis fistulas. J Vasc Interv Radiol. 2002;13:51–9.

29. Turmel-Rodrigues L, Pengloan J, Blanchier D, et al. Insufficient dialysis shunts: improved long term patency rates with close hemodynamic monitoring, repeat percutaneous balloon angioplasty, and stent placement. Radiology. 1993;187:273–8.

30. Miles AM. Upper limb ischemia after vascular access surgery: differential diagnosis and management. Semin Dial. 2000;13:312–6.

31. Leon C, Orozco-Vargas LC, et al. Accuracy of Physical Examination in the Detection of Arteriovenous Graft Stenosis. Seminars in Dialysis. 2008;21(1):85–8

32. National Kidney Foundation. K/DOQI clinical practice guidelines for vascular access, guideline 19: treatment of stenosis without thrombosis in dialysis AV grafts and primary AV fistulae. Am J Kidney Dis. 2002;37(1):S163–4.

33. Beathard GA. Percutaneous transvenous angioplasty in the treatment of vascular access stenosis. Kidney Int. 1992;42:1390–7.

34. Vesely TM, Siegel JB. Use of the peripheral cutting balloon to treat hemodialysis-related stenoses. J Vasc Interv Radiol. 2005;16:1593–603.

35. Tessitore N, Mansueto G, Bedogna V, et al. A prospective controlled trial on effect of percutaneous transluminal angioplasty on functioning arteriovenous fistulae survival. J Am Soc Nephrol. 2003;14:1623–7.

36. Migliacci R, Selli ML, Falcinelli F, et al. Assessment of occlusion of the vascular access in patients on chronic hemodialysis: comparison of physical examination with continuous-wave Doppler ultrasound. Nephron. 1999;82(1):7.

37. Robbin ML, Chamberlain NE, Lockhart ME, et al. Hemodialysis arteriovenous fistula maturity: US evaluation. Radiology. 2002;225:59–64.

38. Robbin ML, Gallichio MH, Deierhoi MH, et al. US vascular mapping before hemodialysis access placement. Radiology. 2000;217:83–8.

39. Nassar GM, Nguyen B, Rhee E, Achkar K. Endovascular treatment of the "failing to mature" arteriovenous fistula. Clin J Am Soc Nephrol. 2006;1:275–80.

40. Falk A, Rajan D. The immature or failure to mature fistula. In: Essentials of percutaneous dialysis interventions. New York: Springer; 2011. p. 323–39.

41. Achkar K, Nassar GM. Salvage of a severely dysfunctional arteriovenous fistula with a strictured and occluded outflow tract. Semin Dial. 2005;18:336–42.

42. Rajan D, Clark TW. Patency of wallstents placed at the venous anastomosis of dialysis grafts for salvage of angioplasty-induced rupture. Cardiovasc Intervent Radiol. 2003;26:242–5.

43. Urbanes AQ. Proper use and indications for stents in vascular access salvage. Quest. 2008;15:15–9.

44. Yevzlin A, Asif A. Stent placement in hemodialysis access: historical lessons, the state of the art and future directions. Clin J Am Soc Nephrol. 2009;4:996–1008.

45. Moossavi S, Reagan J, Pierson ED, Kasey JM, et al. Non-surgical salvage of thrombosed arteriovenous fistulae: a case series and review of the literature. Semin Dial. 2008;20:459–64.

46. Schon D, Mishler R. Salvage of occluded arteriovenous fistulae. Am J Kidney Dis. 2000;36:804–10.

47. Dember LM, Beck GJ, Allon M, et al. Effect of clopidogrel on early failure of arteriovenous fistulas for hemodialysis: a randomized controlled trial. JAMA. 2008;299:2164.

48. Saran R, Dykstra DM, Wolfe RA, Gillespie B, Held PJ, Young EW, Dialysis Outcomes and Practice Patterns Study. Association between vascular access failure and the use of specific drugs: the Dialysis Outcomes and Practice Patterns Study (DOPPS). Am J Kidney Dis. 2002;40:1255–63.

49. Yevzlin AS, Conley EL, Sanchez RJ, Young HN, Becker BN. Vascular access outcomes and medication use: a USRDS study. Semin Dial. 2006;19:535–9.

50. Hasegawa T, et al. Consistent aspirin use associated with improved arteriovenous fistula survival among incident hemodialysis patients in the dialysis outcomes and practice patterns study. Clin J Am Soc Nephrol. 2008;3:1373–8.

51. Nuget HM, Groothuis A, Seifert P, Guerraro JL, Nedelman M, Mohankumar T, Edelman ER. Perivascular endothelial implants inhibit intimal hyperplasia in a model of arteriovenous fistulae: a safety and efficacy study in the pig. J Vasc Res. 2002;39:524–33.

52. Roy-Chaudhury P, Kelly BS, Zhang J, Narayana A, Desai P, Melham M, Duncan H, Heffelfinger SC. Hemodialysis vascular access dysfunction: from pathophysiology to novel therapies. Blood Purif. 2003;21:99–110.

Approach to an Arteriovenous Access with Hyperpulsatile Pulse

Tushar J. Vachharajani

Physical examination of dialysis vascular access is a skill easy to master and implement in clinical practice by everyone involved in the care of dialysis patients [1]. In the USA, the Centers for Medicare and Medicaid Services mandate all dialysis vascular access be examined before each treatment [2, 3]. Arteriovenous fistula (AVF) remains the preferred permanent dialysis vascular access. An established well-functioning AVF generally is less problematic when compared an arteriovenous graft. The common problems associated with an established AVF include (but not limited to) stenosis in the outflow and inflow segments, aneurysm formation in the body of an AVF, central vein stenosis, and infection. Stenosis is a relentless pathology that continues to progress unless diagnosed early for timely intervention with the currently available option of performing percutaneous endovascular angioplasty. Left untreated, stenosis will eventually progress to reduction of blood flow and thrombosis.

In order to perform a detailed physical examination of an AVF, it is essential to understand its basic segments. The different segments of an AVF are described earlier in the chapter – *Approach to Arteriovenous Fistula with Faint Thrill*. In this chapter, the approach to an AVF with hyperpulsatile will be discussed.

14.1 Defining Hyperpulsatile Pulse

The palpation of an AVF involves feeling for the pulsations and thrill. A normal fistula is soft, compressible with a soft continuous thrill all along its outflow segment.

In the presence of stenosis in the outflow segment, the pulsation in the segment distal to the stenosis has a strong bounding character, provided the inflow segment is widely patent (Fig. 14.1). The thrill in a hyperpulsatile outflow segment is diminished or absent.

T.J. Vachharajani, MD, FACP, FASN
Nephrology Section, W. G. (Bill) Hefner Veterans Affairs Medical Center, Salisbury, NC, USA
e-mail: tushar.vachharajani@va.gov

14.2 Etiology of Hyperpulsatile AVF

The hyperpulsatile pulse develops by and large due to the development of stenosis in the outflow segment with a patent inflow segment. The exact pathophysiology behind the development of stenosis is as yet unclear, but neointimal hyperplasia has been implicated in majority of cases [4]. Infrequently, in a high-flow fistula (defined as blood flow more than 2 L/min), the outflow segment may appear to be hyperpulsatile. The strong character to the pulse is because of a large volume of blood flowing through a small-capacity outflow vein. The upper arm AVF is more likely to feel hyperpulsatile due to high flows compared to the forearm AVF.

14.3 Clinical Findings Associated with Hyperpulsatile AVF

The hyperpulsatile AVF is often accompanied by various clinical findings that can assist in the diagnosis of outflow segment stenosis. Table 14.1 summarizes the clinical findings that are described in details below.

14.3.1 Arm Elevation Test

A simple arm elevation test can provide additional clinical finding to confirm outflow segment stenosis. In an AVF with a patent outflow segment with arm elevation, the entire outflow segment collapses. In the presence of outflow segment stenosis, the segment distal to the stenosis remains distended and firm (Fig. 14.2) [3].

14.3.2 Thrill

A thrill is the vibrations that are easily palpable over an AVF. A normal thrill is fine, continuous, and best felt at the arteriovenous anastomosis and transmitted along the outflow

A.S. Yevzlin et al. (eds.), *Interventional Nephrology*,
DOI 10.1007/978-1-4614-8803-3_14, © Springer Science+Business Media New York 2014

Fig. 14.1 Panel **a**: Normal outflow segment with a continuous thrill and soft pulsations. Panel **b**: Stenosis in the outflow segment with hyperpulsatile segment distal to the stenosis (shown with *dashed lines*)

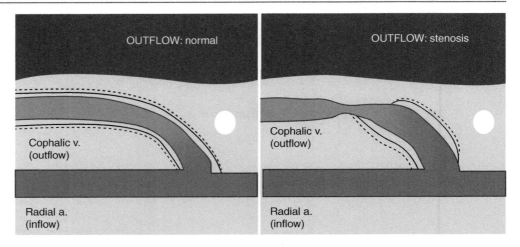

Table 14.1 Clinical findings associated with hyperpulsatile pulse and outflow stenosis

1. Arm elevation test – distended distal segment and flattened proximal segment
2. Thrill – absent over the distal segment and strong over the stenotic segment
3. Bruit – high pitched over the stenosis, occasionally with "whistle-like" character
4. Prolonged bleeding from needle puncture sites
5. Frequent dialysis venous alarms due to high venous pressures
6. Development of aneurysms – if left untreated

segment. The vibrations over the stenosis are strong and easily palpable and tend to disappear as one moves the finger proximally along the outflow segment. The segment distal to the stenosis may not have any vibrations as the segment is firm and pulsatile.

14.3.3 High-Pitched Bruit

A bruit is the sound accompanying a thrill. A normal bruit is soft pitched and continuous during the entire cardiac cycle. In case of outflow stenosis, the bruit tends to be high pitched in character and is primarily heard during the systolic phase of the cardiac cycle. The bruit over a severely stenosed segment may have a "whistle-like" character that is very easy to identify [3].

14.3.4 Prolonged Bleeding

Besides presenting with a bounding pulse in an AVF, patients with outflow segment stenosis can present with prolonged bleeding when the dialysis needles are withdrawn after completion of treatment. The bleeding from the needle puncture site generally stops if adequate and appropriate

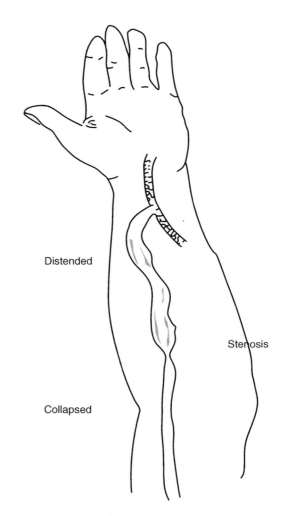

Fig. 14.2 Arm elevation test – outflow stenosis with distal distended segment and proximal collapsed segment (Reprint from www.fistulafirst.org)

pressure is applied for 10–15 min. In the absence of coagulation deficiencies (thrombocytopenia, therapeutic anticoagulation), if the bleeding continues for longer period, one needs to rule out outflow segment stenosis.

14.3.5 High Dialysis Venous Pressures

The venous pressures on the dialysis machine remain elevated despite proper needle placement and in the absence of any kinks in the extracorporeal dialysis circuit. In the USA, the average blood pump speed is maintained at 350–400 mL/min with a well-functioning AVF. The venous pressure recorded with this blood flow is generally less than 200 mmHg. In the presence of stenosis, the high venous pressures cause the venous safety alarm to trip frequently stopping the blood pump.

14.3.6 Development of Aneurysm

The constant elevated back pressure causes the venous segment distal to the stenosis to dilate and lead to formation of an aneurysm.

14.4 Treatment Approach

Stenosis tends to progress unless treated in a timely manner. The progression of stenosis can lead to decrease in blood flow and eventual thrombosis and potential loss of an AVF.

The algorithm in Fig. 14.3 outlines the common clinical approach to manage patients with hyperpulsatile AVF.

Regular and complete physical examination of an AVF before each dialysis therapy remains the corner stone for early diagnosis. Once the outflow stenosis is suspected on clinical examination, close attention to associated clinical findings can help confirm the clinical suspicion. The next step is to refer the patient for a fistulogram for possible endovascular intervention, which remains the current treatment of choice for most patients. Treating stenosis with percutaneous angioplasty involves minimal morbidity as compared to an open surgical treatment. Endovascular procedures can be safely performed in an outpatient setting with patient returning to regular dialysis treatment on the same day.

Venous outflow stenosis tends to recur and needs proper monitoring and surveillance protocols in place to prevent progression to thrombosis. Outflow stenosis that tends to recur at short interval (<3 months) or with significant (>30 %) elastic recoil of intimal tissue may need to be evaluated for possible stent placement. The interventionalist performing these invasive procedures needs to be well versed with the current guidelines from KDOQI regarding the indications for stent placement. An example of recurring stenosis in a

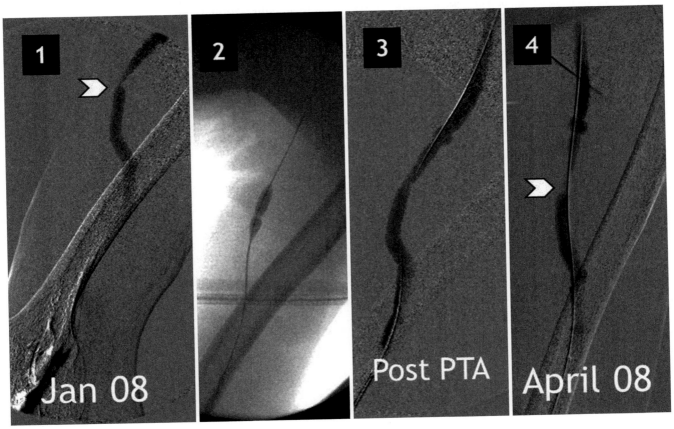

Fig. 14.3 Recurrent outflow stenosis (marked by *white chevron*) in a transposed basilic vein–brachial artery fistula in the right upper arm. *Panels 1, 2,* and *3* show the successful outcome of percutaneous angioplasty. *Panel 4* shows the recurrence of the stenosis in 3 months

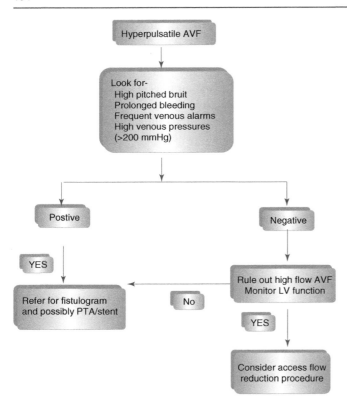

Fig. 14.4 Algorithm for management of hyperpulsatile arteriovenous fistula (AVF). *PTA* Percutaneous angioplasty, *LV* Left ventricular

transposed basilic vein–brachial artery AVF is shown in Fig. 14.4.

An upper arm AVF generally has a higher access blood flow compared to forearm AVF. The average blood flow reported in a study of 96 patients comparing access blood flow in the upper arm and forearm AVF was 1.58 vs. 0.94 L/min. An AVF with flows exceeding 2 L/min is considered to be a high-flow AVF. AVF with flows greater than 2 L/min can increase the risk of developing high-output cardiac failure [5].

Hyperpulsatile AVF without other clinical indications to suspect outflow stenosis can be due to high access flow. The measurement of AVF flow using either Doppler ultrasonography or transonic dilution technique can help confirm the diagnosis of high-flow AVF. Patients with underlying cardiac disease and poor left ventricular function with high-flow AVF may need further intervention to reduce the access blood flow. Patients at high risk of cardiac decompensation may benefit with procedures targeted towards reducing the access blood flow. In rare situation, an AVF may need to be ligated to preserve cardiac function.

References

1. Asif A, Leon C, Orozco-Vargas LC, Krishnamurthy G, Choi KL, Mercado C, Merrill D, Thomas I, Salman L, Artikov S, et al. Accuracy of physical examination in the detection of arteriovenous fistula stenosis. Clin J Am Soc Nephrol. 2007;2(6):1191–4.
2. Abreo K, Allon M, Asif A, Atray N, Besarab A, Dember LM, Dixon BS, DeVita M, Kaufman J, Murray BM, et al. Which direction is right for vascular access surveillance? A debate. Nephrol News Issues. 2010;24(7):30, 32, 34.
3. Fistula First Breakthrough Initiative www.fistulafirst.org/HealthcareProfessionals/FFBIChangeConcepts/ChangeConcept9.aspx; 2013. Accessed on 26 Oct 2013.
4. Lee T, Roy-Chaudhury P. Advances and new frontiers in the pathophysiology of venous neointimal hyperplasia and dialysis access stenosis. Adv Chronic Kidney Dis. 2009;16(5):329–38.
5. Basile C, Lomonte C, Vernaglione L, Casucci F, Antonelli M, Losurdo N. The relationship between the flow of arteriovenous fistula and cardiac output in haemodialysis patients. Nephrol Dial Transplant. 2008;23(1):282.

Approach to an Arteriovenous Access with a Faint Thrill

15

Tushar J. Vachharajani

A well-functioning dialysis vascular access is crucial for providing adequate hemodialysis treatment. Arteriovenous fistula (AVF) remains the preferred vascular access among all the other available options, which include arteriovenous graft (AVG), central venous catheters (CVC), or a hybrid access (combination of AVF-AVG or AVG-CVC). Low incidence of infections and thrombosis and lower maintenance costs are the primary reasons to prefer AVF over other vascular access types [1–4]. Once the initial challenge to attain a mature and functional AVF is overcome, maintaining its patency is relatively easy as compared to AVG.

Arteriovenous fistula is commonly created in the upper extremity either in the forearm or in the upper arm using native vessels. AVF in the lower extremity is uncommon but can be created in select group of patients. The common sites for AVF creation are listed in Table 15.1 [5, 6].

The clinical practice guidelines from the Kidney Dialysis Outcomes and Quality Initiatives recommend establishing a monitoring program for early identification of dysfunctional AVF [7]. Monitoring is defined as performing a detailed physical examination of the vascular access and remains a key component in the evaluation of an AVF. Physical examination is a simple, cost-effective, reproducible, and a validated tool that can be effectively utilized for the assessment of an AVF. Physical examination can be easily performed on every dialysis patient and is mandated in the USA as per 2008 requirements established by the Centers for Medicare and Medicaid Services [6, 8]. An experienced dialysis nurse can diagnose a mature AVF with 80 % accuracy by physical examination alone, a fact validated with ultrasound evaluation of 69 patients with a newly placed AVF [9].

Several studies have confirmed the value of this bedside tool in accurately diagnosing both the inflow and outflow stenoses in an AVF with 85–90 % sensitivity and 75–80 % specificity [10–12]. The physical examination performed by a nephrology fellow after 4 weeks of intense training has been shown to be 100 % sensitive and 78 % specific for inflow stenosis and 76 % sensitive and 68 % specific for outflow stenosis [13].

15.1 Components of an Arteriovenous Fistula

An AVF is a continuous circuit and not merely a surgical anastomosis between an artery and vein. The circuit starts at the heart and ends at the heart, and examining the entire circuit is absolutely essential to evaluate an AVF. Besides the right and left side of the heart, the other components of AVF are the entire arterial and venous system of the extremity and the central veins. An AVF can be examined in three segments (Fig. 15.1): (a) the inflow segment includes the feeding artery, the arteriovenous anastomosis, and the juxta-anastomotic region; (b) the main body includes the cannulation segment that is used to access an AVF during hemodialysis; and (c) the outflow segment includes the veins (including the central veins) proximal to the main body that return the blood to the heart.

15.2 Physical Examination of an Arteriovenous Fistula

15.2.1 Normal Findings

A normal AVF is soft and compressible. A distinct pulse with a continuous thrill is present at the inflow segment and along the majority of the body of the AVF. The thrill tends to dissipate as the palpating finger is moved proximally along the outflow segment. On auscultation the bruit is a low-pitch sound heard during the entire cardiac cycle. The bruit is loudest at the arterial anastomosis and fades along the outflow segment.

T.J. Vachharajani, MD, FACP, FASN
Nephrology Section, W. G. (Bill) Hefner Veterans Affairs Medical Center, Salisbury, NC, USA
e-mail: tushar.vachharajani@va.gov

A.S. Yevzlin et al. (eds.), *Interventional Nephrology*,
DOI 10.1007/978-1-4614-8803-3_15, © Springer Science+Business Media New York 2014

Table 15.1 Common sites for arteriovenous fistula creation

Site	Artery	Vein
Upper extremity – *forearm*		
Snuff-box	Radial	Forearm cephalic
Radiocephalic	Radial	Forearm cephalic
Transposed radio-basilic	Radial	Forearm basilic (transposed to volar surface)
Proximal forearm	Proximal radial	Deep forearm perforating
Transposed brachiocephalic	Brachial	Forearm cephalic (transposed as loop)
Upper extremity – *upper arm*		
Brachiocephalic	Brachial	Upper arm cephalic
Transposed brachiobasilic	Brachial	Transposed basilic
Lower extremity		
Saphenofemoral	Femoral	Saphenous

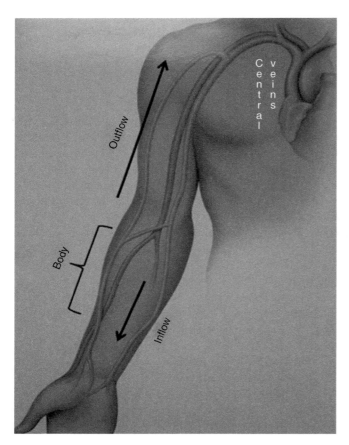

Fig. 15.1 Three segments of an arteriovenous fistula – inflow, body, and outflow

15.2.2 Augmentation Test

A feeble pulse at the inflow segment accompanied by a faint thrill is an abnormal finding that needs further evaluation

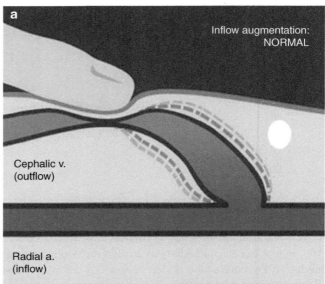

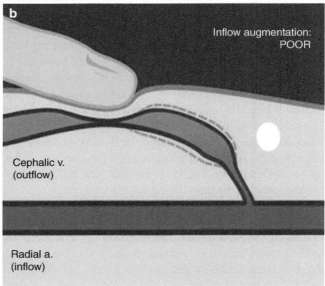

Fig. 15.2 Augmentation test – palpate the segment of the vein between the point of manual occlusion and the anastomosis. Panel **a** – Hyperpulsatile segment shown as distended and dashed segment with patent inflow segment. Panel **b** – Poor augmentation in presence of inflow stenosis

with an "augmentation" test. The test is performed by manually occluding the outflow in the main body of the AVF. The pulse in the inflow segment gets strong and forceful, also called "water hammer pulse" in a normal well-functioning AVF. In a dysfunctional AVF, the manual occlusion of the outflow fails to augment the inflow segment suggestive of inflow pathology. The augmentation test is schematically shown in Fig. 15.2. The thrill and bruit accompanying a feeble pulse are proportionately faint. Additionally, the bruit may be heard only during the systolic phase of the cardiac cycle [14].

Table 15.2 Etiological factors for a faint thrill in an arteriovenous fistula (AVF)

Cardiac
Poor left ventricular function and low ejection fraction
Congestive heart failure
Feeding arteries
Extensive atherosclerotic peripheral arterial disease
Localized stenosis in the proximal arteries
Stenosis at the arteriovenous anastomosis
Poor surgical technique in a new AVF
Neointimal hyperplasia in an established AVF
Stenosis in the juxta-anastomotic segment
"Swing-site" segment stenosis
Neointimal hyperplasia

15.3 Etiology of a Faint Thrill

A faint thrill on physical examination with failed augmentation test localizes the pathology to the inflow segment. The thrill is produced because of the turbulence created by the blood flowing from an artery with high pressure across the arteriovenous anastomosis into a thin-walled vein with low pressure. The high pressure in the artery is maintained by a well-functioning cardiac pump. Any pathology that can compromise any of these components will lead to a physical examination finding of weak pulse and faint thrill. The common etiological factors are listed in Table 15.2.

Hemodynamic status and uremic milieu are key components to maintaining AVF patency. A generally accepted clinical practice dogma is for patients to have a minimum systolic blood pressure of 100 mmHg for AVF to mature. Once an AVF matures, the incidence of AVF dysfunction, especially thrombosis, is frequent with hypotensive episodes during dialysis, highlighting the importance of hemodynamic factors [15].

In a newly created AVF, small vessel size and poor surgical technique often lead to early development of stenosis at the anastomosis site resulting in faint thrill on clinical examination [16]. "Swing site" is the segment of the vessel that is mobilized to create the anastomosis, which for radiocephalic and brachiocephalic fistulas is the juxta-anastomotic region. "Swing site" segment stenosis accounts for 65–70 % of early AVF maturation failures [17].

A fully matured AVF generally needs much less attention compared to AVG. Nevertheless, stenosis remains a major hurdle for long-term patency of AVF. Stenosis is frequently seen at the juxta-anastomotic region secondary to neointimal hyperplasia and smooth muscle cell proliferation. As yet, the exact pathophysiology behind neointimal hyperplasia remains unclear [18, 19].

15.4 Practical Approach for Timely Intervention

Inflow segment pathology can be identified with frequent physical examination of an AVF. A newly created AVF generally matures to support hemodialysis treatment in 8–12 weeks after the surgery. An AVF with blood flow of 500–600 ml/min and luminal diameter of 6 mm is considered to be mature enough to support regular dialysis treatments. KDOQI clinical practice guidelines recommend everyone involved in the care of dialysis patients to be proficient in the physical examination of an AVF. A simple algorithm based on whether an AVF is new or established can assist with identifying the problem sooner for timely intervention.

15.4.1 New AVF

A successful AVF undergoes changes that are predictable with incremental increase in blood flow and vessel size over a 4–6-week period after the surgery. All newly created AVFs need to be examined at least by 6 weeks to identify a failing maturity process. Further management and intervention in a newly created AVF with faint thrill is outlined in Fig. 15.3. The examination of a newly created AVF should be performed by a skilled personnel and include an "augmentation test." If the augmentation test is negative, further testing involving either an ultrasonography or an angiography can help identify the problem for timely intervention. Ultrasound evaluation is a noninvasive test but can help only with confirming the physical examination findings. Moreover, the test adds to the overall cost of care. Angiography is a definitive test that can help identify the stenosis and correct the pathology by simultaneously performing an angioplasty. Inflow stenosis is a very commonly diagnosed problem, and early intervention has helped salvage a great majority of early failed AVF. In a study of 100 cases with early AVF failure, 78 % had significant stenosis identified as an etiology for poor maturation. Percutaneous angioplasty was successful in 98 % of these cases, and 92 % of AVFs were successfully salvaged following intervention [20].

If the augmentation test is positive at 6 weeks, an AVF can be monitored regularly at 1–2-week intervals for a maximum of 12 weeks. If at the end of 12 weeks, an AVF remains immature, then further investigation with fistulography should be considered. Waiting longer than 12 weeks, hoping for an AVF to mature, is generally not in the patient's best interest. Active and aggressive intervention can help salvage these immature fistulas and shorten the duration of alternate vascular access, which is invariably a tunneled central venous catheter. If a fistulogram fails to identify any correctable pathology to assist with AVF maturation process, alternate

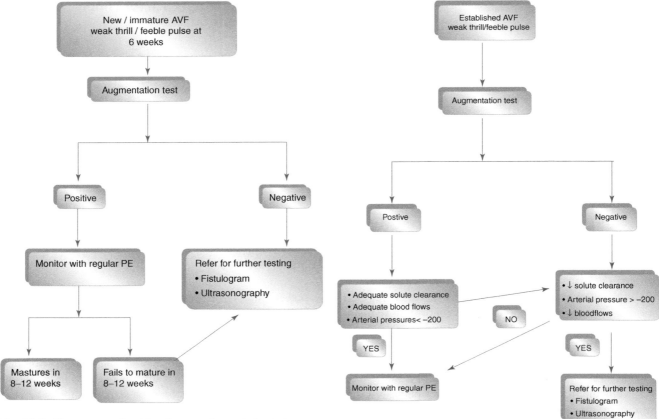

Fig. 15.3 Management algorithm for a newly created arteriovenous fistula with weak thrill or pulse

plans to create another permanent vascular access should be made immediately, and the patient needs to be referred back to the surgeon.

15.4.2 Established AVF

Hemodialysis process is complex and involves constant monitoring of the patient as well as the hemodialysis machine. A complete and thorough physical examination of an established AVF should be performed before each dialysis treatment by skilled dialysis personnel. During the treatment process, various settings on the hemodialysis machines, such as speed of the blood pump, and arterial and venous pressure monitoring are routinely performed by the dialysis staff. The quality of the dialysis treatment is judged by measuring the solute clearance from blood tests performed on a monthly basis. Figure 15.4 outlines the clinical approach for evaluating an established AVF with faint thrill. The algorithm incorporates the physical examination findings and other hemodialysis machine parameters and provides a practical approach to identify a failing AVF. The average blood flow prescribed for hemodialysis treatment in the USA is around 350–400 ml/min.

Fig. 15.4 Management algorithm for an established arteriovenous fistula with weak thrill or pulse

The dialysis arterial pressure recorded with 350–400 ml/min blood flow from a well-functioning AVF is generally less than negative 200 mmHg. Inflow segment stenosis is less than likely, if the prescribed blood flow is not achieved or the arterial pressure is more than negative 200, along with faint thrill at inflow.

A significant inflow segment stenosis is unable to support the high blood flows necessary to provide adequate dialysis treatment. The inability to achieve the prescribed blood flow during treatment leads to high arterial pressures on hemodialysis machine and frequent tripping of arterial alarm limits. The end result is high recirculation rate with inadequate solute clearances on monthly blood tests. Timely identification of these abnormal findings can assist with early intervention of the underlying stenosis. Vascular stenosis is a progressive process that will ultimately culminate in complete occlusion and thrombosis and eventual loss of flow. The next step in the management is confirming the physical examination findings with either an ultrasonography or an invasive angiography. Fistulogram remains the gold standard test to confirm stenosis. Once the diagnosis is confirmed, simultaneous angioplasty can help maintain the access patency.

15.5 Summary

Inflow segment stenosis in both new and established AVF can be diagnosed with a well-performed physical examination by skilled dialysis personnel. Regular monitoring of an AVF can help with early diagnosis for timely intervention to maintain access patency. A simple algorithm utilizing clues obtained from physical examination, blood flows and arterial pressures from dialysis machines, and monthly laboratory test results can effectively help diagnose inflow segment pathology.

References

1. Pisoni RL, Young EW, Dykstra DM, Greenwood RN, Hecking E, Gillespie B, Wolfe RA, Goodkin DA, Held PJ. Vascular access use in Europe and the United States: results from the DOPPS. Kidney Int. 2002;61(1):305–16.
2. Lee H, Manns B, Taub K, Ghali WA, Dean S, Johnson D, Donaldson C. Cost analysis of ongoing care of patients with end-stage renal disease: the impact of dialysis modality and dialysis access. Am J Kidney Dis. 2002;40(3):611–22.
3. Vascular Access Work Group. Clinical practice guidelines for vascular access. Am J Kidney Dis. 2006;48 Suppl 1:S248–73.
4. Allon M. Dialysis catheter-related bacteremia: treatment and prophylaxis. Am J Kidney Dis. 2004;44(5):779–91.
5. Vachharajani TJ. Atlas helps renal staff identify access problems. Nephrol News Issues. 2011;25(2):24.
6. Fistula First Breakthrough Initiative www.fistulafirst.org; 2013. Accessed on 26 Oct 2013.
7. Vascular Access 2006 Work Group. Clinical practice guidelines for vascular access. Am J Kidney Dis. 2006;48 Suppl 1:S176–247.
8. Abreo K, Allon M, Asif A, Atray N, Besarab A, Dember LM, Dixon BS, DeVita M, Kaufman J, Murray BM, et al. Which direction is right for vascular access surveillance? A debate. Nephrol News Issues. 2010;24(7):30.
9. Robbin ML, Chamberlain NE, Lockhart ME, Gallichio MH, Young CJ, Deierhoi MH, Allon M. Hemodialysis arteriovenous fistula maturity: US evaluation. Radiology. 2002;225(1):59–64.
10. Campos RP, Chula DC, Perreto S, Riella MC, do Nascimento MM. Accuracy of physical examination and intra-access pressure in the detection of stenosis in hemodialysis arteriovenous fistula. Semin Dial. 2008;21(3):269–73.
11. Asif A, Leon C, Orozco-Vargas LC, Krishnamurthy G, Choi KL, Mercado C, Merrill D, Thomas I, Salman L, Artikov S, et al. Accuracy of physical examination in the detection of arteriovenous fistula stenosis. Clin J Am Soc Nephrol. 2007;2(6):1191–4.
12. Coentrao L, Faria B, Pestana M. Physical examination of dysfunctional arteriovenous fistulae by non-interventionalists: a skill worth teaching. Nephrol Dial Transplant. 2012;27(5):1993–6.
13. Leon C, Asif A. Physical examination of arteriovenous fistulae by a renal fellow: does it compare favorably to an experienced interventionalist? Semin Dial. 2008;21(6):557–60.
14. Beathard GA. A practitioner's resource guide to physical examination of dialysis vascular access http://fistulafirst.org/Professionals/Literature.aspx; 2013. Accessed on 26 Oct 2013.
15. Chang TI, Paik J, Greene T, Desai M, Bech F, Cheung AK, Chertow GM. Intradialytic hypotension and vascular access thrombosis. J Am Soc Nephrol. 2011;22(8):1526–33.
16. Saran R, Elder SJ, Goodkin DA, Akiba T, Ethier J, Rayner HC, Saito A, Young EW, Gillespie BW, Merion RM, et al. Enhanced training in vascular access creation predicts arteriovenous fistula placement and patency in hemodialysis patients: results from the Dialysis Outcomes and Practice Patterns Study. Ann Surg. 2008;247(5):885–91.
17. Badero OJ, Salifu MO, Wasse H, Work J. Frequency of swing-segment stenosis in referred dialysis patients with angiographically documented lesions. Am J Kidney Dis. 2008;51(1):93–8.
18. Roy-Chaudhury P, Arend L, Zhang J, Krishnamoorthy M, Wang Y, Banerjee R, Samaha A, Munda R. Neointimal hyperplasia in early arteriovenous fistula failure. Am J Kidney Dis. 2007;50(5):782–90.
19. Lee T, Roy-Chaudhury P. Advances and new frontiers in the pathophysiology of venous neointimal hyperplasia and dialysis access stenosis. Adv Chronic Kidney Dis. 2009;16(5):329–38.
20. Asif A, Roy-Chaudhury P, Beathard GA. Early arteriovenous fistula failure: a logical proposal for when and how to intervene. Clin J Am Soc Nephrol. 2006;1(2):332–9.

Approach to an Arteriovenous Access with No Thrill, Bruit, or Pulse

16

Aris Q. Urbanes

16.1 Introduction

The patient with a hemodialysis vascular access that has no palpable thrill or pulse and no audible bruit presents the physician with at least two simultaneously critically important and time-sensitive issues: the resuscitation of the vascular access and the patient's need for ongoing life-sustaining renal replacement. Although it may intuitively appear that the former necessarily leads to the latter, the decision regarding how best to assure the immediate and more crucial need for ongoing dialysis often flavors how one approaches the vascular access. In this regard, the physician must employ his keen clinical sensibilities and judgment, understand the renal patient's history and physiology, and judiciously utilize the most appropriate approach to the problems at hand. The management of the clotted dialysis vascular access can be a most challenging but ultimately uniquely rewarding situation that a clinical interventionalist will face.

16.2 Clinical Considerations

In most circumstances, the patient is referred from the dialysis facility where the health-care professionals assessed the vascular access pre-cannulation and deemed it thrombosed. On occasion, however, they may have attempted cannulation and been unsuccessful in obtaining viable blood return from one or both needles. Invariably, there may have been prodromal symptoms or signs that presaged the clotting of the access. It is useful for the clinical interventionalist to be aware of these because it provides a clue as to the culprit lesion/s that one may anticipate during the procedure. It also aids one to know the duration during which renal replacement has been suboptimal or dysfunctional as this helps stratify procedural and sedation risks based on the patient's

biochemical and fluid disequilibrium. A patient who has been receiving suboptimal dialysis for a week may predictably have more or more severe biochemical derangements than a patient whose dialysis treatments have been uneventful up until the day of access thrombosis.

The clotted vascular access is not difficult to clinically diagnose. A color flow Doppler examination will verify the absence of flow through the access, but this is rarely needed. A sometimes confusing clinical finding is a thrill close to the artery-vein anastomosis in an autologous fistula. If the thrill comes, in fact, from the fistula and not transmitted from the artery, then one's approach might be simplified to a percutaneous angioplasty of a suspected downstream stenosis. Another useful physical finding is whether or not the fistula or the effluent venous drainage of a prosthetic arteriovenous graft is hard or tumescent suggesting extension of clot to this region. A greater length of soft or collapsible fistula portends of a smaller clot burden than a sizeable length of hard or turgid vein. Anticipating the amount and extent of thrombus that one might encounter would be beneficial in planning whether or not to utilize thrombolytics, the approach to removing thrombus, and in anticipating the likelihood of complications such as forward embolization of access thrombi to the pulmonary circulation. The clot burden in a typical AVG is between 1.5 and 4.7 mL [1] but in the fistula can vary from minimal to significantly larger volumes especially in the aneurysmal, serpentine brachiocephalic variety.

It is generally accepted that one's chances of a technical and clinically successful thrombectomy are highest when intervention is performed as soon as possible following the diagnosis. In a chronically thrombosed fistula, gaining entry to the vessel becomes progressively more challenging with time when the absence of blood flow causes it to collapse. This is readily apparent in the case when an angiographically collapsed drainage vein of a thrombosed AVF is found to be widely patent and of large caliber following restoration of flow in the upstream segment without any intervention performed on that specific segment of the collapsed vein.

A.Q. Urbanes, MD
Lifeline Vascular Access, Vernon Hills, IL, USA
e-mail: aris.urbanes@rmslifeline.com

A.S. Yevzlin et al. (eds.), *Interventional Nephrology*,
DOI 10.1007/978-1-4614-8803-3_16, © Springer Science+Business Media New York 2014

Successful endovascular intervention on fistulas thrombosed for as long as 9 days has been reported [2].

Thrombectomy procedures being performed successfully in cases of early graft failures suggest that intervention can be safely done as early as 15 days after creation using straightforward endovascular techniques including thrombolysis with 250,000 units of urokinase [3]. Of the two early occlusion grafts treated in this fashion, they experienced only one episode of extravasation at the tapered arterial end of the graft following thrombolysis and angioplasty with a 4 mm balloon, causing them to abort the procedure. Some investigators report acceptable cumulative patency rates of 74 % at 3 months and 68 % at 12 months; [3, 4] other investigators report dismal findings of median patency rates of 11 days in grafts age $\leq$30 days and 23 days in grafts 31–60 days [5] and 6-month cumulative patency rates of 26 and 44 % for grafts age $\leq$30 days and 31–60 days, respectively [6]. These values fall far below the recommended benchmarks [7] and have caused the authors to question the value of performing endovascular thrombectomy procedures in these early failure grafts. Since the analysis of their results, one group has now opted to channel all early thrombosed prosthetic grafts to surgery for creation of a new access [6].

Extrapolating these observations and conclusions to the native fistula is unwise and fraught with problems. The fistula, of course, requires a maturation process during which flow progressively increases culminating in the thickening of the walls and dilatation of the vessel lumen to accommodate the increased flow and pressure within the circuit. Apart from the surgical anastomoses healing and incorporating into surrounding tissue and the expected perioperative swelling around the tunneled graft, no such maturation process is required. Angiograms done on 1-week-old grafts have demonstrated incorporation of prosthetic into surrounding tissue [3]. The lesions involved in the thrombosis of the graft are different from those in a fistula. While the graft-vein anastomosis is the most common lesion encountered in clotted AVGs [8–11], the clotted fistula can have a variety of lesions or a combination of them [12–16]. In a series of over 100 immature AVF that thrombosed before they were ever used for dialysis, Miller reports a 79 % success rate at endovascular intervention [17]. Although the average age of the fistula at the time of thrombosis was 5.6 months, the average mid-fistula diameter was only 1.5 mm. Regardless of age, these were fistulas that had failed to mature. Following thrombectomy, there was an average maturation time of 46.4 days with 2.64 interventions required to attain maturity, including angioplasties, stent implantation, and coil embolization of side branches. Following maturation, these fistulas required an average of 2.78 interventions/access year to maintain patency and underwent 0.52 thrombectomies/access year. It has previously been reported [18] that fistulas that require two or more interventional procedures to attain suitability

for use behave differently from those that attain this state spontaneously or require only one procedure. Compared to fistulas requiring one or less procedures to attain maturity, those that require two or more have consistently reduced 1-, 2-, and 3-year cumulative survival and require more procedures to maintain patency. For these various different reasons, the experience and practice recommendations with early thrombosed prosthetic grafts should not be translated to fistulas without due caution.

16.3 Precautions

There are two contraindications to percutaneous thrombectomy of the dialysis vascular access: access infection and known right-to-left shunt (e.g., patent foramen ovale).

A known active infection of the thrombosed access could prove to be disastrous by disseminating infection in an otherwise contained area. It should be noted that a nonfunctioning, even chronically thrombosed, prosthetic AVG can be the source of bacteremia and sepsis [19, 20] in up to almost a third of cases seen by surgery for excision of the prosthetic [21].

A patent foramen ovale is seen in about 25 % of the general population over the age of 45 [22] and in 27 % of autopsies of otherwise healthy adults [23]. While right-to-left shunting is not necessarily problematic with a small PFO, the presence of pulmonary hypertension makes the likelihood of significant shunting much more of a concern. With pulmonary hypertension seen in as much as 40 % of hemodialysis patients, 14 % of whom have moderate to severe levels [24], one must be cognizant that a PFO that would otherwise not be problematic could, indeed, prove to be catastrophic. Unfortunately, there is no efficient and cost-effective way to monitor the confluence of these two processes, especially as the natural history of the patient's dialysis unfolds. Pulmonary hypertension is at least 2.7 times more likely to be seen in the hemodialysis patient than in the general population and 1.6 times more likely than the CKD pre-dialysis population [25].

16.4 General Approach

Regardless of specific technical methodology and tools employed, there are some fundamental tenets that one follows in order for the thrombectomy to be successful:

1. Identify and treat all lesions felt to be physiologically significant and have contributed to the dysfunction of the access.
2. Control and minimize risk of peripheral pulmonary or arterial embolization.
3. Keep circuit in the least prothrombotic state as reasonably possible.

Except in few and rare instances of hypercoagulability, insufficiently low perfusion pressures from marginal cardiovascular reserve or function, or an inordinately long access circuit relative to feeding arterial flows, an access will have thrombosed because of an anatomic inflow or outflow abnormality or a combination of these. Unless this pathology is found and fixed, or at the very least mitigated, the thrombectomy will not be technically or clinically successful. It is not enough to remove clot and restore flow without addressing the fundamental reasons why the dysfunction occurred to begin with.

Decisions regarding specific methodology that one will employ for a thrombectomy are flavored, among other things, by how most efficiently to get the job done successfully and in a cost-effective fashion but also how to minimize the risk of complications. One of the complications that one might anticipate is the risk for downstream pulmonary embolization. The risk is generally felt to be minimal because the clots are small in size. Paired pre- and post-procedure scintigraphy scans on 13 patients failed to show any difference [26] although larger studies using similar methodology of thrombectomy and scintigraphy revealed new perfusion defects in about 35–40 % of patients [27, 28]. In these series, all but 1 of 50 patients studied were symptomatic. Another interesting note is that baseline V/Q scan abnormalities were noted in over 70 % of patients [28].

Similar to pulmonary embolism, the incidence of this symptomatic arterial embolism is significantly lower than asymptomatic embolism. The incidence is quoted as between 0.4 and 0.6 % [29, 30]. Treatment is generally limited to the symptomatic patient and/or one whose quality and intensity of peripheral pulses have changed during the course of the procedure.

All implements employed during a thrombectomy procedure are potentially thrombogenic. The trauma of the procedure, especially against the vessel wall, and its attendant biochemical and hormonal effects also contribute to the prothrombotic state of the circuit. Systemic anticoagulation is typically given at the start of a procedure, although we have successfully performed thrombectomies without the benefit of heparin in patients with a heparin-induced thrombocytopenia. The brisk and robust return of blood flow to the circuit has an antithrombotic effect but can be attenuated by small-caliber vessels that are occluded by sheaths and other similar implements and the wall trauma of instrumentation. Once flow is restored, the physician must move quickly but deliberately and decidedly and address all pathologic lesions that are felt to have caused or contributed to the thrombosis.

16.5 Specific Approach

Although there are variations dictated by practice or by the particular case at hand, the approach to the thrombosed prosthetic graft follows the steps in Table 16.1.

Table 16.1 Steps in thrombectomy of a prosthetic dialysis graft

1. Cannulate graft with intent to gain access to the venous effluent tract
2. Cross vein-graft anastomosis
3. Perform central venous angiography ± recanalization/angioplasty of central venous occlusion
4. Administer anticoagulation and sedation analgesics if not already done
5. Treat clot within graft and within effluent vessels
6. Perform venous angioplasty of vein-graft anastomosis
7. Cannulate graft with intent to gain access to the arterial inflow tract
8. Remove arterial fibrin-platelet plug
9. Evaluate and address inflow pathology
10. Evaluate and address outflow pathology
11. Completion angiography of entire circuit

16.5.1 Initial Cannulation

The initial step should be to enter the graft and obtain access to the venous outflow tract and central venous system. While it is fairly easy to determine the direction of the cannulation needle in an open graft, in a straight configuration graft or a graft that has been studied before and for which images and notes are available, one must rely on usual or typical graft architecture. The loop AVG typically has its venous anastomosis/loop at the lateral aspect of the arm, while its arterial anastomosis/loop is at the medial aspect.

16.5.2 Cross the Vein-Graft Anastomosis

If one is unable to cross this anastomosis, then there is no purpose in restoring arterial inflow for which no outflow is available. Several standard endovascular techniques may be called upon if the guidewire will not traverse the anastomosis readily. Remember also that lesions may be eccentric or may have an orifice that allows wire passage more readily from one direction rather than another. It might be necessary to cannulate the predicted draining vein and pass a guidewire through the vein-graft anastomosis in a retrograde fashion. If this approach is necessary, an angioplasty of this area will allow much easier guidewire passage through an antegrade direction should draining or central venous angioplasty be required.

16.5.3 Perform Central Venography

As much as 30 % of dysfunctional dialysis accesses have a physiologically significant central venous stenosis [31–33]. These lesions may be suspected on the basis of clinical history or physical examination. When central occlusions are diagnosed and are felt to be clinically significant based on clinical data, these will need to be treated before restoring flow to the dialysis access; otherwise, the improved/increased flow will cause significant hemodynamic effects centrally that will result in arm, facial, neck, or breast swelling; dilatation of superficial veins; or other similar changes reflective of flow obstruction.

16.5.4 Administer Medications

Depending on the point of service and specific practice setup, the anticoagulation and sedation/analgesia medications may be administered peripherally by the appropriate licensed health-care professional. We have chosen to have the interventionalist administer these medications in an open peripheral or central vein after having been able to cross the vein-graft anastomosis with a guidewire and ensuring that the central veins are not occluded or, if they are, have been successfully treated. This also reduces the oftentimes arduous task of finding and maintaining an intravenous line in the patient's contralateral arm. Standard heparin doses of between 2,000 and 5,000 IU are given at the start of the case, and this can be augmented with additional doses as clinically needed or titrated to a target ACT, generally ≥250 s.

Moderate sedation in the form of midazolam and fentanyl are given. In a series of over 12,000 patients treated, Beathard found the median dose of midazolam to be 3.0 mg and fentanyl 75 μg for most interventional cases, including thrombectomies [34]. These doses were only slightly less when used in combination rather than singly. With these doses, even high-risk patients tolerated the procedures without incident, and pain levels were adequately managed. A trained RN is given the responsibility of monitoring the patient and the response to sedation/analgesia.

16.5.5 Treat Clot

As mentioned earlier, the amount of clot involved in a typical graft thrombectomy is typically around 5 mL. In a graft that is studded with pseudoaneurysms, the clot volume may be larger, but more importantly, the organized clot that is often laminated and adherent to the graft wall is removed only with the use of thrombectomy devices. In the vast majority of cases, maceration of the clot with an angioplasty balloon, thromboaspiration through a sheath or catheter, and use of locally instilled tPA are sufficient for clot removal. But in those cases where tenacious adherent clot remains and the clinical interventionalist feels it is necessary to remove, direct wall contact, rheolytic, or hydrodynamic mechanical devices are available (see Table 16.2). In our experience, these are not often necessary.

Table 16.2 Examples of some mechanical devices for access thrombectomy

Direct wall contact	Argon Medical Cleaner®
	Arrow-Trerotola® percutaneous thrombectomy device (PTD)
	Datascope ProLumen®
	Catañeda® OTW Brush
Hydrodynamic	eV3 Helix Clot Buster® (formerly Amplatz thrombectomy device)
	eV3 X-Sizer®
	Edwards Thromex®
Rheolytic	Boston-Scientific Oasis Thrombectomy System®
	Cordis Hydrolyser®
	Medrad Medical Angiojet® (AVX)
	Spectranetics ThromCat® Thrombectomy Catheter System

Many studies have evaluated the various devices [29, 35–45], and it is apparent that the success and patency rates are unrelated to the device but more to treating the underlying pathology leading up to the stenosis. Some studies have also shown a tendency to higher complication rates when devices are utilized, but this could well be related to a learning curve in the use of the device.

Alteplase (rt-PA, Genentech, South San Francisco, CA) is employed by some, but the indications and doses vary widely. The "lyse-and-wait" first described in 1997 [46] remains popular because it is simple, inexpensive, and easy to follow. We have inconsistently used this method, but when we have the doses have been between 2 and 4 mg of rt-PA. Others have reported similar doses of rt-PA [47, 48]. Using a multipurpose angiographic catheter or via the side arm of the sheath depending on location of cannulation, 2 mg of rt-PA is delivered close to the venous anastomosis and another 2 mg close to the arterial anastomosis. We dilute the drug in only 2 mL of sterile water in order to minimize the volume delivered to a closed circuit and subsequent risk of arterial embolization. A small final volume of flush sterile water is used to empty the catheter or sheath of its "dead space." During injection of the lytic, we ensure that arterial embolization is minimized by digital manual pressure on the arterial inflow. The amount of time that the lytic is allowed to dwell varies, but a "no wait" technique compared to longer dwell times suggests that there is no difference in success or complication rates and similar 3-month primary, primary-assisted, and reanastomosis rates but statistically significant lower procedure and radiation times [49].

Thromboaspiration with or without maceration of the clot with an angioplasty balloon catheter is performed to remove as much clot as possible. Although the exact sequence of when this is performed varies between operators, the aim is to extract as much clot as possible and minimizing downstream embolization. This should therefore be done before there is both free and unimpeded flow of blood from arterial inflow to venous outflow. Some operators would do this after restoring arterial inflow but before addressing the venous anastomotic stenosis, while others would do this after angioplasty of the venous anastomosis but before dislodging the arterial platelet-fibrin plug.

16.5.6 Angioplasty of Vein-Graft Anastomosis

Since most dysfunctional dialysis prosthetic grafts will have the critical culprit lesion at the vein-graft anastomosis [50–53], some operators will preemptively perform an angioplasty in this area before restoring arterial inflow. Most prosthetic grafts used for hemodialysis access are 6 mm diameter, and the appropriately sized angioplasty balloon catheter used will be a 7 or 8 mm diameter.

16.5.7 Remove Arterial Platelet-Fibrin Plug

Following the second cannulation directed towards the arterial inflow, the fibrin plug at the arterial anastomosis is removed using a compliant Fogarty embolectomy catheter. They are both over-the-wire and plain versions of the catheter. The choice of one over the other depends on operator preference but should be flavored by anatomy, amount of manipulation needed to cross the anastomosis, and the security obtained by having a wire across a treated area. The arterial plug is a whitish dense tissue made up of fibrin and platelets and may be aspirated out of the side arm of the arterial sheath. If performed under fluoroscopy, the compliant balloon will be noted to deform as it crosses the anastomosis and dislodges the plug. This motion is performed until the plug is retrieved, until the inflated balloon pulls back with minimal resistance, or until no further clots are aspirated.

16.5.8 Evaluate Arterial Inflow

An antegrade arteriogram is performed in order to evaluate the inflow, the artery-graft anastomosis, the juxta-anastomotic stenosis, and the arterial limb of the graft. Additionally, if the patient develops symptoms consistent with a distal arterial embolus and/or peripheral pulses change in quality, the arteriogram should also evaluate the more distal arterial circulation. Appropriate treatment of the symptomatic embolus should be promptly initiated. How far cephalad the arterial inflow must be evaluated is dictated primarily by one's degree of suspicion based on clinical presentation, history, and physical examination. A recurrently thrombosed or dysfunctional graft without compelling evidence for outflow stenosis and hemodynamic or systemic prothrombotic diathesis should

raise one's suspicion for an inflow pathology. A dedicated and deliberate evaluation of the inflow circuit should then ensue and identified lesions appropriately treated.

16.5.9 Evaluate Venous Outflow

At this point, circulation has been restored to the graft, and attention is turned to the efferent arm of the circuit. Angiography of the entire graft, the vein-graft anastomosis, and the venous effluent tract is performed and identified lesions appropriately treated. High-pressure balloon angioplasty with a 1–2 mm oversize of the balloon relative to the non-stenotic diameter of the vessel is standard. Some lesions will necessitate ultra-high-pressure balloon angioplasty and endovascular stent placement. The indications, methodology, and precautions for stent placement in the setting of an access thrombectomy are no different than in a non-thrombosed access. These are covered in another section of this book.

16.5.10 Perform Completion Angiogram

Once radiologic and clinical parameters indicate that robust flow has been restored to the graft, a final completion angiogram is performed to assure that all physiologically significant lesions have been adequately treated and that there are no complications for which further treatment is required. Based on the completion angiogram, additional studies or surgical referrals may be considered. Endovascular treatment is an essential and important aspect of dialysis vascular access care but should not supplant surgical evaluation and management. Indeed, the most successful vascular access programs have seamlessly integrated endovascular and surgical approaches at all stages of care.

16.6 Autogenous Fistula Thrombectomy

We have described the prototypic thrombectomy approach to a prosthetic dialysis graft. The approach to the thrombosed autogenous fistula, however, is more nuanced and will require a greater degree of operator technical proficiency and clinical acumen.

There are a few important differences between the prosthetic graft and the autogenous fistula that make the approach to thrombectomy different.

16.6.1 Anatomy

While the anatomy of the anastomoses and the inflow/outflow arms are fairly straightforward for a graft, they are variable and may be quite complex for the fistula, for example, the fistula may have a radial arterial anastomosis with a transposed basilic vein or a translocated vein. A proximal radial artery may be anastomosed to the median antebrachial vein which will drain off cephalad and caudad to a number of different veins.

16.6.2 Anastomosis

The prosthetic graft has an artery-graft and a vein-graft anastomoses. Occasionally, one may encounter a graft-graft anastomosis if a patch angioplasty or a bridge graft may have been part of a surgical revision. The autogenous fistula, however, has only the artery-vein anastomosis. In the absence of flow, predicting anatomy of the anastomosis can be daunting.

16.6.3 Lesions

While most dysfunctional grafts will exhibit critical stenosis of the venous anastomosis, the distribution of culprit lesions in the fistula is far more variable [53–55]. A review of the dialysis treatment record with a focused evaluation of laboratory and clinical data may prepare the physician by anticipating the location of the lesions. Nonetheless, even after flow is restored to the fistula, an assessment of the radiologic and clinical record to explain the thrombosis of the fistula may remain challenging.

16.6.4 Thrombectomy

While the graft will almost always require removal of the arterial fibrin-platelet plug in order to restore flow, the fistula may not always require this maneuver. Sometimes, an angioplasty of an occlusive artery-vein or juxta-anastomotic stenosis may be sufficient to restore flow. This is particularly true of the radiocephalic fistula where the arterial inflow pathology tends to be more prominent [53–55].

16.6.5 Angioplasty

Thrombosed fistulas can vary from size from the immature to the mega-fistula. In the absence of flow, it becomes more difficult to predict the diameter of the vessels and makes angioplasty more complicated. One can size the balloons for the central vessels based on expected normal values [56], but there can be a wide variation in the presence of high-flow fistulas.

16.6.6 Clot Volume

The volume of thrombus within the graft is fairly predictable and is fortunately not typically a large amount. However, the clot burden in a fistula can vary widely, especially with the mega-fistulas. In these instances, the risk of embolization to the pulmonary circulation is significantly higher and must factor in one's approach to the thrombectomy. When the clot burden is predicted to be higher, one must attempt to protect the pulmonary circulation by removing as much clot as possible before restoring flow. Use of thrombolytics, with or without a mechanical device, would be an option in this regard.

16.7   HeRO® Graft Thrombectomy

The HeRO® graft (Hemodialysis Reliable Outflow, Hemosphere, Eden Prairie, MN) is a hybrid device approved by the FDA for dialysis-dependent patients whose vascular options have been exhausted. One such indication is central venous stenosis that is poorly responsive to endovascular therapy or is rapidly recurrent and patient is deemed too high risk for surgical bypass. There is a single anastomosis of the 6 mm ID graft to the feeding artery, but the venous end is a length of nitinol-reinforced silicone-coated catheter with an ID of 5 mm and opens to the mid-right atrium. The circuit can thrombose because of poor perfusion pressures but intra-graft or artery-graft stenoses contributing to or causing thrombosis have also been seen.

The findings on examination of a thrombosed HeRO® graft are similar to that of a prosthetic graft. Palpation will show absence of thrill or pulse and auscultation, the absence of bruit. Barring any graft infection, the percutaneous thrombectomy of this device is fairly simple and straightforward and generally follows the same steps as outlined earlier.

The differences in approach between the thrombectomy of the prosthetic graft and the HeRO® graft are the following.

16.7.1 Removal of Thrombus

Using an 80 cm 3 Fr OTW Fogarty catheter of a 5×40 angioplasty balloon catheter, the thrombus is drawn from the tip of the catheter in the mid-RA distally to the venous cannulation site in the graft segment. It is suggested that the balloon be followed under fluoroscopy while being pulled to assure that the untethered end of the HeRO® device is not mobilized out of its intended location. If the tip of the catheter is dragged by the Fogarty or angioplasty balloon, deflating the balloon to less than nominal pressure and size will alleviate this problem.

16.7.2 Angioplasty

Because there is no graft-vein anastomosis, the intra-artery, artery-graft, and intra-graft lesions are the lesions one must evaluate as possibly causing or contributing to the thrombosis. Low flow from marginal cardiac function, poor perfusion pressures, or other similar systemic problems should also be considered.

16.7.3 Anticoagulation

Empirically, the amount of heparin needed for the thrombectomy of this device is typically less than that of a prosthetic graft.

16.8 Summary

The thrombectomy of a dialysis prosthetic graft or autogenous fistula demands of the clinical interventionalist a command of a variety of techniques and tools, coupled with an understanding of the patient's specific clinical history and presentation. The thrombosis of a vascular access is the culmination of progressively critical anatomic and physiologic aberrations that must be identified and corrected if the intervention is expected to be durable. The physician's ability to return the patient to optimum dialysis vascular care depends on a meticulous and assiduous search for and correction of these factors.

References

1. Winkler TA, Trerotola SO, Davidson DD, Milgrom ML. Study of thrombus from thrombosed hemodialysis access grafts. Radiology. 1995;197(2):461–5.
2. Liang H-L, Pan H-B, Chung H-M, et al. Restoration of thrombosed Brescia-Cimino dialysis fistulas by using percutaneous transluminal angioplasty. Radiology. 2002;223(2):339–44.
3. Shemesh D, Goldin I, Berelowitz D, Zaghal I, Olsha O. Thrombolysis for early failure of prosthetic arteriovenous access. J Vasc Surg. 2008;47(3):585–90.
4. Olsha O, Berelowitz D, Goldin I, Zaghal I, Shemesh D. Interventions for maintenance in hemodialysis grafts with early failure. J Vasc Interv Radiol. 2011;22(10):1493.
5. Mudunuri V, O'Neal JC, Allon M. Thrombectomy of arteriovenous dialysis grafts with early failure: is it worthwhile? Semin Dial. 2010;23(6):634–7.
6. Yurkovic A, Cohen RD, Mantell MP, et al. Outcomes of thrombectomy procedures performed in hemodialysis grafts with early failure. J Vasc Interv Radiol. 2011;22(3):317–24.
7. Vascular Access Work Group. Clinical practice guidelines for vascular access. Am J Kidney Dis. 2006;48 Suppl 1:S176–247.
8. Beathard GA. Successful treatment of the chronically thrombosed dialysis access graft: resuscitation of dead grafts. Semin Dial. 2006;19(5):417–20.
9. Chan MG, Miller FJ, Valji K, Kuo MD. Evaluation of expanded polytetrafluoroethylene-covered stents for the treatment of venous outflow stenosis in hemodialysis access grafts. J Vasc Interv Radiol. 2011;22(5):647–53.
10. Green LD, Lee DS, Kucey DS. A metaanalysis comparing surgical thrombectomy, mechanical thrombectomy, and pharmacomechanical thrombolysis for thrombosed dialysis grafts. J Vasc Surg. 2002;36(5):939–45.
11. Kakisis JD, Avgerinos E, Giannakopoulos T, Moulakakis K, Papapetrou A, Liapis CD. Balloon angioplasty vs nitinol stent placement in the treatment of venous anastomotic stenoses of hemodialysis grafts after surgical thrombectomy. J Vasc Surg. 2012;55(2):472–8.
12. Anderson CB, Gilula LA, Sicard GA, Etheredge EE. Venous angiography of subcutaneous hemodialysis fistulas. Arch Surg. 1979;114(11):1320–5.
13. Asif A, Roy-Chaudhury P, Beathard GA. Early arteriovenous fistula failure: a logical proposal for when and how to intervene. Clin J Am Soc Nephrol. 2006;1(2):332–9.
14. Basile C, Ruggieri G, Vernaglione L, Montanaro A, Giordano R. The natural history of autogenous radio-cephalic wrist arteriovenous fistulas of haemodialysis patients: a prospective observational study. Nephrol Dial Transplant. 2004;19(5):1231–6.
15. De Marco Garcia LP, Davila-Santini LR, Feng Q, Calderin J, Krishnasastry KV, Panetta TF. Primary balloon angioplasty plus balloon angioplasty maturation to upgrade small-caliber veins (<3 mm) for arteriovenous fistulas. J Vasc Surg. 2010;52(1):139–44.
16. Coentrão L, Bizarro P, Ribeiro C, Neto R, Pestana M. Percutaneous treatment of thrombosed arteriovenous fistulas: clinical and economic implications. Clin J Am Soc Nephrol. 2010;5(12):2245–50.
17. Miller GA, Hwang W, Preddie D, Khariton A, Savransky Y. Percutaneous salvage of thrombosed immature arteriovenous fistulas. Semin Dial. 2011;24(1):107–14.
18. Lee T, Ullah A, Allon M, et al. Decreased cumulative access survival in arteriovenous fistulas requiring interventions to promote maturation. Clin J Am Soc Nephrol. 2011;6(3):575–81.
19. Nassar GM, Ayus JC. Clotted arteriovenous grafts: a silent source of infection. Semin Dial. 2000;13(1):1–3.
20. Ryan SV, Calligaro KD, Scharff J, Dougherty MJ. Management of infected prosthetic dialysis arteriovenous grafts. J Vasc Surg. 2004;39(1):73–8.
21. Schild AF, Simon S, Prieto J, Raines J. Single-center review of infections associated with 1,574 consecutive vascular access procedures. Vasc Endovascular Surg. 2003;37(1):27–31.
22. Meissner I, Whisnant JP, Khandheria BK, et al. Prevalence of potential risk factors for stroke assessed by transesophageal echocardiography and carotid ultrasonography: the SPARC study. Stroke Prevention: assessment of risk in a community. Mayo Clin Proc. 1999;74(9):862–9.
23. Torbey E, Thompson PD. Patent foramen ovale: thromboembolic structure or incidental finding? Conn Med. 2011;75(2):97–105.
24. Yigla M, Abassi Z, Reisner SA, Nakhoul F. Pulmonary hypertension in hemodialysis patients: an unrecognized threat. Semin Dial. 2006;19(5):353–7.
25. Harp RJ, Stavropoulos SW, Wasserstein AG, Clark TW. Pulmonary hypertension among end-stage renal failure patients following hemodialysis access thrombectomy. Cardiovasc Intervent Radiol. 2005;28(1):17–22.
26. Petronis JD, Regan F, Briefel G, Simpson PM, Hess JM, Contoreggi CS. Ventilation-perfusion scintigraphic evaluation of pulmonary clot burden after percutaneous thrombolysis of clotted hemodialysis access grafts. Am J Kidney Dis. 1999;34(2):207–11.
27. Smits H, Van Rijk P, Van Isselt J, Mali W, Koomans H, Blankestijn P. Pulmonary embolism after thrombolysis of hemodialysis grafts. J Am Soc Nephrol. 1997;8(9):1458–61.
28. Kinney TB, Valji K, Rose SC, et al. Pulmonary embolism from pulse-spray pharmacomechanical thrombolysis of clotted

hemodialysis grafts: urokinase versus heparinized saline. J Vasc Interv Radiol. 2000;11(9):1143–52.

29. Beathard GA, Welch BR, Maidment HJ. Mechanical thrombolysis for the treatment of thrombosed hemodialysis access grafts. Radiology. 1996;200(3):711–6.

30. Kim DH, Goo DE, Yang SB, Moon C, Choi DL. Endovascular management of immediate procedure-related complications of failed hemodialysis access recanalization. Korean J Radiol. 2005;6(3):185–95.

31. Kim CY, Mirza RA, Bryant JA, et al. Central veins of the chest: evaluation with time-resolved MR angiography. Radiology. 2008;247(2):558–66.

32. Kotoda A, Akimoto T, Kato M, et al. Central venous stenosis among hemodialysis patients is often not associated with previous central venous catheters. ASAIO J. 2011;57(5):439–43.

33. Rajan DK, Chennepragada SM, Lok CE, et al. Patency of endovascular treatment for central venous stenosis: is there a difference between dialysis fistulas and grafts? J Vasc Interv Radiol. 2007;18(3):353–9.

34. Beathard GA, Litchfield T. Effectiveness and safety of dialysis vascular access procedures performed by interventional nephrologists. Kidney Int. 2004;66(4):1622–32.

35. Bücker A, Schmitz-Rode T, Vorwerk D, Günther RW. Comparative in vitro study of two percutaneous hydrodynamic thrombectomy systems. J Vasc Interv Radiol. 1996;7(3):445–9.

36. Beathard GA. Mechanical versus pharmacomechanical thrombolysis for the treatment of thrombosed dialysis access grafts. Kidney Int. 1994;45(5):1401–6.

37. Bush RL, Lin PH, Lumsden AB. Management of thrombosed dialysis access: thrombectomy versus thrombolysis. Semin Vasc Surg. 2004;17(1):32–9.

38. Heye S, Van Kerkhove F, Claes K, Maleux G. Pharmacomechanical thrombectomy with the Castañeda brush catheter in thrombosed hemodialysis grafts and native fistulas. J Vasc Interv Radiol. 2007;18(11):1383–8.

39. Littler P, Cullen N, Gould D, Bakran A, Powell S. AngioJet thrombectomy for occluded dialysis fistulae: outcome data. Cardiovasc Intervent Radiol. 2009;32(2):265–70.

40. Rocek M, Peregrin JH, Lasovicková J, Krajíčková D, Slavíoková M. Mechanical thrombolysis of thrombosed hemodialysis native fistulas with use of the arrow-trerotola percutaneous thrombolytic device: our preliminary experience. J Vasc Interv Radiol. 2000;11(9):1153–8.

41. Sahni V, Kaniyur S, Malhotra A, et al. Mechanical thrombectomy of occluded hemodialysis native fistulas and grafts using a hydrodynamic thrombectomy catheter: preliminary experience. Cardiovasc Intervent Radiol. 2005;28(6):714–21.

42. Shatsky JB, Berns JS, Clark TWI, et al. Single-center experience with the Arrow-Trerotola Percutaneous Thrombectomy Device in the management of thrombosed native dialysis fistulas. J Vasc Interv Radiol. 2005;16(12):1605–11.

43. Stainken BF. Mechanical thrombectomy: basic principles, current devices, and future directions. Tech Vasc Interv Radiol. 2003;6(1):2–5.

44. Vorwerk D, Schurmann K, Müller-Leisse C, et al. Hydrodynamic thrombectomy of haemodialysis grafts and fistulae: results of 51 procedures. Nephrol Dial Transplant. 1996;11(6):1058–64.

45. Zaleski GX, Funaki B, Kenney S, Lorenz JM, Garofalo R. Angioplasty and bolus urokinase infusion for the restoration of function in thrombosed Brescia-Cimino dialysis fistulas. J Vasc Interv Radiol. 1999;10(2 Pt 1):129–36.

46. Cynamon J, Lakritz PS, Wahl SI, Bakal CW, Sprayregen S. Hemodialysis graft declotting: description of the "lyse and wait" technique. J Vasc Interv Radiol. 1997;8(5):825–9.

47. Schon D, Mishler R. Pharmacomechanical thrombolysis of natural vein fistulas: reduced dose of TPA and long-term follow-up. Semin Dial. 2003;16(3):272–5.

48. Tseke P, Kalyveza E, Politis E, et al. Thrombolysis with alteplase: a non-invasive treatment for occluded arteriovenous fistulas and grafts. Artif Organs. 2011;35(1):58–62.

49. Almehmi A, Broce M, Wang S. Thrombectomy of prosthetic dialysis grafts using mechanical plus "no-wait lysis" approach requires less procedure time and radiation exposure. Semin Dial. 2011;24(6):694–7.

50. Anain P, Shenoy S, O'Brien-Irr M, Harris LM, Dryjski M. Balloon angioplasty for arteriovenous graft stenosis. J Endovasc Ther. 2001;8(2):167–72.

51. Umphrey HR, Lockhart ME, Abts CA, Robbin ML. Dialysis grafts and fistulae: planning and assessment. Ultrasound Clin. 2011;6(4):477–89.

52. Turmel-Rodrigues L. Stenosis and thrombosis in haemodialysis fistulae and grafts: the radiologist's point of view. Nephrol Dial Transplant. 2004;19(2):306–8.

53. Asif A, Gadalean FN, Merrill D, et al. Inflow stenosis in arteriovenous fistulas and grafts: a multicenter, prospective study. Kidney Int. 2005;67(5):1986–92.

54. Nassar GM, Nguyen B, Rhee E, Achkar K. Endovascular treatment of the "failing to mature" arteriovenous fistula. Clin J Am Soc Nephrol. 2006;1(2):275–80.

55. Beathard GA, Arnold P, Jackson J, Litchfield T. Aggressive treatment of early fistula failure. Kidney Int. 2003;64(4):1487–94.

56. Salik E, Daftary A, Tal MG. Three-dimensional anatomy of the left central veins: implications for dialysis catheter placement. J Vasc Interv Radiol. 2007;18(3):361–4.

Approach to Patient with Arteriovenous Access Presenting with Hand Pain

17

Chieh Suai Tan, Diego A. Covarrubias, and Steven Wu

17.1 Introduction

A dialysis patient presenting with hand pain ipsilateral to the arteriovenous (AV) access has a number of differential diagnoses. The etiology can be broadly divided into neurogenic, vascular, and musculoskeletal in nature (see Table 17.1). A detailed history coupled with physical examination will often reveal the etiology of the hand pain. Additional imaging studies are often required to confirm the diagnosis and planning of treatment. We will focus our discussion on ischemic monomelic neuropathy (IMN) and distal hypoperfusion ischemic syndrome (DHIS), which are two important entities related to vascular access that an interventional nephrologist needs to be aware of.

17.2 History Taking

The chronology of hand pain in relation to AV access creation is paramount in history taking. The type of pain, exacerbating factors, and its associated symptoms are also crucial to elucidating the etiology of hand pain.

C.S. Tan, MBBS • D.A. Covarrubias, MD
Vascular Interventional Radiology,
Massachusetts General Hospital, Harvard Medical School,
55 Fruit Street, Boston, MA 02114, USA

Department of Radiology, Massachusetts General Hospital,
Harvard Medical School, 55 Fruit Street, Boston, MA 02114, USA

S. Wu, MD (✉)
Vascular Interventional Radiology,
Massachusetts General Hospital, Harvard Medical School,
55 Fruit Street, Boston, MA 02114, USA

Department of Medicine, Massachusetts General Hospital,
Harvard Medical School, 55 Fruit Street, Boston, MA 02114, USA

Department of Radiology, Massachusetts General Hospital,
Harvard Medical School, 55 Fruit Street, Boston, MA 02114, USA
e-mail: swu1@partners.org

17.2.1 Neurogenic Pain

Neurogenic pain is usually described as a deep and burning sensation with associated paresthesia and numbness. It can arise as a result of ischemic neuropathy, entrapment, or polyneuropathy. Although each entity has its own distinct characteristics, differentiation of these neuropathies can be difficult in reality as overlapping etiologies may be present in the same patient.

Pain arising from ischemic neuropathy is usually unilateral and can appear to be out of proportion to the physical findings. One of the most feared complications resulting from AV access creation is neurogenic pain secondary to IMN.

The symptoms of IMN classically present immediately after surgery and tend to affect female, diabetic patients with a history of peripheral vascular disease or neuropathy, who have just undergone brachial artery-based access creation [1–4]. In addition to pain, significant sensory loss and dysesthesia in the distribution of all three forearm nerves is usually present, and the impairment is most prominent distally [5]. In severe cases, weakness and paralysis of the muscles of the forearm and hand can also occur [5].

Neurogenic pain secondary to nerve entrapment tends to be better localized and follows the distribution of the affected nerve. Carpal tunnel syndrome is common in chronic dialysis patients. The symptoms are usually bilateral and predate AV access surgery.

Symptoms secondary to uremic and/or diabetic polyneuropathy are usually bilateral and follow a "glove and stocking" distribution. They are usually present before AV access surgery and can confound the diagnosis of IMN.

17.2.2 Vascular Pain

Flow diversion as a consequence of AV creation can result in DHIS or "arterial steal syndrome." This can manifest as ischemic vascular pain. The risk factors for DHIS are largely

A.S. Yevzlin et al. (eds.), *Interventional Nephrology*,
DOI 10.1007/978-1-4614-8803-3_17, © Springer Science+Business Media New York 2014

Table 17.1 Differential diagnosis for hand pain

Neurogenic pain	Vascular pain	Musculoskeletal pain
Ischemic monomelic neuropathy	Ischemic pain secondary to distal hypoperfusion ischemic syndrome	Destructive arthropathy
Peripheral neuropathy	Venous congestion secondary to outflow stenosis[a]	Osteoarthritis
Mononeuropathy secondary to compression, e.g., carpal tunnel syndrome		Autoimmune arthritis, e.g., rheumatoid arthritis
Reflex sympathetic dystrophy syndrome[a]		Tenosynovitis

[a]Associated with limb swelling

similar to IMN, but the symptoms that arise from vascular ischemia are more varied in presentation and depend on the severity of the ischemia. In mild ischemia, the patient may complain of slight numbness and coldness in the hand that occurs only during dialysis [6]. Mild ischemic pain may be self-limiting and resolve without treatment. On the other hand, in severe cases, the patient may complain of severe pain that is associated with numbness and digital cyanosis. Depending on the stage of presentation, patients may present with contractures, gangrene, or even autoamputation of the digits as a consequence of DHIS.

The onset of symptoms can occur immediately or evolve over several weeks and is often exacerbated by dialysis. One study reported that 50–66 % of patients who develop steal syndrome do so within 1 month of surgery [7], while other studies have reported it to be around 8 months [8] after surgery. This difference is probably related to the type of access that was created [9]. Acute DHIS (within 1 day of AV access creation) is strongly correlated with brachial artery AVG creation, while chronic DHIS (occurring more than 1 month post AV access creation) is strongly correlated to a maturing elbow AVF [9, 10].

Pain that occurs in association with arm swelling after AV access creation may suggest the presence of central vein stenosis. The swelling typically affects the entire arm and is secondary to venous congestion. The associated arm swelling is usually gradual and reaches a plateau after a few days. The patient may report a sensation of "heaviness" and purplish discoloration of the affected arm.

17.2.3 Musculoskeletal Pain

Pain secondary to arthropathies is usually over the joints, aggravated by movement and may be associated with morning stiffness and joint swellings.

17.3 Physical Examination

Physical examination in combination with a good history is helpful in establishing the diagnosis in the majority of patients.

The classical textbook teaching of "look, feel, and move" is applicable in the examination of a dialysis patient with hand pain on the side of AV access. It is important to always compare the hand with the AV access with the other hand without the AV access. On inspection, look for the presence of pallor, cyanosis, trophic changes, ulceration, areas of gangrene, and joint swelling. On palpation, compare the temperature of the two hands and examine the joints if there is suspicion of arthropathies. Type (pinprick and/or vibration) and distribution of the sensory loss (mononeuropathy, polyneuropathy, glove, and stocking distribution), if present, should be clearly documented and compared to preoperative physical examination. Examination of both the active and passive movements of the joints is useful for localization of arthropathies and documentation of the power of the intrinsic muscles of the hands.

Palpation of the hand is an important maneuver to differentiate DHIS and IMN. A major diagnostic feature of IMS is the absence of findings to suggest reduction or diversion of arterial flow. The radial pulse is variably present, and the hand is usually warm with no evidence of muscle infarction such as tenderness or pain on passive extension. Active movement of the hand and forearm can be difficult in severe cases and wrist drop may be present [5]. The degree of weakness may appear out of proportion to the physical findings.

In mild cases of DHIS, the physical examination may be normal and the radial pulse is usually present. In severe cases of DHIS, pale or blue-purple discoloration of the fingers can be observed. Ischemic ulcers, trophic changes, and gangrene patches may develop in long-standing cases of DHIS. Classically, the distal pulses are palpable only when the AV access is compressed manually. The value of pulse examination in differentiating patients with or without arterial stenosis in the evaluation of DHIS has also been questioned. In a case series by Asif et al., only 18 % of the patients who showed pulse with access occlusion were found subsequently to be suitable candidates for flow reduction procedure. Furthermore, it is still possible to have hand ischemia despite good radial and ulnar pulses [11]. A lower blood pressure in the access arm when compared to the contralateral arm may be suggestive of the presence of arterial stenosis.

17.4 Differential Diagnosis and Pathophysiology

The differential diagnosis of a patient with AV access presenting with hand pain is broad and can be divided into access-related or non-access-related hand pain. Differential diagnosis for access-related hand pain would include IMN, DHIS, reflex sympathetic dystrophy syndrome, and venous congestion. The non-access-related differentials are various forms of arthropathies (including destructive arthropathy), peripheral neuropathies, or carpal tunnel syndrome. The differentiating features are as summarized in Table 17.2. We will focus our discussion on two important differentials, which are potentially limb threatening.

17.4.1 Ischemic Monomelic Neuropathy

Diagnosis of IMN can be difficult as it is rare, and confounding factors such as diabetic neuropathy (which is common in dialysis patients), effect of anesthesia, poor positioning of arm during surgery, or surgical trauma can delay the diagnosis [3]. Delay in diagnosis can lead to profound loss of function, deformity, and severe neuropathic pain. As interventional nephrologists begin to get involved in access creations [12], awareness of this acute postoperative complication within the nephrology realm is critical to allow for urgent treatment to prevent crippling complications.

The pathogenesis is thought to be secondary to acute transient occlusion of the blood supply to the nerves of the forearm and hand that is severe enough to damage the nerve fibers, but insufficient to produce necrosis of other tissues. The major risk factors are diabetes, female gender, and use of brachial artery for AV access creation. The brachial artery is the main arterial supply to the forearm and hand, and significant diversion of blood in the absence of collaterals around the elbow can result in ischemia of the peripheral nerves. Delay in diagnosis may compromise outcome [13]. Bolton et al. described the absence of neurologic improvement despite the restoration of radial pulses 6 weeks post AV access creation [14]. Even with swift surgical intervention within 4 h of symptom presentation, significant weakness of all intrinsic muscles may remain after surgery [15].

The classical findings of distal sensorimotor neuropathy secondary to axon injuries on electromyography was described by Wilbourn et al. in 1983 [16]. Electrodiagnostic studies can certainly be useful to differentiate the different types of neuropathies, but a high index of suspicion is needed to exclude this devastating condition.

17.4.2 Distal Hypoperfusion Ischemic Syndrome

Arterial steal or shunt is demonstrable in the majority of patients with upper limb AV access when evaluated by Doppler studies [17, 18]. This steal is not unexpected and is secondary to the shunting of blood to the low-resistance area created by AV access surgery. However, not all the patients who have arterial steal on Doppler studies will develop symptoms. Majority of the time, arterial collaterals and compensatory peripheral vasodilatation are sufficient to maintain peripheral tissue perfusion. Symptoms of ischemia only develop in a minority of patients, and this is probably secondary to inadequate compensatory mechanism to maintain tissue perfusion. Therefore, the term "distal hypoperfusion ischemic syndrome" might be more appropriate than "arterial steal syndrome" to describe patients who develop symptoms of ischemia secondary to arterial steal from AV access creation [11].

The incidence of DHIS varies depending on the study, and it can range from 1 to 20 % [11]. The huge variation is probably due to differences in type of anastomosis [19] and anatomical location of the AV access [20]. Some studies have suggested a higher incidence in prosthetic AV access (4–9 %) compared to autogenous AV access (0.25–1.8 %) [4], while others have suggested the contrary [20].

The consistent finding in many studies has been the increased risk of DHIS associated with the use of brachial artery for AV access construction. This is probably related to the higher blood flow rate that is often associated with brachial access. Compared with the radiocephalic (RC) AVF which has a typical flow rate of 500–800 mls/min, the flow in the brachiocephalic/basilic AV access can increase up to 2,000 ms/min over time, and adequate collaterals are necessary to maintain digital pressure above 50 mmHg to avoid ischemia [21]. Inability of the collaterals to maintain digital pressure, either as a consequence of discrete or diffuse arterial stenosis, will result in DHIS.

Discrete arterial stenosis proximal to AV access can also compromise distal tissue perfusion after AV access creation. These proximal lesions may be previously undiagnosed or asymptomatic but will manifest after AV access creation due to increased flow demand. Inability to keep up with the increase in demand can result in distal tissue hypoperfusion. Similarly, if there is an undiagnosed discrete arterial stenosis distal to the AV access, the shunting effects of AV access creation can lead to precipitant fall in distal flow and resultant tissue hypoperfusion.

Diffuse vascular calcification that is associated with chronic kidney disease may also contribute to the development of DHIS. Pre-dialysis chronic kidney disease patients are observed to have a high prevalence of vascular calcification [22]. The prevalence and severity continues to increase with the years on dialysis [23]. Histologically, calcifications affect

Table 17.2 Differentiating features of the etiology of hand pain in dialysis patients

	Ischemic monomelic neuropathy (IMN)	Distal hypoperfusion ischemic syndrome	Venous congestion	Carpal tunnel syndrome	Peripheral neuropathy	Destructive arthropathy
Types of tissue affected	Nerves	Subcutaneous, muscle, and nerves	Subcutaneous	Nerves	Nerves	Joints
Onset of pain in relation to AV access creation	Immediate after access creation	Hours to months after access creation	Days to months after access creation	No relationship to access creation, may predate access creation	No relationship to access creation, may predate access creation	No relationship to access creation.
Etiology	Hypoperfusion injury to the nerves	Hypoperfusion injury to the skin, muscle, and nerves	Outflow stenosis with venous congestion	Compression of nerve from B$_2$-microglobulin deposition	Neuropathy secondary to diabetes mellitus and uremia	Dialysis related with unknown mechanism
Distinguishing features	Acute-onset post surgery + symptoms despite good hand perfusion	Poor perfusion with signs and symptoms of ischemia	Limb swelling	Follows the innervations of the median nerve	"Glove and stocking" sensory loss	Deformities of the joints
Diagnosis	Clinical diagnosis	Clinical diagnosis ± ultrasound, hemodynamic studies, arteriography	Clinical diagnosis ± fistulogram or graftogram	Clinical diagnosis + nerve conduction studies	Clinical diagnosis + nerve conduction studies	Clinical diagnosis + x-ray findings

both the intimal and medial layers of the artery and are thought to originate from chemically diverse nanocrystals [24]. The consequences of vascular calcifications are reduced arterial compliance [25] and impaired microcirculatory functions [26], which have a negative impact on the compensatory vasodilatation that is required to maintain tissue perfusion after AV access creation. In severe cases of diffuse vascular calcification, AV access and tissue perfusion can be compromised.

17.5 Investigations

17.5.1 Ultrasonography

Complex venous runoff and variability of the anastomosis can make evaluation of AVF by Doppler ultrasonography difficult and time-consuming. Success is sometimes dependent on the type of vascular access [27]. Over the years, continuing development and refinement of color Doppler sonography have improved its ability to evaluate the vascular system. Today, Doppler ultrasound can be used in the prevention, diagnosis, and treatment of DHIS.

Doppler ultrasonography can play an important role in the prevention of DHIS. While the benefits of routine arterial Doppler before all AV access creation remain to be elucidated, careful preoperative physical examination in combination with vascular mapping can certainly help to identify the presence of arterial lesions or variant anatomies that may predispose patients to DHIS [28]. Preoperative Doppler assessment of the arterial system in high-risk patients, such as elderly diabetics with a history of peripheral vascular disease, would allow the surgeon to plan for alternative AV access placement sites. In patients who are likely to do poorly in hemodialysis due to vascular access issues, peritoneal dialysis may be an attractive alternative.

Doppler ultrasonography has been shown to be a valuable tool in the evaluation of DHIS [29]. In a study by Middleton et al., ultrasound was able to reveal the etiology of DHIS in 90 % of the patients with ischemic steal syndrome. As mentioned previously, the presence of retrograde flow in the radial artery does not necessarily equate DHIS, and care must be taken to correlate Doppler findings with the overall clinical picture.

Intraoperative Doppler ultrasonography has often been used during banding or flow restricting surgery to help the surgeon control the reduction of flow volume in an objective manner. Various methods on its usage have been described, and the results have been consistently positive [30–33].

17.5.2 Hemodynamic Studies

Numerous hemodynamic studies, including the digital pressure, digital-brachial index (DBI), and transcutaneous oxygen tension (TcO$_2$), have been advocated for confirmation of diagnosis, predicting the risk and management of DHIS after AV access creation.

Digital photoplethysmography is useful for the confirmation of DHIS when the signs and symptoms are nonspecific. A reduction in the amplitude of digital waveforms distal to the proximal AV access is usually seen, but normal pulsatile waveform contours should still be present [34]. Patients with pronounced ischemia from the AV access will have monophasic or flat waveform contours that augment with the compression of the fistula [6].

Digital pressure measurement by digital photoplethysmography has been shown to be excellent in diagnosing DHIS. The accuracy for determining hand ischemia using a threshold-adjusted basal finger pressure of 60 mmHg was shown to have a sensitivity and specificity of 100 and 87 % in a study [35]. The DBI, calculated by dividing the digital pressure by the brachial artery pressure (usually measured by Doppler), is often used in conjunction with finger pressure readings. A value of less than 0.7 is suggestive of the presence of an obstructive lesion. Goff et al. reported that a DBI of less than 0.6 identifies a patient at risk of developing steal syndrome [36]. In a prospective study to examine the value of preoperative DPI, patients with DBI <1.0 were found to be more likely to develop steal syndrome, but there is no DBI threshold below which one can use to predict the occurrence of steal syndrome accurately. Using the DBI cutoff as 1, the sensitivity and specificity were 64 and 69 %, respectively. Decreasing the threshold to <0.8 will increase the specificity to 93 % but sensitivity will decrease to 29 %. The cutoff value of <0.6 was not tested in the study as the only patient with such a value did not develop steal syndrome after access creation [37]. Papasavas et al. did a similar study and found that a DBI of less than 0.6 on the day of surgery can reasonably predict which patients are at risk for the development of symptomatic steal [38].

The digital pressure is increased by decreasing the flow in the AV access. This principle has been used to guide surgical correction of AV access that is causing DHIS. Intraoperative digital photoplethysmography has been used during surgery to guide the amount of banding needed to achieve a digital pressure of 50 mmHg or DBI of more than 0.6 [39, 40].

TcO$_2$ measurement is another noninvasive method for assessing tissue hypoxia. TcO$_2$ of the AV access limb will decrease immediately postoperatively but will recover and stabilize by 1 month. Significant tissue hypoxia, defined as <55 mmHg, may be seen immediately postoperatively. It is observed more frequently in diabetic rather than nondiabetic patients. In most cases, it is transient and will be completely compensated for during the first postoperative month [41].

Although there are no TCPO$_2$ levels below 60 mmHg that will accurately predict if a patient will develop dialysis-associated ischemia [42], TcO$_2$ of less than 30 mmHg can be observed in patients who have severe critical ischemia [43]. Similar to intraoperative digital photoplethysmography, intraoperative use of TcO_2 has been used as a monitoring tool during corrective surgeries for DHIS [44].

The use of the hemodynamic measurements, while useful in providing important collaborative information in the diagnosis of DHIS, can be affected by a variety of factors such as temperature, draft, and emotional stress. The performance of these tests should be done in a controlled environment/laboratory to provide accurate and reproducible results [11].

17.5.3 Catheter-Based Contrast Arteriography

Catheter-based contrast arteriography is often considered the "gold standard" in the evaluation of DHIS. It is very useful to delineate the underlying etiology and develop treatment strategies. As discussed in the earlier section, DHIS can occur as a result of excessive high-flow AV access that overwhelms the normal compensatory mechanism, restriction of blood flow to the hand from discrete arterial stenosis either proximal or distal to the AV access anastomosis, or vascular maladaptation as a consequence of diffuse atherosclerosis or vascular calcification. Frequently, more than one etiology may be present to cause tissue hypoperfusion and angiography with digital subtraction (DSA) is an excellent tool to exclude the presence of arterial stenosis, which can be treated easily with angioplasty. The entire arterial system of the upper limb, from the aorta to the palmar arch, should be visualized. Occasionally, unexpected and interesting causes of DHIS can be identified (Figs. 17.1, 17.2, and 17.3). Either the antegrade approach via the femoral artery or the retrograde approach via the AV access can be employed.

We tend to favor the retrograde approach via the AV access over the femoral approach as it is relatively easy to access and safe and yields good results. For the retrograde approach via the AV access, insert a 5- or 6-French (F) introducer sheath after retrograde puncture of the venous outflow. Avoid puncturing too close to the anastomotic site to avoid damage to the AV anastomosis and to allow sufficient working space for sheath introduction. After the assessment of the

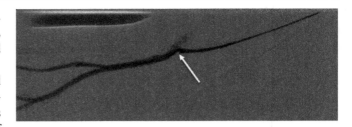

Fig. 17.2 Proximal arterial stenosis from previous arteriovenous graft creation

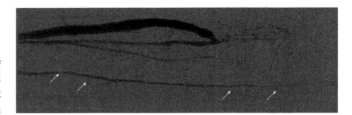

Fig. 17.3 Diffuse arterial disease causing distal hypoperfusion ischemic syndrome. The palmar arch is poorly visualized in this patient

venous outflow is completed, transverse the arterial anastomotic site with a 0.014-in. or 0.035-in. hydrophilic guidewires. Advance a diagnostic catheter (either using a standard 4-Fr straight catheter or pigtail-shaped catheter) into the brachiocephalic trunk (in the case of a right-sided access) or subclavian artery (in the case of a left-sided access), and a complete arteriogram of the inflow can be performed from here. If the most proximal part of the inflow cannot be visualized properly by backflow of contrast with the catheter in the brachiocephalic trunk or subclavian artery, advance the catheter into the aortic arch to visualize this segment. Due to the presence of arterial steal, compression of the AV access is often needed to assess the distal arterial system.

The distinct advantage of arteriography above other imaging modalities such as computed tomography angiography (CTA) and magnetic resonance angiogram (MRA) is the ability to perform intervention in the same setting. After complete diagnostic angiography, retrograde advancement of angioplasty balloons or stents for treatment of upstream stenosis is always feasible. Distal arterial lesions may require an additional puncture, but treatment can be carried out in the same setting.

17.5.4 Imaging Using Computed Tomography Angiography (CTA)

Initial experience with CTA for the evaluation of failing hemodialysis access was performed using single-detector helical CT technology. Despite its limited spatial resolution and anatomic coverage, good correlation to digital subtraction

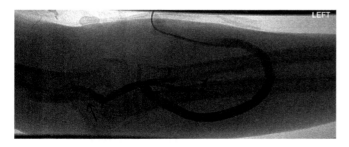

Fig. 17.1 An abandoned AVF causing distal hypoperfusion ischemic syndrome after arteriovenous graft creation

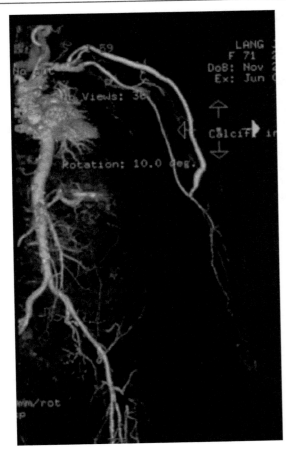

Fig. 17.4 High-quality CTA showing the entire arterial tree and arteriovenous fistula

angiography has been reported [45, 46]. Multi-detector (4, 16, 32, or 64) CT (MDCT) technology offers improved temporal and spatial resolution and greater anatomic coverage, making it a valuable tool for diagnosis of dysfunctional AV access. The reported sensitivity and specificity for lesions detected by a 4-MDCT can be up to 98.7 and 97.5 %, respectively [47].

In view of these, CTA can be a good alternative to DSA to exclude the presence of arterial stenosis in DHIS (Fig. 17.4). This may be useful if high flow through the AV access is the suspected cause of the DHIS and imaging is needed to exclude coexisting arterial stenosis before banding or corrective surgery. The downside to such an approach is the need to schedule a separate intervention procedure if stenotic lesions are detected on CTA. Some surgeons might not be comfortable to perform banding or corrective surgery based on CTA and might request for an angiogram to confirm the CT findings.

Similar to CT angiography, MRA is an excellent tool for diagnosis of dysfunctional AV access without the need for exposure to ionizing radiation. Recent discovery of the association between the use of gadolinium-based contrast agents

(GBCAs) and nephrogenic systemic fibrosis (NSF) in dialysis patients has dampened the enthusiasm for the use of MRA in dialysis patients. Although various strategies have been proposed to decrease the risk of NSF [48], the availability of alternative imaging modalities makes it hard to justify the use of GBCA-enhanced MRA to image the AV access. The use of non-contrast MRA to image the upper limb vasculature has been attempted in healthy volunteers [49]. While it is feasible, the arterial image quality and vessel-to-background ratios were lower [49]; hence, applicability to imaging of AV access is questionable.

17.5.5 Electrophysiology Study

Nerve conduction studies and electromyography (EMG) are valuable in the workup of neuropathy. It should be emphasized that IMN is essentially a clinical diagnosis, and treatment should not be delayed because of the wait for electrophysiological confirmation. In the acute phase, fibrillation potentials and motor unit loss may be demonstrated on EMG. There is usually no evidence of a discrete infarction level, and the characteristic changes revert to normal as one moves proximally in the affected limb. Nerve conduction studies typically reveal decreased amplitudes and low-normal or mildly slowed conduction velocities, but with normal latencies [16].

17.6 Management

The management of IMN and DHIS will be discussed. Due to the potential devastating consequences of IMN, treatment should be initiated immediately. The NKF KDOQI guidelines state that IMN is a clinical diagnosis and immediate closure of the AVF is mandatory [50].

For DHIS, management is dependent on the severity of disease. Various classification has been proposed and summarized in Table 17.3 [10, 21, 30]. The common features are that intervention should be based on clinical symptoms and urgency of intervention is related to the severity of signs and symptoms. Aim of intervention is preservation of limb with salvage of AV access where feasible.

The treatment approach is as shown in Fig. 17.5. Patients with symptomatic DHIS should be screened for the presence of arterial stenosis [8, 51]. Arterial stenosis proximal or distal to the AV access [52] has the potential to cause DHIS, and angioplasty can lead to immediate relief of symptoms [8]. If ischemic symptoms occur in the absence of any arterial lesions or persist despite successful treatment of the arterial lesions, corrective intervention or surgery would be required and various techniques have been described. The interventions can be broadly divided into

Table 17.3 Summary of the classification systems to describe severity and grade of DHIS in the literature

Staging [21]	Severity grading in combination with ultrasound [30]	Grade [10]	Symptoms [10]	Treatment [10]
	Grade 0 (No steal)			
1	Grade 1 (Mild with demonstrable flow augmentation with access occlusion)	1	Signs of ischemia but patient is asymptomatic	No treatment
2	Grade 2 (Moderate)	2a	Symptomatic during dialysis with tolerable pain	Conservative treatment
		2b	Symptomatic during dialysis with intolerable pain	Conservative ± intervention
3	Grade 3 (Severe)	3	Rest pain or loss of motor function	Urgent intervention
4		4a	Limited tissue loss with preservation of hand function after reversal of ischemia	Urgent intervention
		4b	Irreversible tissue loss with loss if significant function	Amputation

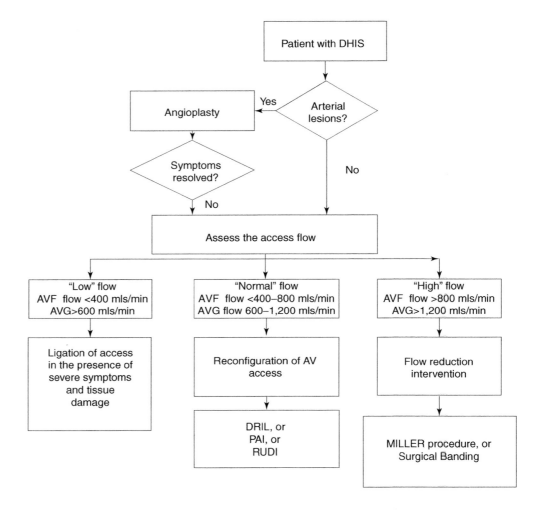

Fig. 17.5 Approach to patient with distal hypoperfusion ischemic syndrome

three categories: flow reduction intervention, reconfiguration of the AV access, or ligation. The underlying principle is to reverse or limit the pathophysiological changes that AV access creation had imposed on the upper limb. Ideally, the interventionist or surgeon would like to ameliorate steal and preserve the AV access for dialysis at the same time. The choice of intervention is often dependent on the baseline AV access flow. If the baseline AV access flow is low (defined as

<400 mls/min in AVF and <600 mls/min in AVG) [43] and is causing steal despite its low flow, ligation of the AV access is probably the best option. On the other hand, a high-flow AV (defined as >800 mls/min in AVF and >1,200 mls/min in AVG) [43] access is probably amendable to flow reduction intervention and still have sufficient flow for dialysis. For AV access that has flows within the "normal range" (defined as between 400 and 800 mls/min in AVF

and 600 and 1,200 mls/min in AVG), reconfiguration of the AV access is probably the best treatment option. In patients who present in advance stages of DHIS where reversal of steal is unlikely to reverse the extensive tissue damage or result in meaningful functional recovery, amputation of the hand rather than ligation of AV access may be considered. The advantages of such a drastic approach would be the preservation of preexisting AV access and protection of the contralateral arm from risk of steal syndrome with new access creation.

17.6.1 Flow Reduction Intervention

Flow reduction intervention can be achieved through the use of open surgical banding techniques or a minimally invasive procedure called the minimally invasive limited ligation endoluminal-assisted revision (MILLER) procedure. The aim is to create a narrow segment around the AV anastomotic site to reduce the flow through the AV access and improve distal perfusion. As alluded to earlier, this type of intervention is best suited if the baseline AV access flow is high. The success rate for banding in a large series was reported to be 86 % for symptom control with a 1-year patency rate of 91 % for AVF [53]. Some forms of objective measurements such as Doppler or TcO_2 are often used intraoperatively to help the surgeon determine the amount of banding that is required to improve tissue perfusion and maintain adequate flow within the AV access. The use of nonabsorbable sutures, polytetrafluoroethylene (PTFE) cuff, and small caliber interposition grafts for surgical bandings is well described in the literature [43].

Interventional nephrologists pioneered the MILLER procedure for treatment of DHIS. The procedure can be performed in the outpatient settings under local anesthesia (1 % Xylocaine) and intravenous conscious sedation. Through a 1–2-cm incision around the AV anastomotic site, the vein or graft is carefully isolated using blunt dissection technique. A nonabsorbable ligature is tied around the isolated segment over an inflated 4- or 5-mm angioplasty balloon to achieve the desired size of the access inflow. The size of the angioplasty balloon is based on the diameter of the distal artery and is usually equal or smaller than the measured diameter. The procedure can be repeated with a second ligature tied approximately 0.5 cm juxtaposed to the first ligature if there is no improvement in the symptoms after the first attempt [54]. The outcomes have been impressive. Symptomatic relief was achieved in 95.6 % of the patients with DHIS, and primary band patency and secondary access patency were 75 and 90 % at 6 and 24 months, respectively [55]. Intra-procedure flow monitoring, if available, may also be used to complement the banding procedure to objectively document the reduction in flow.

17.6.2 Reconfiguration of the AV Access

Three different methods will be described here. The differences in the three approaches are as shown in Fig. 17.6.

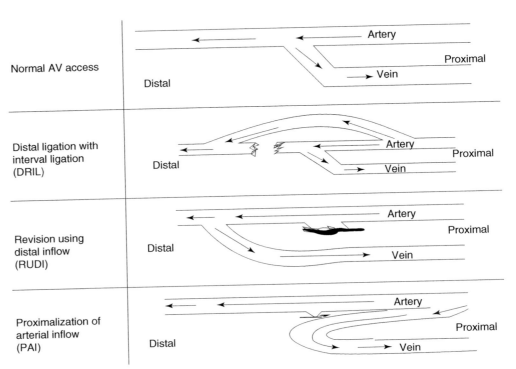

Fig. 17.6 Different surgical techniques for reconfiguration of arteriovenous access

Distal Revascularization with Interval Ligation (DRIL)

Distal revascularization with interval ligation (DRIL) was first described by Schanzer et al. in 1998 for correction of ischemic steal phenomenon and preservation of AV access function [7]. An arterial bypass is created upstream from the anastomosis to the brachial artery just distal to the AV anastomosis using a reversed saphenous vein bypass. The native brachial artery is ligated just distal to the AV access (but before the bypass anastomosis). The success of DRIL was attributed to the ability of the arterial bypass to function as a low-resistance conduit in parallel configuration to the low-resistance conduit created by the AV anastomosis. The net effect is alteration in the ratios of resistance between the AV access and forearm circulation such that the amount of blood shunted through the brachial AV access is decreased and distal perfusion is augmented [6]. Illig et al. measured the intravascular pressure and flow measurements before and after DRIL in nine symptomatic patients with DHIS. He noted an increase in the pressure at the "newly created" junction where the blood flow splits to supply both the hand and AV access. He proposed that the hemodynamic improvement was secondary to the relative increase in the resistance of the fistulae and decreased resistance of the path down the forearm, thus allowing antegrade flow down the new bypass to the forearm [56]. The DRIL procedures has been shown to have a good clinical success rate [57] but does have potential complications such as bypass failure and worsening ischemia [58]. The reported success rates for symptom control and primary patency at 1 year were 77–100 and 29–95.6 %, respectively [57–60].

Revision Using Distal Inflow Procedure (RUDI)

RUDI can be a viable alternative to DRIL, which is a complex surgery. It involves ligating the AV access just after the arterial anastomosis and re-anastomose to a more distal artery such as the radial artery using a bypass graft (which can be autogenous or with PTFE) [61]. It is probably useful for AV access that has "normal" or high flow. This is a simple and useful procedure. If the vein is already well arterialized, the AV access can be used immediately without the need for tunneled dialysis catheter insertion. Another advantage over the DRIL is that the anatomy of the arterial supply to the forearm is intact and there is no risk of forearm ischemia if the bypass graft is occluded.

Proximalization of Arterial Inflow

Proximalization of arterial inflow (PAI) is another good alternative to DRIL. It involves revising the AV anastomosis to a more proximal origin such as the axillary artery using a PTFE bypass graft. The surgery is helpful in relieving ischemic symptoms as the pressure is higher at the proximal arterial anastomosis; therefore, arterial pressure drop distal to the AV anastomosis will be significantly lower at the same access flow. Furthermore, collateral flow begins at a much higher point in the arm, hence, preventing the occurrence of ischemic symptoms. Unlike DRIL, there is no need to ligate the brachial artery, and thrombosis of the bypass graft will only lead to loss of AV access without risk of compromising the distal arterial flow. The reported success rates for symptom control and primary patency at 1 year were 84 and 87 %, respectively [62]. The bypass graft is being used as a conduit and should not be cannulated for dialysis. PAI has been successfully used in the correction of "normal" flow AV access with DHIS [63].

17.6.3 Ligation

Ligation will ameliorate steal and result in improvement of symptoms. This option can be used in the settings of severe limb ischemia where immediate reversal of flow is critical for limb preservation, AV access with low baseline flow, steal syndrome which develops after successful kidney transplant, or failure of flow reduction or reconfiguration surgeries to correct DHIS.

Although uncommon, DHIS have been described to occur in RCAVF as well. In such situation, surgical ligation or endovascular coil embolization [63] of the distal radial artery can be done to ameliorate steal syndrome. It is extremely critical that adequate collateral circulation is confirmed before carrying out the procedure.

17.6.4 Prevention of DHIS

Preoperative assessment can play a key role in the prevention of DHIS. The Allen's test is useful to test the patency of the palmar collaterals. In the presence of risk factors such as advance age, diabetes, and history of peripheral vascular disease, preoperative assessment of the arterial system using Doppler may be useful to diagnosis subclinical lesions. Creation of a radiocephalic AVF should be preferred to elbow AV access as it preserves vascular "real estate" and is associated with a lower risk of DHIS. In cases where creation of BC AVF is necessary, the "extension technique" has been described to be an effective procedure for prevention of DHIS. The surgical approach is similar to BC AVF creation, but instead of anastomosing the vein to the brachial artery, dissection is done beyond the brachial artery bifurcation to expose the proximal radial and ulnar arteries. Either the radial or the ulnar artery is used for anastomosis with the median vein. The added advantage of this technique is concurrent maturation of both cephalic and basilic veins [64].

Conclusion

DHIS can have a wide spectrum of symptoms, and it is important for nephrologists to be cognizant of its presentation, diagnosis, and treatment options. Timely intervention can prevent catastrophic consequences such as loss of hand function and amputation.

References

1. Riggs JE, Moss AH, Labosky DA, Liput JH, Morgan JJ, Gutmann L. Upper extremity ischemic monomelic neuropathy: a complication of vascular access procedures in uremic diabetic patients. Neurology. 1989;39(7):997–8.
2. Morsy AH, Kulbaski M, Chen C, Isiklar H, Lumsden AB. Incidence and characteristics of patients with hand ischemia after a hemodialysis access procedure. J Surg Res. 1998;74(1):8–10.
3. Hye RJ, Wolf YG. Ischemic monomelic neuropathy: an under-recognized complication of hemodialysis access. Ann Vasc Surg. 1994;8(6):578–82.
4. Padberg Jr FT, Calligaro KD, Sidawy AN. Complications of arteriovenous hemodialysis access: recognition and management. J Vasc Surg. 2008;48(5 Suppl):55S–80.
5. Miles AM. Upper limb ischemia after vascular access surgery: differential diagnosis and management. Semin Dial. 2000;13(5):312–5.
6. Wixon CL, Hughes JD, Mills JL. Understanding strategies for the treatment of ischemic steal syndrome after hemodialysis access. J Am Coll Surg. 2000;191(3):301–10.
7. Schanzer H, Skladany M, Haimov M. Treatment of angioaccess-induced ischemia by revascularization. J Vasc Surg. 1992;16(6):861–4; discussion 864–6.
8. Asif A, Leon C, Merrill D, et al. Arterial steal syndrome: a modest proposal for an old paradigm. Am J Kidney Dis. 2006;48(1):88–97.
9. Lazarides MK, Staramos DN, Kopadis G, Maltezos C, Tzilalis VD, Georgiadis GS. Onset of arterial 'steal' following proximal angioaccess: immediate and delayed types. Nephrol Dial Transplant. 2003;18(11):2387–90.
10. Scheltinga MR, van Hoek F, Bruijninckx CM. Time of onset in haemodialysis access-induced distal ischaemia (HAIDI) is related to the access type. Nephrol Dial Transplant. 2009;24(10):3198–204.
11. Leon C, Asif A. Arteriovenous access and hand pain: the distal hypoperfusion ischemic syndrome. Clin J Am Soc Nephrol. 2007;2(1):175–83.
12. Mishler R, Yevzlin AS. Outcomes of arteriovenous fistulae created by a U.S. interventional nephrologist. Semin Dial. 2010;23(2):224–8.
13. Kirksey L. Ischemic monomelic neuropathy: an underappreciated cause of pain and disability following vascular access surgery. J Vasc Access. 2010;11(2):165–8.
14. Bolton CF, Driedger AA, Lindsay RM. Ischaemic neuropathy in uraemic patients caused by bovine arteriovenous shunt. J Neurol Neurosurg Psychiatry. 1979;42(9):810–4.
15. Rogers NM, Lawton PD. Ischaemic monomelic neuropathy in a non-diabetic patient following creation of an upper limb arteriovenous fistula. Nephrol Dial Transplant. 2007;22(3):933–5.
16. Wilbourn AJ, Furlan AJ, Hulley W, Ruschhaupt W. Ischemic monomelic neuropathy. Neurology. 1983;33(4):447–51.
17. Lazarides MK, Staramos DN, Panagopoulos GN, Tzilalis VD, Eleftheriou GJ, Dayantas JN. Indications for surgical treatment of angioaccess-induced arterial "steal". J Am Coll Surg. 1998;187(4):422–6.
18. Kwun KB, Schanzer H, Finkler N, Haimov M, Burrows L. Hemodynamic evaluation of angioaccess procedures for hemodialysis. Vasc Endovascular Surg. 1979;13(3):170–7.
19. Kinnaert P, Struyven J, Mathieu J, Vereerstraeten P, Toussaint C, Van Geertruyden J. Intermittent claudication of the hand after creation of an arteriovenous fistula in the forearm. Am J Surg. 1980;139(6):838–43.
20. van Hoek F, Scheltinga MR, Kouwenberg I, Moret KE, Beerenhout CH, Tordoir JH. Steal in hemodialysis patients depends on type of vascular access. Eur J Vasc Endovasc Surg. 2006;32(6):710–7.
21. Tordoir JH, Dammers R, van der Sande FM. Upper extremity ischemia and hemodialysis vascular access. Eur J Vasc Endovasc Surg. 2004;27(1):1–5.
22. Toussaint ND, Lau KK, Strauss BJ, Polkinghorne KR, Kerr PG. Associations between vascular calcification, arterial stiffness and bone mineral density in chronic kidney disease. Nephrol Dial Transplant. 2008;23(2):586–93.
23. Goldsmith DJ, Covic A, Sambrook PA, Ackrill P. Vascular calcification in long-term haemodialysis patients in a single unit: a retrospective analysis. Nephron. 1997;77(1):37–43.
24. Schlieper G, Aretz A, Verberckmoes SC, et al. Ultrastructural analysis of vascular calcifications in uremia. J Am Soc Nephrol. 2010;21(4):689–96.
25. Toussaint ND, Lau KK, Strauss BJ, Polkinghorne KR, Kerr PG. Relationship between vascular calcification, arterial stiffness and bone mineral density in a cross-sectional study of prevalent Australian haemodialysis patients. Nephrology (Carlton). 2009;14(1):105–12.
26. Sigrist MK, McIntyre CW. Vascular calcification is associated with impaired microcirculatory function in chronic haemodialysis patients. Nephron Clin Pract. 2008;108(2):c121–6.
27. Middleton WD, Picus DD, Marx MV, Melson GL. Color Doppler sonography of hemodialysis vascular access: comparison with angiography. AJR Am J Roentgenol. 1989;152(3):633–9.
28. Malik J, Slavikova M, Maskova J. Dialysis access-associated steal syndrome: the role of ultrasonography. J Nephrol. 2003;16(6):903–7.
29. Davidson I, Chan D, Dolmatch B, et al. Duplex ultrasound evaluation for dialysis access selection and maintenance: a practical guide. J Vasc Access. 2008;9(1):1–9.
30. Shemesh D, Mabjeesh NJ, Abramowitz HB. Management of dialysis access-associated steal syndrome: use of intraoperative duplex ultrasound scanning for optimal flow reduction. J Vasc Surg. 1999;30(1):193–5.
31. Aschwanden M, Hess P, Labs KH, Dickenmann M, Jaeger KA. Dialysis access-associated steal syndrome: the intraoperative use of duplex ultrasound scan. J Vasc Surg. 2003;37(1):211–3.
32. Jackson KL, Charpentier KP. Quantitative banding for steal syndrome secondary to arteriovenous fistulae. Ann R Coll Surg Engl. 2010;92(6):534.
33. Shemesh D, Olsha O, Mabjeesh NJ, Abramowitz HB. Dialysis access induced limb ischemia corrected using quantitative duplex ultrasound. Pediatr Nephrol. 2001;16(5):409–11.
34. Strandness Jr DE, Gibbons GE, Bell JW. Mercury strain gauge plethysmography. Evaluation of patients with acquired arteriovenous fistula. Arch Surg. 1962;85:215–9.
35. Schanzer A, Nguyen LL, Owens CD, Schanzer H. Use of digital pressure measurements for the diagnosis of AV access-induced hand ischemia. Vasc Med. 2006;11(4):227–31.
36. Goff CD, Sato DT, Bloch PH, et al. Steal syndrome complicating hemodialysis access procedures: can it be predicted? Ann Vasc Surg. 2000;14(2):138–44.
37. Valentine RJ, Bouch CW, Scott DJ, et al. Do preoperative finger pressures predict early arterial steal in hemodialysis access patients? A prospective analysis. J Vasc Surg. 2002;36(2):351–6.
38. Papasavas PK, Reifsnyder T, Birdas TJ, Caushaj PF, Leers S. Prediction of arteriovenous access steal syndrome utilizing digital pressure measurements. Vasc Endovascular Surg. 2003;37(3):179–84.
39. Odland MD, Kelly PH, Ney AL, Andersen RC, Bubrick MP. Management of dialysis-associated steal syndrome complicating upper extremity arteriovenous fistulas: use of intraoperative digital photoplethysmography. Surgery. 1991;110(4):664–9. discussion 669–70.

40. van Hoek F, Scheltinga MR, Luirink M, Raaymakers LC, van Pul C, Beerenhout CH. Access flow, venous saturation, and digital pressures in hemodialysis. J Vasc Surg. 2007;45(5):968–73.

41. Harissis H, Koliousi E, Matsagas M, Batsis H, Fatouros M, Siamopoulos K. Measurement of transcutaneous oxygen tension in limbs with arteriovenous hemodialysis access. Dial Transplant. 2008;37:67–70.

42. Lemmon GW, Murphy MP. Dialysis access steal syndromes. Perspect Vasc Surg Endovasc Ther. 2009;21(1):36–9.

43. Mickley V. Steal syndrome – strategies to preserve vascular access and extremity. Nephrol Dial Transplant. 2008;23(1):19–24.

44. Field M, Blackwell J, Jaipersad A, et al. Distal revascularisation with interval ligation (DRIL): an experience. Ann R Coll Surg Engl. 2009;91(5):394–8.

45. Cavagna E, D'Andrea P, Schiavon F, Tarroni G. Failing hemodialysis arteriovenous fistula and percutaneous treatment: imaging with CT, MRI and digital subtraction angiography. Cardiovasc Intervent Radiol. 2000;23(4):262–5.

46. Lin YP, Wu MH, Ng YY, et al. Spiral computed tomographic angiography – a new technique for evaluation of vascular access in hemodialysis patients. Am J Nephrol. 1998;18(2):117–22.

47. Ko SF, Huang CC, Ng SH, et al. MDCT angiography for evaluation of the complete vascular tree of hemodialysis fistulas. AJR Am J Roentgenol. 2005;185(5):1268–74.

48. Zou Z, Zhang HL, Roditi GH, Leiner T, Kucharczyk W, Prince MR. Nephrogenic systemic fibrosis: review of 370 biopsy-confirmed cases. JACC Cardiovasc Imaging. 2011;4(11):1206–16.

49. Bode AS, Planken RN, Merkx MA, et al. Feasibility of non-contrast-enhanced magnetic resonance angiography for imaging upper extremity vasculature prior to vascular access creation. Eur J Vasc Endovasc Surg. 2012;43(1):88–94.

50. Vascular Access Work Group. Clinical practice guidelines for vascular access. Am J Kidney Dis. 2006;48 Suppl 1:S176–247.

51. Guerra A, Raynaud A, Beyssen B, Pagny JY, Sapoval M, Angel C. Arterial percutaneous angioplasty in upper limbs with vascular access devices for haemodialysis. Nephrol Dial Transplant. 2002;17(5):843–51.

52. van den Bosch RP, Crowe PM, Mosquera DA. Endovascular treatment of arterial steal secondary to dialysis fistula. Nephrol Dial Transplant. 2001;16(11):2279–80.

53. Plumb TJ, Lynch TG, Adelson AB. Treatment of steal syndrome in a distal radiocephalic arteriovenous fistula using intravascular coil embolization. J Vasc Surg. 2008;47(2):457–9.

54. Zanow J, Petzold K, Petzold M, Krueger U, Scholz H. Flow reduction in high-flow arteriovenous access using intraoperative flow monitoring. J Vasc Surg. 2006;44(6):1273–8.

55. Goel N, Miller GA, Jotwani MC, Licht J, Schur I, Arnold WP. Minimally invasive limited ligation endoluminal-assisted revision (MILLER) for treatment of dialysis access-associated steal syndrome. Kidney Int. 2006;70(4):765–70.

56. Miller GA, Goel N, Friedman A, et al. The MILLER banding procedure is an effective method for treating dialysis-associated steal syndrome. Kidney Int. 2010;77(4):359–66.

57. Illig KA, Surowiec S, Shortell CK, Davies MG, Rhodes JM, Green RM. Hemodynamics of distal revascularization-interval ligation. Ann Vasc Surg. 2005;19(2):199–207.

58. Huber TS, Brown MP, Seeger JM, Lee WA. Midterm outcome after the distal revascularization and interval ligation (DRIL) procedure. J Vasc Surg. 2008;48(4):926–32. discussion 932–3.

59. Anaya-Ayala JE, Pettigrew CD, Ismail N, et al. Management of dialysis access-associated "steal" syndrome with DRIL procedure: challenges and clinical outcomes. J Vasc Access. 2012;13(3):299–304.

60. Knox RC, Berman SS, Hughes JD, Gentile AT, Mills JL. Distal revascularization-interval ligation: a durable and effective treatment for ischemic steal syndrome after hemodialysis access. J Vasc Surg. 2002;36(2):250–5. discussion 256.

61. Haimov M, Schanzer H, Skladani M. Pathogenesis and management of upper-extremity ischemia following angioaccess surgery. Blood Purif. 1996;14(5):350–4.

62. Minion DJ, Moore E, Endean E. Revision using distal inflow: a novel approach to dialysis-associated steal syndrome. Ann Vasc Surg. 2005;19(5):625–8.

63. Zanow J, Kruger U, Scholz H. Proximalization of the arterial inflow: a new technique to treat access-related ischemia. J Vasc Surg. 2006;43(6):1216–21; discussion 1221.

64. Ehsan O, Bhattacharya D, Darwish A, Al-khaffaf H. 'Extension technique': a modified technique for brachio-cephalic fistula to prevent dialysis access-associated steal syndrome. Eur J Vasc Endovasc Surg. 2005;29(3):324–7.

Central Vein Stenosis

Davinder Wadehra

18.1 Epidemiology

True incidence and prevalence of central vein stenosis are not known as most of CVS is asymptomatic and therefore fails detection. A study done by Schwab et al. estimates prevalence of subclavian stenosis at 25 % [1]. Similarly, another study from the 1980s reported venographic evidence of subclavian stenosis in 18 of 36 (50 %) patients [2, 3]. In a retrospective investigation of symptomatic HD patients undergoing angiography, 19 % of all patients and 27 % of those with a previous history of CVC placement were found to have CVS, similar to the finding of 16 % in a duplex and angiographic study [4, 5].

18.2 Risk Factors Associated with CVS

18.2.1 Prior History of CVC

It is uncommon for CVS to occur in HD patients, without prior history of central venous access placement or intervention. Placement of multiple central venous catheters, with increased duration of catheter dwell times, has been associated with a higher risk of CVS [4, 6, 7].

Study by Hernandez et al. examined 42 consecutive chronic renal failure patients in whom subclavian catheters had been placed as the initial vascular access for hemodialysis. All patients underwent sequential venography studies: at baseline (24–48 h after removal of the catheter) and 1, 3, and 6 months thereafter. Venograms were considered abnormal when there was evidence of unequivocal strictures (more than 30 % narrowing), with or without collateral circulation. At baseline, 52.4 % ($n=22$) of patients showed stenotic vein lesions ($n=19$) or total thrombosis ($n=3$), and identical lesions were also observed after 1 month. Surprisingly, 10 of 22 patients with initial CVS (45.4 %) showed spontaneous recanalization of venous lesions in the venographies performed 3 months after removal. Patients with definitive stenosis at 6 months had a higher number of inserted catheters (1.58 versus 1.2; $p<0.05$), longer time in place (49 versus 29 days; $p<0.05$) than those without CVS or with spontaneous recanalization of venous lesions during follow-up. Furthermore, a higher number of catheter-related infections were observed in patients with definitive CVS (66.6 % versus 33.3 %; $p<0.05$) [8]. Similarly, a study by Macrae et al. found that 55 out of 133 patients (41 %) had evidence of significant CVS on venogram. Patients with CVS had a longer duration on HD and a history of a previous HD catheter insertion [7].

In a prospective study by Oguzkurt et al., 57 patients with temporary dialysis catheters had catheter venography by pulling back the catheter just before removal. This study showed that even short-term catheters result in significantly high rates of pericatheter sleeve and thrombus formation, which are two of the important causes of catheter malfunction. These findings remind us again that we should avoid unnecessary catheter insertion even for short term in these chronically ill patients [9].

18.2.2 Site of CVC Placement

Central venous catheters placed by a subclavian access have a particularly high risk, with a 42 % incidence of CVS compared to a 10 % rate with catheters placed via an internal jugular vein access [2, 6, 10]. This has been reported by Schillinger et al. angiographically, when they compared the subclavian–brachiocephalic vein of 50 patients dialyzed by subclavian catheter to those of 50 patients dialyzed by internal jugular catheters [11].

D. Wadehra, MD, MBBS
LMC Diabetes and Endocrinology,
2130 North Park Dr, Brampton, ON, Canada
e-mail: davinder.wadehra@gmail.com

A.S. Yevzlin et al. (eds.), *Interventional Nephrology*,
DOI 10.1007/978-1-4614-8803-3_18, © Springer Science+Business Media New York 2014

There is also an increased predilection for CVS to occur with left-sided access for catheter placement, which may be related to the more tortuous course catheters that have to traverse from a left-sided access [11–14].

18.2.3 PICC and Ports

Study by Grove et al. showed that the overall thrombosis rate was 3.9 % after PICC placement. Multivariate analysis of the results indicated that only catheter diameter remained significant. There was no thrombosis in catheters 3 F or smaller. The thrombosis rate was 1 % for 4-F catheters, 6.6 % for 5-F catheters, and 9.8 % for 6-F catheters [15]. The smallest acceptable catheter diameter should be used to decrease the incidence of venous thrombosis. New central vein stenosis or occlusion occurred in 7 % of patients following upper arm placement of venous access devices. Patients with longer catheter dwell time were more likely to develop central vein abnormalities. With an increasingly prevalent use of PICC lines, the complication of CVS is likely to become more prevalent. Not only the awareness of this complication needs to be improved, the use of alternative means of intravenous access, such as single-lumen central venous infusion catheters, should be seriously considered to avoid the loss of an arm vein for the future creation of AVF [15–19].

18.2.4 Pacemaker/Defibrillator Wires

CKD/ESRD shares risk factors with cardiovascular disease, and it is not uncommon for these patients to undergo implantation of pacemakers or defibrillators. Thirty consecutive patients with a transvenous defibrillator lead underwent bilateral contrast venography of the cephalic, axillary, subclavian, and brachiocephalic veins as well as the superior vena cava before an elective defibrillator battery replacement. The mean time between transvenous defibrillator lead implantation and venography was 45 ± 21 months. Sixteen patients (>50 %) had more than one lead in the same subclavian vein. No patient had clinical signs of venous occlusion. Subclavian stenosis (defined as more than 50 % stenosis) was found in 50 % of patients, and 13 % of patients had more than 75 % stenosis [20–22]. Total or partial obstruction of the access veins occurs relatively frequently after pacemaker or ICD implantation. Multiple pacing or ICD leads are associated with an increased risk of venous obstruction, whereas antiplatelet/anticoagulant therapy appears to have a preventive effect on the development of access vein thrombosis [23]. If a device is to be placed in a dialysis patient, it should not be placed on the side of the AV access because of the high incidence of CVS. Another study by Bulur et al. studied 86 patients who had undergone biventricular device implantation. Subclavian vein stenosis was

present in 39 % of all participants. Among the patients with subclavian obstruction ($n = 33$), 8 had mild obstruction, 15 had severe obstruction, and 10 had total occlusion [24].

18.2.5 Catheter Composition

A variety of plastic materials including polyvinyl chloride, polyethylene, polyurethane, and silicone has been used in the production of CVC for hemodialysis. In animal experiments, silicone was shown to be less thrombogenic than other materials [25–27]. Trials systematically comparing CVC made from different materials to assess their respective rates of infection or thrombosis in hemodialysis patients have not been published.

In a rabbit model, polyethylene and polytetrafluoroethylene catheters caused more inflammation than silicone and polyurethane. Obstructions of the venous lumen were significantly more frequent with the rigid catheters than with the soft catheters [26].

18.2.6 Idiopathic

A study by Oguzkurt et al. showed that 10 % of hemodialysis patients had stenosis of a central vein without a previous central catheter placement. Central venous stenosis in hemodialysis patients without a history of central venous catheterization tends to occur or be manifested in patients with a proximal permanent vascular access with high flow rates [28].

18.2.7 Catheter Infections

A study by Hernandez et al. retrospectively analyzed 80 catheterizations in a total of 54 chronic HD patients from a single center. Sixteen catheters had to be removed because of a well-documented catheter-related infection. For comparison they matched 14 concurrent catheters, which were electively removed without evidence of infection and with a negative culture of the catheter tip. A venogram of the ipsilateral arm was performed in all the cases after more than 6 months of catheter removal. CVS was three times more common among patients with previous catheter-related infection (75 % versus 28 %; $p < 0.01$) [8, 14, 29, 30].

A group of 479 jugular vein catheterizations, 403 RJVC, and 77 LJVC done in 294 prevalent hemodialysis patients were analyzed. Of the RJVC, 44 (10.9 %) of 403 were removed because of infection compared with 16 (20.8 %) of 77 LJVC ($p < 0.02$). The overall incidence of infections was 1.58 episodes of infection per 1,000 catheter days, 1.57 for RJVC, and 3.72 for LJVC, respectively. Catheter dwell times were not different in this study [14].

18.3 Pathogenesis

The precise mechanism of CVC-associated CVS remains largely undefined. Plausible mechanisms are linked to the CVC-induced trauma to the venous endothelium and the resultant inflammatory response within the vessel wall. Aside from the initial trauma at the time of CVC placement, many factors, including the presence of foreign body in the vein, sliding movement of the catheter with respiration, postural and head movements, and increased flow and turbulence from creation of AVF, alone or in combination, stimulate various processes within the vessel wall. The high blood flow associated with dialysis, turbulence, and vibrations has shown to cause platelet aggregation and deposition and endothelial hyperplasia [31–33].

Histologic examination of specimens from subclavian vein stenosis has corroborated this endothelial hyperplasia hypothesis by demonstrating the presence of fibrous tissue [34]. In addition, the uremic milieu hypothesis has been supported by recent findings of intimal changes in the cephalic vein of renal failure patients even prior to AV fistula construction [35]. Intravascular thrombosis can result from the release of profibrotic cytokines that are associated with platelet–platelet aggregates in this scenario [36]. Furthermore, direct physical damage from the movement of the catheter tip or body against a vessel wall can potentially result in thrombin generation, platelet activation, expression of P-selectin, and an inflammatory response [37, 38].

18.4 Clinical Features

CVS can be asymptomatic, detected on a pre-access placement diagnostic venogram or fistulogram for an immature fistula [1, 39]. One hundred ninety patients, 61 with acute renal failure and 129 with chronic renal failure, underwent hemodialysis using a total of 302 subclavian vein catheters. Local hematomas and sepsis (seven events) were the only acute complications. Subclavian vein stenosis and/or thrombosis had occurred and were shown in 5 of 44 patients who had AV access created distal to the venous outlet obstruction, resulting in the loss of 3 of 5 of these accesses.

In view of the fact that subclavian vein stenosis or occlusion is not associated with any clinical findings and we were unable to identify any predisposing factors associated with the use of the catheters, all patients who have had previous subclavian vein catheters probably should be evaluated to determine the patency of the subclavian vein before creation of a permanent access in that arm [39]. Most occult CVS becomes clinically apparent after development of a functioning AV access in the ipsilateral extremity.

Symptomatology secondary to CVS depends on the anatomical location of the stenosis or obstruction. Narrowing or occlusion of the subclavian vein most commonly presents with edema and/or venous hypertension of the corresponding extremity and breast. Innominate vein stenosis or occlusion affects blood flow from the same side of the face as well as the upper extremity and breast leading to ipsilateral extremity and possible facial edema. Approximately, only 50 % of patients with significant CVS will develop ipsilateral upper extremity edema. In study by Schwab et al., 47 patients underwent upper arm venography to evaluate fistula dysfunction. Subclavian vein stenosis was documented in 12. Eleven of twelve had elevated venous dialysis pressure (196 ± 8.9 mmHg), and six had arm edema [1].

Edema is much more common once a functional ipsilateral upper extremity AV access is created [40]. Use of this access for HD can lead to further exacerbation of the edema, with acute swelling, tenderness, pain, and associated erythema, which can mimic cellulitis. Associated edema of the breast on the ipsilateral side along with pleural effusions may develop [41, 42]. See Fig. 18.1 below.

CVS may lead to aneurysmal dilation and tortuosity of an AV access. Progression may be prevented with prompt treatment of the inciting central lesion. Marked aneurysmal dilation may have to be treated with surgical revision or ligation of the AV access. CVS leads to the development of collaterals, which divert blood centrally via enlarged collateral veins. The collateral veins are often evident on physical examination of the neck, chest, and ipsilateral extremity. Rarely, the collaterals can bypass sufficient blood flow centrally, leading to improvement or stabilization of the CVS symptoms. See Fig. 18.2 below.

Superior vena cava syndrome is a very uncommon but feared complication of superior vena cava stenosis or

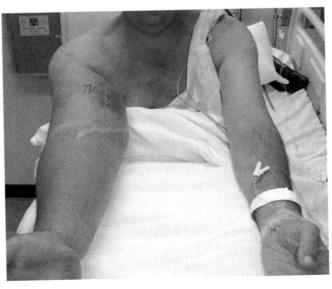

Fig. 18.1 R arm swelling due to CVS (Image courtesy of Dr. Vachhrajani)

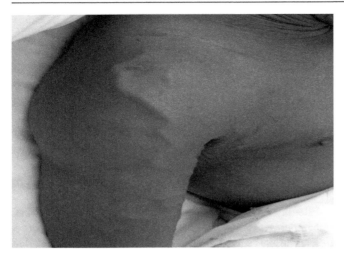

Fig. 18.2 Visible distended veins on arm and shoulder (Image courtesy of Dr. Vachhrajani)

obstruction or bilateral innominate vein narrowing or occlusion [43, 44]. This clinical syndrome is comprised of edema of the upper extremities, face, and neck, along with multiple dilated collateral veins over the chest and neck. Acute emergent treatment of superior vena cava syndrome is sometimes required.

CVS may also decrease access blood flow, leading to access recirculation and inadequate dialysis. This may also present as elevated venous pressure during HD and prolonged bleeding from needle sites after dialysis. If there is a significant decline in access blood flow, the AV access may become occluded secondary to thrombosis. Thrombolysis techniques will be ineffective or lead to recurrent thrombosis, unless the CVS is also treated.

Positioning of the central venous catheter tip low down in the superior vena cava or in the right atrium has been advocated to improve dialysis adequacy and to reduce the incidence of catheter thrombosis. However, placement of the catheter tip within the right atrium may be associated with an increased risk of right atrial thrombus.

18.5   Diagnosis

An asymptomatic CVC is usually detected by angiography performed either in preparation of access placement or after the placement of AV access.

The diagnosis of the CVS can most often be made or suspected based upon a careful history and clinical examination. History of previous CVC placement, especially if multiple, should alert one to the possibility of CVS. Presence of pacemakers or automatic cardioverter defibrillators should prompt careful investigation to look for the presence of CVS and its resolution prior to placing a vascular access on the

ipsilateral side. Extrinsic causes of CVS should also be considered and investigated.

Examination revealing numerous dilated collaterals in the neck or chest and arm edema on the ipsilateral side indicates obstruction to outflow. In case of bilateral CVS, a clinical picture of SVC syndrome can be seen, with facial edema. The direction of blood flow in collateral veins can be ascertained by careful examination. Central vein stenosis can often be confirmed by color-flow duplex venous ultrasound. A normal respiratory variation in the diameter of central veins and polyphasic atrial waves are present in most patients with patent central veins [45]. The presence of numerous collaterals in the neck is usually indicative of CVS. However, Doppler may mistake a dilated collateral vein as a patent central vein, unless attention is paid to the absence of respiratory variation [46]. It may be difficult to visualize central veins with ultrasound in those with significant muscle mass or obesity.

Central venography is the gold standard for the diagnosis of CVS. In a series of 141 patients, 54 stenoses were diagnosed in 41 patients by color-flow duplex and 64 stenoses were diagnosed by angiography [47]. There were 13 CVS (20.3 %), with 9 of the 13 CVS diagnosed by angiography only. Digital subtraction angiography is more sensitive than color duplex sonography in the evaluation of dialysis access. The DOQI guidelines recommend venography prior to placement of a permanent access in patients with previous subclavian catheterization [48]. See Figs. 18.3 and 18.4 below.

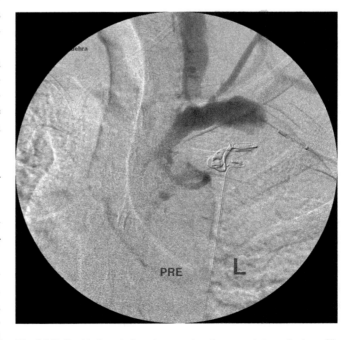

Fig. 18.3 L-sided central angiogram showing complete occlusion of L brachiocephalic vein with back flow into L IJV and presence of collaterals

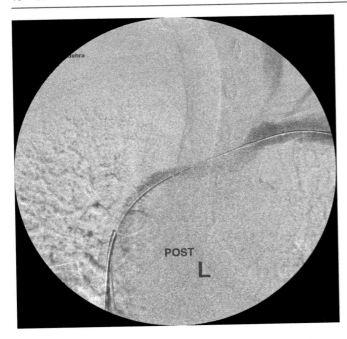

Fig. 18.4 Post-PTA disappearance of collaterals with forward flow

Magnetic resonance venogram permits avoidance of radiocontrast in a patient with advanced chronic kidney disease (CKD), where preservation of residual renal function is important [49]. This may also be useful in those with radiocontrast allergy. However, it should be noted that patients with decreased glomerular filtration rate (GFR) are at risk of developing nephrogenic systemic fibrosis [50].

18.6 Treatment

The treatment of CVS is indicated when symptoms are present. Some patients with asymptomatic CVS have adequate development of collaterals, which allow continuation of dialysis from the access without the development of symptoms or signs. These individuals need close monitoring and intervention if there is deterioration.

18.6.1 Conservative

The conservative treatment of CVS that is non-emergent involves elevation of the extremity and anticoagulation to prevent thrombosis associated with CVS. This strategy may be effective as a bridge to more definitive therapy and relies on the development of relatively adequate collaterals. In one study of high-grade (>50 %) CVS in 35 asymptomatic HD patients with 38 AVGs, 86 venograms were reviewed [51]. No intervention was done in 28 %, and none of these patients deteriorated or need further interventions. In contrast, 72 %

of the patients who underwent percutaneous angioplasty (PTA) had escalation of CVS after PTA in 8 %, which required further interventions. PTA of asymptomatic CVS greater than 50 % in the setting of hemodialysis access maintenance procedures was associated with more rapid stenosis progression and escalation of lesions, compared with a conservative approach. These observations are consistent with the empiric observation that stenosis often accelerates after PTA [52].

The appropriate use of prophylactic PTA can reduce thrombosis rates and possibly prolong access life [53–55], but injudicious use of the same technique may accelerate stenosis formation and access failure. This is not surprising as the mechanism of venous PTA is endothelial disruption and intimal stretching. Damage to these sensitive vessel layers can trigger immune reactions, myointimal proliferation, and fibromuscular hyperplasia, processes that together may ultimately accelerate stenosis formation [56].

In their study, not only did CVS progress at a greater rate in treated individuals, but PTA also may have triggered adverse events such as new stenosis formation, stent requirement, and progression to symptomatic arm swelling. Along with being detrimental to the long-term patency of the central veins, the treatment of asymptomatic CVS with PTA had a low technical success rate in this cohort. A mean of 40 % residual stenosis was left after treatment with PTA despite aggressive use of large high-pressure balloons. While this degree of residual stenosis following PTA is higher than that in other studies in which PTA and/or stent placement for CVS has been described, restenosis is always the rule when this treatment modality is implemented.

On the other hand, it can be argued that the 40 % residual stenosis in the aforementioned study left the lesion essentially untreated, so there is no surprise that the outcomes in the intervention group were worse. This observation is especially meaningful in light of the Society of Interventional Radiology (SIR) guidelines' definition of a "refractory lesion" as postintervention stenosis of >30 % [52]. Some authors have even suggested that central venous lesions represent a primary indication for stent placement due to the poor outcome usually found with balloon dilation alone and the relatively small diameters that can be achieved with PTA [57, 58].

18.6.2 Percutaneous Transluminal Angioplasty

Glanz et al. first reported PTA for CVS in 1984, with 100 % technical success rate [57]. A subsequent study by Trerotola et al. in 1986 demonstrated similar technical and clinical success rates [60]. PTA is the first-generation technology and the first-line treatment for CVS. Unfortunately, at the time of the preliminary PTA studies, there were no clear defined reporting standards in place, leading to variable study methodology and endpoints. There are no large randomized control level one studies to assess PTA for CVS, making it difficult to draw conclusions on the outcomes of PTA, and make comparisons to alternative technologies.

The work of Gerald Beathard set the tone for the debate in the early 1990s. In his pivotal study, stenoses were identified by venography in patients who met a set of clinical criteria indicating the need for evaluation. The lesions were classified by location and type. Central lesions had the worst secondary patency with only 28.9 % of all lesions remaining patent at 180 days, compared with a secondary patency 61.3 % for peripheral lesions treated with PTA alone ($p < 0.01$) [61]. PTA has demonstrated a variable technical success rate ranging from 70 to 90 % [31, 61–66]. A PTA study by Kovalik et al. in 1994 [60] made some interesting observations, including a technical failure rate of 7 %, with greater than 50 % improvement (nonelastic lesions) in 70 % of patients with CVS, and less than 50 % improvement (elastic lesions) in 23 % of patients with CVS. The study concluded that there were two types of central venous lesion: nonelastic lesions, which responded well to PTA, and elastic lesions, which were unresponsive or poorly responsive to PTA. It was felt the histology of the two types of lesions were different based on observations on intravascular ultrasound [62].

Overall, the PTA patency results for CVS demonstrate a wide range of variability. There is a 6-month primary patency range of 23–63 % and a cumulative patency range of 29–100 %. There is a 12-month primary patency range of 12–50 % and a cumulative patency range of 13–100 % [31, 61–66]. One of the largest studies to date on PTA for CVS by Bakken et al. in 2007, comprising of 47 patients, demonstrated a technical success rate of 77 %. There was a primary patency rate at 3 months of 58 %, 6 months of 45 %, and 12 months of 29 %. There was a cumulative patency rate at 3 months of 76 %, 6 months of 62 %, and 12 months of 53 % [66].

Technical failures will occur in a minority of patients when treating CVS with PTA in the range of 10–30 %. There

is clearly a subgroup of CVS patients with elastic lesions, unresponsive to PTA. It is also apparent that multiple repeated interventions with close surveillance are required with PTA for CVS, to maintain patency and prevent occlusion over the long term.

Guideline 20 of K/DOQI recommends percutaneous transluminal balloon angioplasty (PTA), with or without stent placement and is considered the preferred approach to CVS [67]. PTA usually provides excellent initial results, but the long-term primary patency is not optimal. Among 50 CVS in a series of 862 venous stenoses, an initial success rate of 89 % was followed by primary 6-month patency of only 25 % [61]. In contrast, peripheral venous angioplasty had an initial success rate of 94 % and a 6-month primary patency of 77 % indicating a different response of central veins to angioplasty. This is probably due to their greater elasticity and recoil than peripheral veins. Postoperative surveillance, either by clinical examination or by angiography, is necessary to detect recurrence of the lesion. Multiple procedures are usually needed.

It is important to note that in patients with a pacemaker, angioplasty can be successfully performed with pacemaker wires in place [20–22]. In a study by Asif et al. 28 consecutive patients underwent PTA procedure. Technical success was 95 %. Postprocedure clinical success was achieved in 100 % of the cases where the procedure was successful. The primary patency rates were 18 and 9 % at 6 and 12 months, respectively. The secondary patency rates were 95, 86, and 73 % at 6, 12, and 24 months, respectively. On average, 2.1 procedures/year were required to maintain secondary patency. There were no procedure-related complications. This study finds PTA to be a viable option in the management of PM/ICD lead-induced CVS.

The histologic basis for recurrent stenosis after PTA has been studied in stenotic AVF but not in CVS. Immunohistochemical measurement of proliferating cell nuclear antigen showed a very high proliferative index in 20 restenotic AVF, when compared with 10 primary stenotic AVF [68]. The process was even more significant in diabetic individuals. However, the process of neointimal hyperplasia seen in AVF stenosis may not be applicable to the process of smooth muscle hyperplasia in CVS (Table 18.1).

Table 18.1 Comparing patency rates of PTA

Angioplasty			Primary patency		Secondary patency	
Study	Year	Number	6 month	12 month	6 month	12 month
Beathard [59]	1992	27	29	–	–	–
Quinn et al. [61]	1995	28	81	23	100	100
Surowiec et al. [63]	2004	35	55	43	–	80
Bakken et al. [64]	2007	49	–	29	77	73

18.6.3 Bare-Metal Stents

Bare-metal stents (BMS) were first placed in the dialysis access circuit, for refractory stenoses by Gunther et al. in 1989 [67]. BMS are the second-generation technology and second-line treatment for CVS. BMS provide mechanical support to a site of stenosis which is resistant or unresponsive to PTA. BMS are potentially useful in CVS in the setting of the following: kinked stenoses, elastic stenosis post-PTA, sealing dissections or circumscribed perforations post-PTA, establishing and maintaining patency of chronic central vein occlusions, and post-PTA of highly resistant stenoses.

However, there are significant limitations to BMS. Post-deployment, BMS may migrate, shorten, or fracture on a subacute or delayed basis. BMS placement may preclude future endovascular procedures or surgical revision. It is also clearly evident that all BMSs incite intimal hyperplasia, leading to recurrent stenoses and multiple repeat interventions to maintain patency.

The use of BMS in HD access PTA interventions has significantly increased from 0 % in 1991 to over 9 % in 2001 according to the United States Renal Data System [69, 70]. The exponential increase in BMS usage in HD access procedures has led to the development of guidelines for its applications. The Society of Interventional Radiology Quality Improvement Guidelines recommend BMS be reserved for central vein lesions in which PTA has failed or that recur within 3 months after initially successful PTA or rupture after PTA [52]. Similarly, the consensus guidelines of the National Kidney Foundation Dialysis Outcomes Quality Initiative recommend that the use of stents be reserved for surgically inaccessible stenoses in which PTA fails [71–73].

Stent structure and composition may be a factor in the initial technical success rate and long-term patency, although this has not been clearly demonstrated in the literature to date. As a general rule, self-expanding stents have been utilized for CVS. The first-generation self-expanding stent is the Wallstent™ (Boston Scientific). The Wallstent™ is constructed of 18 filaments of Elgiloy woven into a mesh. The advantages of this stent include low profile, flexibility, and radiopacity. The disadvantages of this stent include foreshortening at the time of placement, eccentric loading (stenosis) which can lead to concentric narrowing and decreased radial strength, and rare delayed shortening and migration [74–78].

The second-generation self-expanding stents are the nitinol stents. Nitinol is an alloy of nickel and titanium. It has a crystalline structure, which exists in two types of temperature-dependent forms. Nitinol undergoes a reversible shape transformation, which is preset by the ratio of nickel and titanium and high-temperature heating. When nitinol transforms to its higher temperature crystalline form (28–33 °C), it will expand to its preset size and become relatively more rigid.

Nitinol also has the characteristic of superelasticity, which will cause an applied external force to deform it but attempt to return to its original shape over time, or if the external force is removed [77–80].

The results for BMS demonstrate a wide range of variability. The vast majority of the literature demonstrates a very high technical success rate, in the range of 100 %. There is a 3-month primary patency range of 63–100 % and a secondary patency range of 72–100 %. There is a 6-month primary patency range of 42–89 % and a secondary patency range of 55–100 %. There is a 12-month primary patency range of 14–73 % and a secondary patency range of 31–91 % [57, 58, 62–66, 81–86]. One of the largest retrospective studies to date on BMS with Wallstent™ for CVS by Haage et al. published in 1999 with 50 patients demonstrated a 3-month primary patency rate of 92 % and 6- and 12-month primary patency rates of 84 and 56 %, respectively. There was a secondary patency rate at 6 and 12 months of 97 % [84]. Unfortunately, these results have not been replicated elsewhere in the literature. Another retrospective study on nitinol BMS for CVS by Vogel et al. in 2004 [79] with 16 patients demonstrated 3-, 6-, and 12-month primary patency rates of 81, 74 and 67 %, respectively. Secondary patency rates were not reported in this study [81].

There are no randomized control trials to date, comparing PTA and BMS in the setting of CVS. Another retrospective study by Bakken et al. [64] published in 2007 comparing PTA and BMS for CVS demonstrated 3-, 6-, and 12-month primary patency rates with PTA of 58, 25, and 29 % in comparison with 3-, 6-, and 12-month primary patency rates with BMS of 65, 54, and 45 %. There were 3-, 6-, and 12-month secondary patency rates with PTA of 76, 62, and 53 % in comparison with 3-, 6-, and 12-month secondary patency rates with BMS of 72, 55, and 46 %. There was no significant difference in patency results between the PTA and BMS group.

In summary, it appears BMS for CVS demonstrate a high technical success rate. There is clearly a group of CVS patients, who are unresponsive to PTA and will require BMS to achieve technical success. However, there is no literature to date demonstrating the superiority of BMS over PTA in the setting of CVS. Future randomized control trials will be needed to determine the appropriate role of BMS for CVS. See Figs. 18.5, 18.6, and 18.7 below.

18.6.4 Covered Stents

Covered stents (CS) also known as peripheral endografts have been proposed as a new treatment option for CVS. The potential advantages of a CS would include providing a relatively inert and stable intravascular matrix for endothelialization while providing the mechanical advantages of a

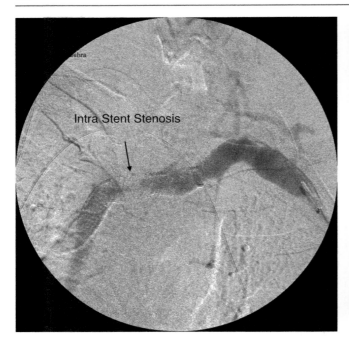

Fig. 18.5 Intrastent stenosis in L brachiocephalic vein

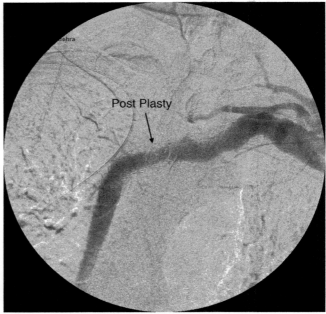

Fig. 18.7 Post-PTA result of intrastent stenosis

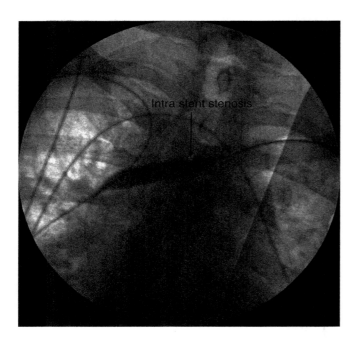

Fig. 18.6 PTA of intrastent stenosis

BMS. This could potentially reduce the intimal hyperplastic response, causing restenosis post-PTA or BMS placement. CSs are available in balloon expandable or self-expanding platforms. In practical terms, a self-expanding platform would be preferred, given the rigidity of the balloon expandable platforms. There is minimal literature on CS usage in the HD access circuit. Most of the literature to date has been

on the treatment of graft or outflow vein aneurysms and refractory venous outflow stenosis. A recent study by Jones et al. looked into the role of CS in CVS. Their results indicated primary patency of 67 and 45 % at 12 and 24 months, respectively. Secondary patency rates reported were 80 and 75 % at 12 and 24 months [14]. Another recent study by Anaya-Ayala et al. also reported 100 % technical success like Jones study. Their 12-month primary and secondary patency rates were 56 and 100 %, respectively [39]. These studies have shown superiority over BMS and PTA and are the steps in the right direction. Further randomized studies are needed to confirm these findings. One of the concerns with covered stents is the risk of jailing other central veins (Table 18.2).

18.6.5 Surgery

Access Abandonment

The simplest surgical solution for access-associated CVS is ligation of the access, which results in immediate relief of symptoms [87–90]. At the same time ligation is the most frustrating option as the vascular pathology causing the patient's problem is not corrected and the respective extremity is rendered unsuitable for further access procedures. Access abandonment requires placement of further catheter, while new access is being planned resulting in increased morbidity of these patients. This may result in development of CVS on contralateral side as well, which may preclude further access creation on contralateral side. Therefore

Table 18.2 Comparing patency rates of stents

| Study | Year | Number | Primary patency | | Secondary patency | | Stent type |
			6 month	12 month	6 month	12 month	
Stent after angioplasty failure							
Quinn et al. [61]	1995	28	67	11	100	89	Gianturco
Haage et al. [82]	1999	50	84	56	97	97	Wall
Vogel et al. [79]	2004	15	74	67	–	–	Smart
Jones et al. [85]	2011	30	81	67	100	80	Viabahn
Anaya-Ayala et al. [86]	2011	25	–	56	–	100	Viabahn
Primary stent placement							
Bakken et al. [64]	2007	26	–	21	–	46	Wall

access ligation should be considered as the last resort, only when interventional or other surgical therapy of CVS is unreasonable or has failed.

Surgical Reconstruction

Based on data obtained from the few reports in the literature [91–96], the results of surgical reconstruction of mediastinal veins in ESRD patients are better than those of interventional procedures with primary patency rates of 80–90 % at 12 months. These procedures, however, always mean major surgery. Patch angioplasty of a subclavian or brachiocephalic veins or orthotropic bypass surgery [93–96] requires clavicular division or sternotomy (and general anesthesia) and is associated with high rates of postoperative morbidity and mortality. Extra-anatomical bypass (such as axillary-to-internal jugular vein) [91, 92, 96] is less distressing to the patient, but this results in the loss of another central vein for further access.

Advanced Procedures

When the central venous drainage of all four extremities is compromised, construction or maintenance of AV access can be difficult or impossible. In low-risk patients fit for median sternotomy, a subclavian artery-to-right atrial appendix bridge graft [97] can be constructed, or an axillary vein-to-right atrial bypass [94] be performed. In patients unfit for major surgery, fashioning an arterio-arterial loop graft [98, 99] can be considered as an alternative to the insertion of a translumbar, transhepatic, or transthoracic, cuffed tunneled catheter [69, 70, 100].

Future Directions

Future treatments may include coated drug-eluting stents with rapamycin or paclitaxel to prevent development of neo-intimal hyperplasia inside stent. Other alternatives may include brachytherapy with beta radiation, which has shown some benefit in coronary circulation.

The greatest impact will be achieved as we evolve our understanding of various hemodynamic, molecular, pathologic, and genetic factors of CVS. This might result in the development of newer treatments and preventative strategies that may be critical to improve the patency of CVS lesions.

Conclusion

Prevention of CVS in HD patients is paramount like any other condition. Central venous catheter placement is the most important risk factor for CVS. Central venous catheter placement should be avoided if at all possible, particularly in the subclavian vein. The use of other peripheral lines should be minimized to preserve future peripheral and central venous capital as potential access sites. This would need close collaboration between nephrologists and internists. Policies need to be created for CKD patients specifically dealing with this issue.

All of the current treatment options for CVS will lead to recurrent stenosis or occlusion requiring multiple repeat interventions to maintain patency. Further randomized control trials with long-term follow-up for the currently available treatment options are essential in the future to develop appropriate treatment algorithms. Further advancements in treatment technique, technology, and the mechanisms of CVS with proper scientific evaluation will be essential to continue to improve the long-term results for this arduous problem.

References

1. Schwab SJ, Quarles LD, Middleton JP, et al. Hemodialysis-associated subclavian vein stenosis. Kidney Int. 1988;33:1156–9.
2. Barrett N, Spencer S, Mcivor J, Brown EA. Subclavian stenosis: a major complication of subclavian dialysis catheters. Nephrol Dial Transplant. 1988;3:423–5.
3. Surratt RS, Picus D, Hicks ME, Darcy MD, Kleinhoffer M, Jendrisakm M. The importance of preoperative evaluation of the subclavian vein in dialysis access planning. AJR Am J Roentgenol. 1991;156:623–5.
4. Agarwal AK, Patel BM, Farhan NJ. Central venous stenosis in hemodialysis patients is a common complication of ipsilateral central vein catheterization. J Am Soc Nephrol. 2004;15:368A–9.

5. Macdonald MJ, Martin LG, Hughes JD, et al. Distribution and severity of stenoses in functioning arteriovenous grafts: A duplex and angiographic study. J Vasc Tech. 1996;20:131–6.

6. Vanherweghem JL, Yasine T, Goldman M, et al. Subclavian vein thrombosis: a frequent complication of subclavian cannulation for hemodialysis. Clin Nephrol. 1986;26:235–8.

7. Macrae JM, Ahmed A, Johnson N, Levin A, Kiaii M. Central vein stenosis: a common problem in patients on hemodialysis. ASAIO J. 2005;51:77–81.

8. Hernandez D, Diaz F, Rufino M, et al. Subclavian vascular access stenosis in dialysis patients: Natural history and risk factors. J Am Soc Nephrol. 1998;9:1507–10.

9. Oguzkurt L, Tercan F, Torun D, Yildirim T, Zümrütdal A, Kizilkilic O. Impact of short-term hemodialysis catheters on the central veins: a catheter venographic study. Eur J Radiol. 2004;52: 293–9.

10. Cimochowski GE, Worley E, Rutherford WE, Sartain J, Blondin J, Harter H. Superiority of the internal jugular vein over the subclavian access for temporary dialysis. Nephron. 1990;54:154–61.

11. Schillinger F, Schillinger D, Montagnac R, Milcent T. Post catheterization venous stenosis in hemodialysis: comparative angiographic study of 50 subclavian and 50 internal jugular accesses. Nephrol Dial Transplant. 1991;6:722–4.

12. Schon D, Whittman D. Managing the complications of long-term tunneled dialysis catheters. Semin Dial. 2003;16:314–22.

13. Moss AH, Vasilaksi C, Holley HL, Foulks CJ, Pillai K. mcdowell DE. Use of a silicon dual-lumen catheter with a Dacron cuff as a long-term vascular access for hemodialysis patients. Am J Kidney Dis. 1990;16:211–5.

14. Salgado OJ, Urdaneta B, Comenares B, García R, Flores C. Right versus left internal jugular vein catheterization for hemodialysis: complications and impact on ipsilateral access creation. Artif Organs. 2004;28:728–33.

15. Grove JR, Pevec WC. Venous thrombosis related to peripherally inserted venous catheters. J Vasc Interv Radiol. 2000;11:837–40.

16. Gonsalves CF, Eschelman DJ, Sullivan KL, Dubois N, Bonn J. Incidence of central vein stenosis and occlusion following upper extremity PICC and port placement. Cardiovasc Intervent Radiol. 2003;26:123–7.

17. Trerotola SO, Kuhn-Fulton J, Johnson MS, Shah H, Ambrosius WT, Kneebone PH. Tunneled infusion catheters: increased incidence of symptomatic venous thrombosis in subclavian versus internal jugular venous access. Radiology. 2000;217:89–93.

18. Wu X, Studer W, Skarvan K, et al. High incidence of intravenous thrombi after short-term central venous catheterization of the internal jugular vein. J Clin Anesth. 1999;11:482–5.

19. Ryder MA. Peripherally inserted central venous catheters. Nurs Clin North Am. 1993;28:937–71.

20. Arif A, Salman L, Carrillo RG, Garisto JD, et al. Patency Rates for Angioplasty in the Treatment of Pacemaker-Induced Central Venous Stenosis in Hemodialysis Patients: Results of a Multi-Center Study. Semin Dial. 2009;22(6):671–6.

21. Chuang C, Tarng D, Yang W, et al. An occult cause of arteriovenous access failure: Central vein stenosis from permanent pacemaker wire. Am J Nephrol. 2001;21:406–9.

22. Sticherling C, Chough SP, Baker RL, et al. Prevalence of central venous occlusion in patients with chronic defibrillator leads. Am Heart J. 2001;141:813–6.

23. Haghjoo M, Nikoo MH, Fazelifar AF, Alizadeh A, Emkanjoo Z, Sadr-Ameli MA. Predictors of venous obstruction following pacemaker or implantable cardioverter-defibrillator implantation: a contrast venographic study on 100 patients admitted for generator change, lead revision, or device upgrade. Europace. 2007;9(5): 328–32.

24. Bulur S, Vural A, Yazıcı M, Ertaş G, Özhan H, Ural D. Incidence and predictors of subclavian vein obstruction following biven-

tricular device implantation. J Interv Card Electrophysiol. 2010;29(3):199–202.

25. Agraharkar M, Isaacson S, Mendelssohn D, et al. Percutaneously inserted silastic jugular hemodialysis catheters seldom cause jugular vein thrombosis. ASAIO J. 1995;41:169–72.

26. Di Costanzo J, Sastre B, Choux R, Kasparian M. Mechanism of thrombogenesis during total parenteral nutrition: role of catheter composition. JPEN J Parenter Enteral Nutr. 1988;12:190–4.

27. Beenen L, Van Leusen R, Deenik B, Bosch FH. The incidence of subclavian vein stenosis using silicone catheters for hemodialysis. Artif Organs. 1994;18:289–92.

28. Oguzkurt L, Tercana F, Yıldırım S. DilekTorun: Central venous stenosis in haemodialysis patients without a previous history of catheter placement. European Journal of Radiology. 2005;55:237–42.

29. Hernandez D, Diaz F, Suria S, Machado M, Lorenzo V, Losada M, Gonzalez-Posada JM, DeBonis E, Dominguez ML, Rodriguez AP. Subclavian catheter related infection is a major risk factor for the late development of subclavian vein stenosis. Nephrol Dial Transplant. 1993;8:227–30.

30. Davis D, Peterson J, Feldman R, Cho C, Stevick CA. Subclavian venous stenosis. A complication of subclavian dialysis. JAMA. 1984;252:3404–6.

31. Glanz S, Gordon DH, Lipkowitz GS, Butt KM, Hong J, Sclafani SJ. Axillary and subclavian vein stenosis: percutaneous angioplasty. Radiology. 1988;168:371–3.

32. Fillinger MF, Reinitz ER, Schwartz RA, Resetarits DE, Paskanik AM, Bruch D, Bredenberg CE. Graft geometry and venous intimal-medial hyperplasia in arteriovenous loop grafts. J Vasc Surg. 1990;11:556–66.

33. Middleton WD, Erickson S, Melson GL. Perivascular color artifact: pathologic significance and appearance on color Doppler US images. Radiology. 1989;171:647–52.

34. Gray RJ, Dolmatch BL, Buick MK. Directional atherectomy treatment for hemodialysis access: early results. J Vasc Interv Radiol. 1992;3:497–503.

35. Wali MA, Eid RA, Dewan M, Al-Homrany MA. Intimal changes in the cephalic vein of renal failure patients before arterio-venous fistula (AVF) construction. J Smooth Muscle Res. 2003;39:95–105.

36. Weiss MF, Scivittaro V, Anderson JM. Oxidative stress and increased expression of growth factors in lesions of failed hemodialysis access. Am J Kidney Dis. 2001;37:970–80.

37. Palabrica T, Lobb R, Furie BC, Aronovitz M, Benjamin C, Hsu YM, Sajer SA. Leukocyte accumulation promoting fibrin deposition is mediated by P-selectin on adherent platelets. Nature. 1992;359:848–51.

38. Agarwal AK, Patel BM, Haddad NJ. Central vein stenosis: a nephrologist's perspective. Semin Dial. 2007;20:53–62.

39. Clark DE, Albina JE, Chazan JA. Subclavian stenosis and thrombosis: a potential serious complication in chronic hemodialysis patients. Am J Kidney Dis. 1990;15:265–8.

40. Nakhoul F, Hashmonai M, Angel A, Bahous H, Green J. Extreme swelling of a limb with AV shunt for hemodialysis resulting from subclavian vein thrombosis due to previous catheterization. Clin Nephrol. 1998;49:134–6.

41. Gadallah MF, El-Shahawy MA, Campese VM. Unilateral breast enlargement secondary to hemodialysis arteriovenous fistula and subclavian vein occlusion. Nephron. 1993;63:351–3.

42. Wright RS, Quinones-Baldrich WJ, Anders AJ, Danovitch GM. Pleural effusion associated with ipsilateral breast and arm edema as a complication of subclavian vein catheterization and arteriovenous fistula formation for hemodialysis. Chest. 1994;106:950–2.

43. Baker GL, Barnes HJ. Superior vena cava syndrome: etiology, diagnosis, and treatment. Am J Crit Care. 1992;1:54–64.

44. Kanna S, Sniderman K, Simons M, et al. Superior vena cava stenosis associated with hemodialysis catheters. Am J Kidney Dis. 1992;21:278–81.

45. Rose SC, Kinney TB, Bundens WP, Valji K, Roberts AC. Importance of Doppler analysis of transmitted atrial waveforms prior to placement of central venous access catheters. J Vasc Interv Radiol. 1998;9:927–34.

46. Middleton WD, Picus DD, Marx M, Melson GL. Color Doppler sonography of hemodialysis vascular access: comparison with angiography. Am J Roentgenol. 1989;152:633–9.

47. Levit RD, Cohen RM, Kwak A, et al. Asymptomatic central venous stenosis in hemodialysis patients. Radiology. 2006;238:1051–6.

48. National Kidney Foundation. National Kidney Foundation – dialysis outcomes quality i: clinical practice guidelines for vascular access. New York: National Kidney Foundation; 1997. p. 20–1.

49. Haage P, Krings T, Schmitz-Rode T. Nontraumatic vascular emergencies: imaging and intervention in acute venous occlusion. Eur Radiol. 2002;12:2627–43.

50. Aruny JE, Lewis CA, Cardella JF, et al. Society of Interventional Radiology Standards of Practice Committee: Quality improvement guidelines for percutaneous management of the thrombosed or dysfunctional dialysis access. J Vasc Interv Radiol. 2003;14:S247–53.

51. Dember LM, Holmberg EF, Kaufman JS. Randomized controlled trial of prophylactic repair of hemodialysis arteriovenous graft stenosis. Kidney Int. 2004;66:390–8.

52. McCarley P, Wingard RL, Shyr Y, Pettus W, Hakim RM, Ikizler TA. Vascular access blood flow monitoring reduces access morbidity and costs. Kidney Int. 2001;60:1164–72.

53. Tessitore N, Mansueto G, Bedogna V, et al. A prospective controlled trial on effect of percutaneous transluminal angioplasty on functioning arteriovenous fistulae survival. J Am Soc Nephrol. 2003;14:1623–7.

54. Swedberg SH, Brown BG, Sigley R, Wight TN, Gordon D, Nicholls SC. Intimal fibromuscular hyperplasia at the venous anastomosis of PTFE grafts in hemodialysis patients: clinical, immunocytochemical, light and electron microscopic assessment. Circulation. 1989;80:1726–36.

55. Vorwerk D, Guenther RW, Mann H, Bohndorf K, Keulers P, Alzen G, Sohn M, Kistler D. Venous stenosis and occlusion in hemodialysis shunts: followup results of stent placement in 65 patients. Radiology. 1995;195:140–6.

56. Aytekin C, Boyvat F, Yag˘Murdur MC, Moray G, Haberal M. Endovascular stent placement in the treatment of upper extremity central venous obstruction in hemodialysis patients. Eur J Radiol. 2004;49:81–5.

57. Glanz S, Gordon D, Butt KMH, Hong J, Adamson R, Sclafani SJ. Dialysis access fistulas: treatment of stenoses by transluminal angioplasty. Radiology. 1984;152:637–42.

58. Trerotola SO, McLean GK, Burke DR, et al. Treatment of subclavian venous stenoses by percutaneous transluminal angioplasty. J Vasc Interv Radiol. 1986;1:15–8.

59. Beathard GA. Percutaneous transvenous angioplasty in the treatment of vascular access stenosis. Kidney Int. 1992;42:1390–7.

60. Kovalik EC, Newman GE, Suhocki P, Knelson M, Schwab SJ. Correction of central venous stenoses: use of angioplasty and vascular wallstents. Kidney Int. 1994;45:1177–81.

61. Quinn SF, Schuman ES, Demlow TA, et al. Percutaneous transluminal angioplasty versus endovascular stent placement in the treatment of venous stenoses in patients undergoing hemodialysis: intermediate results. J Vasc Interv Radiol. 1995;5:851–5.

62. Dammers R, de Haan MW, Planken NR, van der Sande FM, Tordoir JH. Central vein obstruction in hemodialysis patients: Results of radiological and surgical intervention. Eur J Vasc Endovasc Surg. 2003;26:317–21.

63. Surowiec SM, Fegley AJ, Tanski WJ, et al. Endovascular management of central venous stenoses in the hemodialysis patient: results of percutaneous therapy. Vasc Endovascular Surg. 2004;38: 349–54.

64. Bakken AM, Protack CD, Saad WE, Lee DE, Waldman DL, Davies MG. Long-term outcomes of primary angioplasty and primary stenting of central venous stenosis in hemodialysis patients. J Vasc Surg. 2007;45:776–83.

65. Guideline 20. NKF-K/DOQI clinical practice guidelines for vascular access, 2000. Am J Kidney Dis. 2001;37:s137–81.

66. Chang CJ, Ko PJ, Hsu LA, Ko YS, Ko YL, Chen CF, Huang CC, Hsu TS, Lee YS, Pang JH. Highly increased cell proliferation activity in the restenotic hemodialysis vascular access after percutaneous transluminal angioplasty: Implication in prevention of restenosis. Am J Kidney Dis. 2004;43:74–84.

67. Gunther RW, Vorwerk D, Bohndorf K, et al. Venous stenosis in dialysis shunts: treatment with self-expanding metallic stents. Radiology. 1989;170:401–5.

68. USRD System. USRD 2003 annual data report: atlas of end-stage renal disease in the United States. Bethesda: National Institutes of Health, National Institute of Diabetes and Digestive and Kidney Diseases; 2003.

69. NKF-K/DOQI clinical practice guidelines for vascular access. Am J Kidney Dis. 2001;37:s137–81.

70. National Kidney Foundation Dialysis Outcomes Quality Initiative. NKF-DOQI clinical practice guidelines for vascular access. Am J Kidney Dis. 1997;30(Suppl):s150–91.

71. Clark TWI. Nitinol stents in hemodialysis access. J Vasc Interv Radiol. 2004;15:1037–40.

72. Flueckiger F, Sternthal H, Klein GE, Aschauer M, Szolar D, Kleinhappl G. Strength, elasticity, and plasticity of expandable metal stents: in vitro studies with three types of stress. J Vasc Interv Radiol. 1994;5:745–50.

73. Rogers C, Edelman ER. Endovascular stent design dictates experimental restenosis and thrombosis. Circulation. 1995;91:2995–3001.

74. Trerotola SO, Fair JH, Davidson D, Samphilipo Jr MA, Magee CA. Comparison of Gianturco Z stents and Wallstents in a hemodialysis access graft animal model. J Vasc Interv Radiol. 1995;6:387–96.

75. Dyet JF, Watts WG, Ettles DF, Nicholson AA. Mechanical properties of metallic stent: how do these properties influence the choice of stent for specific lesions? Cardiovasc Intervent Radiol. 2000;23:47–54.

76. Verstandig AG, Bloom AI, Sasson T, Haviv YS, Rubinger D. Shortening and migration of Wallstents after stenting of central venous stenoses in hemodialysis patients. Cardiovasc Intervent Radiol. 2003;26:58–64.

77. Shabalovskaya SA. On the nature of the biocompatibility and on medical applications of NiTi shape memory and superelastic alloys. Biomed Mater Eng. 1996;6:267–89.

78. Duda SH, Wiskirchen J, Tepe G, et al. Physical properties of endovascular stents: an experimental comparison. J Vasc Interv Radiol. 2000;11:645–54.

79. Vogel PM, Parise CP. SMART stent for salvage of hemodialysis access grafts. JVIR. 2004;15:1051–60.

80. Chen CY, Liang HL, Pan HB, et al. Metallic stenting for treatment of central venous obstruction in hemodialysis patients. J Chin Med Assoc. 2003;66:166–72.

81. Oderich GS, Treiman GS, Schneider P, Bhirangi K. Stent placement for treatment of central and peripheral venous obstruction: A long-term multi-institutional experience. J Vasc Surg. 2000;32:760–9.

82. Haage P, Vorwerk D, Piroth W, Schuermann K, Guenther RW. Treatment of hemodialysis-related central venous stenosis or occlusion: results of primary wallstent placement and follow-up in 50 patients. Radiology. 1999;212:175–80.

83. Vesely TM, Hovsepian DM, Pilgram TK, Coyne DW, Shenoy S. Upper extremity central venous obstruction in hemodialysis patients: Treatment with wallstents. Radiology. 1997;204:343–8.

84. Gray RJ, Horton KM, Dolmatch BL, et al. Use of wallstents for hemodialysis access-related venous stenoses and occlusions untreatable with balloon angioplasty. Radiology. 1995;195:479–84.

85. Jones RG, Willis AP, Jones C, McCafferty IJ, Riley PL. Long-term results of stent-graft placement to treat central venous stenosis and occlusion in hemodialysis patients with arteriovenous fistulas. J Vasc Interv Radiol. 2011;22(9):1240–5.

86. Anaya-Ayala JE, Smolock CJ, Colvard BD, Naoum JJ, Bismuth J, Lumsden AB, Davies MG, Peden EK. Efficacy of covered stent placement for central venous occlusive disease in hemodialysis patients. J Vasc Surg. 2011;54(3):754–9.

87. Hwang SM, Lee SH, Ahn SK. Pincer nail deformity and pseudo-Kaposi's sarcoma: complications of an artificial arteriovenous fistula for haemodialysis. Br J Dermatol. 1999;141:1129–32.

88. Okadome K, Komori K, Fukumitsu T, Sugimachi K. The potential risk for subclavian vein occlusion in patients on haemodialysis. Eur J Vasc Surg. 1992;6:602–6.

89. Wisselink W, Money SR, Becker MO, Rice KL, Ramee SR, White CJ, et al. Comparison of operative reconstruction and percutaneous balloon dilatation for central venous obstruction. Am J Surg. 1993;166:200–5.

90. Money S, Bhatia D, Daharamsy S, Mulingtapang R, Shaw D, Ramee S. Comparison of surgical by-pass, percutaneous balloon dilatation (PTA) and PTA with stent placement in the treatment of central venous occlusion in the dialysis patient. One-year follow-up (Abstract). Int Angiol. 1995;14:176.

91. Gradman WS, Bressman P, Sernaque JD. Subclavian vein repair in patients with an ipsilateral arteriovenous fistula. Ann Vasc Surg. 1994;8:549–56.

92. El-Sabrout RA, Duncan JM. Right atrial bypass grafting for central venous obstruction associated with dialysis access: Another treatment option. J Vasc Surg. 1999;29:472–8.

93. Haug M, Popescu M, Vonderbank E, Kruger G. Die Rekonstruktion mediastinaler Venen beim gleichseitigen Dialyseshunt. Zentralbl Chir. 1999;124:2–6.

94. Mickley V. Stent oder Bypass? Behandlungsergebnisse zentralveno ser Obstruktionen. Zentralbl Chir. 2001;126:445–9.

95. Mickley V. Subclavian artery to right atrium haemodialysis bridge graft for superior vena caval occlusion. Nephrol Dial Transplant. 1996;11:1361–2.

96. Bunger CM, Kroger J, Kock L, Henning A, Klar E, Schareck W. Axillary-axillary interarterial chest loop conduit as an alternative for chronic hemodialysis access. J Vasc Surg. 2005; 42:290–5.

97. Zanow J, Kru¨ Ger U, Petzold M, Petzold K, Miller H, Scholz H. Arterioarterial prosthetic loop: A new approach for hemodialysis access. J Vasc Surg. 2005;41:1007–12.

98. Kinney TB. Translumbar high inferior vena cava access placement in patients with thrombosed inferior vena cava filters. J Vasc Interv Radiol. 2003;14:1563–7.

99. Smith TP, Ryan JM, Reddan DM. Transhepatic catheter access for hemodialysis. Radiology. 2004;232:246–51.

100. Wellons ED, Matsuura J, Lai KM, Levitt A, Rosenthal D. Transthoracic cuffed hemodialysis catheters: a method for difficult hemodialysis access. J Vasc Surg. 2005;42:286–9.

Approach to a Patient with Pseudoaneurysm

19

Marius C. Florescu and Troy J. Plumb

19.1 Definition

The pseudoaneurysm is caused by a tear through all the layers of a vessel, allowing a blood collection to form outside the blood vessel, but remaining in continuity with the vessel lumen. The blood is contained by the surrounding tissues and flows in and out of the pseudoaneurysm's cavity during systole and diastole. The pseudoaneurysm has two components: a cavity and a neck by which the cavity communicates with the lumen of the vessel. Figure 19.1 presents an angiogram of an arteriovenous graft with pseudoaneurysm.

The pseudoaneurysm should be differentiated from an aneurysm, the latter being a dilatation of a blood vessel without the blood leaving the lumen of the vessel and from a hematoma when the collection of extraluminal blood is contained by the surrounding tissues, but it is not communicating anymore with the blood vessel lumen.

The interventional nephrologist will encounter and will have to manage pseudoaneurysms in the following situations:

1. Arteriovenous graft (AVG) pseudoaneurysm
2. Arteriovenous fistula (AVF) pseudoaneurysm
3. Arterial pseudoaneurysm caused by erroneous cannulation of an artery with the hemodialysis needles or after arterial puncture to access the arterial system for diagnostic or therapeutic procedures

19.2 AVG Pseudoaneurysm

The AVG pseudoaneurysms can develop over time as a result of repeated punctures by hemodialysis needles in a limited area of the graft leading to the graft material deterioration and from inadequate hemostasis after needle removal. The presence of a proximal venous stenosis can accelerate the pseudoaneurysm's growth by increasing the intra-access pressure [1]. Early cannulation of the AVG, less than 2 weeks after its creation, might increase the risk of pseudoaneurysm formation due to insufficient graft incorporation into the surrounding tissues.

The pseudoaneurysm's progressive enlargement produces thinning of the overlying skin potentially leading to skin necrosis, poor eschar healing, prolonged bleeding after needles removal, possible spontaneous bleeding, and, finally, acute graft rupture with severe blood loss.

Figure 19.2 presents an arteriovenous graft pseudoaneurysm with necrosis and bleeding of the overlying skin.

Hemodialysis needles should not be inserted into pseudoaneurysms irrelevant of their size [2]. Because of that, large pseudoaneurysms limit the availability of AVG cannulation sites.

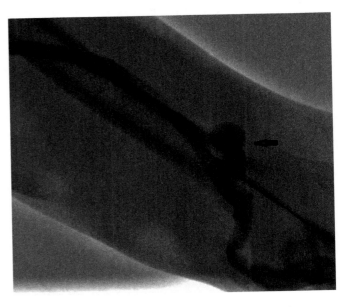

Fig. 19.1 Arteriovenous graft with pseudoaneurysm (*arrow*)

M.C. Florescu, MD (✉) • T.J. Plumb, MD
Division of Nephrology, Department of Internal Medicine,
University of Nebraska Medical Center, Omaha, NE, USA
e-mail: mflorescu@unmc.edu

A.S. Yevzlin et al. (eds.), *Interventional Nephrology*,
DOI 10.1007/978-1-4614-8803-3_19, © Springer Science+Business Media New York 2014

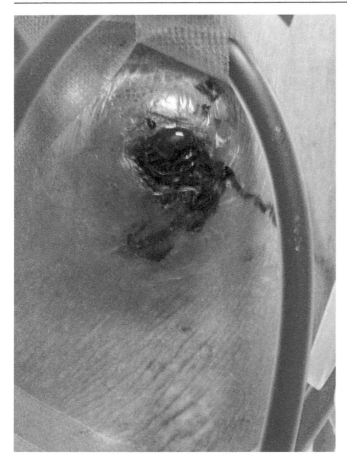

Fig. 19.2 Arteriovenous graft with large pseudoaneurysm with skin necrosis and bleeding

Pseudoaneurysm formation is a well-known complication of AVG, and its incidence rates range between 2 and 10 % [3–5]. Because the repeated needle insertion in a limited portion of the graft is an important determinant of AVG pseudoaneurysm formation, we assume that the incidence of this complication might vary according to the pattern of needle insertion in different hemodialysis units.

19.2.1 Diagnosis

The pseudoaneurysm is readily diagnosed clinically by the presence of a dilated area of the graft that is growing in size. They are pulsatile, but sometimes the pulsations are difficult to palpate because of possible stenoses located upstream of the aneurysm and scarring of the overlying tissue. The skin overlying the aneurysm can be normal at the beginning, and as the aneurysm is growing in size, the skin will become thinner and eventually can develop areas of necrosis.

Duplex ultrasound can detect the presence of the dilated pseudoaneurysm, can measure its size, can detect the presence of a possible thrombus, and can document the movement of blood between the pseudoaneurysm and the lumen of the AVG.

AVG angiogram is more invasive than the ultrasound evaluation but can easily diagnose, measure, and treat suitable pseudoaneurysms and their associated abnormalities, like venous anastomosis stenosis.

A patient with a suspected pseudoaneurysm should be referred for evaluation and treatment if signs of increased risk of rupture, prolonged bleeding, rapid growth, pain, skin necrosis, or spontaneous bleeding, are present [2].

19.2.2 Management

Small, asymptomatic pseudoaneurysms can be followed if they are stable and painless, the overlying skin is normal, and there are adequate sites available on the graft for needle insertion. Even small, stable pseudoaneurysms should not be stuck with hemodialysis needles [2].

National Kidney Foundation Kidney Disease Outcomes Quality Initiative (NKF KDOQI) guidelines [2] established indications for revision/repair of pseudoaneurysms:

1. The cannulation sites are limited by the presence of the pseudoaneurysm.
2. The pseudoaneurysm threatens the viability of the overlying skin.
3. The pseudoaneurysm is symptomatic (pain, throbbing).
4. Infection.

The treatment can be surgical or endovascular. Obviously, an infected pseudoaneurysm should be surgically treated. The surgical approach is recommended by the KDOQI guidelines [2] in cases where the pseudoaneurysm is rapidly expanding, when the pseudoaneurysm diameter exceeds twice the graft's diameter, and when the integrity of the skin overlying the pseudoaneurysm is broken increasing the risk of graft infection. The surgical treatment consists of resection of the affected segment of the graft followed by graft segment interposition [6].

Infected AVG pseudoaneurysms can be treated with interposition bypass graft tunneled through noninfected tissues and connected end to end with the noninfected segments of the old graft, followed by excision of AVG's infected portion. Graft patency and wound healing has been achieved using this approach in 74 % of infected AVGs whose infection was not affecting their entire length [7–9].

The outcome of the AVG surgical revision, performed specifically to treat pseudoaneurysms, has not been well documented in the literature. In one study [6], involving a total of 189 polytetrafluoroethylene (PTFE) AVGs implanted in 131 end-stage renal disease (ESRD) patients, 49 required surgical revision extending their survival to a rate similar to that of nonrevised grafts. In this particular study [6], the assisted patency rates for all grafts were 76 % at 12 months,

50 % at 36 months, and 40 % at 60 months. We have to mention that pseudoaneurysm repair was not the indication for surgical revision, but the revision consisted in partial excision of the graft and segment interposition, the same surgical management used for pseudoaneurysm treatment. Despite our best efforts we could not find any studies reporting graft patency after surgical revision for pseudoaneurysm repair, but we can assume that it is close to the one reported above.

The surgical revision of the AVGs for the treatment of pseudoaneurysms has not been directly compared with the endovascular treatment using stent grafts nor were their indications thoroughly studied. KDOQI indications for surgical revision were based more on expert opinions than on hard data. It is obvious that shin necrosis overlying the pseudoaneurysm and an infected pseudoaneurysm are indications for surgical revision. KDOQI also recommends that aneurysms with a diameter that exceeds twice the diameter of the graft should be surgically corrected. However, there are numerous reports [10–13] of large pseudoaneurysms surpassing the size limits suggested by KDOQI, which were endovascularly treated with stent grafts with immediate success and good long-term patency. These reports are challenging the recommendation for surgical revision of all pseudoaneurysms larger than twice the graft's diameter.

Currently there are three available stent grafts for the treatment of AVG pseudoaneurysms.

Wallgraft endoprosthesis (Boston Scientific Corporation, Natick, MA) has an outer layer made of polyethylene terephthalate and an inner layer of Elgiloy stent with platinum tracer wires. It is Food and Drug Administration (FDA) approved for tracheobronchial applications.

Viabahn endoprosthesis (Gore & associates, Flagstaff, AZ) has an expanded polytetrafluoroethylene (ePTFE) inner structure with a nitinol self-expanding external stent. It is approved by FDA for the treatment of superficial femoral artery lesions.

Fluency (Bard, Tempe, AZ) is a self-expanding nitinol stent encapsulated into an ePTFE graft material. It is FDA approved for tracheobronchial applications.

All the stents are used off-label for the AVG pseudoaneurysm endovascular treatment and for hemodialysis needles punctures.

19.2.3 Technique of Endovascular Treatment of AVG Pseudoaneurysms

Stent grafts have been used in the percutaneous treatment of noninfected AVG pseudoaneurysms. Before the procedure, it is paramount to perform a thorough AVG's physical examination to exclude skin necrosis or infection, both being contraindications for the endovascular treatment.

After gaining access to the graft in an adequate location for stent deployment, the angiogram will assess the pseudoa-

neurysm's size and location. If the lesion is deemed treatable with the stent graft, a large enough vascular sheath to allow the passage of the stent delivery system should be placed. The diameter of the graft portions adjacent to the pseudoaneurysm should be measured. The manufacturer recommends using endograft devices with a diameter 15–20 % larger than the graft diameter adjacent to the lesion. Before the stent deployment some authors are recommending to administer 3,000 units of intravenous heparin to prevent thrombosis [1]. We should consider the stent to overlap 10 mm of normal graft on both sides in order to prevent endoleaks [14]. In order to preserve a maximum length of un-stented AVG, we should choose the shortest stent that can appropriately cover the pseudoaneurysm without excessively overlapping with the normal graft. The stent is deployed in the usual manner. A repeated angiogram is performed to check for the successful exclusion of the pseudoaneurysm.

After the stent placement, the blood still present in the now isolated pseudoaneurysm should be percutaneously aspirated if possible. According to Barshes et al. [1], who presented a series of 26 patients with AVG pseudoaneurysms treated with covered stents, pulsatility was still presented within the pseudoaneurysms for at least 24 h after the procedure in all patients despite the successful pseudoaneurysm isolation on the final angiogram, but it disappeared at subsequent follow-up visits.

Figure 19.3 depicts successful isolation of arteriovenous graft pseudoaneurysm presented in Fig. 19.1 using a stent graft.

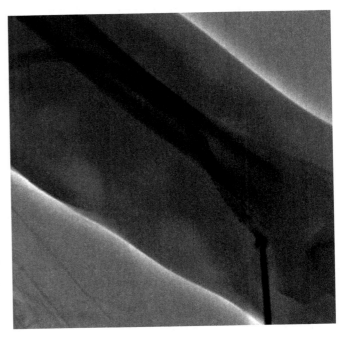

Fig. 19.3 Arteriovenous graft pseudoaneurysm treated with a stent graft

19.2.4 Outcomes

Barshes et al. [1], in their 26 patient series, using mostly Wallgraft stent grafts (18 out of 26 patients) had 100 % technical success rate in deploying stents and excluding the AVG pseudoaneurysms. All patients had hemodialysis within 48 h of intervention with the needles placed through the graft. Seventy-three percent of patients developed complete resolution or significant decrease in pseudoaneurysms size. Out of 26 patients 13 had pseudoaneurysms with mean diameters of 4.8 cm. Out of the entire group, 4 patients (15 %) required surgical revision between postoperative day 21 and 49 for return of the pulsatility or persistently large pseudoaneurysms. The mean pseudoaneurysm diameter in this group was 4.3 cm. For the entire group, the primary patency rate was 82 % at 30 days and 28 % at 6 months following endograft placement. The results are similar with the 11 patient's series presented by Vesely et al. [15] who used Viabahn endografts for AVG pseudoaneurysms repair and had a primary patency of 71 % at 3 months and 20 % at 6 months.

Moszkowicz et al. [16], using Fluency Plus stent grafts in 16 patients with AVG pseudoaneurysms, obtained good immediate results but did not report a long-term patency rate. He reported that true pseudoaneurysms with narrow mouths responded well to the placement of only one stent compared with areas of graft degenerations with widemouthed pseudoaneurysms that required more than one stent and despite that had more endoleaks.

In a series of ten patients [12] with AVG pseudoaneurysms with a mean diameter of 3 cm treated with Wallgraft stent grafts, all patients have successful exclusion of the pseudoaneurysms. At 2 weeks nine out of ten AVG remained functional, and at 6 months duplex scan showed complete pseudoaneurysms exclusion in seven patients (out of initial ten).

The stents were not compared head to head to assess which model offer the best outcomes in isolating AVG pseudoaneurysms or which stent is better suited to withstand the effects of long-term hemodialysis needle cannulations, so we cannot make any recommendation in regard to which stent model should be used.

19.2.5 Pseudoaneurysm Size

KDOQI recommends that AVG pseudoaneurysms with diameters that exceed twice the AVG diameter should be treated by surgical revision, not endovascularly. However, the case series reporting good outcomes obtained with the endovascular repair of large AVG pseudoaneurysms are challenging this recommendation.

Pseudoaneurysm's size might be an important determinant of successful initial endovascular treatment and the long-term results. Out of the 26 patients presented by Barshes et al. [1], 4 required surgical revisions for failed treatment, and in this group the mean pseudoaneurysm's diameter was 4.3 cm. However, out of 26 patients, 13 patients had a mean pseudoaneurysm diameter of 4.8 cm and most of them fared well. In the 11 patient series presented by Vesely [15], the 2 patients requiring surgical revision had large pseudoaneurysms. Currently, there is no well-established pseudoaneurysm size above which the endovascular treatment is ineffective and should be avoided.

As Moszkowicz et al. [16] suggested, the width of the pseudoaneurysm mouth might play an important role. They are reporting that true pseudoaneurysms with narrow mouths can be easily treated, whereas widemouthed pseudoaneurysms that are rather graft degenerated than pseudoaneurysms require more than one stent and are more prone to endoleaks.

The use of stent-graft devices is less invasive compared with the surgical revision and permits continuous hemodialysis using the same AVG without the need for a new catheter placement. If unsuccessful, the surgical revision option is still available as demonstrated by Barshes et al. [1] who reported an AVG pseudoaneurysm excision and bypass graft interposition to treat a stent-graft separation which occurred 6 weeks after the initial successful stent-graft pseudoaneurysm exclusion.

The role of the surgical intervention in the treatment of AVG pseudoaneurysms has not been directly compared with the endovascular treatment.

19.2.6 Stent-Graft Cannulation for Hemodialysis

Rhodes et al. [13] describe good results after regular needle punctures of the Wallstent grafts used to treat pseudoaneurysms. Their studies of 6 patients comparing stent needle punctures initiated few days after stenting or waiting 2–3 weeks before cannulating the stents did not show any significant differences between the approaches. The outcomes presented by Barshes et al. [1] also support the safety of placing needles through the covered stents. However, graft stent infection is possible to occur when cannulation is performed through these devices [17]. A stent strut protrusion through the skin that posed a risk of stent infection and also a risk of injury to the hemodialysis staff has been recently described [18] and required surgical intervention to remove the stent. At this time, it is unclear which covered stent model offers the best outcomes for long-term needle use. None of them are approved for hemodialysis needle puncture.

The safety of repeated stent-graft cannulation has not been adequately studied. It is a good practice to inform the patient, the nephrologist, and the hemodialysis unit of the stent placement and its location and to make suggestions where the needles should be placed. Efforts should be made to avoid placing the needles through the stents. As described before, protrusion of a broken strut through patient's skin is possible and can pose a risk not only for the patient but also for the hemodialysis staff taking care of that patient.

19.2.7 Infection and AVG Pseudoaneurysms

An AVG infection can weaken the graft wall and can be the primary cause for pseudoaneurysm formation or can affect an existing pseudoaneurysm. Differentiating between infected pseudoaneurysms from noninfected ones can be challenging because of the local erythema and increased skin temperature induced by the presence of the pseudoaneurysm. Blood culture results and fever are useful in differentiating the presence of infection. Identifying an infected pseudoaneurysm is important because this is a contraindication for endovascular intervention and surgical revision should be performed instead.

19.2.8 Pseudoaneurysm and Thrombosis

Many times AVG pseudoaneurysms are diagnosed incidentally during thrombectomy procedures. It is difficult to determine if the pseudoaneurysm has a role in triggering the thrombosis or it is just an innocent bystander. We can hypothesize that the turbulent, stagnant blood in the pseudoaneurysm can predispose to thrombosis. If the thrombosed part of the pseudoaneurysm can be isolated with the stent graft, there is no need to remove an old thrombus located in the pseudoaneurysm.

19.2.9 Daily Hemodialysis and the Risk of Pseudoaneurysm Formation

We consider that AVG pseudoaneurysms are caused by the cumulative damage inflicted to the graft integrity by the repeated needle punctures in a limited area of the graft, and we can assume that daily hemodialysis requiring a double number of needle punctures might favor the development of AVG pseudoaneurysms. Published studies assessing the vascular access in daily hemodialysis did not show that AVF or AVG outcomes are any worse in daily HD patients compared with conventional, 3 times/week hemodialysis [19–22]. Contrary to our expectations those outcomes seem to be slightly better in daily HD patients. The most common reported complication of AVF was stenosis and thrombosis. No cases of AVG pseudoaneurysms were reported, but the published studies included a very small number of AVG – 22 in 3 studies [20–22]. As of now, the available data does not show any evidence of increased risk of pseudoaneurysm formation in daily hemodialysis patients with AVGs, but probably we do not have enough information to draw a definitive conclusion.

19.2.10 Prevention of AVG Pseudoaneurysms

Prevention of AVG pseudoaneurysms formation consists of strict adherence to needle puncture site rotation, thorough hemostasis after needle removal, and avoiding needle sticks 2 weeks after AVG creation to allow enough time for AVG material to be encapsulated by the surrounding tissues. Avoiding needle puncture in all pseudoaneurysms even small and stable and prompt treatment of venous stenosis that is increasing intragraft pressure might delay pseudoaneurysm growth.

Although, to our knowledge, no cases were reported, we advise against using the Trerotola thrombectomy device for the thrombectomy procedures performed in AVG or AVF with previously implanted stents that were used for needle insertions. The device might get caught in a disrupted strut or it might dislodge the stent.

19.3 AVF Pseudoaneurysm

AVF pseudoaneurysms arise from the body of the AVF, not from the feeding artery. Five such cases were reported [23–25]. The pseudoaneurysms formed during or a few hours after the hemodialysis session as new pulsating, painful, masses arising over an AVF puncture sites. Their size ranged from 15 to 40 mm [23] and 26 mm for the case presented by Reichle et al. [25]. All the reported cases were successfully treated by ultrasound-guided compression. In the three case series presented by Witz et al. [23], the compression was applied manually over the pseudoaneurysm, and the Doppler ultrasound was used to ensure the lack of blood flow into the pseudoaneurysm's cavity and continuation of the blood flow in the AVF's feeding artery as well as in AVF's body. The compression time ranged between 20 and 45 min, all the pseudoaneurysms were successfully thrombosed, and AVF's patency was preserved in all cases. No recurrences were noted afterwards. The cases presented suggest that ultrasound-guided compression is effective in inducing pseudoaneurysm thrombosis while preserving AVF's patency and is preserving the critically important "AVF's real estate." The compression should be Doppler ultrasound guided to ensure isolation of the pseudoaneurysm and blood flow preservation in the AVF and the feeding artery. We consider that ultrasound-guided compression should be tried first on all AVF pseudoaneurysms before proceeding to more invasive interventions.

Najibi et al. [12] described two cases of AVF pseudoaneurysms successfully treated with covered stents (Wallgraft). One had a diameter of 3.5 and the other 3 cm. Both were successfully excluded by using covered stents (7 mm and, respectively, 8 mm in diameter). One fistula failed at 3 months and the other continued to be used successfully at 6 months without requiring any additional intervention.

We were unable to identify any cases of the AVF pseudoaneurysms treated with thrombin injection.

19.4 Arterial Pseudoaneurysm

A pseudoaneurysm can arise from any artery. ESRD patients are at increased risk for developing arterial pseudoaneurysms secondary to inadvertent hemodialysis needle placement, inadvertent arterial placement of large diameter hemodialysis catheters, and numerous diagnostic and interventional vascular procedures they require because of increased prevalence of peripheral arterial and coronary artery diseases.

19.5 Arterial Pseudoaneurysms Formed After Inadvertent Arterial Hemodialysis Needle Placement

19.5.1 Clinical Presentation

Cases of brachial artery pseudoaneurysms developed after inadvertent puncture with hemodialysis needles were described [26–31]. The brachial artery is most commonly affected because of its proximity to the basilic vein or cephalic vein and can be easily confounded with the body of the AVF and inadvertently cannulated. The pseudoaneurysms presented 1–7 days after the inadvertent cannulation, and most of them had a history of prolonged bleeding from the puncture site at the end of hemodialysis treatment. They present as pulsatile masses with a systolic bruit on auscultation, located over the brachial artery. Their diameters tend to be larger than the pseudoaneurysms arising from the AVFs, being in the range of 5–6 cm [26, 27]. They can be associated with neuropathy and venous thrombosis caused by compression of the adjacent structures by the pseudoaneurysm's mass [26, 27]. Duplex ultrasound and arteriography confirm the nature, size, and location of the lesion. Complications include rupture with severe hemorrhage, infection, or distal vascular insufficiency.

Most of the cases were treated surgically with draining of the blood collection and repairing the arterial wall defect with suture of the arterial wall or venous patch repair. In one case ultrasound-guided compression was attempted without success and turned out that the arterial defect was very large [26].

Covered stents can be used to treat arterial pseudoaneurysms. A femoral artery covered stent was successfully used to treat the pseudoaneurysm associated with a femoral artery to femoral vein fistula that developed after femoral vein catheterization for placement of a hemodialysis catheter for acute hemodialysis [32].

19.6 Pseudoaneurysms Formed After Arterial Puncture for Diagnostic and Interventional Procedures

The interventional nephrologists are more and more involved in vascular access procedures involving the arterial system. Femoral artery cannulation is frequently used to gain access to the arterial system for diagnostic and interventional procedures, and femoral artery pseudoaneurysm is the most common complication of femoral artery catheterization [33].

The pseudoaneurysm occurs as a pulsatile mass with a systolic bruit located over the catheter insertion site, and the duplex ultrasound confirms its presence by identifying the blood collection, the in and out movement of the blood inside the pseudoaneurysm, and the presence of the neck that connects the pseudoaneurysm with the artery. Most of the pseudoaneurysms develop within 3 days of the arterial sheath removal [34].

An important risk factor for pseudoaneurysm formation is the inadequate period of manual compression after vascular sheath removal. According to Katzenschlager et al. [35], the incidence of pseudoaneurysms noted after femoral artery catheterization decreased significantly if manual pressure was applied for at least 5 min after local bleeding had stopped. Large sheaths, administering antiplatelets and anticoagulant medications during or after procedure, obesity, age above 65 years, peripheral artery disease, hypertension, and end-stage renal disease are additional risk factors for arterial pseudoaneurysm formation [34–36].

Surgical intervention is indicated if the pseudoaneurysm occurs at the site of a vascular anastomosis; there is an associated arteriovenous fistula; the diameter is very large; the pseudoaneurysm causes skin necrosis, is rapidly growing, and is infected; and there is failure of the minimally invasive procedures to control the pseudoaneurysm [36]. Table 19.1 summarizes the indications for surgical treatment.

Small pseudoaneurysms with diameters of 1.8–2 cm and not growing, asymptomatic, and occurring in not anticoagulated patients can be safely observed [33]. Kent et al. [37] found that pseudoaneurysms with a mean size of less than 1.8 cm would spontaneously thrombose and the average time to thrombosis was 22 days. If an intervention is needed, the most commonly used minimally invasive procedures to treat arterial

Table 19.1 Arterial pseudoaneurysm, surgical indications

Large aneurysm
Rapidly growing
Associated arteriovenous fistula
Located at the site of arterial anastomosis
Skin necrosis
Infection
Failure of the minimally invasive procedures

pseudoaneurysms are ultrasound-guided pseudoaneurysm compression and direct percutaneous thrombin injection.

Ultrasound-guided pseudoaneurysm compression (UGPC) can be performed in non-anticoagulated patients with small pseudoaneurysms with long necks. The skin overlying the lesion should be intact. Contraindications consist of all the surgical indications mentioned before. The success rate is 80 % [33]. Before the procedure, it is very important to rule out skin necrosis and infection. Pre-procedure duplex ultrasound examination should evaluate the size, position, relation with the feeding artery, presence of a possible arteriovenous fistula, and location of the neck and determine the best location and direction to apply pressure in order to occlude the blood flow into the pseudoaneurysm's sac without applying pressure over the pseudoaneurysm or the artery. The compression can be performed using the ultrasound transducer or by manual digital compression.

The patients need local anesthesia and conscious sedation because the pseudoaneurysm compression is a painful maneuver. The ultrasound probe is positioned over the pseudoaneurysm's neck, and pressure is applied until the blood flow into the aneurysm stops. Ideally, we should avoid compressing the femoral artery, but this cannot be achieved in all patients. The pressure is applied for intervals between 6 and 20 min at the time. Pseudoaneurysm thrombosis with the cessation of the blood flow into the body of the pseudoaneurysm documented by Doppler ultrasound means the procedure was successful and can be stopped. If there is still blood flow, an additional compression is needed. In average the total compression time is 40 min divided in 3 to 4 compression sessions [33].

Ultrasound-guided thrombin injection is highly effective, 97 % success rate [33], and reasonably safe, 1.4 % incidence of complications [33]. The procedure can be performed in all the cases not carrying a surgical indication. Another contraindication is the known allergic reaction to bovine thrombin developed from previous procedures.

Pre-procedure evaluation should exclude the presence of skin necrosis or infection as those are contraindications for injection. Baseline distal arterial pulses need to be established. Duplex ultrasound should determine the pseudoaneurysms size, possible presence of multiple lobes, location

of the neck, the relation with the supplying artery, and very importantly the presence of an arteriovenous fistula that represents an absolute contraindication to thrombin injection because of the danger that some thrombin might spill into the venous circulation with potentially dangerous consequences. Thrombin affects the final pathway of the clotting cascade, and it is not affected by heparin or Coumadin treatment. However, in the general circulation, the thrombin can be inactivated by the presence of plasma antithrombin.

The needles used for thrombin injection can be 21–25 gauge attached to a 3 ml syringe. The ultrasound probe on gray scale is used to guide the needle insertion into the pseudoaneurysm's sac. Gray scale or Doppler ultrasound can be used to monitor the thrombin injection. The thrombin should be injected as far away as possible from the pseudoaneurysm's neck. The ultrasound will document the instant formation of hyperechoic thrombus as the fibrin is injected. The rate of thrombin injection should be kept between 0.1 and 0.3 ml/s and should ensure a gradual filling of the pseudoaneurysm's cavity with thrombus. Many times the complete thrombosis can be achieved in seconds. Gray scale ultrasound and Doppler can be switched intermittently to monitor thrombosis, since acute thrombus can, at times, be hypoechoic and hence difficult to detect on gray scale. Compression following partial thrombosis of the pseudoaneurysm may be effective in inducing thrombosis but also can expel thrombus fragments into the artery with possible severe consequences. Resuming thrombin injection is a safer alternative in case of partial thrombosis. Cases unresponsive to thrombin injection require surgical intervention. An arterial laceration is the most likely cause of unsuccessful thrombin injection, and surgery is the treatment of choice for this large arterial lesion [38].

At the end of the procedure use ultrasound to confirm the thrombosis and the lack of blood flow into the pseudoaneurysm, and clinically assess the distal pulses for signs of possible embolization. The patient can be kept on bed rest for 4–6 h or, in cases of large pseudoaneurysms, admitted for observation. Moderate pressure dressings can be used. If discharged, another clinical examination and Doppler ultrasound to confirm the pseudoaneurysm's thrombosis and the femoral artery patency is indicated. The follow-up time vary at different institutions from the next day to 3–10 days post procedure. The patient should avoid strenuous activity for 2–3 days. Complications can be distal embolization that can occur in 1 % of cases, but only 30 % of them will require surgery [33] and bleeding, usually caused by the rupture of the pseudoaneurysm and can manifest as external bleeding or rapid expansion of the pseudoaneurysm. Severe embolization and bleeding require surgical intervention.

References

1. Barshes NR, Annambhotla S, Bechara C, et al. Endovascular repair of hemodialysis graft-related pseudoaneurysm: an alternative treatment strategy in salvaging failing dialysis access. Vasc Endovascular Surg. 2008;42(3):228–34.
2. NKF KDOQI guidelines. Clinical practice guidelines and clinical practice recommendations 2006 updates. Clinical practice guidelines for vascular access. Guideline 6: Treatment of arteriovenous graft complications.
3. Chen CY, Teoh MK. Graft rescue for haemodialysis arterio-venous grafts: is it worth doing and which factors predict a good outcome? J R Coll Surg Edinb. 1998;43(4):248–50.
4. Gross GF, Hayes JF. PTFE graft arteriovenous fistulae for hemodialysis access. Am Surg. 1979;45(11):748–9.
5. Vogel KM, Martino MA, O'Brien SP, Kerstein MD. Complications of lower extremity arteriovenous grafts in patients with end-stage renal disease. South Med J. 2000;93(6):593–5.
6. Rizzuti RP, Hale JC, Burkart TE. Extended patency of expanded polytetrafluoroethylene grafts for vascular access using optimal configuration and revisions. Surg Gynecol Obstet. 1988;166(1): 23–7.
7. Schwab DP, Taylor SM, Cull DL. Isolated arteriovenous dialysis access graft segment infection: the results of segmental bypass and partial graft excision. Ann Vasc Surg. 2000;14(1):63–6.
8. Hallett JW, Mills JL, Earnshaw JJ, Reekers JA. Comprehensive vascular and endovascular surgery. 2nd ed. Philadelphia: Mosby/Elsevier; 2009. p. p. 454.
9. Ryan SV, Calligaro KD, Scharff J, Dougherty MJ. Management of infected prosthetic dialysis arteriovenous grafts. J Vasc Surg. 2004;39(1):73–8.
10. Hausegger KA, Tiessenhausen K, Klimpfinger M, Raith J, Hauser H, Tauss J. Aneurysms of hemodialysis access grafts: treatment with covered stents: a report of three cases. Cardiovasc Intervent Radiol. 1998;21(4):334–7.
11. Sapoval MR, Turmel-Rodrigues LA, Raynaud AC, Bourquelot P, Rodrigue H, Gaux JC. Cragg covered stents in hemodialysis access: initial and midterm results. J Vasc Interv Radiol. 1996;7(3): 335–42.
12. Najibi S, Bush RL, Terramani TT, et al. Covered stent exclusion of dialysis access pseudoaneurysms. J Surg Res. 2002;106(1):15–9.
13. Rhodes ES, Silas AM. Dialysis needle puncture of wallgrafts placed in polytetrafluoroethylene hemodialysis grafts. J Vasc Interv Radiol. 2005;16(8):1129–34.
14. Pandolfe LR, Malamis AP, Pierce K, Borge MA. Treatment of hemodialysis graft pseudoaneurysms with stent grafts: institutional experience and review of the literature. Semin Intervent Radiol. 2009;26(2):89–95.
15. Vesely TM. Use of stent grafts to repair hemodialysis graft-related pseudoaneurysms. J Vasc Interv Radiol. 2005;16(10):1301–7.
16. Moszkowicz A, Behrens G, Gueyikian S, Patel NH, Ferral H. Occlusion of a rapidly expanding hemodialysis graft pseudoaneurysm with placement of a stent graft. Semin Intervent Radiol. 2007;24(1):34–7.
17. Gadalean F. Covered stent outcomes for arteriovenous hemodialysis access salvage [abstract]. J Am Soc Nephrol. 2008;19:899A.
18. Salman L, Asif A. Stent graft for nephrologists: concerns and consensus. Clin J Am Soc Nephrol. 2010;5(7):1347–52.
19. Steven W, Jennifer J, Deborah B. Vascular access concerns in home haemodialysis. Eur Nephrol. 2011;5(1):45–8.
20. Lindsay RM, Leitch R, Heidenheim AP, Kortas C, London Daily/Nocturnal Hemodialysis Study. The London Daily/Nocturnal Hemodialysis Study – study design, morbidity, and mortality results. Am J Kidney Dis. 2003;42(1 Suppl):5–12.
21. Piccoli GB, Bermond F, Miez E, et al. Vascular access survival and morbidity on daily dialysis: a comparative analysis of home and limited care haemodialysis. Nephrol Dial Transplant. 2004;19(8):2084–94.
22. Kjellstrand C, Twardowski Z, Bower J, et al. A comparison of CV-catheters, grafts, and fistulae in quotidian hemodialysis, abstract. Hemodial Int. 2003;7(1):73–104.
23. Witz M, Werner M, Bernheim J, Shnaker A, Lehmann J, Korzets Z. Ultrasound-guided compression repair of pseudoaneurysms complicating a forearm dialysis arteriovenous fistula. Nephrol Dial Transplant. 2000;15(9):1453–4.
24. Zehnder T, Chatterjee T, Mahler F, Do DD. Successful ultrasonographically guided compression repair of a dialysis fistula pseudoaneurysm. J Ultrasound Med. 2000;19(5):329–31.
25. Reichle J, Teitel E. Sonographically guided obliteration of multiple pseudoaneurysms complicating a dialysis shunt. AJR Am J Roentgenol. 1998;170(1):222.
26. Yildirim S, Nursal Z, Yildirim T, Tarim A, Caliskan K. Brachial artery pseudoaneurysm: a rare complication after haemodialysis therapy. Acta Chir Belg. 2005;105(2):190–3.
27. Cina G, De Rosa MG, Viola G, Tazza L. Arterial injuries following diagnostic, therapeutic, and accidental arterial cannulation in haemodialysis patients. Nephrol Dial Transplant. 1997;12(7): 1448–52.
28. Lapus TP, Trerotola SO, Savader SJ. Radial artery pseudoaneurysm complicating a Brecia-Cimino dialysis fistula. Nephron. 1996;72(4):673–5.
29. Corso R, Rampoldi A, Vercelli R, Leni D, Vanzulli A. Percutaneous repair of radial artery pseudoaneurysm in a hemodialysis patient using sonographically guided thrombin injection. Cardiovasc Intervent Radiol. 2006;29(1):130–2.
30. Clark TW, Abraham RJ. Thrombin injection for treatment of brachial artery pseudoaneurysm at the site of a hemodialysis fistula: report of two patients. Cardiovasc Intervent Radiol. 2000;23(5): 396–400.
31. Wongwanit C, Ruangsetakit C, Sermsathanasawadi N, Chinsakchai K, Mutirangura P. Treatment of iatrogenic pseudoaneurysm of brachial artery with percutaneous ultrasonographically guided thrombin injection (PUGTI): a case report and a literature review. J Med Assoc Thai. 2007;90(8):1673–9.
32. Brümmer U, Salcuni M, Salvati F, Bonomini M. Repair of femoral postcatheterization pseudoaneurysm and arteriovenous fistula with percutaneous implantation of endovascular stent. Nephrol Dial Transplant. 2001;16(8):1728–9.
33. Dogra VS, Saad WEA, Menias CO. Ultrasound – guided procedures. New York: Thieme Medical Publishers Inc.; 2010. p. 305.
34. Krueger K, Zaehringer M, Strohe D, Stuetzer H, Boecker J, Lackner K. Postcatheterization pseudoaneurysm: results of US-guided percutaneous thrombin injection in 240 patients. Radiology. 2005;236(3):1104–10.
35. Katzenschlager R, Ugurluoglu A, Ahmadi A, et al. Incidence of pseudoaneurysm after diagnostic and therapeutic angiography. Radiology. 1995;195(2):463–6.
36. Webber GW, Jang J, Gustavson S, Olin JW. Contemporary management of postcatheterization pseudoaneurysms. Circulation. 2007; 115(20):2666–74.
37. Kent KC, McArdle CR, Kennedy B, Baim DS, Anninos E, Skillman JJ. A prospective study of the clinical outcome of femoral pseudoaneurysms and arteriovenous fistulas induced by arterial puncture. J Vasc Surg. 1993;17(1):125–33.
38. Sheiman RG, Mastromatteo M. Iatrogenic femoral pseudoaneurysms that are unresponsive to percutaneous thrombin injection: potential causes. AJR Am J Roentgenol. 2003;181(5): 1301–4.

Approach to Chest Pain During Dialysis

20

Chieh Suai Tan, Diego A. Covarrubias, and Steven Wu

20.1 Introduction

A patient who complains of chest pain during dialysis represents an immediate challenge. The symptoms may be of benign etiology, but occasionally, they may also be a harbinger of a potential catastrophe. Although mild chest pain or discomfort is reported to occur in 1–4 % of dialysis treatments [1], in light of the high incidence of cardiovascular events and sudden cardiac deaths in dialysis patients, any acute onset of chest pain in a patient on hemodialysis should be attended to promptly.

20.2 Initial Evaluation of Chest Pain

The initial evaluation should begin with the consideration of immediately life-threatening causes such as acute coronary syndrome (ACS), arrhythmia, aortic dissection, and pulmonary and air embolism. The dialysis should be terminated immediately and patient reclined to a recumbent position on the dialysis chair. Immediately check the venous bloodline; the presence of foaming is suggestive of air within the dialysis system, and port-wine appearance of blood is suggestive of hemolysis.

C.S. Tan, MBBS • D.A. Covarrubias, MD
Vascular Interventional Radiology, Massachusetts General Hospital, Harvard Medical School, 55 Fruit Street, Boston, MA 02114, USA

Department of Radiology, Massachusetts General Hospital, Harvard Medical School, 55 Fruit Street, Boston, MA 02114, USA

S. Wu, MD (✉)
Vascular Interventional Radiology, Massachusetts General Hospital, Harvard Medical School, 55 Fruit Street, Boston, MA 02114, USA

Department of Medicine, Massachusetts General Hospital, Harvard Medical School, 55 Fruit Street, Boston, MA 02114, USA

Department of Radiology, Massachusetts General Hospital, Harvard Medical School, 55 Fruit Street, Boston, MA 02114, USA
e-mail: swu1@partners.org

If present, clamp the bloodlines and stop the pump to prevent the return of blood to the patient. If the patient is unstable, activation of an ambulance equipped with a defibrillator to an emergency department should be done immediately.

Stabilization of such patients should begin immediately in the dialysis center. The dialysis needles may be left in situ after disconnection from the dialysis circuit. In the absence of peripheral venous access, in an emergency situation, the venous dialysis needle may be used for intravenous access. Dialysis catheter, if present, can also be used during resuscitation.

Concurrently, placement of a cardiac monitor and supplemental oxygen should be done. Noninvasive monitoring of oxygen saturation should be set up. A 12-lead electrocardiogram and a blood sample for cardiac enzyme measurement should be obtained if possible.

Patients who are thought to be experiencing an ACS, which includes ST-segment elevation myocardial infarction, non ST-segment elevation myocardial infarction, and unstable angina, should be given a 325 mg aspirin tablet. Sublingual nitroglycerin can be given for chest pain unless the patient has relatively low blood pressure.

Once a life-threatening etiology has been excluded, attempts can be made to identify the specific cause of the chest pain.

20.3 History Taking

The purpose of history taking and physical examination is to identify the specific causes of chest pain. As vascular disease accounts for 42 % of all deaths in dialysis patients [2], exclusion of cardiovascular etiology of chest pain is of paramount importance.

20.3.1 Nature and Location of Pain

The nature and location of the chest pain often give a clue to the underlying etiology. The patient with myocardial ischemia typically describes the chest pain as a diffuse

A.S. Yevzlin et al. (eds.), *Interventional Nephrology*,
DOI 10.1007/978-1-4614-8803-3_20, © Springer Science+Business Media New York 2014

discomfort that is squeezing, tight, constricting, strangling, or aching in nature. In some cases, the "Levine sign" (clenched fist held over the chest) may be demonstrated to describe ischemic chest pain. Patients with a history of coronary heart disease tend to have similar pain with recurrent ischemic episodes. Unfortunately, dialysis patients with acute myocardial infarction (AMI) often have atypical presentation. The prevalence of chest pain in dialysis patients with AMI was reported to be only 44 % versus 68.4 % in non-dialysis patients [3]. As such, suspicion should be raised if associated symptoms such as acute diaphoresis and dyspnea occur during dialysis, especially if the patient has a history of ischemic heart disease. Acute chest pain with a classically ripping or tearing quality may be suggestive of acute aortic dissection. Chest pain that is pleuritic in nature may be secondary to acute or uremic pericarditis, pulmonary embolism, or pneumonia.

20.3.2 Radiation of Chest Pain

The pain of myocardial ischemia may radiate to the neck, lower jaw, upper extremity, or shoulder. Chest pain that radiates between the scapulae may be due to aortic dissection, while the pain of pericarditis typically radiates to the trapezius ridges.

20.3.3 Timing of Chest Pain

The time course of the onset of chest pain is very important. Each dialysis session is akin to a cardiac "stress test." Chest pains that occur during dialysis and similar in nature to those that occur on physical exertion are highly suggestive of myocardial ischemia. Pain that resolves with exertion or with cessation of dialysis is also suggestive of ischemia. Postprandial chest pain, if present, can be a marker of severe coronary heart disease or may be suggestive of gastrointestinal disease.

20.3.4 Associated Symptoms

The occurrence of chest pain may be secondary to intradialytic hypotension. The common causes of intradialytic hypotension include excessive ultrafiltration, targeting the dry weight too low, relative lack of vasoconstriction (e.g., autonomic neuropathy in diabetic patients), and use of antihypertensive medications before dialysis. Recurrent intradialytic hypotension, if untreated, can lead to myocardial stunning, development of regional wall movement abnormalities (RWMA) on echocardiography, and increased mortality. On the other hand, cardiac factors such as myocardial ischemia,

diastolic dysfunction, and failure to increase cardiac output may manifest as intradialytic hypotension. Hence, cardiac evaluation is often warranted to determine the cause of intradialytic hypotension.

Diaphoresis and exertional dyspnea are strongly associated with myocardial ischemia. Patients with ischemia may also complaint of palpitations secondary to ventricular ectopy and atrial fibrillation.

20.3.5 Vascular Access

Intradialysis chest pain that occurs in patients who have recently undergone dialysis catheter placement should alert the physician to the possibility of perforation. Routine X-ray after insertion of a temporary dialysis catheter may not detect perforation of the vessels, and delay perforation has been reported [4, 5]. A high index of suspicion coupled with good clinical judgment is needed to exclude this complication.

The background history of the creation and location of the arteriovenous (AV) access is an important aspect that is often overlooked. High-output cardiac failure and myocardial ischemia can occur in patients with arteriovenous fistula (AVF) that have undergone dilation with large increases in flow. Risk factors for AVF-induced high-output cardiac failure include upper arm AVF, male gender, upper arm AVF in the same arm with a previously functioning forearm AVF, and baseline heart disease [6].

A patient who has a history of arterial disease causing poor flow, slow maturation of access, or steal syndrome may have concurrent coronary lesions that are causing myocardial ischemia and chest pain during dialysis. AV access that is created on the same side of the internal mammary artery that is used for coronary artery bypass grafting may cause coronary-subclavian steal syndrome resulting in chest pain during dialysis [7].

20.4   Physical Examination

Complete cardiac examination including palpation and auscultation should be done in a patient who has chest pain during dialysis. Localized tenderness on palpation of the chest wall may be suggestive of musculoskeletal pain. The presence of a pulse deficit together with a history of tearing chest pain may be suggestive of aortic dissection. Pericardial rub and murmurs are suggestive of pericarditis and valvular heart disease, respectively. Examination of the respiratory system and abdomen is also important to exclude noncardiac causes of chest pain.

The examination of the vascular access is a rarely practiced skill among nephrologists, but it can provide important information for the physician. In a patient with chest pain during dialysis, the presence of a severely dilated and ecstatic AVF with exaggerated bruit and thrill is suggestive of a high-flow AVF, which may contribute to high-output cardiac failure and myocardial ischemia. Poor peripheral pulses and cold extremity on the side of the AV access might be suggestive of arterial stenosis and significant atherosclerotic disease of the cardiovascular system. The presence of a systolic bruit in the axillary artery between the subclavian artery and AV access raises the possibility of disease of the aortic arch vessels. Improvement of symptoms after temporary occlusion of the AV access is suggestive of the contributory effects of the AV access to the pathogenesis of chest pain.

20.5 Differential Diagnosis and Pathophysiology

The differential diagnosis for chest pain is summarized in Table 20.1.

Dialysis patients are at increased risk of cardiovascular death when compared to the general population. Although the percentage of deaths in the prevalent dialysis patient attributable to cardiovascular disease has declined over the last decade in the USA, vascular disease remained the primary cause for almost 42 % of all deaths of dialysis patients between 2007 and 2009. Specifically, cardiac arrest was the single most common cause of death and accounted for more than half of all cardiac deaths [2].

Although coronary atherosclerosis is more common and severe in dialysis patients, the pathophysiological process may not be the same as in the general population. As illustrated in A Study to Evaluate the Use of Rosuvastatin in Subjects on Regular Hemodialysis: An Assessment of Survival and Cardiovascular Events (AURORA) and Die Deutsche Diabetes Dialyze (4D) studies, there are limited benefits for dialysis patients on statin therapy compared to the general population [8, 9]. In addition to the traditional risk factors for cardiovascular disease such as hypertension, diabetes mellitus, and left ventricular hypertrophy which are commonly present in a dialysis patient, "uremic-specific" risk factors such as secondary hyperparathyroidism, anemia, volume overload, and vascular calcifications are also

important in the progression of cardiovascular disease. It was suggested that the uremic environment in a dialysis patient could potentiate vascular calcification [10]. While it is unclear if vascular calcification itself is a risk or a causal factor, the associated increase in mortality with severe coronary artery calcification at the time of initiation of hemodialysis [11] is suggestive of some role in increasing cardiovascular events in dialysis patients. Vascular access calcification has also been shown to be an independent mortality predictor and is a cost-effective method to identify patients at increased mortality risk [12].

The creation of an AV access is a nonphysiological process that could add to cardiovascular stress. Cardiac output (CO) increases immediately after the creation of an AV access; this increase is achieved via the reduction of peripheral resistance and increased cardiac contractility to increase stroke volume [13]. The adjustment of stroke volume and cardiac output is vital to maintain a constant blood pressure [14]. A prospective study utilizing echocardiographic evaluation of cardiac parameters showed increases in left ventricular end-diastolic volume (LVEDV) (+4 %), fractional shortening (+8 %), and CO (+15 %) 14 days after the placement of AVFs [15]. In a seminar paper by Korsheed et al., patients with high-flow AV access(Qa), defined as Qa > 1,000 mL/min (but less than 1,500 mL/min), were found to have a lower prevalence of left ventricular hypertrophy (55 % vs. 76 %, $P = 0.01$) and dialysis-induced myocardial stunning [16]. One can therefore hypothesize that some sort of myocardial and arterial adaptation are required to sustain the lifelong increase in CO to maintain a well-functioning access. On the other hand, if the access flow is very high (Qa > 2,000 mL/min), the risk of occurrence of high-output heart failure is increased. This is because the increase in Qa is not accompanied by a parallel increase of CO, suggestive of a limit in myocardial reserve and ability to adapt to the presence of very high-flow AV access [17].

The process of dialysis can exert significant acute stress upon the cardiovascular system. McIntyre et al. demonstrated that hemodialysis is associated with significant reductions in myocardial blood flow and that dialysis stress-induced myocardial ischemia results in the development of regional

Table 20.1 Differential diagnosis of chest pain during dialysis

Cardiovascular	Pulmonary	Dialysis related	Access related	Gastrointestinal	Musculoskeletal disorder
Acute coronary syndrome	Pulmonary embolism	Air embolism	Coronary-subclavian steal syndrome	Peptic ulcer disease	Costochondritis
Stable angina	Pneumonia	Hemolysis	High-flow AV access	Esophageal disorder	Rib fracture
Aortic dissection	Pneumothorax	Catheter malposition			Renal osteodystrophy
Pericarditis		Intradialytic hypotension			Herpes zoster
Valvular heart disease		Type B dialyzer reaction			
Arrhythmia					

wall movement abnormalities (RWMA) [18]. Of note, these findings occurred in the absence of large-vessel epicardial coronary disease. Such episodes of ischemia are associated with long-term loss of systolic cardiac function, increased cardiac events, and reduced patient survival. In multivariate analysis, intradialytic reduction in blood pressure and ultrafiltration (UF) volume both independently determined the propensity to suffer dialysis-induced cardiac injury [19]. Dasselaar et al. reported similar intradialytic reduction in myocardial blood flow but noted that the decrease occurred early during dialysis [20]. The early occurrence of reduced myocardial blood flow is postulated to be due to acute dialysis-related factors such as electrolyte shifts, acid–base shifts, or temperature changes.

Other important differential diagnosis of chest pain during dialysis would include acute pericarditis, pleuritis, air embolism, gastroesophageal reflux, hemolysis, and musculoskeletal disorders.

In patients on chronic hemodialysis via an upper extremity arteriovenous (AV) access in whom the ipsilateral internal mammary artery (IMA) was used for coronary artery bypass grafting (CABG), angina can occur because of the coronary-subclavian steal syndrome.

Reivich et al. first described subclavian steal syndrome in two patients with vertebrobasilar insufficiency and vertebral artery flow reversal [21]. It involved a proximal subclavian artery obstruction, reversed flow in the vertebral artery with resultant siphoning of blood from the brain, and symptoms of cerebral ischemia. Coronary-subclavian steal syndrome was subsequently described in patients who had undergone CABG using the IMA [22]. The pathophysiology is similar to a proximal subclavian artery stenosis or occlusion, but the steal consists of siphoning of blood from the IMA graft to the subclavian artery with resulting myocardial ischemia and symptoms of angina.

Similarly, coronary-subclavian steal syndrome can also occur if there is a high-flow AV access draining the ipsilateral IMA graft [7, 23, 24]. Crowley et al. postulated that the AV fistula represents a low-resistance bed that draws flow away from the relatively higher-resistance zone where the IMA graft is anastomosed to the coronary artery. The resistance is lowered further during dialysis as blood is withdrawn from the fistula, and this can cause symptoms of angina in vulnerable patients [7].

In an elegant study by Gaudino et al., blood flow in the IMA graft ipsilateral to the AV fistula was compared to the contralateral mammary artery by means of transthoracic echo-color Doppler at baseline and during hemodialysis. A marked reduction of peak systolic and end-diastolic velocities and time average mean velocity and flow in the IMA graft ipsilateral to the fistula at the onset of hemodialysis was demonstrated. There was no substantial hemodynamic modification in the contralateral IMA. The reduction in flow was

accompanied by evidence of hypokinesia of the anterior left ventricular wall [23].

20.6 Diagnostic Approach to Chest Pain

The diagnostic approach to chest pain during dialysis is as outlined in Fig. 20.1. Due to the high risk of cardiac events in a dialysis patient, chest pains during dialysis should be thoroughly investigated after initial stabilization and evaluation. Relevant laboratory tests such as serial cardiac enzymes and electrocardiogram, complete blood count, blood urea nitrogen, creatinine, and electrolytes should be conducted. Chest radiography is needed to exclude pulmonary causes of chest pain and reassess position of indwelling catheter if present. Echocardiography is very useful for assessment of the left ventricular ejection fraction, valvular lesions, and pericardial disease such as pericardial effusion.

Stress tests using echocardiography or nuclear imaging are useful to identify the presence of myocardial ischemia. Invasive coronary angiogram remains the most definitive way to diagnose coronary artery disease.

Intradialytic echocardiography may be performed to identify patients who remain symptomatic despite a normal cardiac evaluation. The presence of RWMA during dialysis should prompt the alteration of dialysis technique. Conversion to nocturnal dialysis, shorter daily dialysis, or peritoneal dialysis should be considered. Use of biofeedback technique or decreasing the temperature of the dialysate can also be used if the patient chose to remain on conventional hemodialysis.

If the symptoms persist, rare causes such as a high-flow AV access or even coronary-subclavian steal syndrome should be considered in a patient whose IMA ipsilateral to the AV access had been used for CABG.

It is essential to exclude the presence of a concomitant subclavian artery stenosis before attributing the steal syndrome to the AV access [25]. On physical examination, the presence of a systolic bruit in the axillary artery between the subclavian artery and AV access raises the possibility of disease of the aortic arch vessels [26]. Doppler ultrasound with color flow findings of monophasic changes, color aliasing, and increased blood velocities at stenotic sites is suggestive of significant obstruction. Computed tomography angiography has the advantage of revealing the anatomy of the aortic truck and supra-aortic vessels, including the subclavian artery. Contrast angiography with table hemodynamic measurements of the subclavian lesion can confirm the diagnosis of subclavian stenosis.

The diagnosis of coronary-subclavian steal syndrome secondary to AV access can be made using pulsed Doppler or an aortogram. A reduction in the flow velocity of the IMA graft at the initiation of dialysis would be strongly suggestive

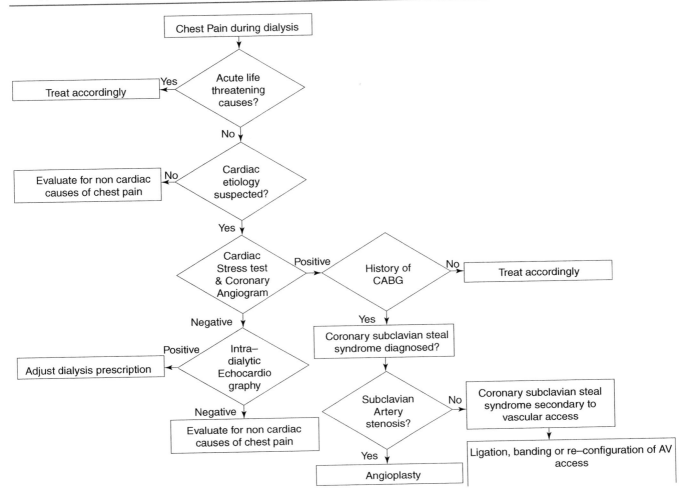

Fig. 20.1 Diagnostic approach for evaluation of chest pain during dialysis

of hemodynamically evident flow steal [23]. Angiographically, retrograde flow of the IMA graft during diastole may be demonstrated. On table, restoration of the antegrade flow in the IMA graft during diastole with occlusion of the AV access would be highly suggestive of significant steal syndrome [24].

20.7   Management

20.7.1 Coronary Artery Disease

Interventional Therapy for Coronary Artery Disease

In the presence of coronary artery disease (CAD), coronary revascularization can be performed either with percutaneous coronary intervention (PCI) or with CABG to improve myocardial perfusion. The optimal method of coronary revascularization in dialysis patients is unclear as there are no randomized studies that have directly compared the outcomes

of the two methods. Furthermore, there are also no randomized prospective trials that have compared drug-eluting stents (DES) with bare-metal stents (BMS) in dialysis patients. There is some evidence in dialysis patients that PCI with DES has higher patency rates compared to BMS [27] although long-term outcome appears to be inferior to CABG [28, 29].

The downside to using DES in dialysis patients is the long duration required for dual antiplatelet therapy, which reduces the risk of stent thrombosis. Premature discontinuation of therapy is associated with increased risk of thrombosis. The 2011 American College of Cardiology Foundation/American Heart Association Task Force on Practice Guidelines and the Society for Cardiovascular Angiography and Intervention recommended that for non-ACS intervention, clopidogrel, in combination with aspirin, should be given for at least 12 months and 1 month for DES and BMS, respectively, if patients are not at high risk of bleeding [30]. The longer duration of dual antiplatelet therapy required for DES can pose a challenge in dialysis patients who are already at increased risk for bleeding. Furthermore, combination therapy with aspirin and clopidogrel has been shown to be associated with increased bleeding risk in dialysis patients in the Veterans Affairs Cooperative Study Group on Hemodialysis Access Graft Thrombosis study [31]. Nevertheless, these should not be taken as contraindications to having DES, but rather, careful patient selection, monitoring for bleeding, or even decreasing the anticoagulant dose during dialysis can be taken into consideration to optimize the therapy for CAD in dialysis patients.

Medical Therapy for Coronary Artery Disease

Optimal medical therapy for coronary artery disease in dialysis patients has predominantly been extrapolated from studies done in the general population. Antiplatelet therapy should be started in the absence of any contraindications. The controversy generated by the 4D and AURORA trial has been discussed in the earlier section. The decision to initiate, continue, or stop statin therapy should be individualized. Lifestyle modifications such as smoking cessation and regular exercise may be beneficial in decreasing the risk for cardiovascular morbidity and mortality.

The use of nitrates, beta-blockers, or calcium channel blockers is useful in the control of angina. The presence of coexisting medical conditions such as hypertension and peripheral vascular disease might influence the choice of antianginal medications. Regardless of the choice, the potential hypotensive effects of these drugs during dialysis and clearance by dialysis should be taken into consideration when adjusting the dosage and timing of the medications.

The optimal blood pressure in dialysis patient is unclear as excessively lowering of blood pressure is associated with increased mortality. Lower blood pressures are also associated with increased risk of vascular access failure. Hence, blood pressure targets should be individualized, taking into account the comorbidities and intradialytic fluctuations in the blood pressure. Control of the blood pressure can be achieved via optimization of the dry weight and use of antihypertensive agents.

The target hemoglobin level with erythropoietin-stimulating agents is between 11 and 12 g/dL. Normalization of hemoglobin in dialysis patient is associated with higher mortality [32].

20.7.2 Subclavian Coronary Steal Syndrome

When creating a new AV access post CABG, care should be taken to avoid using the arm ipsilateral to the side where the IMA is used. In a situation where an arteriovenous (AV) access was created ipsilateral to the side where the IMA was used for CABG, whereby the steal syndrome is attributable solely to the AV access, ligation of the AV access would abolish the steal but result in a loss of dialysis access. In centers where expertise is available, creation of a new arterial conduit from the contralateral subclavian artery to the existing AV access would salvage the AV access and abolish the steal syndrome [33].

If the subclavian coronary steal syndrome occurs as a consequence of subclavian artery stenosis, the culprit lesion should be treated. The therapeutic options include bypass procedures and endovascular stenting [34].

The high technical success rates (91–100 %) with minimal complication rates (0.9–1.4 %) [34] of endovascular treatment of subclavian artery stenosis have made it an attractive alternative to open surgical repair, especially for dialysis patients who are already at increased surgical risk. Reported complications, while minimal, include stroke, transient ischemic attack, distal embolization, thrombosis, and access site hematoma. Patel et al. reported a large case series of 170 patients who underwent endovascular stenting of the subclavian (94 %) or innominate (6 %) arteries over a 13-year period. The primary patency at 12 months and 5 years was 93 and 84 %, respectively, and secondary patency at 12 months and 4 years was 99 % and 98, respectively [35].

Technical Details

In preparation for the procedure, both the femoral and brachial access sites should be made available as both may be needed to gain access to the subclavian artery in difficult situation. The decision to employ the femoral or brachial approach is dependent on a few factors. The common femoral route is generally used because of familiarity with the approach, experience, and lower risk of hematoma complications than the brachial approach. The brachial approach is favored in the presence of severe aortoiliac disease, steep angulation of the subclavian artery from the aorta, or if the origin of the subclavian artery is not well defined. For the femoral approach, a 5- to 6-F short sheath is deployed initially, while the 5-F short sheath is used for the brachial approach. Once arterial access is obtained, 5,000 units of heparin is administered to maintain patency and prevent thrombosis.

The arch aortogram is then performed using a 5-F pig tail catheter in the aortic arch (see Fig. 20.2). The patient needs to be placed in a 30° left anterior oblique (LAO) position to obtain a reasonable image of the aortic arch and great vessels. Choice of guidewire depends on the lesion characteristics, sheath, and guide catheter that is required. The lesion can be crossed with a .035 in. Wholey wire in moderate stenosis or a .035 regular-angled Glidewire for high-grade stenosis. A 5-F, 100 cm hockey stick-shaped diagnostic catheter is used for support. Once the lesion is crossed, exchange the diagnostic catheter for a long sheath (6-F to 7-F) or guide catheter (7-F to 8-F) just proximal to the lesion.

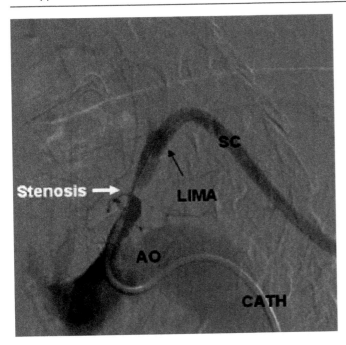

Fig. 20.2 Subclavian artery stenosis causing coronary-subclavian steal syndrome (note the absence of flow in the left internal mammary artery graft)

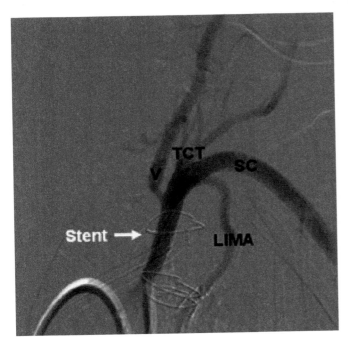

Fig. 20.3 Reestablishment of flow in the internal mammary artery after stenting of the subclavian artery stenosis

Balloon angioplasty is subsequently performed to predilate the lesion to decrease risk of stripping and facilitate the passage of a balloon-mounted stent. In general, balloon-expandable stents are preferred as they allow precise placement with greater radial strength and lower risk of stent

migration than self-expanding stents. The balloon-mounted stents are frequently 7–8 mm in diameter and 15–20 mm in length. Appropriate sizing is needed to ensure that the ipsilateral internal mammary and vertebral artery are not obstructed. Deployment of the stent can be affected by large movement from the aortic arch pulsation, therefore, hold the balloon carefully and rapidly deploy the stent to approximately 8 atm. Avoid overdilation as it can result in subclavian artery rupture and catastrophic consequences. After stent placement, a selective subclavian arteriogram is taken to confirm the technical success of the procedure (see Fig. 20.3).

Conclusion

Chest pain during dialysis can be a diagnostic challenge. In addition to the "usual" differential diagnoses, the dialysis vascular access can sometimes be contributory to the symptoms that the patient is experiencing. Awareness of the physiological impact of AV access creation on the cardiovascular system can help to unearth diagnoses which could otherwise be overlooked in the evaluation of chest pain during dialysis.

References

1. Daugirdas JT, Blake PG, Ing TS. Handbook of dialysis. 4th ed. Philadelphia: Lippincott Williams & Wilkins; 2007. xx, 774 pp.
2. U S Renal Data System. USRDS 2011 annual report: atlas of chronic kidney disease and end-stage renal disease in the United States. Bethesda: National Institutes of Health, National Institute of Diabetes and Digestive and Kidney Diseases; 2011.
3. Herzog CA, Littrell K, Arko C, Frederick PD, Blaney M. Clinical characteristics of dialysis patients with acute myocardial infarction in the United States: a collaborative project of the United States Renal Data System and the National Registry of Myocardial Infarction. Circulation. 2007;116(13):1465–72.
4. Modi KS, Gross D, Davidman M. The patient developing chest pain at the onset of haemodialysis sessions – it is not always angina pectoris. Nephrol Dial Transplant. 1999;14(1):221–3.
5. Kielstein JT, Abou-Rebyeh F, Hafer C, Haller H, Fliser D. Right-sided chest pain at the onset of haemodialysis. Nephrol Dial Transplant. 2001;16(7):1493–5.
6. Begin V, Ethier J, Dumont M, Leblanc M. Prospective evaluation of the intra-access flow of recently created native arteriovenous fistulae. Am J Kidney Dis. 2002;40(6):1277–82.
7. Wanner C, Krane V, März W, et al. Atorvastatin in patients with type 2 diabetes mellitus undergoing hemodialysis. N Engl J Med. 2005;353(3):238–48.
8. Fellstrom BC, Jardine AG, Schmieder RE, et al. Rosuvastatin and cardiovascular events in patients undergoing hemodialysis. N Engl J Med. 2009;360(14):1395–407.
9. Chen NX, O'Neill KD, Duan D, Moe SM. Phosphorus and uremic serum up-regulate osteopontin expression in vascular smooth muscle cells. Kidney Int. 2002;62(5):1724–31.
10. Block GA, Raggi P, Bellasi A, Kooienga L, Spiegel DM. Mortality effect of coronary calcification and phosphate binder choice in incident hemodialysis patients. Kidney Int. 2007;71(5):438–41.
11. Schlieper G, Krüger T, Djuric Z, et al. Vascular access calcification predicts mortality in hemodialysis patients. Kidney Int. 2008;74(12):1582–7.

12. Guyton AC, Sagawa K. Compensations of cardiac output and other circulatory functions in a reflex dogs with large A-V fistulas. Am J Physiol. 1961;200:1157–63.

13. London GM, Guerin AP, Marchais SJ. Hemodynamic overload in end-stage renal disease patients. Semin Dial. 1999;12(2):77–83.

14. Girerd X, London G, Boutouyrie P, Mourad JJ, Safar M, Laurent S. Remodeling of the radial artery in response to a chronic increase in shear stress. Hypertension. 1996;27(3 Pt 2):799–803.

15. Korsheed S, Burton JO, McIntyre CW. Higher arteriovenous fistulae blood flows are associated with a lower level of dialysis-induced cardiac injury. Hemodial Int. 2009;13(4):505–11.

16. Basile C, Lomonte C, Vernaglione L, Casucci F, Antonelli M, Losurdo N. The relationship between the flow of arteriovenous fistula and cardiac output in haemodialysis patients. Nephrol Dial Transplant. 2008;23(1):282–7.

17. McIntyre CW, Burton JO, Selby NM, et al. Hemodialysis-induced cardiac dysfunction is associated with an acute reduction in global and segmental myocardial blood flow. Clin J Am Soc Nephrol. 2008;3(1):19–26.

18. Burton JO, Jefferies HJ, Selby NM, McIntyre CW. Hemodialysis-induced cardiac injury: determinants and associated outcomes. Clin J Am Soc Nephrol. 2009;4(5):914–20.

19. Dasselaar JJ, Slart RH, Knip M, et al. Haemodialysis is associated with a pronounced fall in myocardial perfusion. Nephrol Dial Transplant. 2009;24(2):604–10.

20. Reivich M, Holling HE, Roberts B, Toole JF. Reversal of blood flow through the vertebral artery and its effect on cerebral circulation. N Engl J Med. 1961;265:878–85.

21. Harjola PT, Valle M. The importance of aortic arch or subclavian angiography before coronary reconstruction. Chest. 1974;66(4):436–8.

22. Crowley SD, Butterly DW, Peter RH, Schwab SJ. Coronary steal from a left internal mammary artery coronary bypass graft by a left upper extremity arteriovenous hemodialysis fistula. Am J Kidney Dis. 2002;40(4):852–5.

23. Gaudino M, Serricchio M, Luciani N, et al. Risks of using internal thoracic artery grafts in patients in chronic hemodialysis via upper extremity arteriovenous fistula. Circulation. 2003;107(21):2653–5.

24. Kato H, Ikawa S, Hayashi A, Yokoyama K. Internal mammary artery steal in a dialysis patient. Ann Thorac Surg. 2003;75(1):270–1.

25. Lee PY, Ng W, Chen WH. Concomitant coronary and subclavian steal caused by ipsilateral subclavian artery stenosis and arteriovenous fistula in a hemodialysis patient. Catheter Cardiovasc Interv. 2004;62(2):244–8.

26. Schoenkerman AB, Gimelli G, Yevzlin AS. An interesting case: retrograde blood flow from a LIMA sustaining hemodialysis via an AVF. Semin Dial. 2009;22(5):566–8.

27. Abdel-Latif A, Mukherjee D, Mesgarzadeh P, Ziada KM. Drug-eluting stents in patients with end-stage renal disease: meta-analysis and systematic review of the literature. Catheter Cardiovasc Interv. 2010;76(7):942–8.

28. Manabe S, Shimokawa T, Fukui T, et al. Coronary artery bypass surgery versus percutaneous coronary artery intervention in patients on chronic hemodialysis: does a drug-eluting stent have an impact on clinical outcome? J Card Surg. 2009;24(3):234–9.

29. Sunagawa G, Komiya T, Tamura N, Sakaguchi G, Kobayashi T, Murashita T. Coronary artery bypass surgery is superior to percutaneous coronary intervention with drug-eluting stents for patients with chronic renal failure on hemodialysis. Ann Thorac Surg. 2010;89(6):1896–900; discussion 1900.

30. Levine GN, Bates ER, Blankenship JC, et al. 2011 ACCF/AHA/SCAI Guideline for Percutaneous Coronary Intervention: a report of the American College of Cardiology Foundation/American Heart Association Task Force on Practice Guidelines and the Society for Cardiovascular Angiography and Interventions. Circulation. 2011;124(23):e574–651.

31. Kaufman JS, O'Connor TZ, Zhang JH, et al. Randomized controlled trial of clopidogrel plus aspirin to prevent hemodialysis access graft thrombosis. J Am Soc Nephrol. 2003;14(9):2313–21.

32. Besarab A, Bolton WK, Browne JK, et al. The effects of normal as compared with low hematocrit values in patients with cardiac disease who are receiving hemodialysis and epoetin. N Engl J Med. 1998;339(9):584–90.

33. Ginzburg V, Margulis G, Greenberg G, et al. Preserving the left arm vein in cases of hemodialysis access generating left internal mammary artery steal syndrome. J Vasc Access. 2004;5(3):133–5.

34. Ochoa VM, Yeghiazarians Y. Subclavian artery stenosis: a review for the vascular medicine practitioner. Vasc Med. 2011;16(1):29–34.

35. Patel SN, White CJ, Collins TJ, et al. Catheter-based treatment of the subclavian and innominate arteries. Catheter Cardiovasc Interv. 2008;71(7):963–8.

Approach to Cyanotic Digits and Hand Paresis

21

Arif Asif

Arterial stenoses, vascular calcification, and true arterial steal can all play a critical role in the pathogenesis of peripheral hypoperfusion [1]. In contrast, the exact mechanism of nerve injury (ischemic monomelic neuropathy) sustained after the creation of an arteriovenous access is not entirely known [1]. This chapter would address hand ischemia and nerve injury as two separate entities and discuss the current strategies to combat the two situations.

21.1 Cyanotic Digits

While there are multiple etiologies of digital cyanosis, in a patient with an ipsilateral arteriovenous access, distal ischemia assumes a more central causative role. There are multiple mechanisms that can cause cyanotic digits due to hand ischemia in a dialysis patient with ipsilateral arteriovenous access. (a) True steal can produce peripheral ischemia ("true steal"). It is important to note, however, that in a great majority of forearm as well as proximal arteriovenous accesses, clinically silent retrograde flow can be seen [1]. In this context, demonstration of retrograde flow alone does not predict nor indicate the existence of hand ischemia. (b) Vascular calcification and diabetes is an important factor that may also contribute to the development of symptoms of hand ischemia [1]. Vascular calcification affects both intimal and media layers. Disturbance in mineral metabolism in the uremic milieu, calcium-containing phosphate binders and vitamin D treatment of secondary hyperparathyroidism, increased oxidized low-density lipoprotein cholesterol, increased oxidative stress, and hyperhomocysteinemia may contribute to the pathogenesis. (c) Arterial stenotic disease is a major mechanism that can cause hand ischemia.

Arterial stenoses play a major role in the pathogenesis of hand ischemia in hemodialysis (HD) patients with an arteriovenous access. Recent data have emphasized that significant (≥50 %) arterial stenoses are commonly seen in dialysis patients presenting with symptoms of hand ischemia or vascular access dysfunction [2–8]. These lesions can occur anywhere within the arteries of the upper extremities including the proximal arteries and have been demonstrated to cause peripheral ischemia in hemodialysis patients [2–4]. Using arteriography, the incidence of arterial stenosis in patients with peripheral ischemia has been reported to occur in a significant number of patients. In one study [2], complete arteriography from the aortic to the palmar arch was performed to assess the presence of arterial stenosis in HD patients presenting with symptoms of peripheral ischemia ($n = 13$). It was found that 62 % of the 13 patients referred for the evaluation of symptoms of hand ischemia syndrome demonstrated a significant (≥50 %) arterial stenosis. In another report of patients with hand ischemia [4], stenosis in the inflow circulation was found in over 80 % of the patients who underwent complete arteriography ($n = 12$).

It is important to mention that the goal for managing hand ischemia must focus on augmenting blood flow distal to the access to relieve ischemia while preserving the lifeline of the patient. A variety of percutaneous interventions including percutaneous balloon angioplasty, intravascular coil insertion and endovascular stent placement are available to achieve this goal. Use of one or a combination of these interventions has made access ligation the procedure of last resort for patients with hand ischemia. However, this procedure might still be used when the symptoms are apparent immediately after access creation and for those cases which are unresponsive to other treatments and demonstrate advancing ischemia.

Arterial stenoses can have a significant effect on the surgical procedure performed to correct distal ischemia. Recognition of these stenoses before planning a surgical procedure is very important. For example, in the presence of a significant arterial stenosis proximal to the anastomosis, a

A. Asif, MD, FASN, FNKF
Division of Nephrology and Hypertension, Albany Medical College, 25 Hackett Blvd, MC 69, Albany, NY 12206, USA
e-mail: aasif@med.miami.edu, asifa@mail.amc.edu

A.S. Yevzlin et al. (eds.), *Interventional Nephrology*,
DOI 10.1007/978-1-4614-8803-3_21, © Springer Science+Business Media New York 2014

banding procedure applied to correct arterial steal can result in a critical decline in access blood flow culminating in access thrombosis.

Because arterial stenosis is an important cause of distal ischemia, the percutaneous approach is gaining popularity in the management of hand ischemia. In one study, arteriography was performed to evaluate patients with symptoms of hand ischemia [2]. The entire arterial tree from the aortic arch to the palmar arch was evaluated. Seven of the ten patients with hand pain revealed arterial stenoses while three were found to have excessive flow into the access through the anastomosis. Five of the seven patients with arterial stenosis were amenable to angioplasty. Of these, four demonstrated resolution of symptoms post treatment. Of the three patients with excessive flow, two cases with radiocephalic fistulae were treated by coil embolization of the efferent radial artery to abolish the steal. The authors concluded that transcatheter therapy can be very successful in selected case of hand ischemia. In another report, eight of ten patients with advanced limb ischemia became symptom free after the application of percutaneous balloon angioplasty (PTA) [3]. In a recent report of 12 patients presenting with hand ischemia, 10 were found to have arterial stenosis and 8 were successfully treated with PTA [4]. There were no procedure-related complications reported in any of these studies.

Many reports have focused on the use of surgical interventions including banding/plication, tapered graft insertion, distal revascularization-interval ligation (DRIL), and revision using distal inflow procedure to correct steal resulting in distal ischemia [9–15]. However, a minimally invasive percutaneous technique designed to limit excessive flow (true steal) through the anastomosis causing distal ischemia has been reported recently [16]. This technique is based upon the application of a ligature around an inflated angioplasty balloon to create a stenosis of a defined size. According to this technique, the body of the access is punctured and entered in a retrograde direction. A complete arteriography (with and without occlusion) to ascertain the presence of stenosis or aberrant anatomy is performed. Under local anesthesia, a small (1–2 cm) incision is made over the access some 2–3 cm from the arterial anastomosis. At this point, blunt dissection is performed so that that a ligature (nylon, Prolene) can be passed around the access. An angioplasty balloon is then positioned at the inflow. The size of the balloon is based on the size of the artery just distal to the arterial anastomosis (4–5 mm balloon for elbow fistulae); the goal is to create a significant stenosis once the ligature has been applied. The balloon is then inflated in the juxta-anastomotic region and a ligature is snugly applied on the external surface of the access to create a stenotic lesion. The balloon is deflated and the symptoms are assessed. In the absence of resolution of symptoms, another ligature juxtaposed to the first one to cre-

ate a segment of high resistance can be applied. All 16 patients treated in this manner demonstrated immediate symptomatic and angiographic improvement of flow to the forearm post procedure. The study did not provide information regarding quantification of the reduction of access flow or augmentation of perfusion to the hand.

The advantages of the percutaneous approach include demonstration of arterial anatomy as well as clarification of the etiology of hand ischemia. Both angioplasty of an occlusive lesion and reduction of flow into the access can be performed using minimal invasive techniques. Other benefits include performance of the procedures on an outpatient basis, utilization of local anesthesia, and reduced incidence of procedure-related complications. It is important to note, however, that the outcome of these interventions depends strongly on the experience and persistence of the interventionalist. The advantage of surgical approach is that surgical interventions can still be successful where endovascular approaches have failed. In summary, a team approach would only result in benefits for the patient.

21.2 Hand Paresis

Nerve injury leading to hand paresis is also observed in patients undergoing arteriovenous access creation. Such injuries are usually seen immediately postoperatively and often in diabetics. Patients with upper arm accesses are at increased risk compared to those with a forearm fistula. In simple terms, ischemic monomelic neuropathy (IMN) is a nerve injury sustained after the creation of an arteriovenous access. It is a complication of vascular access that is observed almost exclusively in diabetics particularly those with preexisting neuropathy [16, 17]. This entity is characterized by the development of acute pain, weakness, and paralysis of forearm and hand muscles often associated with sensory changes. IMN occurs very early (minutes to hours) after the creation of an arteriovenous access. It is caused by ischemic infarction of the vasa nervosa. It is most commonly seen in cases of upper arm accesses [16, 17]. IMN can be diagnosed clinically based on an acute onset of pain following access creation with a history of diabetes and dominant neurologic symptoms and signs. Typically, the hand is warm and the radial pulse variably present. Prompt ligation of the access and rehabilitation of the decrease in hand and upper extremity function have been the traditional approaches to combat this situation.

Diabetes mellitus can be associated with limb pain due to isolated nerve involvement [18]. However, this neuropathy is generally symmetrical. Carpal tunnel syndrome is due to entrapment of the median nerve. Diagnostic clues include pain in both hands as median nerve entrapment is bilateral in a large proportion of cases. Wasting of the lateral thenar

Table 21.1 Causes, presentation, and management of dialysis access-associated cyanotic digits and hand paresis

	Cyanotic digits	Hand paresis
Clinical feature	Cold hand with pain on or off dialysis	Weakness and paralysis of muscles with prominent sensory loss
Presentation	Acute and chronic	Acute
Access type	Common with upper arm but also seen with forearm accesses	Only with upper arm accesses
Tissue involved	Skin>muscle>nerve	Nerves
Etiology	Vascular insufficiency leading to distal hypoperfusion	Vascular insufficiency causing nerve damage
Radial pulse	Usually diminished	Usually present
Diagnostic evaluation	Thorough history, physical examination, and arteriography	History and the clinical features
More prevalent in	Diabetics, peripheral vascular disease, smokers	Diabetics, peripheral vascular disease
Management strategies	Percutaneous and surgical interventions	Access ligation

muscles is often present at diagnosis, denoting advanced nerve compression [19–21]. An EMG showing reduction of motor conduction can help establish the diagnosis [20].

21.3 Summary

Cyanotic digits causing hand pain and nerve injury leading to hand paresis can result from ischemic events in patients with ipsilateral arteriovenous access. Prompt diagnosis is needed to optimally manage both conditions (Table 21.1). For cyanotic digits and hand ischemia, multiple interventions are available. In this context, ligation of the access has become a last resort to combat hand ischemia. On the other hand, access ligation may be required to limit ongoing nerve injury. Hand paresis also requires rehabilitation therapy to improve hand function.

References

1. Leon CA, Asif A. Arteriovenous access and hand pain: the distal hypoperfusion ischemic syndrome. Clin J Am Soc Nephrol. 2007;2:175–83.
2. Valji K, Hye RJ, Roberts AC, Oglevie SB, Ziegler T, Bookstein JJ. Hand ischemia in patients with hemodialysis access grafts: angiographic diagnosis and treatment. Radiology. 1995;196:697–701.
3. Guerra A, Raynaud A, Beyssen B, Pagny JY, Sapoval M, Angel C. Arterial percutaneous angioplasty in upper limbs with vascular access devices for haemodialysis. Nephrol Dial Transplant. 2002;17:843–51.
4. Asif A, Leon C, Merrill D, Bhimani B, Ellis R, Ladino M, Gadalean FN. Arterial steal syndrome: a modest proposal for an old paradigm. Am J Kidney Dis. 2006;48:88–97.
5. Asif A, Gadalean FN, Merrill D, Cherla G, Cipleu CD, Epstein DL, Roth D. Inflow stenosis in arteriovenous fistulas and grafts: a multicenter, prospective study. Kidney Int. 2005;67:1986–92.
6. Khan FA, Vesely TM. Arterial problems associated with dysfunctional hemodialysis grafts: evaluation of patients at high risk for arterial disease. J Vasc Interv Radiol. 2002;13:1109–14.
7. Lockhart ME, Robbin ML, McNamara MM, Allon M. Association of pelvic arterial calcification with arteriovenous thigh graft failure in haemodialysis patients. Nephrol Dial Transplant. 2004;9:2564–9.
8. Duijm LEM, Liem YS, van der Rijt RHH, et al. Inflow stenosis in dysfunctional hemodialysis access fistulae and grafts. Am J Kidney Dis. 2006;48:98–105.
9. DeCaprio JD, Valentine RJ, Kakish HB, Awad R, Hagino RT, Claggett GP. Steal syndrome complicating hemodialysis access. Cardiovasc Surg. 1997;5:648–53.
10. Schild AF, Pruett CS, Newman MI, Raines J, Petersen F, Konkin T, Kim P, Dickson C, Kirsch WM. The utility of the VCS clip for creation of vascular access for hemodialysis: long-term results and intraoperative benefits. Cardiovasc Surg. 2001;9:526–30.
11. Schaffer D, Schaffer D. A prospective, randomized trial of 6-mm versus 4-7-mm PTFE grafts for hemodialysis access in diabetic patients. In: Henry ML, Ferguson RM, Gore WL, Associates, Inc, editors. Vascular access for hemodialysis-V. Chicago: Precept Press; 1997. p. 91–4.
12. Schanzer H, Schwartz M, Harrington E, Haimov M. Treatment of ischemia due to "steal" by arteriovenous fistula with distal artery ligation and revascularization. J Vasc Surg. 1988;7:770–3.
13. Berman SS, Gentile AT, Glickman MH, et al. Distal revascularization-interval ligation for limb salvage and maintenance of dialysis access in ischemia steal syndrome. J Vasc Surg. 1997;26:393–404.
14. Minion DJ, Moore E, Endean E. Revision using distal inflow: a novel approach to dialysis-associated steal syndrome. Ann Vasc Surg. 2005;19:625–8.
15. Goel N, Miller GA, Jotwani MC, et al. Minimally invasive limited ligation endoluminal-assisted revision for dialysis access associated steal. Kidney Int. 2006;70:765–70.
16. Riggs JE, Moss AH, Labosky DA, Liput JH, Morgan JJ, Gutmann L. Upper extremity ischemic monomelic neuropathy: a complication of vascular access procedures in uremic diabetic patients. Neurology. 1989;39:997–8.
17. Miles AM. Vascular steal syndrome and ischaemic monomelic neuropathy: two variants of upper limb ischaemia after haemodialysis vascular access surgery. Nephrol Dial Transplant. 1997;14:297–300.
18. Bansal V, Kalita J, Misra UK. Diabetic neuropathy. Postgrad Med J. 2006;82:95–100.
19. Vellani G, Dallari D, Fatone F, Martella D, Bonomini V, Gualtieri G. Carpal tunnel syndrome in hemodialyzed patients. Chir Organi Mov. 1993;78:15–8.
20. Bartova V, Zima T. Diagnosis and treatment of carpal tunnel syndrome. Ren Fail. 1993;15:533–7.
21. Asencio G, Rigout C, Ramperez P, et al. Hemodialysis-related lesions of the hand. Rev Rhum Engl Ed. 1995;62:233–40.

Approach to an Abnormal Surveillance Measurement

22

Loay Salman

22.1 Introduction

Hemodialysis vascular access dysfunction still significantly contributes to hemodialysis patients' hospitalization and adds to the cost of delivering care to dialysis patients [1, 2]. While hemodialysis access dysfunction can have various manifestations such as prolonged bleeding, edema, high recirculation, low dialysis adequacy, or frequently alarming dialysis machine, access thrombosis is the most feared complication as it requires urgent intervention due to the loss of the lifeline of the dialysis patient, and thrombosis by itself may affect the longevity of the access even after a successful thrombectomy procedure.

Vascular stenosis induced by neointimal hyperplasia is the most common cause of hemodialysis vascular access dysfunction. Vascular stenosis is seen in almost all patients with clotted arteriovenous access [3]. A high percentage of hemodialysis patients will develop vascular stenosis [4].

Unexplained low Kt/V can be a result of dysfunctional vascular access. It is clear now that for every 0.1 decrease in Kt/V, there is a significant increase in hospitalizations, hospital days, and Medicare cost [5]. The detection of the presence of vascular stenotic lesions might be helpful as this stenosis can be treated successfully by an outpatient procedure which is percutaneous balloon angioplasty [6]. Additionally there is evidence that treatment of stenotic lesions might decrease vascular access thrombosis [7, 8].

Regular vascular access evaluation can be beneficial for early detection of abnormalities such as stenotic lesions. This evaluation can be performed by two main means which are monitoring and surveillance.

L. Salman, MD
Interventional Nephrology, University of Miami Miller
School of Medicine, Miami, FL, USA
e-mail: lsalman@med.miami.edu

22.2 Vascular Access Monitoring

Vascular access monitoring is by definition performing a physical examination by a qualified individual on regular basis. It is recommended that monitoring be performed on monthly basis [9]. Vascular access physical examination will be discussed in detail in another chapter in this book.

22.3 Vascular Access Surveillance

Vascular access surveillance by definition means the use of additional tools and instrumentations to perform regular periodic evaluation of the hemodialysis vascular access for early detection of stenotic lesions. Surveillance not only involves the use of additional tools and instruments but also requires trained staff to perform it. This translates into additional cost and burden on the health-care system. The biggest obstacle in front of performing surveillance is the fact that Medicare does not reimburse surveillance due to the lack of well-designed studies to show its benefit on vascular access thrombosis or other morbidity parameters.

There are a number of surveillance methods that have been developed to detect vascular stenosis. The main types of vascular access surveillance that has been recommended for use are intra-access flow measurement by an outlined method, directly measured or derived static venous dialysis pressure by an outlined method, and duplex ultrasound. These methods are categorized by KDOQI as preferred or acceptable. While intra-access flow measurement is preferred for both arteriovenous fistulae and arteriovenous grafts, directly measured or derived static venous dialysis pressure is preferred for arteriovenous graft and categorized as only acceptable for arteriovenous fistulae [9].

A.S. Yevzlin et al. (eds.), *Interventional Nephrology*,
DOI 10.1007/978-1-4614-8803-3_22, © Springer Science+Business Media New York 2014

Table 22.1 Indications for referral for arteriovenous access angiogram. Based on access blood flow measurement [1]

Arteriovenous fistula (AVF)	Arteriovenous graft (AVG)
Access flow rate less than 400–500 ml/min	Access flow rate less than 600 ml/min in grafts
	If access flow is 1,000 ml/min that has dropped 25 % over 4 months
Prospective trend analysis of the test parameter has greater power to detect dysfunction than isolated values alone	
Persistent abnormalities in any of the monitoring or surveillance parameters should prompt referral for access angiogram	

Table 22.2 Arteriovenous access pressure measurement interpretation and indications for referral for angiogram [1]

		AV graft		AV fistula	
		Arterial segment	Venous segment	Inflow	Outflow
Less than 50 % stenosis (not significant stenosis)		0.35–0.74	0.15–0.49	0.13–0.43	0.08–0.34
More than 50 % stenosis (significant stenosis)	Venous outflow	>0.75	Or >0.5	>0.43	Or >0.35
	Intra-access	≥0.65	And <0.5	>0.43	And ≤0.35
	Arterial inflow	<0.3	Clinical findings	<0.13 + clinical finding	Clinical findings

22.3.1 Intra-access Flow Measurement

There are a number of techniques that have been used to measure intra-access blood flow: Duplex Doppler ultrasound (DDU), magnetic resonance angiography (MRA), variable flow Doppler ultrasound (VFDU), ultrasound dilution (Transonics)(UDT), Crit-Line III (OABF), Crit-Line III (TQA), glucose pump infusion technique (GPT), urea dilution (UreaD), differential conductivity (GAMBRO) (HDM), and in-line dialysance (Fresenius) (DD) [9]. However, most of these have significant limitations. Duplex Doppler ultrasound is operator dependent and requires skilled personnel and vascular cross-sectional measurement. Additionally it is not available in the hemodialysis units. The cost of others and inability to perform the measurement during dialysis also are significant obstacles in front of their routine use. Additionally the description of nephrogenic systemic fibrosis (NSF) in dialysis patients made the use of gadolinium in hemodialysis patients a contraindication [10]. An ideal surveillance method would be the one that can be performed during hemodialysis treatment. This, theoretically, will enable regular periodic measurements and more compliance from patients as no additional appointments will be needed.

The National Kidney Foundation Kidney Disease Outcomes Quality Initiative (KDOQI) recommends when measuring access blood flow with ultrasound dilution, conductance dilution, thermal dilution, Doppler or other technique to be performed monthly. The assessment also should be performed during the first 1.5 h of the treatment to eliminate error caused by decrease in cardiac output or blood pressure related to ultrafiltration or hypotension [1]. The official KDOQI recommendation indicates that an access flow of less than 600 ml/min in arteriovenous graft and less 400–500 ml/min in arteriovenous fistula or if the access flow is 1,000 ml/min that has decreased by more than 25 % over 4 months the patient should be referred for hemodialysis access angiogram for further evaluation for

the presence of stenotic lesions [1]. Table 22.1 summarizes the indication of referral of arteriovenous fistula and graft for angiogram as set by KDOQI guidelines [1].

22.3.2 Access Pressure

Static access pressure is measured during dialysis treatment by using a manometer connected to the dialysis needles. The ratio of intra-graft pressure to the systemic pressure is used. This ratio has established parameters that are categorized as normal or abnormal.

Table 22.2 shows the pressure ratios and the indications for referral for dialysis access angiogram based on these ratios. This table is adapted from the KDOQI guidelines [1].

Static pressure measurement is within the preferred methods by KDOQI guidelines when used for arteriovenous graft surveillance. However, it is only acceptable method when used for the arteriovenous fistula surveillance [1]. This might be simply due to the fact that fistula would have additional paths for blood flow (collateral veins) when outflow stenosis develops. These collateral veins will affect the intra-access pressure increase (as a consequence of the outflow stenosis). Additionally the magnitude of the pressure change as result of the same outflow stenosis would be affected by the number and size of these collaterals. Therefore, static pressure measurement would be theoretically less valuable when used for arteriovenous fistulae surveillance.

22.3.3 Duplex Ultrasonography

Arteriovenous access surveillance can also be done by the use of duplex ultrasonography. This is performed by measuring peak systolic velocity on both sides of the detected stenotic lesion. Then the ratio of the two peak systolic velocity measurements is calculated. A ratio of more than two is suspicious for significant vascular stenosis [11].

One major limitation of this method is that it is not available in hemodialysis units. This mean it cannot be performed during dialysis treatment. Patients have to be scheduled for an additional visit. Duplex ultrasonography is operator dependent.

22.4 Vascular Access Surveillance Evidence

A number of observational studies have been performed evaluating various surveillance methods reported a substantial decrease in the graft thrombosis after implementing a surveillance program [12–16]. Based on this evidence the National Kidney Foundation Kidney Disease Outcomes Quality Initiative (KDOQI) VA guidelines have emphasized that hemodialysis units should implement graft surveillance programs and refer patients with suspected graft stenosis for preemptive angioplasty [1].

There is paucity in randomized control studies that were conducted to evaluate hemodialysis access surveillance. These randomized studies raised serious doubts regarding the validity of this approach [17–25]. However, the available randomized trials have significant limitations. Table 22.3 summarizes these trials.

In one of the randomized [17], controlled trial, 101 patients were assigned to control ($n=34$), access flow ($n=32$), or duplex ultrasound to diagnose significant vascular stenosis ≥50% ($n=35$). The control group underwent physical examination. Access flow was determined by ultrasound dilution test on a monthly basis in the access flow group. Duplex ultrasound was performed quarterly to assess the percentage of stenosis in the duplex ultrasound group. Referral for angiography was based on an established criteria {Control group ($n=34$), flow group ($n=32$), blood flow

<600 ml/min or clinical criteria; and stenosis group ($n=35$)}. Stenosis of >50 % was corrected by percutaneous transluminal angioplasty. This study found that graft thrombosis was the lowest in the duplex ultrasound group at 28 months while the 2-year graft survival was similar (62 %), (60 %) and (64 %) for the control , access flow , and duplex ultrasound groups respectively ($P=0.89$). Flow monitoring and duplex ultrasound were not superior to clinical examination.

Robbin et al. [18] randomized 126 patients to clinical monitoring (control group) and surveillance with ultrasound (ultrasound group) in patients with AVG. Ultrasound surveillance was for graft stenosis and clinical monitoring included detailed physical examination of abnormalities related to dialysis session (prolonged bleeding, cannulation difficulties, clot aspiration, inability to achieve the prescribed blood flow). Ultrasound surveillance for graft stenosis was performed every 4 months. This study showed that there was no difference in the frequency of thrombosis between the two groups (control 0.78; ultrasound group 0.67; $P=0.37$). The median time to permanent graft failure did not differ between the two groups (38 versus 37 months; $P=0.93$). The authors concluded that the addition of ultrasound surveillance to clinical monitoring increased the frequency of invasive procedures but failed to decrease the likelihood of graft thrombosis or failure.

Although these studies failed to show an advantage, others emphasized a beneficial effect of surveillance and improved graft survival [21, 22]. Tonelli et al. [23] conducted a randomized clinical trial comparing access surveillance (using access blood flow or ultrasound-based surveillance) with standard care. This study did not show any decrease in the risk for graft thrombosis or access loss in the access screening group. Although there was a significant reduction in thrombosis rates in AVF, there was no difference in the risk for fistula loss or resource use. Therefore, this study also showed no evidence that screening with either access blood

Table 22.3 Randomized clinical trials comparing surveillance to monitoring

Study	Number of patients	Surveillance method	Type of access	Primary outcome	Results
Sands et al. [23]	103	Access flow Static venous pressure	68 AVF 35 AVG	AV access thrombosis	Positive (in favor of access flow measurement)
Moist et al. [19]	112	Access flow Dynamic venous pressure	AVG	AV access thrombosis or loss	Negative
Ram et al. [17]	101	Access flow Stenosis	AVG	AV access thrombosis or access survival	Negative
Polkinghorne et al. [24]	137	Access flow	AVF	Significant stenosis	Negative
Mayer et al. [25]	70	Duplex scan (ultrasound)	AVG	AVG survival	Positive
Malik et al. [21]	192	Duplex scan (ultrasound)	AVG	AVG patency	Positive
Robbin et al. [18]	126	Duplex scan (ultrasound)	AVG	AVG survival	Negative

flow or Doppler ultrasound is of benefit in patients with AVG; however, it did have a number of limiting factors such as small sample size and inadequate power. In light of these confounding factors, the role of surveillance at best remains controversial.

Beathard et al. [26] conducted a study where a 101 patients were assigned to control, flow (<600 ml/min by ultrasound dilution), or stenosis (luminal narrowing $\geq$50% by ultrasound). Patients were followed for up to 28 months. The access-related hospitalizations and costs of care were assessed in the three groups. The study also looked into the use of tunneled dialysis catheter among the three groups. The results showed that hospitalization rates were significantly higher in the control and flow groups than in the stenosis group (0.50, 0.57, and 0.18 per patient-year, respectively; P=0.01). The costs of care were the highest in the control and flow groups than in the stenosis group (P=0.015).

Conclusion

The National Kidney Foundation Kidney Disease Outcomes Quality Initiative (KDOQI) recommends an organized monitoring/surveillance approach with regular assessment of clinical parameters of the AV access and HD adequacy. Data from the clinical assessment and HD adequacy measurements should be collected and maintained for each patient's access and made available to all staff. The data should be tabulated and tracked within each HD center as part of a quality assurance (QA)/CQI program [1].

There is some evidence that implementing such program might be beneficial in regard to access thrombosis, hospitalization, and cost burden. But this benefit might be on the expense of increasing procedure numbers. However, due to the conflicting results of other studies that looked at the same and other variables, the health care is in need of a well-designed randomized controlled trial adequately powered to evaluate multiple variables like access thrombosis, cumulative access patency, need for tunneled dialysis catheters, hospitalizations, and cost. Such a study need to cover both arteriovenous fistulae and arteriovenous grafts.

References

1. National Kidney Foundation. K/DOQI clinical practice guidelines in vascular access: 2006 update. Am J Kidney Dis. 2006;48(Suppl 1):S176–306.
2. US Renal Data System. Annual data report: atlas of chronic kidney disease and end-stage renal disease in the United States. Bethesda: National Institutes of Health, National Institute of Diabetes and Digestive and Kidney Diseases; 2007.
3. Turmel-Rodrigues L, Pengloan J, Rodrigue H, Brillet G, Lataste A, Pierre D, Jourdan JL, Blanchard D. Treatment of failed native arteriovenous fistulae for hemodialysis by interventional radiology. Kidney Int. 2000;57(3):1124.
4. Asif A, Gadalean FN, Merrill D, Cherla G, Cipleu CD, Epstein DL, Roth D. Inflow stenosis in arteriovenous grafts and fistulae: result of a prospective study. Kidney Int. 2005;67:1986–92.
5. Sehgal AR, Snow RJ, Singer ME, Amini SB, DeOreo PB, Silver MR, Cebul RD. Barriers to adequate delivery of hemodialysis. Am J Kidney Dis. 1998;31(4):593–601.
6. Beathard GA. The treatment of vascular access graft dysfunction: a nephrologist's view and experience. Adv Ren Replace Ther. 1994;1:131–47.
7. Gruss E, Portolés J, Jiménez P, Hernández T, Rueda JA, del Cerro J, Lasala M, Tato A, Gago MC, Martínez S, Velayos P. Prospective monitoring of vascular access in hemodialysis by means of a multidisciplinary team. Nefrologia. 2006;26(6):703–10.
8. Schwab SJ, Oliver MJ, Suhocki P, McCann R. Hemodialysis arteriovenous access: detection of stenosis and response to treatment by vascular access blood flow. Kidney Int. 2001;59:358–62.
9. http://www.kidney.org/professionals/kdoqi/guideline_uphd_pd_va/va_guide4.htm.
10. http://www.fda.gov/Drugs/DrugSafety/PostmarketDrugSafetyInformationforPatientsandProviders/ucm142884.htm. Accessed Mar 2012.
11. Robbin ML, Oser RF, Allon M, Clements MW, Dockery J, Weber TM, Hamrick-Waller KM, Smith JK, Jones BC, Morgan DE, Saddekni S. Hemodialysis access graft stenosis: US detection. Radiology. 1998;208(3):655.
12. Schwab SJ, Raymond JR, Saeed M, Newman GE, Dennis PA, Bollinger RR. Prevention of hemodialysis fistula thrombosis: early detection of venous stenosis. Kidney Int. 1989;36:707–11.
13. Besarab A, Sullivan KL, Ross RP, Moritz MJ. Utility of intraaccess pressure monitoring in detecting and correcting venous outlet stenosis prior to thrombosis. Kidney Int. 1995;47:1364–73.
14. Safa AA, Valji K, Roberts AC, Ziegler TW, Hye RJ, Oglevie SB. Detection and treatment of dysfunctional hemodialysis access grafts: effects of surveillance program on graft patency and incidence of thrombosis. Radiology. 1996;199:653–7.
15. Cayco AV, Abu-Alfa AK, Mahnensmith RL, Perazella MA. Reduction in arteriovenous graft impairment: results of a vascular access surveillance protocol. Am J Kidney Dis. 1998;32:302–8.
16. McCarley P, Wingard RL, Shyr Y, Pettus W, Hakim RM, Ikizler TA. Vascular access blood flow monitoring reduces access morbidity and costs. Kidney Int. 2001;60:1164–72.
17. Ram SJ, Work J, Caldito GC, Eason JM, Pervez A, Paulson WD. A randomized control trial of blood flow and stenosis surveillance of hemodialysis grafts. Kidney Int. 2003;64:272–80.
18. Robbin ML, Oser RF, Lee JY, Heudebert GR, Mennemeyer ST, Allon M. Randomized comparison of ultrasound surveillance and clinical monitoring on arteriovenous graft outcomes. Kidney Int. 2006;69:730–5.
19. Moist LM, Churchill DN, House AA, Millward SF, Elliott JE, Kribs SW, DeYoung WJ, Blythe L, Stitt LW, Lindsay RM. Regular monitoring of access flow compared with monitoring of venous pressure fails to improve graft survival. J Am Soc Nephrol. 2003;14:2645–53.
20. Dember LM, Holmberg EF, Kaufman JS. Randomized controlled trial of prophylactic repair of hemodialysis arteriovenous graft stenosis. Kidney Int. 2004;66:390–8.
21. Malik J, Slavikova M, Svobodova J, Tuka V. Regular ultrasonographic screening significantly prolongs patency of PTFE grafts. Kidney Int. 2005;67:1554–8.
22. Tessitore N, Lipari G, Poli A, Bedogna V, Baggio E, Loschiavo C, Mansueto G, Lupo A. Can blood flow surveillance and pre-emptive repair of subclinical stenosis prolong the useful life of arteriovenous fistulae? A randomized controlled study. Nephrol Dial Transplant. 2004;19(9):2325–33.

23. Sands JJ, Jabyac PA, Miranda CL, Kapsick BJ. Intervention based on monthly monitoring decreases hemodialysis access thrombosis. ASAIO J. 1999;45(3):147–50.

24. Polkinghorne KR, Lau KK, Saunder A, Atkins RC, Kerr PG. Does monthly native arteriovenous fistula blood-flow surveillance detect significant stenosis—a randomized controlled trial. Nephrol Dial Transplant. 2006;21(9):2498–506.

25. Mayer DA, Zingale RG, Tsapogas MJ. Duplex scanning of expanded polytetrafluoroethylene dialysis shunts: impact on patient management and graft survival. Vasc Surg. 1993;27(9): 647–58.

26. Beathard GA, Welch BR, Maidment HJ. Mechanical thrombolysis for the treatment of thrombosed hemodialysis access grafts. Radiology. 1996;200:711–6.

23

Arterial Stenosis Affecting Arteriovenous Fistulae and Grafts in Hemodialysis Patients: Approach to Diagnosis and Management

Diego A. Covarrubias, Chieh Suai Tan, and Steven Wu

23.1 Introduction

Adequate arterial inflow is an essential requirement of a successfully functioning arteriovenous (AV) access for hemodialysis (HD). Patients with end-stage renal disease (ESRD) on HD have a high incidence of peripheral artery disease (PAD) and vascular derangements in general. The arteries utilized for AV access creation are subject to similar pathologic processes as those of the lower extremities in this population, leading to the potential for AV access dysfunction. Arterial disease is a relatively underappreciated cause of AV access dysfunction. This chapter will provide an overview of the approach to the patient with suspected arterial stenosis leading to AV access dysfunction.

23.2 Definition, Epidemiology, and Pathophysiology

23.2.1 Definition of Arterial Stenosis

The precise definition of arterial stenosis in the setting of HD AV access is somewhat variable. An acceptable working definition is an arterial stenosis of 50 % or greater decrease

D.A. Covarrubias, MD • C.S. Tan, MBBS
Vascular Interventional Radiology, Massachusetts
General Hospital, 55 Fruit Street, Boston, MA 02114, USA

Department of Radiology, Massachusetts General Hospital,
55 Fruit Street, Boston, MA 02114, USA

S. Wu, MD (✉)
Vascular Interventional Radiology, Massachusetts
General Hospital, 55 Fruit Street, Boston, MA 02114, USA

Department of Medicine, Massachusetts General Hospital,
Harvard Medical School, 55 Fruit Street, Boston, MA 02114, USA

Department of Radiology, Massachusetts General Hospital,
55 Fruit Street, Boston, MA 02114, USA
e-mail: swu1@partners.org

in luminal diameter as compared with adjacent normal caliber artery occurring in the arterial inflow to the AV access anywhere from the anastomosis to the ascending aorta. This will be the definition used for the purposes of this chapter. Some authors specifically choose to exclude the juxta-anastomotic region in their definition of arterial stenosis; however, lesions in specific locations will be addressed later in the discussion.

23.2.2 Epidemiology of Arterial Stenoses

Traditionally, arterial inflow stenoses were considered to be a rare cause of dysfunctional AV access, especially when compared to lesions of the venous outflow. Early estimates cited occurrence of arterial stenoses in 0–4 % of patients [1], while recent publications have provided evidence of an incidence ranging from 14 to 42 % [2]. The majority of lesions are juxta-anastomotic in location, with up to one third involving the more proximal feeding arteries. A higher incidence of inflow stenoses is seen in forearm AV access compared to the upper arm location [3]. Also, a higher incidence of these lesions is seen in fistulas than grafts [4]. Most commonly, non-anastomotic stenoses are seen in the subclavian artery, followed by the radial artery [5]. The likelihood of arterial lesions increases with increasing age [6]. Venous stenoses coexist with arterial lesions up to 54 % of the time in patients with fistulas and up to as high as 100 % of the time in patients with grafts [7].

23.2.3 Pathophysiology of Arterial Stenoses

The pathogenesis of arterial inflow stenosis is unclear likely multifactorial in etiology. In a proportion of patients, some degree of underlying arterial disease was inevitably present prior to surgical creation of AV access. The high-flow state the vessels endure under regular hemodialysis is also likely a contributory causal factor [8]. Unfortunately, no clinical

A.S. Yevzlin et al. (eds.), *Interventional Nephrology*,
DOI 10.1007/978-1-4614-8803-3_23, © Springer Science+Business Media New York 2014

studies specifically address how or when the high-flow state of HD causes its effects on healthy native arteries. Precursors to arterial stenoses include neointimal hyperplasia and atherosclerotic plaques, both calcified and noncalcified [9]. The altered physiologic state of HD contributes to both initiation and accelerated progression of these lesions, likely due to its inflammatory nature [10]. As these lesions develop and advance in severity, they lead to luminal narrowing and eventually stenosis.

23.3 Initial Evaluation

The presence of limb ischemia during hemodialysis may prompt a search for a specific cause. While the differential diagnosis may be broad, an arterial lesion should be considered and ruled out as this may represent a curable etiology.

23.3.1 History

Evaluation should begin with the taking of a thorough history. This would include questioning regarding the occurrence of relevant symptoms such as claudication, the presence of cold hands or feet, and rest pain. The relationship of these symptoms to hemodialysis sessions should also be determined, with careful recording of number of occurrences, nature/character of symptoms, as well as duration and whether or not the limb affected contains the AV access. Patients should also be questioned concerning a history of previous surgery, trauma, or prior failed AV access. The goal of history taking is to attempt to elucidate a specific cause of the symptoms in question. Admittedly, in the setting of an arterial stenosis as the causal factor, the history is limited in contributing to actually arriving at the diagnosis.

23.3.2 Physical Examination

Physical examination in combination with a detailed history will increase diagnostic confidence. The physical exam should obviously be focused on the area of symptomatology. In the hemodialysis patient, this is most commonly in the limb containing the AV access. Palpation for thrill and tension is the first step in evaluating the AV access. However, abnormality in flow through the access on palpation is a nonspecific finding. Other basic initial maneuvers involve evaluation of the radial and ulnar blood supply as well as comparison of bilateral blood pressures. The Allen's test can be utilized to evaluate the adequacy of the dual blood supply to the hand. Blood pressures in the extremity containing the AV access typically are 10–20 mmHg higher than in the contralateral extremity. If the blood pressure in the access extremity is lower than that in the contralateral extremity, this suggests the presence of arterial stenosis. Additional assessment of the extremity for stigmata of vascular compromise should also be undertaken. The presence of pain, sensory deficits, skin discoloration, and ulceration should be noted. If hand pain is present and relieved by occlusion of the AV access, distal hypoperfusion ischemic syndrome (DHIS) may be considered. This entity is commonly due to arterial stenosis and is specifically addressed in a separate chapter on hand pain. Additionally, loss of hair or nail bed changes should be sought. The physical examination may need to be repeated during a hemodialysis session, as the symptoms may only occur at such times.

23.3.3 Hemodynamic Parameters During Hemodialysis

Measurement of certain hemodynamic parameters during hemodialysis is an important component of AV access maintenance. Problems during HD are often the first manifestation of access dysfunction. Recent studies have found that when measurement of access blood flow (Qa) is less than 650 ml/min, this represents a relatively sensitive and specific sign of inflow stenosis [11]. A full discussion of hemodialysis parameters is beyond the scope of this chapter.

23.3.4 The Importance of Prior Imaging Studies

A thorough initial evaluation should not only include history and physical exam but also a review of pertinent prior imaging studies. The increasingly widespread acceptance of electronic medical records and picture archiving and communications systems (PACS) allows for a wealth of patient information to remain readily available to the physician. This information should be maximally utilized. A hemodialysis patient with symptomatology and history and physical exam findings suggestive of the presence of arterial stenosis may have a prior imaging study on file that could provide a clue as to the etiology. Such possible findings may include the presence of either central or peripheral vascular lesions or abnormalities. If prior imaging studies are not available or unhelpful, dedicated imaging of the central vasculature supplying the AV access may be advisable.

23.3.5 Diagnosis Requires a High Index of Suspicion

The signs and symptoms of arterial stenosis are usually nonspecific, rendering diagnosis by history and physical exam difficult. The challenge is compounded by the fact that commonly arterial and venous outflow lesions coexist. A high index of suspicion is necessary to pursue a diagnosis of arterial inflow stenosis. After successful and complete treatment of the venous disease, persistence of clinical features of inadequate arterial inflow or observation of sluggish flow on post-angioplasty angiogram warrants further investigation of the arterial tree. Clinical assessment can raise the index of suspicion for the presence of arterial stenosis, but the mainstay of diagnosis is via imaging.

23.3.6 Preventative Measures

Finally, preventative measures undertaken when planning placement of the AV access will ensure adequate future function. Ideally, the entire arterial tree supplying the intended site of AV access should be thoroughly evaluated prior to surgical creation. An arterial stenosis involving the inflow of the planned AV access may represent a subclinical preexisting condition which is only unmasked following surgical placement of a low vascular resistance AV access. Arterial lesions like these are extremely important to recognize because they can lead to poor AV access maturation and function as well as being the direct cause of symptoms such as hand ischemia. Again, it is imperative to evaluate the entire arterial inflow prior to surgical creation of an AV access in order to decrease the probability of clinically significant issues involving the arterial side of the access arising in the future. Discovery of a significant arterial stenosis or lesion during presurgical work-up does not preclude placement of AV access, as many of these lesions can be successfully treated using endovascular techniques, such as percutaneous transluminal angioplasty (PTA) and/or stenting (Table 23.1 Evaluation).

Table 23.1 Evaluation of patients with suspected arterial stenosis affecting an AV access

1. History
Inquire regarding claudication, "cold" hands, rest pain, relationship of symptoms to HD, previous surgery, trauma, or failed AV access
2. Physical exam
Palpate for thrill and tension
Comparison of bilateral blood pressures (AV access extremity typically 10–20 mmHg higher)
Search for stigmata of vascular compromise: skin discoloration, ulceration, loss of hair, nail bed changes
3. Assess hemodynamic parameters during hemodialysis
4. Review prior imaging studies
5. Obtain diagnostic studies

23.4 Differential Diagnosis

The differential diagnosis of AV access dysfunction includes lesions of both the venous outflow and arterial inflow, as well as the access itself. When evaluating hemodialysis AV access problems, the practitioner should visualize the access as a portion of a circuit, which includes the heart, arterial inflow, AV access, and venous outflow. The circuit model allows for a systematic approach to potential clinical issues that may arise with an AV access. Each component of the circuit should be carefully evaluated, which will ensure a thorough assessment. For example, once other causes such as venous outflow obstruction, heart failure, and thrombosis are excluded, logically, the arterial inflow must be the culprit. Perhaps the major challenge in diagnosing and treating arterial stenoses lies in the lack of a standardized algorithmic approach to evaluation. Whenever a patient presents with a problematic AV access, the concept of the vascular circuit should be kept in mind, as rendered treatments may be insufficient if only one portion of the circuit is addressed. A highly specific and sensitive sign of arterial stenosis is when poor blood flow persists after adequate treatment of the venous outflow [7].

23.5 Diagnostic Studies

23.5.1 Overview

Assessment of the arterial tree in patients with problematic AV access can be performed with various modalities. The modalities differ in accuracy, effectiveness, and specific advantages and disadvantages. Noninvasive studies may provide an accurate diagnosis; however, treatment will typically require either endovascular intervention or surgery. Conventional angiography in the form of a fistulogram or graftogram is an acceptable first option for evaluation of dysfunctional AV access as it provides both a diagnosis and the potential to render treatment simultaneously.

23.5.2 Noninvasive Studies

Noninvasive modalities include sonography, computed tomographic (CT) angiography, and magnetic resonance (MR) angiography.

Ultrasound

Ultrasound is a widely available low-cost imaging modality uniquely suited to examination of vascular structures. The superficial location of HD AV access facilitates sonographic visualization. Sonography has the ability to quantify flow velocity and direction in real time and can depict morphologic abnormalities such as stenoses or thrombus [12]. Disadvantages of ultrasound include an inability to evaluate the central vasculature and significant dependence on the skill of the operator.

CT Angiography

CT angiography provides a rapid, well-tolerated means of evaluating the entire arterial tree as well as the venous outflow. Other advantages include excellent spatial resolution and the ability to post-process acquired data, for example, creation of three-dimensional reconstructions. CT is also widely available and technically does not depend on the operator for high-quality images. The major disadvantages of CT include the use of ionizing radiation and intravenous contrast material. Growing acceptance of low-dose CT protocols has somewhat lessened patient radiation exposure [13]. In the HD population, use of IV contrast does not pose a problem as renal function is not a concern.

MR Angiography

MR angiography is similar to CT in that it has the ability to depict the entire AV access circuit, including the central vasculature. An advantage is the lack of ionizing radiation. MR can be performed without intravenous contrast using certain parameters; however, the acquired data sets with these techniques are not as accurate as their contrast-enhanced counterparts, and diagnostic confidence is potentially decreased by multiple artifacts. Contrast-enhanced MR angiography is an excellent study for evaluation of vascular structures. Unfortunately, the recognition of the association of NSF with poor clearance of gadolinium has limited the use of contrast-enhanced MR in the HD population [14]. Other disadvantages of MR include longer image acquisition times, which may not be well tolerated by patients. Additionally, many HD patients have comorbid conditions that may preclude exposure to a magnetic field, such as an indwelling pacemaker. Patients with vascular stents pose a significant problem for evaluation with MRA as the stents will create artifacts limiting evaluation of patency and adjacent vascular segments.

23.5.3 Conventional Angiography

Conventional angiography is the gold standard method for evaluation of AV access dysfunction. It is highly accurate and can be used to evaluate the entire access circuit. A major advantage of angiography is that it allows for concurrent diagnosis and treatment, via endovascular techniques such as PTA and/or stenting (Fig. 23.1). Disadvantages include the invasive

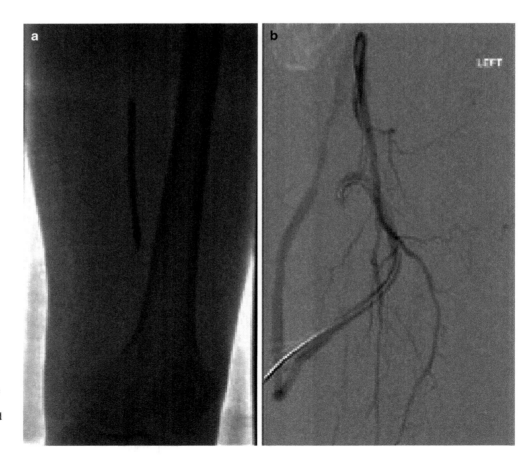

Fig. 23.1 Fluoroscopic image shows an angioplasty balloon inflated in the left superficial femoral artery (**a**). This was the feeding artery of a lower extremity AV access, which had occluded but was successfully recanalized (**b**)

nature of the procedure, use of iodinated contrast and ionizing radiation, relative cost, need for patient sedation and monitoring, and the potential occurrence of associated complications. Complications of conventional angiography include bleeding, infection, and vascular injury. Major complications, though rare, do occur, and patients may require emergent surgery.

Common interventional practice is to use the fistula or graft itself as the point of access for diagnosis or treatment (fistulogram/graftogram). This approach facilitates assessment of the venous outflow and anastomosis and allows for relatively simple and straightforward treatment of lesions on the venous side of the AV access circuit. Complete evaluation of the arterial inflow then requires crossing the anastomosis and placing a diagnostic catheter centrally. Noninvasive imaging studies may allow for detection of central lesions prior to fistulogram/graftogram. Armed with this knowledge, the operator could then consider a different approach to assist in treatment if necessary, such as the common femoral artery route (Table 23.2 Diagnostic studies).

23.6 Classification of Arterial Lesions

23.6.1 Overview

Arterial stenoses can be classified according to location and type. Locations include central, feeding arteries, juxta-anastomotic, and distal. These lesions can be due to intrinsic

Table 23.2 Diagnostic studies: advantages and disadvantages

1. Noninvasive:
   - (a) Ultrasound
     Pro: widely available, low cost, ability to quantify flow velocity and direction in real time, can depict stenoses or thrombus
     Con: Inability to evaluate central vasculature, highly operator dependent
   - (b) CT angiography
     Pro: fast, evaluate entire arterial tree/venous outflow, excellent spatial, post-processing, widely available, no operator dependence for high-quality images
     Con: ionizing radiation, intravenous contrast material
   - (c) MR angiography
     Pro: similar advantages to CT with additional lack of ionizing radiation
     Con: longer image acquisition times, artifacts of non-contrast sequences, NSF, pacemakers and stents contraindicated
2. Invasive:
   - (a) Conventional angiography
     Pro: gold standard method for evaluation of AV access, highly accurate, evaluate entire access circuit, concurrent diagnosis and treatment (PTA/stent)
     Con: iodinated contrast, ionizing radiation, relative cost, need for sedation/anesthesia, potential complications

vascular factors such as underlying atherosclerosis or due to external factors such as compression by adjacent anatomic structures. The degree of stenosis can be described as mild, moderate, or severe. A severe stenosis is usually hemodynamically significant. The significance of mild to moderate stenoses is generally not so easily qualifiable, with such lesions not necessarily associated with a hemodynamic abnormality. In the non-dialysis population, clinically insignificant mild to moderate stenoses may be the norm [15]. In HD patients, even a mild arterial stenosis can be problematic if it limits the inflow to the AV access or causes limb ischemia.

23.6.2 Anastomotic and Juxta-anastomotic Lesions

Up to 50 % of lesions in patients with AV access for HD are located in the anastomotic and juxta-anastomotic regions, by far the most common location [16]. Fortunately, these lesions are typically easily diagnosed at fistulogram/graftogram via retrograde injection with manual occlusion of the venous outflow, allowing for treatment.

23.6.3 Central and Feeding Artery Lesions

In contrast, central or feeding artery stenoses present a diagnostic challenge, as lesions in these locations are not usually identified during the typical fistulogram/graftogram (Fig. 23.2). Stenoses in these locations can account for up to roughly 30–40 % of lesions and are not uncommon [17]. If the index of suspicion for a central lesion is high, diagnosis may require retrograde cannulation of the aorta through the AV access to perform arteriography and runoff or an antegrade approach via arterial puncture at a site other than the access.

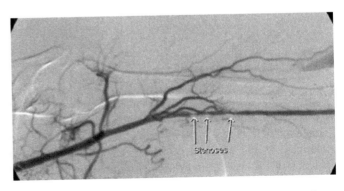

Fig. 23.2 Digital subtraction angiogram demonstrates segmental stenoses (labeled) of the left brachial artery in the inflow of the forearm AVF. This led to AVF dysfunction. Note no catheter is seen within the vessel, denoting that the arterial system was not accessed through the AV access

23.6.4 Distal Artery Lesions

Distal arterial stenoses are less frequently encountered than juxta-anastomotic and central lesions. The association of peripheral arterial disease and general vasculopathy with the HD patient population predisposes these patients to diffuse arterial disease. Although a distal arterial stenosis will not have a direct affect on AV access function, it has the potential to induce devastating clinical consequences. These include hand ischemia or tissue loss in the extremity containing the AV access. For this reason, if there are symptoms attributed to arterial stenosis and the more common locations for disease demonstrate no evidence of disease, the distal arteries should be thoroughly evaluated. Another caveat that must be kept in mind is that distal arterial stenoses often coexist with abnormalities of the venous outflow. Treatment of venous outflow disease without addressing a distal arterial stenosis can inadvertently trigger a steal phenomenon. This occurs because the low resistance to flow in the treated AV access preferentially shunts blood away from the vascular territories beyond the high-resistance distal arterial lesion. A thorough retrograde angiogram should demonstrate at least the immediate distal arterial segments and allow for avoidance of this scenario.

23.6.5 Lesions Due to External Compression

External compression of the arterial inflow by adjacent anatomic structures is a rare cause of AV access dysfunction. Examples of potential situations are compression of the subclavian artery by a thoracic aortic aneurysm or a cervical rib. Endovascular treatment of these lesions alone is futile, as the underlying compression must be addressed. Surgical decompression is required. Occasionally, an arterial stenosis at the anastomotic or juxta-anastomotic region of a previous failed AV access in the same extremity acts as the direct cause of dysfunction of a downstream AV access and/or hand ischemia.

23.7   Management

Endovascular techniques are the mainstay of management of AV access dysfunction for both venous and arterial lesions. This approach allows for confirmation of the diagnosis and treatment in the same session and can lead to continued patency of the access. Endovascular treatments are safe and effective, can be performed on an outpatient basis in most instances, and can be repeated as needed should future problems arise [18]. In rare cases, recanalization of severe occlusive arterial stenosis with a guidewire fails, making surgical bypass a second-line treatment option. Especially in the case of arterial inflow disease, primary patency rates are excellent, with multiple studies documenting no requirement for additional treatment following successful angioplasty or stenting [19].

23.7.1 Percutaneous Transluminal Angioplasty

Percutaneous transluminal angioplasty is the main form of endovascular treatment. PTA is used in both venous and arterial structures. Interventionalists that regularly perform evaluation of HD AV access should have a definite familiarity with endovenous PTA, as it is commonly performed. PTA of arterial lesions varies somewhat from its venous counterpart, due to the underlying physiologic differences between artery and vein. Depending on the unique training pathway of the interventionalist, some individuals may not be as comfortable or familiar with arterial PTA. For example, common practice of endovenous PTA usually requires an oversized balloon under high pressure with a relatively long duration of inflation to achieve acceptable results. In contrast, for arterial angioplasty, a balloon appropriately sized to the vessel diameter is used, lower pressures are required, and less inflation time is necessary [20]. PTA of arterial lesions is associated with more potential complications than venous angioplasty. Potential complications include arterial dissection, occlusion, thrombosis, distal embolization, and rupture [21]. Despite the higher complication rate, successful angioplasty of arterial lesions carries a higher primary patency rate than venous treatments, which often require multiple repeated sessions to maintain a patent outflow. Complication rates, though higher than venous angioplasty, are nevertheless acceptable in light of the usually complicated medical comorbidities present in the HD population. Operator experience also plays a role in complication rates, and as evaluation and treatment of the arterial portion of the AV access circuit become more routine, interventionalists will continue to become more adept at their performance.

23.7.2 Stents

Stents are a treatment option available as an adjunct to PTA. Following PTA, a significant residual stenosis may be seen. Also, lesions resistant to balloon dilatation are sometimes encountered during angioplasty (Fig. 23.3). In these cases, stenting would allow for effective restoration and preservation of adequate luminal diameter. Other cases in which stents are useful are in the setting of angioplasty complications. Should arterial dissection or rupture arise due to PTA, stents can be used to quickly and safely treat these lesions while preserving the native vascular channels and the AV access.

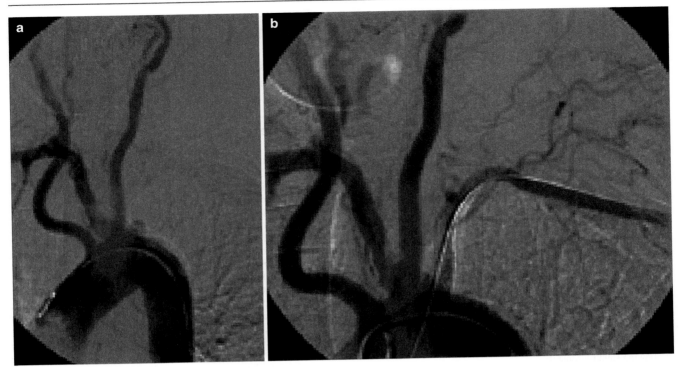

Fig. 23.3 (**a**) Digital subtraction angiogram demonstrates complete occlusion of the left subclavian artery. The patient has a left upper extremity AVF and presented with ischemic signs in the left upper extremity as well as AV access dysfunction. (**b**) The occlusion was successfully crossed, and a stent was placed across the closed segment, restoring patency and inflow to the left upper extremity

Stent Varieties

Stents are available in a wide variety of types. These include variations in external design such as bare metal or covered as well as variations in delivery methods, such as self-expanding or balloon-mounted. Each of the available systems offers its own advantages and disadvantages, such as specific safety profile, limitations, patency rates, and precision of delivery. Self-expanding stents generally have greater tensile and radial strength, while balloon-mounted stents allow for very precise delivery. There is a higher potential for stent fracture/malfunction when using balloon-mounted stents. Self-expanding stents may be preferred in the more central arterial tree. Newer stents have been designed with greater flexibility, and placement across joints or points of flexion has become more commonplace. This should, however, be avoided whenever possible as the risk of stent occlusion and fracture increases in such locations. Covered stents are preferred in the treatment of venous lesions due to higher patency rates in comparison to bare-metal stents [22]. Bare-metal stents are effective for treatment of arterial lesions and are commonly used for resistant or recoiling stenosis [23].

23.7.3 Angiographic Approach

As mentioned previously, common practice for angiography is to cannulate the AV access. Again, for treatment of arterial lesions, this requires retrograde cannulation across the anastomosis. This approach has been proven to be safe and effective and eliminates some potential complications associated with arterial puncture at other sites, such as pseudoaneurysm formation. The interventionalist can choose to access the arterial tree through a variety of routes, including the common femoral artery, the axillary artery, the brachial artery, and the radial artery. Studies have demonstrated that an antegrade approach is associated with increased rates of detection of the presence of inflow lesions relative to the retrograde approach [24]. Regardless of the approach, the basic principles of angiography should be practiced. This entails gaining arterial access and using a guidewire and catheter system to cannulate the vessel of interest under fluoroscopic guidance, allowing for injection of contrast material. Of import, when treatment is planned, guidewire access across the lesion undergoing PTA or stenting should be maintained at all times (Table 23.3 Management).

23.7.4 Anticoagulation

The use of anticoagulants during diagnostic and therapeutic angiography varies by institution. Although anticoagulation therapy with heparin is usually not required, the interventionalist may choose to administer a dose prior to angio-

Table 23.3 Endovascular management

1. Access

   Commonly through AV access

   If site of arterial lesion known from prior noninvasive imaging, common femoral or other approach may be useful

2. Diagnosis

   Depiction of the venous outflow, AV access, and arterial anatomy

   Depending on access route, retrograde cannulation of central/feeding arteries may be necessary

3. Treatment

   Guidewire access across lesion to be treated maintained at all times

   (a) PTA

      Appropriately sized balloon based on vessel diameter; lower pressures/shorter inflation than venous PTA

   (b) Stents

      Used for resistant or recoiling stenoses; generally self-expanding type preferred

Table 23.4 Anticoagulation recommendations

During PTA:

   Use of heparin varies by institution

   3,000 units IV a reasonable dose, with titration to ACT >250 s

Following stent placement:

   Immediate loading dose of clopidogrel (300 mg) followed by 75 mg daily for 6 months

   Aspirin 81–325 mg daily

plasty. If stents are placed, standard antiplatelet therapy with aspirin and clopidogrel should be initiated following the procedure (Table 23.4 Anticoagulation recommendations).

Conclusion

Arterial stenoses are an underappreciated significant contributor to AV access dysfunction. The HD population has a high degree of associated vasculopathy, which emphasizes the prevalence of arterial lesions in this setting. Interventions, including PTA and stent placement, performed on arterial lesions typically have excellent results, with an up to 20 % increase of flow in 90 % of cases as well as superb long-term patency rates. However, diagnosis still poses a significant challenge, as many interventionalists do not visualize the entire arterial tree at fistulogram/graftogram. Noninvasive imaging may facilitate diagnosis in certain cases, but the gold standard remains angiography. Complete evaluation of the arterial tree, including the central arteries and feeding arteries as well as the juxta-anastomotic region, is crucial; however, this may be a time-consuming endeavor that also increases procedural risk. The exceptional clinical results obtained with endovascular treatment warrant a thorough evaluation in at least patients who are likely to have an arterial lesion. A combination of clinical and noninvasive imaging findings may allow for stratification of patients in this regard. The interventionalist should be familiar with the available approaches to arterial diagnosis, potential complications, and benefits of treatment in order to deliver the best possible care while minimizing adverse outcomes.

References

1. Long B, Brichart N, Lermusiaux P, Turmel-Rodrigues L, Artru B, Boutin JM, Pengloan J, Bertrand P, Bruyère F. Management of perianastomotic stenosis of direct wrist autogenous radial-cephalic arteriovenous accesses for dialysis. J Vasc Surg. 2011;53(1):108–14. Epub 2010 Sep 22.
2. Kumakura H, Kanai H, Aizaki M, Mitsui K, Araki Y, Kasama S, Iwasaki T, Ichikawa S. The influence of the obesity paradox and chronic kidney disease on long-term survival in a Japanese cohort with peripheral arterial disease. J Vasc Surg. 2010;52(1):110–7. Epub 2010 May 15.
3. Bonforte G, Rossi E, Auricchio S, Pogliani D, Mangano S, Mandolfo S, Galli F, Genovesi S. The middle-arm fistula as a valuable surgical approach in patients with end-stage renal disease. J Vasc Surg. 2010;52(6):1551–6. Epub 2010 Aug 25.
4. Schild AF, Perez E, Gillaspie E, Seaver C, Livingstone J, Thibonnier A. Arteriovenous fistulae vs. arteriovenous grafts: a retrospective review of 1,700 consecutive vascular access cases. J Vasc Access. 2008;9(4):231–5.
5. Hong HP, Kim SK. Usefulness of percutaneous intervention with transarterial approach in the salvage of nonmaturing native fistulas status-post transvenous approach failure: transarterial approach in the salvage of nonmaturing native fistulas. Cardiovasc Intervent Radiol. 2009;32(6):1252–6. Epub 2009 Jul 31.
6. Escobar C, Blanes I, Ruiz A, Vinuesa D, Montero M, Rodríguez M, Barbera G, Manzano L. Prevalence and clinical profile and management of peripheral arterial disease in elderly patients with diabetes. Eur J Intern Med. 2011;22(3):275–81. Epub 2011 Mar 15.
7. Asif A, Gadalean FN, Merrill D, et al. Inflow stenosis in arteriovenous fistulas and grafts: a multicenter, prospective study. Kidney Int. 2005;67:1986–92.
8. Rattanasompattikul M, Chanchairujira K, On-Ajyooth L, Chanchairujira T. Evaluation of atherosclerosis, arterial stiffness and related risk factors in chronic hemodialysis patients in Siriraj Hospital. J Med Assoc Thai. 2011;94 Suppl 1:S117–24.
9. Puntmann VO, Bigalke B, Nagel E. Characterization of the inflammatory phenotype in atherosclerosis may contribute to the development of new therapeutic and preventative interventions. Trends Cardiovasc Med. 2010;20(5):176–81.
10. Swaminathan S, Shah SV. Novel inflammatory mechanisms of accelerated atherosclerosis in kidney disease. Kidney Int. 2011;80:453–63.
11. Tessitore N, Bedogna V, Melilli E, Millardi D, Mansueto G, Lipari G, Mantovani W, Baggio E, Poli A, Lupo A. In search of an optimal bedside screening program for arteriovenous fistula stenosis. Clin J Am Soc Nephrol. 2011;6:819–26.
12. Grogan J, Castilla M, Lozanski L, Griffin A, Loth F, Bassiouny H. Frequency of critical stenosis in primary arteriovenous fistulae before hemodialysis access: should duplex ultrasound surveillance be the standard of care? J Vasc Surg. 2005;41:1000–6.
13. Marin D, Nelson RC, Schindera ST, Richard S, Youngblood RS, Yoshizumi TT, Samei E. Low-tube-voltage, high-tube-current multidetector abdominal CT: improved image quality and decreased radiation dose with adaptive statistical iterative reconstruction algorithm–initial clinical experience. Radiology. 2010;254(1):145–53.

14. Coelman C, Duijm LEM, Liem YS, et al. Stenosis detection in failing hemodialysis access fistulas and grafts: comparison of color Doppler ultrasonography, contrast-enhance magnetic resonance angiography and digital subtraction angiography. J Vasc Surg. 2005;42:739–46.

15. Khan FA, Vesely TM. Arterial problems associated with dysfunctional hemodialysis grafts: evaluation of patients at high risk for arterial disease. J Vasc Interv Radiol. 2002;13(1109–1114):12.

16. Kanterman RY, Vesely TM, Pilgram TK, et al. Dialysis access grafts: anatomic location of venous stenosis and results of angioplasty. Radiology. 1995;195:135–9.

17. Duijm LE, Liem YS, van der Rijt RH, Nobrega FJ, van den Bosch HC, Douwes-Draaijer P, Cuypers PW, Tielbeek AV. Inflow stenosis in dysfunctional hemodialysis access fistulae and grafts. Am J Kidney Dis. 2006;48(1):98–105.

18. Duijm LEM, van der Rijt RHH, Cuypers PWM, et al. Outpatient treatment of arterial inflow stenoses of dysfunctional hemodialysis access fistulas by retrograde venous access puncture and catheterization. J Vasc Surg. 2008;47:591–8.

19. Guerra A, Raynaud A, Beyssen B, et al. Arterial percutaneous angioplasty in upper limbs with vascular access device for haemodialysis. Nephrol Dial Transplant. 2002;17:843–51.

20. Yevzlin AS, Asif A. Arterial stenoses in patients with arteriovenous dialysis access. US Nephrology 2.

21. Duijm LE, Overbosch EH, Liem YS, et al. Retrograde catheterization of haemodialysis fistulae and grafts: angiographic depiction of the entire vascular access tree and stenosis treatment. Nephrol Dial Transplant. 2009;24:539–47.

22. Shemesh D, Goldin I, Zaghal I, Berlowitz D, Raveh D, Olsha O. Angioplasty with stent graft versus bare stent for recurrent cephalic arch stenosis in autogenous arteriovenous access for hemodialysis: a prospective randomized clinical trial. J Vasc Surg. 2008;48(6):1524–31, 1531.e1–2. Epub 2008 Oct 1.

23. Beathard GA. Angioplasty for arteriovenous grafts and fistulae. Semin Nephrol. 2002;22:202–10.

24. Chan MR, Chhokar VS, Young HN, et al. Retrograde occlusive arteriography of hemodialysis access: failure to detect inflow lesions? Semin Dial. 2010;24:452–5.

Approach to the Patient with Suspected Renal Artery Stenosis

24

Alexander S. Yevzlin and Micah R. Chan

24.1 Introduction

Atherosclerosis is the underlying mechanism of 90 % of all renal artery stenosis (RAS) [1]. In the Cardiovascular Health Study (CHS), the prevalence of significant RAS was detected by renal duplex sonography in 6.8 % of subjects [2–4]. Renovascular disease was independently associated with age, hyperlipidemia, and hypertension. In a series of nearly 4,000 patients undergoing coronary angiography, aortography demonstrated ≥75 % renal artery stenosis in 4.8 % of patients [5]. In 3.7 % of patients, the renal arteries were affected bilaterally [6]. In patients with aortic aneurysms, aorto-occlusive or lower-extremity occlusive disease greater than 50 % stenosis was present in more than 30 % of patients [7]. The increased prevalence of RAS in patients with coronary or peripheral arterial disease reflects the systemic nature of atherosclerosis and the overlapping existence of the disease in multiple vascular beds.

Atherosclerotic RAS is a progressive disease. In a series of 295 kidneys followed by renal artery duplex scans, the 3-year cumulative incidence of renal artery disease progression stratified by initial degree of stenosis was 18, 29, and 49 % for renal artery classified as normal, with <60 % stenosis and with ≥60 % stenosis, respectively [8]. In this study, there were nine occlusions, which occurred in patients who had ≥60 % stenosis at the time of initial evaluation. Schreiber et al., however, have reported progression to total occlusion in 39 % of patients with ≥75 % stenosis at renal arteriography [7]. In the Dutch Renal Artery Stenosis Intervention Cooperative study, a randomized trial of medical therapy versus balloon angioplasty for the treatment of hypertension in RAS patients, progression to complete occlusion occurred in 16 % of patients treated medically [9, 10].

24.2 Ischemic Nephropathy

The term *ischemic nephropathy* refers to the deterioration of renal function that is thought to occur as a result of renovascular disease and which may lead to ESRD in 14–20 % of affected patients [11, 12]. The nature of ischemic nephropathy is complex and multifactorial. As the main function of the kidney is filtration, renal blood flow is among the highest of all organs, and only 10 % is necessary for this organ's metabolic needs [13]. Furthermore, the kidney is capable of autoregulating blood flow in the presence of renal artery stenosis of up to 75 % diameter reduction, and in conditions of impaired perfusion, oxygen delivery can be maintained by the development of collaterals from the adrenal and lumbar arteries [14].

Proposed pathways activated in chronic renal hypoperfusion and which can lead to parenchymal injury and interstitial fibrosis involve the complex and interrelated effects of angiotensin II, nitric oxide, endothelin, vasodilating and vasoconstrictive prostaglandins, and a variety of cytokines [15]. Angiotensin II maintains glomerular filtration pressure and GFR by constricting the efferent arterioles, but its effects in the kidney also include local inflammatory responses, cell hypertrophy, and hyperplasia, which are mostly mediated by AT1 receptors [15]. Other angiotensin II effects also include vascular smooth muscle proliferation, mesangial cell growth, platelet aggregation, activation of adhesion molecules and macrophages, induction of gene transcription for proto-oncogenes, and oxidation of low-density lipoproteins [16, 17].

A.S. Yevzlin, MD (✉)
Division of Nephrology,
Department of Medicine (CHS),
University of Wisconsin,
Madison, WI 53705, USA
e-mail: asy@medicine.wisc.edu

M.R. Chan
Division of Nephrology, Department of Medicine,
University of Wisconsin College of Medicine and Public Health,
Madison, WI, USA

A.S. Yevzlin et al. (eds.), *Interventional Nephrology*,
DOI 10.1007/978-1-4614-8803-3_24, © Springer Science+Business Media New York 2014

These and other mechanisms, such as the generation of free oxygen radicals, interact with each other, eventually resulting in renal scarring even in the absence of "true" renal ischemia [18]. The complexity and variability of these interactions in different individuals are another factor that makes predictions on the recovery of kidney function after revascularization difficult and explains why patients with impaired renal function before revascularization may have no significant increase in their GFR after percutaneous or surgical interventions [19, 20].

Since hypertension associated with RAS is mediated by renal parenchymal ischemia and subsequent activation of the renin-angiotensin-aldosterone axis, hypertension in the setting of RAS may be thought of as a form of ischemic nephropathy. For the remainder of the chapter, we will use the term ischemic nephropathy to mean either a deterioration of renal function in the setting of RAS or severe hypertension in the setting of RAS, or both.

24.3 Defining the Controversy

The impact of RAS and resulting ischemic nephropathy on kidney function has been well described. Based on several recent randomized, multicenter trials that revealed limitations to the utility of nonselective renal artery intervention, the general nephrology community has recently taken a conservative stance on this disease state. This conservative position is largely a reaction to the inappropriate overutilization of what has come to be known as the "drive-by angiogram" by interventional specialists. A recent report from the California Technology Assessment Forum (CTAF) entitled "Renal Artery Stents for the Treatment of Hypertension" attempts to evaluate the literature for RAS intervention in terms of pre-defined criteria and to articulate a recommendation. The paper concludes:

> Renal artery stenting is widely used, although the evidence supporting its use is limited. Observational studies have shown that stenting can reduce blood pressure and can improve renal function. However, in randomized trials that have compared renal artery stenting with medical therapy, renal artery stenting was not associated with an improvement in clinical outcomes, and there were significant associated complications. It is recommended that renal artery stenting for severe hypertension does not meet CTAF criteria 4 or 5 for safety, efficacy and improvement in health outcomes.

The interaction of the atherosclerotic lesion and the putatively consequent ischemic nephropathy is complex and multifactorial [21]. As a result, a renal artery lesion does not categorically imply ischemic nephropathy (There may be physiologic compensation from other blood flow sources.). Likewise, ischemic nephropathy does not necessarily entail renal artery stenosis. The etiology of ischemia may be small-vessel disease. It is for this reason that the "drive-by angiogram" is not effective and should be discouraged.

As the CTAF report suggests, several recent prospective, randomized, multicenter studies have failed to show improvement in outcomes related to RAS following an intervention compared to medical therapy [22]. In the Stent Placement in Patients With Atherosclerotic Renal Artery Stenosis and Impaired Renal Function (STAR) trial [23], 140 patients with eGFR <80 ml showed no clear effect on progression of impaired renal function after intervention but led to a small number of significant procedure-related complications. Similarly, in the Angioplasty and Stenting for Renal Artery Lesions (ASTRAL) trial [24], the change in renal function over time as assessed by the mean slope of the reciprocal of the serum creatinine showed no evidence of a change in chronic kidney disease course after revascularization. Finally, the Dutch Renal Artery Stenosis Intervention Cooperative (DRASTIC) trial [8], consisting of more than 100 patients, showed no significant advantage of angioplasty over medical therapy.

There are several fundamental limitations associated with these clinical trials. For instance, in the ASTRAL trial, patients were enrolled based on physician's discretion and perhaps suffered from selection bias. In this context, patients who were thought to benefit from angioplasty (based on their physician's opinion) were excluded from the study. In the presence of this confounding factor, it might be difficult to conclusively establish the role of angioplasty or medical therapy in the management of RAS. An additional recognized drawback of clinical treatment trials is the intermixture of high-risk and low-risk patients into the "average" of the entire cohort. A possible explanation for the findings of the STAR, ASTRAL, and DRASTIC trials is that these studies included patients who had a minimal chance to improve. Quite simply, if you intervene on RAS that is not causing ischemia, then there is unlikely to be benefit from the intervention. Similarly, if there is another reason for the chronic kidney disease besides RAS, then fixing the RAS will not improve the ischemic process. An ongoing trial, CORAL [25], has been slow to enroll largely because of the pervasive belief by the referring community (general nephrologists) that RAS intervention is, at best, not beneficial and, at worst, unsafe.

Are we, as nephrologists, justified in the belief that RAS intervention should no longer be offered to our patients as a therapeutic option? The key to the management of RAS is to identify patients who are most likely to benefit from intervention. Good medical practice is to then intervene only on those that meet the supposed intervention criteria. But how is this to be done? Unfortunately, prior efforts to identify predictive factors that could differentiate between responders and non-responders to RAS intervention using several functional and imaging techniques have been disappointing. None of the previously investigated techniques could individually fulfill a satisfactory role as an outcome predictor.

Nevertheless, there are a few studies that can guide patient selection. Pre-intervention GFR, initial size of the treated kidney, vascular resistive index, and patient age have all been shown in separate studies to predict outcomes, although no single test is adequate individually [26, 27]. None of the studies evaluated in the CTAF report attempted to evaluate the potential of end-organ recovery after RAS intervention.

24.4 Approach to Diagnosis and Intervention

Rather than rejecting RAS intervention out of hand based on the aforementioned, flawed studies, we recommend assessing the probability of each patient with known RAS to benefit from intervention. A recent observational study by Hegde et al. [28] witnessed improvement in renal function in 10 % and stabilization in 60 % of the subjects. Estimated glomerular filtration rate (eGFR) improved significantly in bilateral RAS, and eGFR improved or stabilized in 75.5–81 % of the subjects. The authors noted a >90 % technical success rate.

Figure 24.1 presents a diagnostic algorithm that attempts to identify whether a patient, based on known epidemiologic and diagnostic data, is likely to benefit from intervention [29]. The data used in the algorithm includes the stage of CKD, kidney size, age, and resistive indices as a measure of small-vessel disease. Using this algorithm, Yevzlin et al. report

excellent patient outcomes, though in a small set of patients. This selective approach to RAS leads to a rejection of the vast majority of all those patients that are referred for intervention as unlikely to benefit; only 10 % of the patients referred in the above report went on to receive an intervention [29].

24.5 Diagnostic Angiography

Once a patient is judged to be a likely candidate to benefit from intervention, angiogram is scheduled. Contrast angiography remains the gold standard for diagnosis and the assessment of the severity of both atherosclerotic and fibrodysplastic RAS. The value of this diagnostic modality has been buoyed by the recently described association of nephrogenic systemic fibrosis (NSF) with magnetic resonance contrast agents, such as are required for MR angiography [30]. Angiography, further, allows evaluation of the abdominal aorta, renal arteries and branch vessels, the presence of accessory renal arteries, as well as cortical blood flow and renal dimensions. Moreover, pressure gradients across a renal artery stenosis can be obtained to evaluate its hemodynamic significance. Digital subtraction angiography (DSA) has become available in many institutions, and although its resolution is inferior to film, it permits the use of lower concentrations of iodinated contrast as well as of alternative contrast agents such as CO_2 [31].

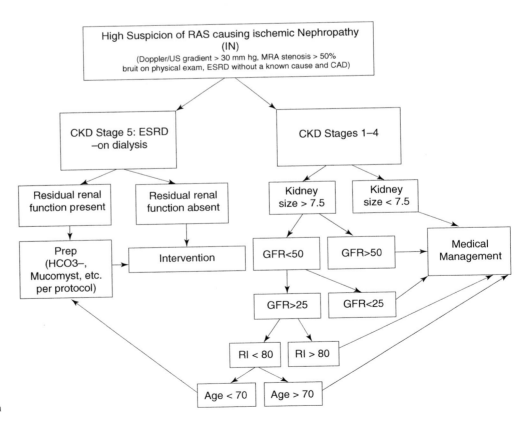

Fig. 24.1 RAS algorithm for patient selection for intervention

Typically, an abdominal aortogram is performed prior to selective catheterization of the renal artery, usually positioning a pigtail catheter at the lower edge of the first lumbar vertebra and power injecting 15–20 ml of dye at 20 ml/s. The abdominal aortogram will provide information regarding the aorta itself, the position of the renal arteries, and the presence of accessory arteries as well as of aortic or renal artery calcification. In most instances, the aortogram provides adequate visualization of the renal arteries, but if optimal imaging or pressure gradient measurement are needed, selective catheterization becomes necessary. This can be achieved with a variety of different 4–6 F diagnostic catheters. Whatever catheter shape is used, the goal is to achieve selective cannulation of the renal artery without excessive catheter manipulation, especially when evaluating atherosclerotic RAS, as aortic atheromas are often adjacent or contiguous to the renal artery lesion and distal embolization can occur. In visualizing the renal arteries, it is important to recognize that they originate posteriorly from the aorta; therefore, it may be necessary to obtain ipsilateral oblique projections (15–30°) to optimally outline the ostium and the proximal segments of the vessels. Furthermore, angiography should be performed long enough to image the renal cortex and assess renal size and perfusion [32].

24.6 Intervention

Percutaneous therapy for renovascular disease has largely supplanted surgery; it is associated with a lower incidence of adverse events, equivalent outcome in terms of hypertension control, and lower cost compared to surgery [33–35]. The first description of balloon angioplasty for renovascular disease was provided by Gruntzig et al. in 1978 [36]. Balloon angioplasty remains the treatment of choice in patients with uncontrolled hypertension and renovascular disease secondary to fibromuscular dysplasia [37].

Stenting has largely supplanted balloon angioplasty in the catheter-based treatment of renovascular disease. A randomized trial of stenting versus balloon angioplasty in 84 patients with ostial renovascular disease demonstrated improved procedural success and patency rates with stenting; however, there were no significant differences in HTN control or improvement in renal function [38]. Two meta-analyses have analyzed the success and durability of renal artery stenting [39]. Initial angiographic success rates were significantly improved compared to balloon angioplasty at 96–100 % with no significant difference in complication rates. The ability of renal artery stenting to improve blood pressure control and renal function has been studied in multiple series. A meta-analysis demonstrated an overall HTN cure rate of 20 % and improved HTN control in 49 % and improvement in renal function in 30 % with stabilization of renal function in 38 %

of patients [40]. With similar complication rates and improved initial and long-term angiographic success, it is safe to say that renal artery stenting is the percutaneous treatment of choice in patients with renal artery stenosis.

Although not necessarily true in the past, modern procedural techniques for percutaneous renal intervention utilize much the same equipment as coronary interventions. The choice of guide catheter is determined by the angle with which the renal artery arises off the aorta. Most commonly, retrograde access via the femoral artery is used. A very sharp caudal angle of origin of the renal artery may, however, require an antegrade approach using the radial or brachial arteries to achieve optimal guide-catheter engagement. Interventions are usually performed using a 6- or 7-French system with commonly used guide catheters with shapes such as the Judkins-Right series, the "renal standard curve," "renal double curve," and "hockey stick." Engagement of the guide catheter can be performed directly or using a telescoping technique.

High-grade ostial lesions with concomitant aortic plaque can increase the risk for atheroembolism. The recently proposed "no-touch" technique attempts to minimize trauma to the vessel ostium, at least theoretically lessening the risk of atheroembolism to the renal parenchyma [41]. With this technique, a 0.035-in. "J-tip" guidewire is advanced just past the guide-catheter tip, to lean against the abdominal aorta above the renal artery, thus keeping the catheter away from the aortic wall. Once the guide catheter is directed toward the ostium of the renal artery, visualization of the renal artery is

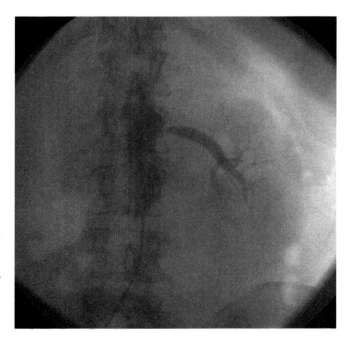

Fig. 24.2 Catheter-directed renal angiogram revealing severe left ostial renal artery lesion

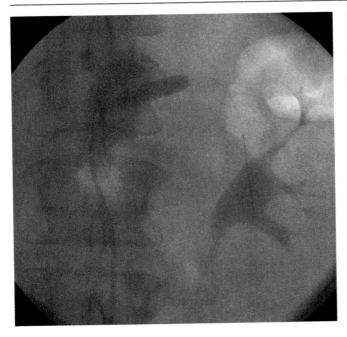

Fig. 24.3 Angioplasty balloon-expandable stent deployment in ostial left renal artery lesion

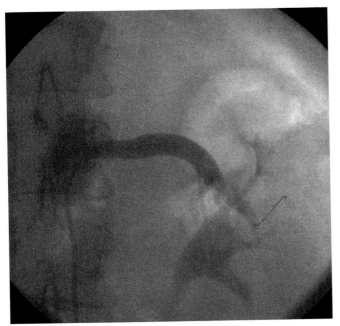

Fig. 24.4 Post-intervention directed renal angiogram revealing no residual stenosis

obtained by subselective injection of contrast (Fig. 24.2); a 0.014-in. guidewire is navigated past the target lesion into the distal renal vessel. The 0.035-in. guidewire is then withdrawn from the catheter, allowing it to gently slide into or adjacent to the ostium of the renal artery over the 0.014-in. wire. Predilatation of the target lesion is especially recommended

in aorto-ostial atherosclerotic lesions and is typically performed with a balloon approximately 1 mm less than the measured diameter of the vessel.

The two balloon-expandable stents specifically approved by the FDA for use in failed renal angioplasty are the Palmaz stent (Cordis Corp., Miami Lakes, FL) and the Double Strut stent (Medtronic Corp., Santa Rosa, CA), but the most frequently used stents have been approved for biliary tree interventions (Fig. 24.3). In ostial lesions, after the stent is deployed, its proximal portion can be "flared" with a slightly oversized balloon protruding into the aorta. Stent placement should be confirmed with post-intervention angiography (Fig. 24.4). Careful attention to contrast dye load is required, especially in patients at high risk for contrast nephropathy. As mentioned above, CO_2 can be used as alternative contrast agents at least during some parts of the intervention.

Adjuvant pharmacology before and after renal artery percutaneous intervention has not been systematically studied. Heparin to maintain an ACT of 250–300 s is frequently used as the anticoagulant of choice during interventional procedures; most interventionists are quite familiar with its use, and it can be easily reversed with protamine. Patients are usually pretreated with aspirin, which is continued indefinitely. The use of clopidogrel seems theoretically necessary following percutaneous intervention; however, there are no controlled studies exploring its use in the renal artery. Other possible intra-procedural anticoagulants, such as glycoprotein 2B3A receptor antagonists and direct thrombin inhibitors such as bivalirudin, have not been formally studied in renal interventions.

Conclusion

There remains a great variability in response in blood pressure control and/or kidney function with percutaneous RAS intervention. Patient selection to determine those who will benefit the most from renal revascularization is the key to correct management of this complex disease state.

References

1. Safian RD, Textor SC. Renal-artery stenosis. N Engl J Med. 2001;344:431–42.
2. Hansen KJ, Edwards MS, Craven TE, Cherr G, Jackson S, Appel R, Burke G, Dean R. Prevalence of renovascular disease in the elderly: a population-based study. J Vasc Surg. 2002;36:443–51.
3. Conlon PJ, Little MA, Pieper K, Mark DB. Severity of renal vascular disease predicts mortality in patients undergoing coronary angiography. Kidney Int. 2001;60:1490–7.
4. Rihal CS, Textor SC, Breen JF, McKusick MA, Grill DE, Hallett JW, Holmes DR. Incidental renal artery stenosis among a prospective cohort of hypertensive patients undergoing coronary angiography. Mayo Clin Proc. 2002;77:309–16.

5. Olin JW, Melia M, Young JR, Graor RA, Risius B. Prevalence of atherosclerotic renal artery stenosis in patients with atherosclerosis elsewhere. Am J Med. 1990;88:46N–51N.

6. Caps MT, Perissinotto C, Zierler RE, Polissar NL, Bergelin RO, Tullis MJ, Cantwell-Gab K, Davidson RC, Strandness Jr DE. Prospective study of atherosclerotic disease progression in the renal artery. Circulation. 1998;98:2866–72.

7. Schreiber MJ, Pohl MA, Novick AC. The natural history of atherosclerotic and fibrous renal artery disease. Urol Clin North Am. 1984;11(3):383–392.

8. Van Jaarsveld BC, Krijnen P, Pieterman H, Derkx FH, Deinum J, Postma CT. The effect of balloon angioplasty on hypertension in atherosclerotic renal-artery stenosis. Dutch Renal Artery Stenosis Intervention Cooperative Study Group. N Engl J Med. 2000;342:1007–14.

9. Dean RH, Kieffer RW, Smith BM, Oates JA, Nadeau JHJ, Hollifield JU, DuPont WD. Renovascular hypertension: anatomic and renal function changes during drug therapy. Arch Surg. 1981;116:1408–15.

10. Scoble JE, Maher ER, Hamilton G, Dick R, Sweny P, Moorhead JF. Atherosclerotic renovascular disease causing renal impairment—a case for treatment. Clin Nephrol. 1989;31:119–22.

11. Simon P, Benarbia S, Charasse C, Stanescu C, Boulahrouz R, Le Cacheux P, Ang KS, Ramée MP. Ischemic renal diseases have become the most frequent causes of end stage renal disease in the elderly. Arch Mal Coeur Vaiss. 1998;91:1065–8.

12. Epstein FH. Oxygen and renal metabolism. Kidney Int. 1997;51:381–5.

13. Yune HY, Klatte EC. Collateral circulation to an ischemic kidney. Radiology. 1976;119:539–46.

14. Kontogiannis J, Burns KD. Role of AT1 angiotensin II receptors in renal ischemic injury. Am J Physiol. 1998;274(1 Pt 2):F79–90.

15. Lerman L, Textor SC. Pathophysiology of ischemic nephropathy. Urol Clin North Am. 2001;28:793–803, ix.

16. Matsusaka T, Hymes J, Ichikawa I. Angiotensin in progressive renal diseases: theory and practice. J Am Soc Nephrol. 1996;7:2025–43.

17. Lerman LO, Nath KA, Rodriguez-Porcel M, Krier JD, Schwartz RS, Napoli C. Increased oxidative stress in experimental renovascular hypertension. Hypertension. 2001;37(2 Part 2):541–6.

18. Garovic VD, Textor SC. Renovascular hypertension and ischemic nephropathy. Circulation. 2005;112:1362–74.

19. Sadowski EA, Bennett LK, Chan MR, Wentland AL, Garrett AL, Garrett RW, Djamali A. Nephrogenic systemic fibrosis: risk factors and incidence estimation. Radiology. 2007;243:148–57. Epub 2007 Jan 31.

20. Textor SC, Wilcox CS. Renal artery stenosis: a common, treatable cause of renal failure? Annu Rev Med. 2001;52:421–42.

21. Yevzlin AS, Schoenkerman AB, Gimelli G, Asif A. Arterial interventions in arteriovenous access and chronic kidney disease: a role for interventional nephrologists. Semin Dial. 2009;22:545–56.

22. Hegde U, Rajapurkar M, Gang S, Khanapet M, Durugkar S, Gohel K, Aghor N, Ganju A, Dabhi M. Fifteen years experience of treating atherosclerotic renal artery stenosis by interventional nephrologists in India. Semin Dial. 2012;25:97–104.

23. Bax L, Woittiez AJ, Kouwenberg HJ, Mali WP, Buskens E, Beek FJ, Braam B, Huysmans FT, Schultze Kool LJ, Rutten MJ, Doorenbos CJ, Aarts JC, Rabelink TJ, Plouin PF, Raynaud A, van Montfrans GA, Reekers JA, van den Meiracker AH, Pattynama PM, van de Ven PJ, Vroegindeweij D, Kroon AA, de Haan MW, Postma CT, Beutler JJ. Stent placement in patients with atherosclerotic renal artery stenosis and impaired renal function: a randomized trial. Ann Intern Med. 2009;150(12):840–8, W150–1.

24. The ASTRAL, Investigators T. Revascularization versus medical therapy for renal-artery stenosis. N Engl J Med. 2009;361:1953–62.

25. Cooper CJ, Murphy TP, Matsumoto A, et al. Stent revascularization for the prevention of cardiovascular and renal events among patients with renal artery stenosis and systolic hypertension: rationale and design of the CORAL trial. Am Heart J. 2006;152:59–66.

26. Zeller T, Muller C, Frank U, Burgelin K, Horn B, Schwarzwalder U, Cook-Bruns N, Neumann FJ. Stent angioplasty of severe atherosclerotic ostial renal artery stenosis in patients with diabetes mellitus and nephrosclerosis. Catheter Cardiovasc Interv. 2003;58:510–5.

27. Radermacher J, Chavan A, Bleck J, Vitzthum A, Stoess B, Gebel MJ, Galanski M, Koch KM, Haller H. Use of Doppler ultrasonography to predict the outcome of therapy for renal artery stenosis. N Engl J Med. 2001;344:410–7. Krijnen P, van Jaarsveld BC, Deinum J, Steyerberg EW, Habbema JD. Which patients with hypertension and atherosclerotic renal artery stenosis benefit from immediate intervention? J Hum Hypertens. 2004;18:91–6.

28. Hegde U, Rajapurkar M, Gang S, Khanapet M, Durugkar S, Gohel K, Aghor N, Ganju A, Dabhi M. Fifteen years experience of treating atherosclerotic renal artery stenosis by interventional nephrologists in India. Semin Dial. 2012;25(1):101–4.

29. Yevzlin AS. Comprehensive renal artery stenosis management by nephrology: a more selective approach. Semin Dial. 2012;25(1):105–7.

30. Fisher JEE, Olin JW. Renal artery stenosis: clinical evaluation. In: Creager MA, Loscalzo J, editors. Vascular medicine: a companion to Braunwald's heart disease. 1st ed. Philadelphia: Saunders/Elsevier; 2006. p. 335–47.

31. Mukherjee D, Bhatt DL, Robbins M, Roffi M, Cho L, Reginelli J, Bajzer C, Navarro F, Yadav JS. Renal artery end-diastolic velocity and renal artery resistance index as predictors of outcome after renal stenting. Am J Cardiol. 2001;88(9):1064–6.

32. Schreier DZ, Weaver FA, Frankhouse J, Papanicolaou G, Shore E, Yellin AE, Harvey F. A prospective study of carbon dioxide-digital subtraction vs standard contrast arteriography in the evaluation of the renal arteries. Arch Surg. 1996;131:503–7; discussion 507–8.

33. Weibull H, Bergqvist D, Bergentz SE, Jonsson K, Hulthen L, Manhem P. Percutaneous transluminal renal angioplasty versus surgical reconstruction of atherosclerotic renal artery stenosis: a prospective randomized study. J Vasc Surg. 1993;18:841–50; discussion 850–2.

34. Xue F, Bettmann MA, Langdon DR, Wivell WA. Outcome and cost comparison of percutaneous transluminal renal angioplasty, renal arterial stent placement, and renal arterial bypass grafting. Radiology. 1999;212:378–84.

35. Bettmann MA, Dake MD, Hopkins LN, Katzen BT, White CJ, Eisenhauer AC, Pearce WH, Rosenfield KA, Smalling RW, Sos TA, Venbrux AC. Atherosclerotic vascular disease conference: Writing Group VI: revascularization. Circulation. 2004;109:2643–50.

36. Gruntzig A, Kuhlmann U, Vetter W, Lutolf U, Meier B, Siegenthaler W. Treatment of renovascular hypertension with percutaneous transluminal dilatation of a renal-artery stenosis. Lancet. 1978;1: 801–2.

37. Tegtmeyer CJ, Elson J, Glass TA, Ayers CR, Chevalier RL, Wellons Jr HA, Studdard Jr WE. Percutaneous transluminal angioplasty: the treatment of choice for renovascular hypertension due to fibromuscular dysplasia. Radiology. 1982;143:631–7.

38. Van De Ven PJ, Kaatee R, Beutler JJ, Kaatee R, Beek FJ, Mali WP, Koomans HA. Arterial stenting and balloon angioplasty in ostial atherosclerotic renovascular disease: a randomised trial. Lancet. 1999;353:282–6.

39. Leertouwer TC, Gussenhoven EJ, Bosch JL, Van Jaarsveld BC, Van Dijk LC, Deinum J. Stent placement for renal arterial stenosis: where do we stand? A meta-analysis. Radiology. 2000;216:78–85. Isles CG, Robertson S, Hill D. Management of renovascular disease: a review of renal artery stenting in ten studies. QJM. 1999;92:159–67.

40. Rocha-Singh K, Jaff MR, Rosenfield K. Evaluation of the safety and effectiveness of renal artery stenting after unsuccessful balloon angioplasty: the ASPIRE-2 study. J Am Coll Cardiol. 2005;46: 776–83.

41. Feldman RL, Wargovich TJ, Bittl JA. No-touch technique for reducing aortic wall trauma during renal artery stenting. Catheter Cardiovasc Interv. 1999;46:245–8.

Rajiv Dhamija

25.1 Introduction

Vascular ruptures encountered during vascular access interventions are potentially fatal adverse events. Vascular complications account for 70–75 % of all such procedure-related complications. A majority of these ruptures can be handled effectively by the performing interventionalist in the interventional suite. Appropriately managed perforations and ruptures can avoid escalating further morbidity and mortality.

Vascular ruptures are most often due to cannulation technique and direct endothelium compromise from foreign device placements such as guidewire passage or coil perforation through the vessel wall. Other causes can be angioplasty related or even from forceful vessel manipulation or forceful contrast injection in an otherwise weakened vessel. Proper patient selection including a thorough history and physical examination as well as advanced anatomical and pathophysiological knowledge are vital to prevent and treat vascular ruptures. Patient outcomes after rupture are time dependent and need to be managed urgently.

Management techniques include conventional manual compression, endovascular methods utilizing balloon tamponade, stent placement, and open surgical methods. Skilled performance of endovascular techniques as well as establishing proper procedures and protocols for higher level of care management are vital for quality of care purposes. The availability of technologically advanced equipment, high-quality imaging and medical devices, as well as a well-trained interdisciplinary team help ensure technical success.

25.2 Historical Perspective

The first reported vascular rupture management techniques were described open surgical methods on trauma patients. Open repair techniques such as direct vessel repair, patch placement, interposition graft, and stent revisions were some of the management strategies. Vessel ligation and the use of vascular clamps when indicated were effective.

However, it was also noted that the emergent surgical exposure of certain injuries including axillo-subclavian injuries could cause potential iatrogenic injury to surrounding neurovascular structures, blood loss, and prolonged operative times. In the presence of significant hemorrhage, exposures including paraclavicular approach, or clavicle resection, could compromise the brachial plexus and other proximity nerves as well as damage other structures including the thoracic duct or the underlying pleura. Remote access to these injuries with endovascular techniques can help decrease the morbidity associated with open surgical exposure. In fact, current trauma clinical management combines an endovascular approach with traditional open surgical techniques [1–5].

Endovascular historical experiences for rupture management come from interventional procedures related to cardiology, peripheral vascular disease, and interventional neurology. Early vascular rupture encountered during cardiac catheterization and peripheral vascular interventions most often deals with direct arterial vessel wall rupture. Much literature is also available in arterial models both in vivo and in vitro. Adequate volume replacement, appropriate use of anticoagulation, and an interdisciplinary team approach are some of the outcome findings. Some of the conclusions from these arterial studies are applicable for hemodialysis arteriovenous access vascular rupture management. In addition, arterial rupture models describing hemostasis, flow dynamics, vessel remodeling, as well as the clinical viability of the procedure [6] are similarly encountered amongst the various endovascular procedure disciplines.

R. Dhamija, MD
Division of Nephrology, Rancho Los Amigos National
Rehabilitation Center, Downey, CA, USA

Internal Medicine, Western University of Health Sciences,
Pomona, CA, USA
e-mail: rdhamija@dhs.lacounty.gov

A.S. Yevzlin et al. (eds.), *Interventional Nephrology*,
DOI 10.1007/978-1-4614-8803-3_25, © Springer Science+Business Media New York 2014

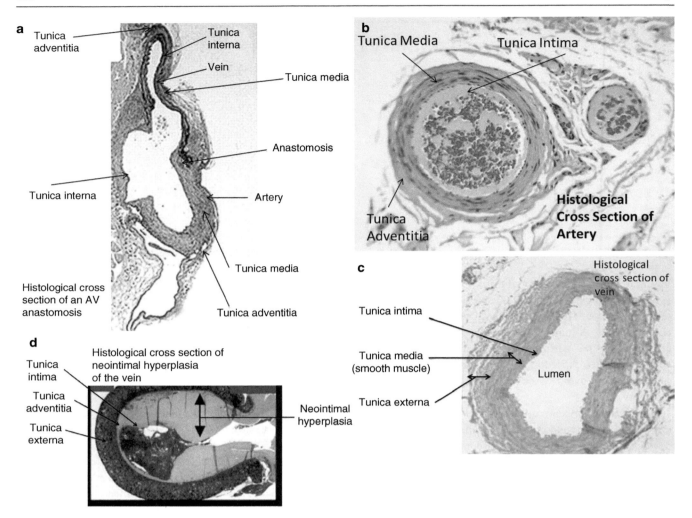

Fig. 25.1 (**a**) Anastomosis histological section including artery and vein segments. (**b**) Histological section of an artery. (**c**) Histological section of a vein. (**d**) Histological cross section of a vein displaying neointimal hyperplasia and compromised lumen size (Images courtesy of Nicholas Hanna and Brian T. Moy)

Table 25.1 Types of complications: ASDIN classification [7]

Type I	Access site hematoma
Type II	Vascular rupture
Type III	Arterial complications
Type IV	Stent-related complications
Type V	Catheter insertion complications
Type VI	Adverse reactions to medications
Type VII	Oxygen saturation and apnea
Type VIII	Hypotension/hypertension
Type IX	Cardiac arrhythmia
Type X	General clinical status

In hemodialysis vascular access procedures, many times the cannulation site as well as the target vessel to be intervened upon is of venous origin. Although arterial ruptures can also be encountered, the biophysical profiles of the artery, juxta-anastomotic region, as well as venous outflow and central veins need to be separately considered for optimal clinical management (Fig. 25.1a–c). For example, the histological stenotic lesion which is targeted for intervention differs in the type of vessel being intervened upon. Arterial stenotic lesions may be due to atheromatous plaque rupture. Vulnerable sites for such arterial rupture include plaque dissection in those areas where there is a transition from atheromatous plaque to normal vessel and the transition between calcified and noncalcified areas. However, the hemodialysis access stenotic lesion may be due to neointimal hyperplasia commonly seen in the venous juxta-anastomotic region as well as in the venous outflow vessels (Fig. 25.1d). The types of complications encountered as well as the classification of grades of vascular rupture and their clinical management are described in regard to hemodialysis access interventions (Tables 25.1 and 25.2) [7–9].

Table 25.2 Grades of vascular rupture requiring therapy [7]

Grade 1	Nominal therapy
	Localized extravasation
	Stable hematoma—no alteration in blood flow through vascular access
Grade 2	Minimal therapy
	Hemorrhage controlled by balloon tamponade
	Hemorrhage controlled by stent/graft insertion
	Hematoma causing reduction in blood flow
Grade 3	Major therapy
	Persistent hemorrhage requiring surgery, blood transfusion
	Unstable expanding hematoma
	Thrombosis of vascular access (spontaneous or intentional)
	Hospitalization for continued observation or therapy
Grade 4	Permanent impairment—loss of limb/function >30 days

25.3 Epidemiology

Currently, there are over 600,000 end-stage renal disease patients in the USA with the majority undergoing renal replacement therapy by hemodialysis [10]. On average, these patients require multiple access-related interventions per year. In general, 70–75 % of all intervention-related complications are due to vascular perforation and rupture [11, 12]. Many of these complications are type I of insignificant clinical correlation. However, there can be associated morbidity and mortality with higher stage (types II and III) vascular rupture reported around 1–14 % in interventional procedures [13]. Arterial or venous rupture can occur at the site of intervention or anywhere along the path back to the access site.

Type I rupture includes micro-perforations of vascular endothelium without clinical sequelae and does not require clinical intervention.

Type II rupture includes those micro- and macro-perforations with evident clinical compromise as well as partial rupture of the vessel requiring clinical intervention including endovascular techniques.

Type III rupture includes those partially or completely ruptured vessels requiring advanced clinical interventions which are not otherwise controlled by endovascular techniques and require higher levels of care and even open surgical management/ligation.

With interventional procedures more often being performed in the elective outpatient setting, rapid recognition and management of vascular rupture is needed. End-stage renal disease patients traditionally have high rates of cardiac morbidity. Coronary artery disease continues to be the leading cause of death in end-stage renal disease patients [10]. Disorders of calcium and phosphate metabolism encountered in advanced renal disease as well as uremia are known cardiovascular risk factors for coronary artery disease and

vascular pathology. Calcium deposition in vasculature is often visible during ultrasound and radiography imaging. Ideally, initial cannulation should be attempted at a readily accessible site with a superficial vessel location whenever possible. Patients in whom access thrill and peripheral pulses are difficult to determine, real-time ultrasound guidance of the vessel to be punctured may be beneficial to avoid perforations and rupture.

Moreover, hemorrhagic complications may be propagated from preexisting medical conditions. Many dialysis patients are already anticoagulated with heparin, Coumadin, and other antiplatelet therapy or are given thrombolytic medications. These medications can increase the incidence of bleeding from intervention-associated vascular ruptures. Cardiac and anesthesia risk stratification as well as sound history and physical including comorbid conditions should be considered. Such conditions may be seen in diabetics, elderly, obese patients, and other subgroups in which access placement may be initially difficult. These patients may then require repeat interventions and potentially associated vascular perforations and rupture. Additionally genetics, race, and/or sex may be contributing factors to a friable vascular anatomy [14].

25.4 Pathophysiology

Vascular interventions require the identification of suitable patients to undergo intervention for a treatable pathology such as stenotic lesions and flow compromising collateral vessels. A successful vascular procedure entails the management of a particular pathology (stenosis, collateral vessels) and then the achievement of hemostasis afterwards. The coagulation cascade plays a vital role in achieving hemostasis (Fig. 25.2a). Likewise, on occasion need for thrombolysis may be encountered when treating embolus and thrombosis (Fig. 25.2b). Patient outcomes after vascular injury are time dependent, and a continued sense of urgency is required in such management.

A thorough understanding of anatomy and histology of vessels is important. The histological and biophysical properties of arteries vary from those found at the arterial inflow versus the surgically created juxta-anastomotic region. Likewise, the biophysical profile of surgically manipulated venous segments found at the juxta-anastomotic region may differ from that found in the native outflow vein and from those veins eventually draining into the large central veins. Potentially the calcified vessels and uremic inflammatory milieu in end-stage renal disease patients may predispose these patients to vascular perforations and ruptures [15].

In general, the caliber of flow directly relates to the potential for serious consequences from vascular rupture. Upper arm accesses tend to have higher blood flows than forearm

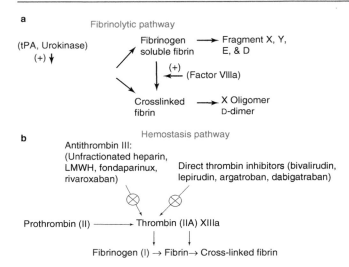

a

Fibrinolytic pathway

(tPA, Urokinase)
(+) ↓

Fibrinogen ⟶ Fragment X, Y,
soluble fibrin   E, & D

(+)
← (Factor VIIIa)

Crosslinked ⟶ X Oligomer
fibrin   D-dimer

b

Hemostasis pathway

Antithrombin III:
(Unfractionated heparin,
LMWH, fondaparinux,   Direct thrombin inhibitors (bivalirudin,
rivaroxaban)   lepirudin, argatroban, dabigatraban)

⊗   ⊗

Prothrombin (II) ⟶ Thrombin (IIA) XIIIa

Fibrinogen (I) → Fibrin→ Cross-linked fibrin

Fig. 25.2 (a) Fibrinolytic Pathway. (b) Hemostasis Pathway (Images courtesy of Brian T. Moy and Nicholas Hanna)

accesses. Therefore, brachial artery ruptures have a potential for greater exsanguination than would a rupture of the distal radial or ulnar arteries. It has also been reported that the location of venous access predisposes to rupture with cephalic arch and transposed upper arm access being more commonly ruptured than forearm arteriovenous access [16]. Also, the incidence of complications is greater during recanalization of total occlusions, compared with the treatment of nonocclusive lesions [17].

When a vascular rupture occurs during intervention, the vascular injury inflammatory cascade and modified response to injury can determine the severity of such complication. Hemorrhage and vascular injury can cause end-organ ischemia of the vascular bed fed by the injured vessel. Factors to consider include complete versus incomplete disruption, the adequacy of collateral blood flow, and the underlying metabolic state. Also, the sensitivity of the end organ to ischemia and the time required to repair the injury will affect tissue viability. Tissue ischemia causes anoxic cell death. Restoration of oxygen-rich blood flow after ischemic injury can produce a reperfusion injury mediated by free radicals and pro-inflammatory mediators. This can further damage the microvasculature and result in increased permeability and edema formation. This in turn can ultimately lead to worsening ischemia, microvascular stasis, and cell lysis. The resultant tissue destruction from this vicious cycle may be fatal.

Arteries have an inherent vasospastic tendency with a large amount of smooth muscle in the intima media. Common vascular rupture etiologies include angioplasty related and guidewire related. Angioplasty with or without cutting balloons may rupture atherosclerotic plaques and can even render the host vessel weakened. Guidewire manipulation may also cause direct endothelial damage or even subintimal pen-

etration leading to vascular perforation or vascular rupture. Imaging catheters and sheaths may inadvertently be advanced over subintimal cannulations further complicating the vascular rupture.

The juxta-anastomotic region in hemodialysis vascular access creation encompasses the 2 cm proximal arterial inflow, the arteriovenous anastomosis, as well as the 2 cm distal venous outflow region. This site may also be prone to vascular rupture when interventions with high-pressure angioplasty inflations are needed for stenosis from neointimal hyperplasia or can be directly damaged from vessel trauma during surgical technique, guidewire manipulations, forceful retrograde contrast injection, or large-bore cannulations often required for upper am and central vein angioplasty or coil/stent placement.

The treatment of neointimal hyperplasia often requires high pressures to inflate the angioplasty balloon completely. These high inflation pressures may directly cause a tear or perforation in the vascular wall. On occasion, vascular ruptures may also result indirectly from bursting of the angioplasty balloon during high pressure dilatations [13].

Percutaneous transluminal angioplasty increases the lumen size by barotrauma with cracking, splitting, and endothelial denudation of stenotic lesions and also affecting the adjacent vessel layers (Fig. 25.1). These alterations in morphology dilate the vessel lumen for blood flow with increased caliber size and flows for hemodialysis. However, the acute traumatic angioplasty process of endothelial and vascular dilation may leave the vessel weakened and damaged with evident perforations or ruptures [11–14].

25.5 Differential Diagnosis

Symptoms of vascular rupture may present with the "Ps" pulselessness, pain, pallor, paralysis, poikilothermia, and paresthesia. Other diagnostic signs include an expanding hematoma felt on physical exam, palpable thrill, audible bruit, or bruising near the ruptured vessel site. Further workup should be documented when clinical signs suggest a suspected rupture. In such circumstances, contrast extravasation seen on imaging studies or Doppler evidence of active hematoma formation or distal lack of perfusion may be evident (Fig. 25.3). Pseudoaneurysm formation and changes in sizing can also be diagnostic signifying vascular rupture and compromised vessel integrity. Peripheral pulses should be compared from one side versus the other. However, rupture may still be suspected because distal pulses can be intact in some cases of proximal vascular injury [14].

In addition to exsanguination and ischemia, the surrounding structures may be compromised from a rapidly expanding enclosed space hematoma formation. Compartment syndrome and nerve impingement are potentially serious

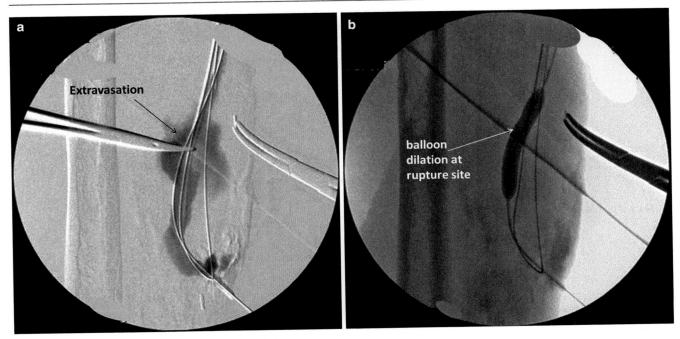

Fig. 25.3 (**a**) Contrast extravasation from rupture site. (**b**) Balloon tamponade at rupture site

adverse outcomes which need to be managed appropriately. Compartment syndrome does not preclude endovascular techniques, but the fact that surgical exposure is necessary diminishes the potential advantages of endovascular management [18].

The skilled interventionalist should consider the commonly encountered causes include the cannulation technique, guidewire vessel perforation, angioplasty-associated vessel perforation, intra-procedural use of anticoagulant/thrombolytic therapy, and large-bore cannulation sheaths with inability to achieve hemostasis post-procedure [19]. Forceful post-angioplasty angiograms have been reported to potentially cause vascular perforation and rupture in otherwise weakened vessel segments [20]. Exposure to high blood flows and pressures may promote vascular rupture after a planned angioplasty intervention for otherwise diseased friable stenotic vascular segments [21]. Successful management by the performing interventionalist using manual and endovascular techniques can successfully tackle a great majority of such vascular rupture complications.

25.6 Clinical Management

Most vascular ruptures encountered during intervention can routinely be managed by the performing interventionalist. Proper patient selection including a thorough history and physical examination as well as advanced anatomical and pathophysiological knowledge are vital to prevent and treat vascular rupture. Cardiac risk stratification should be determined and

considered prior to attempting vascular procedures and also when attempting management of clinically significant vascular ruptures. Stratification of patients may also help determine which treatment algorithm to pursue (Fig. 25.4).

For instance, at times coil embolization and/or proximal vessel balloon dilation may be preferred to thrombose/ligate those ruptured accesses deemed otherwise unsalvageable. In such cases, advanced management techniques to salvage an access may not be required [22] and rapid ligation can be pursued.

The skill of the interventionalist is paramount to prevent vascular ruptures. Good tactile perception as well as using high-quality medical devices and imaging equipment are required. Newer hydrophilic atraumatic guidewires, imaging catheters, micro-introducer sets as well as introducer sheaths should be used. Appropriate catheters and guidewires should be used with preformed angles and shapes to aid in gentle manipulation to the desired target vessels. Proper imaging allows the physician to better perform the procedure and can also help identify complications should they occur. Proper radiographic attenuation utilizing appropriate power, field of vision, as well as digital subtraction angiography and road mapping features may help improve diagnostic and therapeutic interventions [16].

Care should be taken to avoid forceful manipulations of medical devices and also avoid the forceful manipulation of vessels including the surgically created juxta-anastomotic region during interventions. When cannulating an access, good pulsatile blood return and careful guidewire advancement are some methods of rupture prevention.

Treatment algorithms include determining the site and severity of rupture (Fig. 25.4).

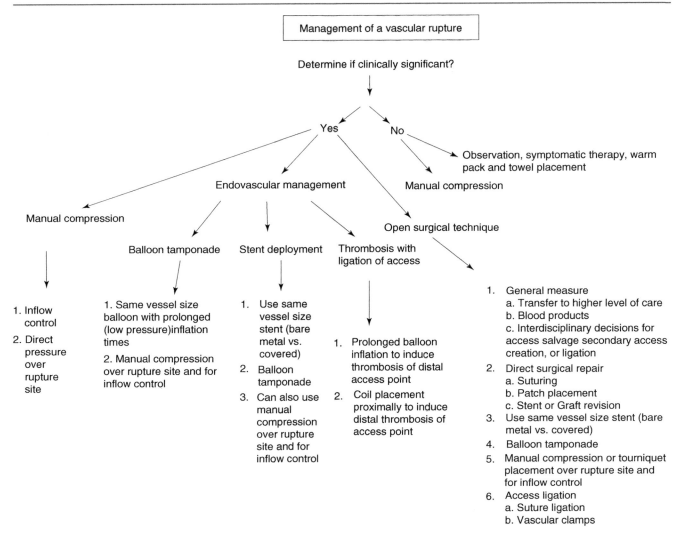

Fig. 25.4 Clinical management flow chart for intervention-related vascular rupture

Type I perforations and ruptures of no clinical significance can be observed or require minimal therapy. Type II ruptures including partial tears of vessels can be managed by manual compression, endovascular techniques, and open surgical methods. Type III ruptures include complicated partial tears as well as complete tears; may not be amenable to endovascular therapy and may require open surgical repair. The complicated type II vascular rupture patients along with type III patients should be quickly identified, and higher level of care as well as surgical support protocols should be activated when appropriate.

25.6.1 Manual Therapy

Manual therapy includes direct manual compression over the rupture site. Use of special dressing materials or pressure dressings may be beneficial adjuvant therapy. Warm compresses as well as dressing using Xeroderm, Vaseline, and other procoagulant therapies over rupture site have been reported as good synergistic therapy along with manual compression. Procoagulant therapy including bandages and sure seal band aids along with manual control of the arterial inflow can also help limit the amount of blood loss and avoid higher pressures within the access. In addition, manual compression directly above the rupture with or without arterial inflow control may help facilitate rapid resolution of the vascular rupture in type I and some type II perforations.

Additional management with tourniquets or manual compression strategically placed to control the inflow to the arteriovenous access may help facilitate a more rapid hemostasis. Inflow control theoretically serves two purposes including limiting the amount of blood loss as well as controlling the high flow pressures in the vascular access to promote platelet plug formation and hemostasis. Other manual techniques to consider are utilizing a figure of eight or purse string suture to help in closure of large-bore cannulations. Additionally, closure devices can be used for similar purposes. Although not commonly utilized in vascular access procedures, anecdotal data from cardiac and peripheral arterial disease management studies is available on closure devices. These devices may be suture mediated or may involve placement of topical hemostatic devices at the arterial puncture site. Time and cost of the procedure are additional variables that may be considered when routinely selecting closure devices [7, 8, 11–13].

25.6.2 Endovascular Management

Endovascular management includes balloon tamponade or stent deployment. The key principle in endovascular management is maintaining guidewire placement across the ruptured vessel (Fig. 25.3a). If guidewire placement is lost, attempted balloon tamponade or stent deployment may potentially enlarge the vascular rupture site or even cause a complete tear to the otherwise compromised vessel. Proper Seldinger technique can maintain guidewire placement across the vascular rupture site.

Balloon-assisted tamponade theoretically helps control rupture by decreasing blood loss as well as by promoting hemostasis. The angioplasty balloon when inflated will prevent high access pressures and high blood flows in proximity to the rupture site. In addition, the inflated angioplasty balloon provides over the guidewire structural integrity to the vessel and lumen [20]. The balloon can also help with direct apposition of the vessel wall and rupture site especially with subintimal dissections, flap dissections, and other perforations. Hemostasis with platelet plug creation can then ensue to control the rupture and commence vascular remodeling.

In general, sizing of venous angioplasty balloons tends to be same or 1 mm larger than the measured venous diameter of the vessel (Fig. 25.3a, b). This type of sizing is commonly employed when performing interventions in the venous juxta-anastomosis as well as venous outflow stenotic lesions. In the arterial segment and the arterial juxta-anastomotic region, sizing of angioplasty balloons should generally be same size or 1 mm undersized balloons. When managing ruptures with balloon expansion, low-pressure inflations approximating the operating pressure of the balloon may facilitate balloon-assisted tamponade. Prolonged inflation times along with manual compression of the inflow vessel may be required in order to achieve effective hemostasis [11, 12].

When an expanding hematoma or contrast extravasation is not completely managed by balloon tamponade, stent deployment can be attempted. Granted stent deployment may require a larger introducer sheath and thus potential for an additional vascular rupture site, risk versus benefit must always be considered. Stents deployed for rupture management are generally of two types: bare metal and covered. When collateral vessels are present, bare metal stents may be preferable to covered stents to avoid jailing those vessels. Covered stents are also effective in the treatment of vascular rupture. Stents can help maintain vessel patency for continued use of the dialysis access.

Stent sizing generally follows that of balloon sizing with same size or slightly enlarged sizing used in the venous outflow and juxta-anastomotic venous segments and same size or slightly smaller stent sizing used in the arterial inflow and juxta-anastomotic arterial segments. Stents may require balloon expansion for deployment. Stent deployment in a region of mobility may preclude this option for other alternative management techniques [7, 8, 11–13, 18, 23–25].

25.6.3 Open Surgical Techniques

When an expanding hematoma does not resolve with endovascular techniques and manual compression, higher levels of care as well as open surgical techniques should be initiated. Protocols and procedures should already be in place to facilitate transfer of the patient to a higher level of care in a monitored setting with the active assistance of surgical backup available. Proper agreements between transferring and receiving institutions and physicians should be established. Placement of large-bore IVs with volume repletion and or blood products may be required. Appropriate laboratory tests should be ordered. Tourniquet placement and or manual compression at the rupture site and inflow may prevent large volume blood loss while in transit. Anticoagulation therapy especially in arterial rupture should be evaluated and implemented when appropriate.

An interdisciplinary team may be required to control morbidity and mortality in unresolved ruptures and type III ruptures. Location of the rupture should also be stratified. Rapid control of hemorrhage, rapid restoration of blood flow to an ischemic vascular bed, and prevention of further injury such as extremity compartment syndrome are the goals of therapy. Those vascular ruptures occurring within the chest bony cavity may lead to hemothorax. This may be seen during central catheter placements or central stenosis endovascular management. In such case, drainage with a chest tube may be required especially when continuous hemorrhage of over 1,500 ml is present or when continuous hemorrhage occurs of over 200 ml for more than 3 h [26]. Although rare, vascular rupture during central catheter placement can lead to cardiac tamponade with the traditional Beck's triad of hypotension, distended neck and muffled heart sounds. Knowledge of anatomical venous segments including superficial versus deep versus perforating veins can help determine appropriate therapy. In regard to the extremity, vascular rupture control with primary amputation protocol scoring may need to be assessed in order for limb salvage.

Specific open surgical techniques include direct vessel repair utilizing suturing, patch placement, and stent and/or graft placement. Indeed open surgical procedure may utilize balloon tamponade therapy and coil embolization or ligature placement to control the inflow and pressure flows to the diseased ruptured segment. Secondary AV fistula or graft creation may also be a viable option at time of rupture repair. Communication between the nephrologist, performing interventionalist as well as vascular surgeon can help guide choice of therapy and determine which accesses to abandon and ligate and which to promote advanced therapies in hope of access salvage ability.

Surgical repairs of vascular injury are generally determined by the damaged vessel circumference percent and defect size. For instance, direct lateral repair might be attempted when the vessel circumference is compromised less than 25 %, and patch angioplasty can be used when less than 50 %. Primary end-to-end anastomosis might be achievable when less than 2 cm defects are present with favorable mobilizing ends that spatulate. When defects are greater than 2 cm, interposition grafts with reversed vein polytetrafluoroethylene are most commonly done. In cases where there is extensive defect, an extra-anatomic bypass repair is possible. In otherwise uncontrolled rupture, suture ligation with consideration for distal embolectomy, anticoagulation, and even prophylactic fasciotomy to prevent compartment syndrome might be indicated [1].

When the access is determined to be unsalvageable or if the vascular rupture is not otherwise controllable with other measures, access ligation may be necessary. Balloon occlusive therapy, manual obstructive therapy, or suture ligations are common techniques used for access ligation.

In such techniques, a proximal area is identified, and sutures can be placed to interrupt flow through the ruptured vascular segment. These situations are not uncommon in patients with recoiling central stenosis and advanced peripheral vascular disease. Care should be taken to preserve perfusion to collateral vessels supplying the distal segment to prevent extending ischemia. Distal extremity Doppler flow and assessment for pulse, pallor, pain, and paresthesia can be observed prior to tying off or ligating the desired vascular segment.

An interdisciplinary approach is of utmost importance in the management of the unstable vascular rupture to prevent further morbidity and mortality. Good follow-up management includes evaluating for post-procedure pulse, pallor, paresthesia, and pain. Patients should be monitored for hemodynamic instability and followed up periodically for hemodynamically significant blood losses [1, 4, 5].

25.7 Outcomes

Successful management of type I and type II ruptures by the interventionalist is reported in the literature above 90 % [11, 12, 27]. The complicated rupture cases encountered during interventional procedures need to be avoided and properly managed when encountered. The incidence of access site complications varies from 1 to 10 %. Clinically evident hematoma occurs in 2–8 % of patients with previously reported rates of incidence range from 0.7 to 4.5 %. Historically, the Standards of Practice Committee of the Society of Cardiovascular and Interventional Radiology (SCVIR), in their Quality Improvement Guidelines for Percutaneous Management of the Thrombosed or Dysfunctional Dialysis Access, recommends a threshold rate of 0.5 % for major complications associated with vascular rupture or perforation. Additionally, the SCVIR Quality Improvement Guidelines suggest threshold rates of 0.5 % for major bleeding, venous rupture, acute respiratory arrest, and death and a threshold of 2 % for arterial emboli [8, 12, 13, 27–31].

In another reported series, venous perforation or rupture occurred during or after the percutaneous treatment of thrombosed or failing hemodialysis accesses in 11 of 1,242 procedures (0.9 %) [24]. Benchmarking and quality care indicators should be promoted across all disciplines to improve the quality of care and promote the practice methods of highly skilled physicians utilizing proper facilities and technologies.

The American Society of Diagnostic Interventional Nephrology (ASDIN) has recently initiated data collection for benchmarking studies (www.ASDIN.org) to promote quality of care improvements.

25.7.1 Newer Gene and Pharmaceutical Management

Gene therapy has the potential to reduce neointimal hyperplasia and also reduce restenosis by targeting the proliferating cells thereby hopefully reducing the number of interventions needed and failed access maturations. The cells found in vessels with neointimal hyperplasia lesions have been genetically traced to originate from the juxta-anastomotic venous vasculature as opposed to arterial or even bone marrow stem cell origination [32]. Pharmaceutical agents including anticoagulant and antiplatelet medications including argatroban and lepirudin and cilostazol as well as thrombolytic therapies will help direct and advance management and research in the field of vascular biology to help improve management options for intervention-related vascular rupture [6, 16, 33].

Conclusion

Vascular rupture encountered during vascular access intervention is a potentially serious adverse event which needs to be managed appropriately to avoid escalating morbidity and mortality. A majority of vascular ruptures encountered during interventions can be handled effectively by the performing interventionalist.

Proper patient selection including a thorough history and physical examination as well as advanced anatomical and pathophysiological knowledge are vital to prevent and treat vascular rupture. Management techniques include conventional manual compression, endovascular methods including balloon tamponade, stent placement, and open surgical techniques. Skilled performance of endovascular techniques as well as establishing proper procedures and protocols for higher level of care assistance when appropriate are vital. The availability of technologically advanced equipment with high-quality medical devices as well as a well-trained interdisciplinary team can help ensure technical success.

References

1. Mulholland MW, Lillemoe KD, Doherty GM, Maier RV, Al E. Greenfield's surgery scientific principles and practice. 5th ed. New York: Lippincott Williams and Wilkins; 2011.
2. Johnson CA. Endovascular management principles in peripheral vascular trauma. Semin Interv Radiol. 2010;27(1):38–44.
3. Saleh HA. Iatrogenic vascular injuries in western Saudi Arabia. Cardiovasc Surg. 1995;3(1):39–41.
4. Moore W. Vascular surgery a comprehensive review. 4th ed. Philadelphia: WB Saunders Company; 1993.
5. Rutherford R. Vascular surgery. 4th ed. Philadelphia: WB Saunders Company; 1995.
6. Werner GS, Ferarri M, Figulla HR. Superficial femoral artery rupture after balloon angioplasty: Treatment with implantation of a balloon expandable endovascular graft. Journal of vascular interventional radiology. 1999;8:1115–7.
7. Vesely T, Beathard G, Ash S, Hoggard J, Schon D. Classification of complications associated with hemodialysis vascular access procedures. Semin Dial. 2007;20(4):359–64.
8. Beathard GA, Litchfield T. Effectiveness and safety of dialysis vascular access procedures performed by interventional nephrologists. Kidney Int. 2004;66:1622–32.
9. Sofocleous CT, Schur I, Koh E, Hinrichs C, Cooper SG, Welber A, Brountzos E, Kelekis D. Percutaneous treatment of complications occurring during hemodialysis graft recanalization. Eur J Radiol. 2003;47:237–46.
10. US Renal Data System. USRDS 2010 annual data report: Atlas of chronic kidney disease and end-stage renal disease in the United States. Bethesda: National Institutes of Health, National Institutes of Diabetes and Digestive and Kidney Diseases; 2010.
11. Beathard GA. Management of complications of endovascular dialysis access procedures. Semin Dial. 2003;16:309–13.
12. Beathard GA. ASDIN core curriculum for interventional nephrology. RMS lifeline training manual for interventional nephrology. 13th ed. Mississippi: ASDIN;2007.
13. Falk A, Towne J, Hollier H. Complications in vascular surgery. 2nd ed. New York: Marcel Dekker; 2004. p. 557–69.
14. Wilson SE. Complications of vascular access procedures: thrombosis, venous hypertension, arterial steal and neuropathy. In: Vascular access principles. New York: Lippincott Williams & Wilkins; 1996. p. 212–25.
15. Chen SM, Hang CL, Yip HK, Fang CY, Wu CJ, Yang CH, Hsieh YK, Guo GB. Outcomes of interventions via a transradial approach for dysfunctional Brescia-Cimino fistulas. Cardiovascular Interventional Radiology. 2009;32:952–9.
16. Zev Noah Kornfield BA. Incidence and management of percutaneous transluminal angioplasty–induced venous rupture in the "fistula first" era. J Vasc Interv Radiol. 2009;20:744–51.
17. Casserly IP, Sachar R, Yadav JS. Manual of peripheral vascular intervention. 1st ed. New York: Lippincott Williams and Wilkins; 2005.
18. Zelenock GB, Huber TS, Messina LM, Lumsden AB, Moneta GL. Mastery of vascular and endovascular surgery: an illustrated review (Mastery of vascular). Philadelphia: Lippincott Williams and Wilkins; 2008.
19. Miyayama S, Matsui O. Occluded Brescia–Cimino hemodialysis fistulas: endovascular treatment with both brachial arterial and venous access using the pull-through technique. Cardiovasc Interv Radiol. 2005;28:806–12.
20. Jacco LG, Steenhuijsen JM. Rupture of the arterial wall causes deflection in pressure. Cathet Cardiovasc Diagn. 1997:92–101.
21. Bunt TJ, Manship L, Moore W. Iatrogenic vascular injury during peripheral vascularization. Journal of vascular surgery. 1985;2:491–8.
22. Raynaud A, Novelli L, Bourquelot P, Stolba J. Low-flow maturation failure of distal accesses: Treatment by angioplasty of forearm arteries. 2009;49(4):995–9.
23. Hemodialysis Adequacy Work Group. Clinical practice guidelines for hemodialysis adequacy, update 2006. Am J Kidney Dis. 2006;48 Suppl 1:S2–90.
24. Bittl JA. Venous rupture during percutaneous treatment of hemodialysis fistulas and grafts. Catheter Cardiovasc Interv. 2009;74:1097–101.
25. Asif A, Agarwal A, Yevzlin A, Wu S, Wu S, Beathard G, et al. Interventional nephrology. New York: McGraw-Hill; 2012.
26. DeVirgilio C. Review of surgery for ABSITE and boards. Philadelphia: Saunders; 2012.
27. Raynaud AC, Angel CY, Sapoval MR, Beyssen B, Pagny JY, Auguste M. Treatment of hemodialysis access rupture during PTA with Wallstent implantation. J Vasc Interv Radiol. 1998;9:437–42.
28. Turmel-Rodrigues L, Pengloan J, Baudin S, et al. Treatment of stenosis and thrombosis in haemodialysis fistulas and grafts by interventional radiology. Nephrol Dial Transplant. 2000;15:2029–36.
29. Vesely TM. Complications related to percutaneous thrombectomy of hemodialysis grafts. J Vasc Access. 2002;3:49–57.
30. Rajan DK, Platzker T, Lok CE, et al. Ultrahigh-pressure versus high-pressure angioplasty for treatment of venous anastomotic stenosis in hemodialysis grafts: is there a difference in patency? J Vasc Interv Radiol. 2007;18:709–14.
31. National Kidney Foundation. Clinical practice guidelines for vascular access. Am J Kidney Dis. 2006;48 Suppl 1:176–247.
32. Skartsis N, et al. Origin of neointimal cells in arteriovenous fistulae: bone marrow, artery, or the vein itself? Semin Dial. 2011;24(2):242–8.
33. Apple S, Lindsay Jr J. Principles and practice of interventional cardiology. 1st ed. Maryland: Lippincott Williams and Wilkins; 2000.

Pulmonary Embolism Associated with Dialysis Access Procedure

Gerald A. Beathard

26.1 Introduction

When an arteriovenous shunt, either a fistula (AVF) or a synthetic graft (AVG) is used and maintained as a dialysis access, recurrent bouts of pulmonary embolism (PE) are possible. These emboli range from those that are small and cause no recognizable immediate effect to those that can have fatal consequences. It is also possible for a pulmonary embolus to occur with a dialysis catheter removal. Although this probably occurs quite frequently, it is difficult to document, and there have been no studies reporting the incidence. However, one may occasional encounter a catheter patient in whom symptoms occur which are suggestive. A massive embolus is unlikely.

26.2 Pulmonary Protective Features

The lungs have two features that allow them to be somewhat resistant to the deleterious effects of a PE: the presence of a double circulation and the existence of a vigorous fibrinolytic system.

26.2.1 Double Circulation

Two separate vascular networks support the lung parenchyma. The primary pulmonary circulation flows forward from the main pulmonary artery, passes throughout the pulmonary interstitium and airways, and reconstitutes itself into pulmonary veins before entering the left atrium. The bronchial circulation, the second system, draws approximately 1 % of the systemic cardiac output and transmits blood at six times the pressure of the pulmonary circulatory system. The bronchial arteries (Fig. 26.1) supply blood to the bronchi and connective tissue of the lungs. They travel and branch with the bronchi, ending at about the level of the respiratory bronchioles [1–3]. These vessels anastomose with branches of the pulmonary arteries, and together, they supply the visceral pleura of the lung. Much of the blood supplied by the bronchial arteries is returned via the pulmonary veins rather than the bronchial veins via several microvascular interconnections [1].

The bronchial circulation responds to decreased pulmonary flow and ischemia with enlargement, hypertrophy, and focal proliferation across mesh-like anastomotic channels [1, 4]. This serves to protect the viability of lung parenchyma in the case of an embolus. Bronchial blood flow has been shown to increase by as much as 300 % in the weeks following pulmonary artery embolization [5].

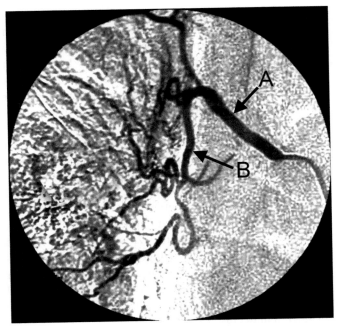

Fig. 26.1 Bronchial artery. (*A*) Intercostobrachial artery. (*B*) Right bronchial artery

G.A. Beathard, MD, PhD, FASN
Department of Internal Medicine,
University of Texas Medical Branch,
Galveston, TX, USA
e-mail: gbeathard@msn.com

A.S. Yevzlin et al. (eds.), *Interventional Nephrology*,
DOI 10.1007/978-1-4614-8803-3_26, © Springer Science+Business Media New York 2014

Despite the protective effect of the bronchial circulation, pulmonary infarction can occur. It is least likely to develop in cases of central pulmonary arterial occlusion, in which massive bronchial collateral flow is easily accommodated by the pulmonary arterial circuit [1, 6–8]. The likelihood of infarction increases when a more distal medium- or small-sized (approximately 3 mm or less) artery is obstructed, and the high-pressure collateral bronchial influx must be accommodated within a smaller intravascular volume. This reperfusion by the bronchial circulation, combined with locally increased vascular permeability due to tissue ischemia and capillary endothelial injury, causes the intra-alveolar extravasation of blood cells. This is generally followed by regression and a return to normal architecture as the blood is absorbed. Localized pulmonary hemorrhage tends to progress to infarction in settings of underlying malignancy, high embolic burden, diminished bronchial flow (due to shock, hypotension, or impaired circulation as in chronic disease), vasodilator use, elevated pulmonary venous pressure, or interstitial edema (typically due to heart failure) [1, 6–10]. Heart failure is generally considered the single most important predisposing condition in the development of pulmonary infarction [7].

26.2.2 Fibrinolysis

Once fresh thrombus forms (or embolizes), it is cleared from the vascular structure, at least to some degree, by endogenous thrombolysis. This is initiated by plasminogen being converted by plasminogen activators to plasmin, an enzyme that degrades the fibrin within the clot resulting in its dissolution. This process appears to occur more rapidly in the lungs than in other areas, presumably because of a higher blood flow in pulmonary arteries that exposes thrombi to more plasminogen and, possibly, a greater thrombolytic capacity of pulmonary arteries than peripheral veins [11].

Urokinase is the primary endogenous plasminogen activator active in this situation. Evidence indicates that the normal bronchoalveolar surface is functionally saturated with urokinase. Bronchoalveolar fluid recovered from normal individuals contains this factor [12, 13]. The cellular sources of alveolar urokinase are multiple. Alveolar macrophages synthesize urokinase [14], and recently reported evidence suggests that alveolar epithelial cells do also [15, 16]. This is consistent with prior observations that urokinase is associated with epithelial cells lining body surfaces such as the renal pelvis, urinary bladder, and ductus arteriosus [17].

26.3 Types of Emboli

During the course of a patient's sojourn on hemodialysis therapy, there is the potential for exposure to recurrent bouts of PE. These vary in size from micro to massive and in frequency from those associated with each dialysis treatment to those that occur only as a consequence of an access salvage procedure such as a thrombectomy.

26.3.1 Microemboli

The fact that microembolization occurs during dialysis has been well documented using ultrasound detection of microembolic signals (MES) over the subclavian artery during the course of a treatment [18–21]. It is presumed that most of these are gaseous due to air bubbles either already within the hemodialysis device or caused by cavitation resulting from pressure gradients within the device [20]. Oxygen inhalation has been shown to reduce the number of MES originating from cavitation bubbles by replacing the blood's physically dissolved nitrogen with oxygen, which has a lower tendency to form gaseous bubbles. In one study [20] that looked at this phenomenon, however, the number of MES was not significantly reduced by oxygen inhalation suggesting that at least in some cases, they are not all gaseous.

Paradoxical Emboli: Microemboli

The microemboli occurring during dialysis are generally felt to be of no consequence. However, studies [21] demonstrating the presence of microemboli within the common carotid artery as well as the dialysis access during dialysis indicate that these small emboli can actually pass through the lung barrier and may cause ischemic lesions in organs such as the brain that are supported by the affected arterial circuit.

26.3.2 Macro-emboli

The time of greatest risk for significant pulmonary embolization in the hemodialysis patient is in conjunction with a thrombectomy procedure performed upon an arteriovenous access. Although generally well tolerated, both percutaneous [22–25] and surgical thrombectomies [26] can result in a significant incidence of pulmonary embolism (PE).

The actual volume of clot that is present within a thrombosed arteriovenous graft (AVG) is frequently overestimated. If one calculates the maximum clot volume that is possible, it is found to be rather small (Fig. 26.2). It has been determined from surgical specimens that the total clot volume for grafts measuring 30 to more than 50 cm

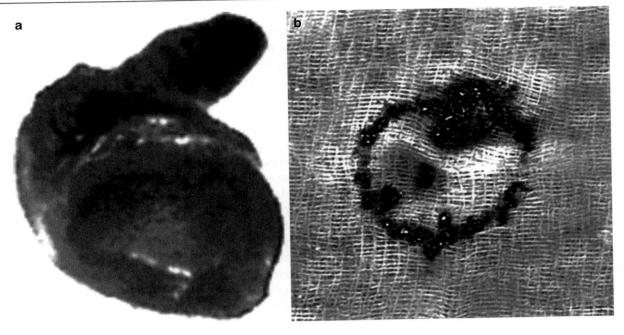

Fig. 26.2 Thrombus from thrombosed graft. (**a**) Arterial plug. (**b**) Clot aspirated from graft

(mean, 42 cm) averages only 3.2 ml in volume; this includes the arterial plug [27].

Several investigators have performed pulmonary scans to determine the occurrence and frequency of PE after percutaneous thrombectomy [25, 26, 28, 29]. Swan et al. [28] studied 43 thrombosed hemodialysis graft cases undergoing percutaneous thrombectomy using pulse-spray pharmacomechanical thrombolysis with urokinase. Perfusion lung scans were obtained in 22 patients after the procedure; none were studied prior to the event. These scans were interpreted as consistent with PE in 59 % of those studied, but no clinical signs or symptoms were present in 41 of the 43 cases (95 %). However, two patients developed both signs and symptoms of acute PE in the post-procedural period and died. One had underlying pulmonary disease, and the other had chronic heart disease. Both patients were oxygen dependent. Unfortunately, it is not known how many of the cases in this study actually had pulmonary defects prior to the procedure.

Beathard et al. [25] obtained pulmonary perfusion scans in six patients selected at random from a cohort of 1,176 cases of thrombosed dialysis access grafts in which percutaneous thrombectomy was performed mechanically without the use of a lytic agent. Scans were obtained immediately before the thrombectomy procedure and 48 h afterward. If the 48-h image showed positive results, a third scan was obtained at 2 weeks. No clinical signs or symptoms of pulmonary embolization were noted in any of the total cohort in this series. In no instance was the oxygen saturation at the end of the procedure lower than it was at the beginning. All pre-procedure scans were negative. In five of the patients with lung scans (83 %), multiple small defects were present at 48 h. All of the positive scans were negative 2 weeks after treatment.

Smits et al. [26] performed a study designed to determine the incidence of pulmonary embolization following percutaneous thrombectomy in 23 patients with occluded hemodialysis grafts. Mechanical (MT) was performed in 12 cases and pharmacomechanical percutaneous thrombolysis (PMT) in 11. Pulmonary perfusion scans were performed within a few hours before and within 24 h after thrombolysis in all cases. In eight patients (8 of 23, 35 %), perfusion defects were seen on the second scan, which were absent on the first and were consistent with the presence of PE. Only one of these cases was symptomatic. In five of the eight patients who had PE, a third pulmonary perfusion scan was performed 3–4 months after the procedure. In four patients, the perfusion defects were completely resolved, and in one they were substantially diminished.

In 1999, Petronis et al. [30] conducted a study on 13 patients to determine if pulmonary perfusion defects were detectable by ventilation–perfusion scintigraphy after percutaneous thrombolysis of clotted hemodialysis access grafts in their program. Four patients underwent pharmacomechanical thrombolysis with urokinase, and the remainder had only mechanical thrombolysis. Pre- and post-thrombolysis scintigraphic studies were performed on all patients. In only one patient did a study show a new nonvascular perfusion defect and this case had a matching ventilation abnormality. The defect was believed to be caused by mucus plugging. The patient had no evidence of pulmonary embolism.

In another study reported in 2000, Kinney, et al. [29] studied 25 cases in a prospective, randomized, double-blind study evaluating PE with two pulse-spray pharmacomechanical thrombolysis protocols. Eleven patients were treated with urokinase and 14 with heparinized saline only. Nuclear medicine perfusion lung scans were performed before treatment and after graft declotting procedures. Baseline nuclear medicine perfusion lung scan results were abnormal (≥ 20 % segmental perfusion defect) in 19 patients (70.4 %). A new PE (one or more pulmonary segments) occurred in two patients treated with urokinase (18.2 %) and nine patients treated with heparinized saline (64.3 %; $P = .04$). All cases of embolism were asymptomatic. The post-intervention primary patency rates for the dialysis access were similar between groups.

These studies taken together suggest that PE does occur with some percutaneous thrombectomy procedures. However, they are generally small, asymptomatic, and completely clear with time. The exceptions to this are not common, but may occur in cases with significant cardiopulmonary comorbidity. However, there is a high incidence of pulmonary hypertension in dialysis patients [31], and the possibility that recurrent pulmonary emboli resulting from repeated episodes of treated thrombosis might play a causative role has been raised [26, 32]. However, using an anatomically based theoretical model of perfusion in the pulmonary acinar blood vessels, Clark et al. [33] produced evidence to indicate that distal microemboli were not as likely to cause pulmonary hypertension as more proximal emboli and that occlusion alone was not sufficient.

Harp et al. [34] evaluated the incidence of pulmonary hypertension in a group of 88 cases with a hemodialysis vascular access that had been treated with percutaneous thrombectomy. These cases were compared with two control groups, one consisting of cases without end-stage renal disease and a second with end-stage renal disease who had not had a percutaneous thrombectomy. The incidence of pulmonary hypertension was higher in both ESRD groups than in normal controls. However, the difference between those who had had and those who had not had a percutaneous thrombectomy was not significant. This result suggests that microembolization associated with this procedure is not an issue in the etiology of pulmonary hypertension in these patients.

Paradoxical Emboli: Macro-emboli

Normal fetal circulation is dependent upon the foramen ovale, which provides a communication for oxygenated blood flow between the right and left atria during lung maturation. At birth, decreased pulmonary vascular resistance and increased left atrial pressure promote closure of the foramen ovale. However, a probe patent foramen ovale (Fig. 26.3) has been reported to be present in 27 % of the general population at autopsy [35, 36], meaning that a probe can be passed across the opening although its flap-valve-like architecture is such that it normally prevents the passage of blood.

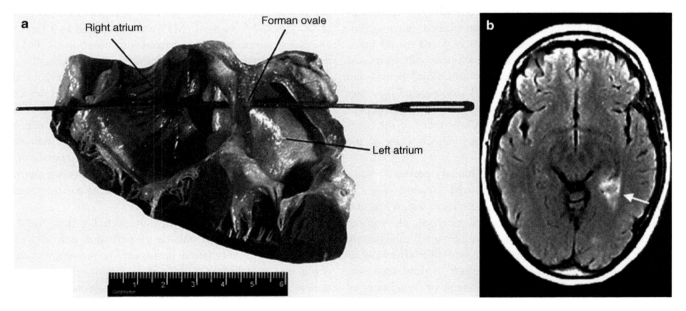

Fig. 26.3 Paradoxical embolus. (**a**) Probe patent foramen ovale. (**b**) Cerebral infract from embolus (*arrow*)

Although thought to be uncommon, there are instances in which the potential for right-to-left shunting is actually realized. The pulmonary hypertension that develops in the dialysis patient can result in this phenomenon [36–39]. A Valsalva maneuver or even a strong cough can also result in right-to-left shunting. This occurs because upon release of the Valsalva maneuver, right atrial pressure momentarily exceeds left atrial pressure due to the sudden rush of blood into the right ventricle [36]. This maneuver has been used to diagnose of a right-to-left shunt, and in the presence of a PFO, it has been reported to result in a paradoxical embolus (PDE) [40].

Basically, four elements are required to make a diagnosis of PDE: (1) systemic embolism confirmed by clinical, angiographic, or pathologic findings without an apparent source in the left area of the heart or proximal arterial tree; (2) an embolic source within the venous system; (3) an abnormal intracardiac or intrapulmonary communication between right and left circulations; and (4) a pressure gradient that promotes right-to-left shunting at some point in the cardiac cycle.

There is strong evidence that there is a causal relationship between a PFO and embolic strokes. Despite extensive workup, 40 % of cerebral infarcts have no known underlying cause [36]. In one study [41], it was found that the prevalence of a patent foramen ovale in 40 stroke patients under the age of 40 years was 50 % as compared with 15 % in control subjects. In the same study, 56 % of patients with stroke and no identifiable cause had a patent foramen ovale. In another study [42], the prevalence of PFO among young ischemic stroke patients was twice as high as that of the normal population.

It is easy to see that the requirements for such an event can occur with a thrombectomy procedure performed on a dialysis vascular access. Clots are being released into the circulation, a PFO is statistically present in a significant proportion of patients, and there is a high incidence of pulmonary hypertension [31]. Several such episodes have been reported [39, 43–45]; however, the paucity with which the phenomenon has been reported would suggest that its occurrence is not common. In a large series in which a comprehensive review of complications associated with interventional dialysis access procedures was reported [46], no episodes of stroke were encountered following 4,899 thrombectomy procedures (228 on fistulas). This too would suggest that PDE is uncommon.

PDE has also been reported with catheter exchange [44] and associated with an air embolus occurring during a manipulation of a hemodialysis catheter [47–49]. Additionally, since blood passing through an arteriovenous access is being shunted from the arterial to the venous circulation without passing through a capillary bed, it is possible for an inverse paradoxical embolus (embolus from the arterial to the venous circulation) to occur. In one report [50], a case with aortic vegetations secondary to endocarditis, a septic pulmonary embolus occurred 4 weeks after the removal of a dialysis catheter which was infected.

26.3.3 Massive Emboli

Some AVGs have pseudoaneurysms. These anomalous structures are frequently lined with laminated, organized thrombus. In a patient with large pseudoaneurysms that are very firm, the clot load within the thrombosed AVG may be quite large. The amount of clot in a thrombosed AVF varies considerably [51]. In most instances, it is rather small, but in some cases the thrombus load can be quite large (Fig. 26.4). This is more likely to be seen in the upper arm AVFs and in what has come to be referred to as a "mega-fistula," i.e., one that is markedly dilated, tortuous, with multiple aneurysms. In addition to pseudoaneurysms and aneurysms, the presence of a central venous stenosis can promote the development of a large clot load. In these unusual cases an embolus may be large enough to lead to serious problems. Unfortunately, physicians dealing with these cases are reticent to publish them; however, the author is familiar with two cases which experienced a fatal PE following an attempted thrombectomy in the face of a large clot load.

26.4 Concerns Related to PE

The performance of a thrombectomy carries with it the risk of a pulmonary embolus. Since the interventional nephrologist is generally performing these procedures in a free-standing facility, there are several questions that should be considered [32]. What makes an embolus lethal, and how much pulmonary embolization (clot load) is safe?

26.4.1 What Makes an Embolus Lethal?

The clinical presentation of a PE varies from asymptomatic (incidentally diagnosed) to fatal. Development of symptoms depends on the embolic burden and the severity of any underlying cardiopulmonary disease. The severe physiologic consequences of a PE are due to two factors that lead to a cascade of hemodynamic and respiratory events that can end in death of the patient – mechanical obstruction and the release of vasoactive mediators (Fig. 26.5). Of these two, mechanical obstruction of the pulmonary arteries and their segmental and subsegmental branches is predominant [52–54]. Angiographic studies suggest that, in the absence of prior cardiopulmonary disease, approximately 25 % of pulmonary arteries become occluded before there is any increase in pulmonary arterial pressure [55]. Most people who die of PE have sustained multisegmental or main pulmonary arterial occlusion [56].

Fig. 26.4 Massive thrombus (**a**) Vessels filled with thrombus. (**b**) Mega thrombus that is thrombosed

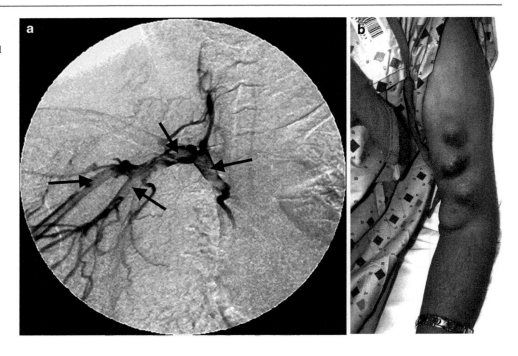

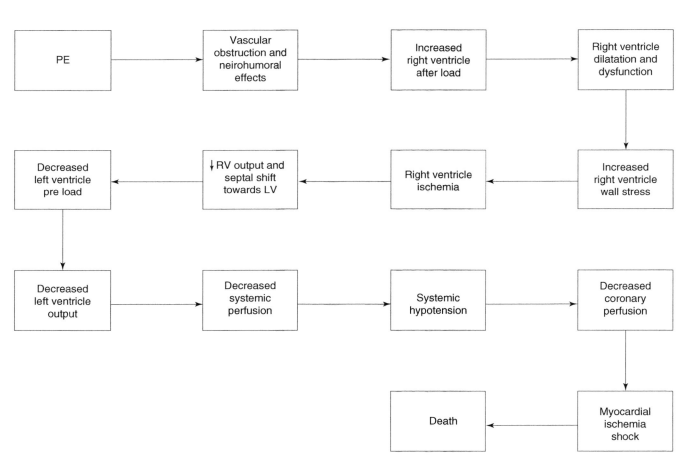

Fig. 26.5 Sequence of events leading to death from PE

In order to determine whether quantification of PE could be used as a predictor of patient outcome, 59 cases were studied using computed tomographic (CT) pulmonary angiography by Wu et al. [57] studies that were performed on hospitalized patients with PE. A pulmonary arterial obstruction index was derived for each set of images on the basis of embolus size and location. By using logistic regression, PE indexes were calculated using the technique originally described by Qanadli et al. [58]. This index is defined as the product of N X D, where N is the value of the proximal pulmonary artery clot site, equal to the number of segmental arterial branches arising distally, and D is the degree of obstruction, defined as 1 for partial obstruction and 2 for total obstruction. Wu et al. then compared the calculated index with patient outcome, survival or death, to determine if there was a correlation between PE volume and survival. One of 53 patients (1.9 %) with an index of less than 60 % died. The cause of death in this case was end-stage malignancy. Five of six patients (83 %) with an index of 60 % or higher died. All five deaths were related to the presence of PE. The one survivor with a PE index higher than 60 % received thrombolytic therapy. By using a cutoff of 60 %, the PE index was used to identify 52 of 53 (98 %) patients who survived and five of six (83 %) patients who died.

The importance of CT-derived clot volume was also demonstrated in a subsequent study of 125 consecutive patients with acute PE [59]. Ten patients (8 %) died of PE within 30 days following CT. The authors of this report developed a central clot score which was used to evaluate clot volume. This scoring system was very similar to that described by Qanadli et al. [58] except that while the proximal artery was given a score equal to the number of segmental arteries arising distally as in the study described above, the degree of occlusion was graded 0–5. They showed that a central clot index of 53 % had 100 % sensitivity, 76.5 % specificity, 23.5 % positive predictive value, and 98 % negative predictive value for 30-day PE death.

A number of observations have challenged the concept that the hemodynamic manifestations of PE are due solely to mechanical obstruction [38, 60, 61]. Additionally, a strictly mechanical obstruction of the left or right pulmonary artery during a surgical procedure produced by cross-clamping, or by unilateral balloon occlusion, causes only a modest rise in pulmonary artery pressure and almost never results in right-sided heart failure [38, 62], whereas PE with obstruction of only 25 % of the pulmonary vascular tree can cause marked pulmonary hypertension [63]. Published studies indicate that this discrepancy is largely explained by pulmonary vasoconstriction caused by vasoactive mediators, released primarily by activated platelets. Thromboxane-A$_2$ and serotonin are the two most important pulmonary vasoconstrictors

in this context [64]. Antagonizing their effects has been shown to dramatically increase tolerance to experimental pulmonary embolism in animals [64].

Acute right-sided heart failure due to increased pulmonary vascular resistance resulting from mechanical obstruction and vasoconstriction is the prime cause of death in PE [55]. The rapid rise in afterload causes dilatation of the right ventricle, which, together with systemic hypotension, compromises coronary perfusion, and causes ischemia and sometimes even myocardial infarction. A septal shift resulting from right ventricle dilatation further reduces left ventricular preload, and the patient enters a "vicious cycle" of acute right-sided heart failure [65, 66]. The terminal event is systemic hypotension related to acutely elevated pulmonary pressures, right ventricular failure [52, 67] and hypoxemia [68] (Fig. 26.5).

Comorbidity plays an important role in the lethal effects of a PE, especially underlying cardiopulmonary disease. This can make an otherwise well-tolerated PE life-threatening and may render a smaller volume of PE lethal [38, 55, 56, 69, 70].

26.4.2 How Much Is Too Much?

The volume of thrombus in an access can vary considerable in the face of different predisposing factors, but when should it be considered a large or excessive clot load? There are no standards by which to make this judgment. It seems appropriate to answer this question based upon the size of thrombus that would be sufficient to be considered a serious medical risk.

The clot volume quantification studies quoted above suggest that if the cross-sectional area of the pulmonary vascular bed is reduced by 50–60 %, there is risk of death from the episode. In a study of 19 cases, Milnor et al. [71] determined total vascular volume of the pulmonary bed using a dye dilution method. They found the average volume to be 365 cc/m^2. Which means that for a 70-kg individual who is 70 in. tall, the total pulmonary vascular volume would be in the range of 683 cc. According to the studies described above, an embolus of 340–410 cc (50–60 % reduction) would be expected to have a fatal effect. In order to minimize the risk of such an occurrence and be totally safe (to the degree possible), it would seem that one should avoid situations that would have the possibility of creating a volume of embolus that would exceed 50 % of this amount, something that could be thought as an LCV-50 (50 % of the lethal clot volume). This would mean avoiding situations that might generate a clot load exceeding approximately 200 cc. While this is certainly speculative, it does offer a possible threshold value for concern that has some basis in established evidence.

To place this in perspective, an acute thrombus in an aneurysm that is 8 cm × 12 cm in a patient with a hematocrit of 35 %

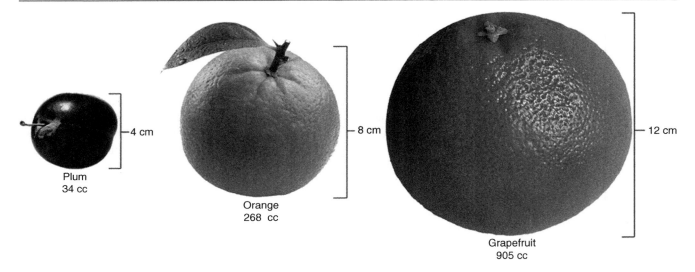

Fig. 26.6 Size comparisons for clot volume (for fresh clot, multiply by percent hematocrit)

equals 200 cc. Using the time-honored practice of equating pathology to food (Fig. 26.6), an average plum is 4 cm in diameter with a volume of 33.5 cc; an average orange is about 8 cm in diameter and represents 268 cc. A grapefruit averages 12 cm in diameter, and an equivalent volume would be 905 cc. This comparison would suggest that an acute thrombus within an aneurysm the size of an orange in a patient with a hematocrit of 35 % or less would be relatively safe to attack. However, one must realize that chronic, laminated clot may fill the defect in some of these dilated access. These clot volumes would not be affected by the patient's hematocrit. However, this type of thrombus is generally attached to the wall and difficult to embolize.

26.4.3 How Should Excessive Clot-Load Case Be Managed?

If one accepts the concept of excessive clot load, then it follows that these cases must receive special consideration in their management. The first issue to consider is whether the access should be salvaged. Cases with excessive clot burdens frequently have significantly severe structural defects. Although individualization is important, surgical revision or access replacement might be in the patient's best interest. If a thrombectomy is felt to be necessary, it should be done using appropriate precautions in the hospital setting rather than a free-standing dialysis access facility.

26.4.4 What Happens to the Embolic Thrombus?

In many instances, fresh thrombus is cleared from the pulmonary arterial system by endogenous thrombolysis. This process starts relatively quickly following embolization. However, 50 % of patients with PE have persistent defects on follow-up scan 4–6 months [72–74] after diagnosis. There is a wide variation in resolution of thrombi in individual patients. As many as a third of patients will show no clot lysis [73, 75–78]. Cardiopulmonary disease adversely affects clearance of thrombotic emboli [73, 75, 78]. Lysis of a PE is also reduced in older patients [78] and in patients who do not undergo anticoagulant therapy after the acute event [72, 77]. Eventually, complete resolution of PE occurs in about two thirds of patients, with partial resolution in the remainder [79–81]. One report [74] compiled the results of four studies dealing with the resolution of PE. Two studies [82, 83] used V/Q (ventilation–perfusion) lung scintigraphy as the follow-up test, and two studies [84, 85] used helical CT. These reports showed that the percentage of patients with residual pulmonary thrombi averaged 87 % at 8 days after diagnosis, 68 % at 6 weeks, 65 % at 3 months, 57 % at 6 months, and 52 % after 11 months.

Embolic material that has not been cleared by thrombolysis undergoes organization and conversion into firm fibrotic deposits that become adherent to the pulmonary arterial wall [75]. These organized deposits can obstruct pulmonary arterial flow and can lead to chronic pulmonary arterial hypertension and eventually cor pulmonale [86, 87]. Pulmonary artery pressure of over 50 mmHg at the time of presentation of a PE and age ≥70 years are frequently associated with persistent pulmonary hypertension [88]. It has been shown that 4–5 % [85, 89] of first-time, symptomatic PE patients acquire symptomatic chronic thromboembolic pulmonary hypertension (CTPH) within 2 years. Surgical thromboendarterectomy can be a highly effective treatment for CTPH in such patients [90, 91].

26.5 Management of PE

Typically, a discussion of the management of PE includes those of all sizes: however, for our purposes we will restrict this review to the situation as it might present itself in the interventional facility, dealing with a patient with a dialysis vascular access, basically a massive PE.

26.5.1 Risk Stratification

While PE is common with thrombectomy of an arteriovenous access, these emboli are generally of such a size that adverse effects are rarely seen: however, with a large clot load, a massive PE is possible, and emergency management may be critical to the patient's survival. The 30-day mortality rate for massive PE has been reported to be approximately 30 % [92], and in a significant number, death is immediate. Shock or systemic hypotension at presentation represents the most important clinical sign of poor prognosis in patients with acute PE [93, 94]. The presence of shock in these patients defines a three- to sevenfold increase in mortality, with a majority of deaths occurring within 1 h of occurrence [95].

A risk stratification tool that accurately quantifies the prognosis of patients with PE is useful in guiding the intensity of initial treatment of these cases. Derived primarily from work done in associated with deep vein thrombosis, multiple clinical models for determining prognosis in patients with PE have been developed. Of these the Pulmonary Embolism Severity Index (PESI) has been extensively validated internally and externally [96, 97]. This index is based upon the assessment of 11 clinical variables.

Multiple studies have shown that patients with acute PE who have elevated serum levels of cardiac biomarkers such as troponin and brain natriuretic peptide, or evidence of right-heart dysfunction on either echocardiography or CT angiography, have a worse short-term survival than those without these features [98–101]. However, these tests take time and require the immediate availability of a facility capable of doing the testing. The PESI is based upon the assessment of clinical variables which are objective and easily identifiable factors that can be ascertained within minutes of a patient's presentation and do not require laboratory or imaging assessment. The value of this index is felt to lie primarily in the identification of patients with a low mortality risk who might be suitable for home management of their acute PE [96, 97, 102, 103]. However, It has also been found to have a strong correlation with mortality rate following PE [96, 104].

A simplified version (sPESI) has been described [105]. This version eliminates factors that are not significantly associated with 30-day mortality. It is based upon the

Table 26.1 Clinical features of PE [106]

Variable	Massive PE	Non-massive PE
Systolic pressure	75 ± 10	131 ± 23
Heart rate	117 ± 28	98 ± 21
Chest pain	41 (40)	1,127 (50)
Dyspnea	86 (81)	1,876 (82)
Syncope	41 (39)	271 (12)
Cough	10 (9)	483 (21)
Hemoptysis	2 (2)	160 (7)

Numbers in () represent percentages of total group

determination of age ≤ 80 years and absence of systemic hypotension, tachycardia, hypoxia, cancer, heart failure, and lung disease to produce its risk stratification score. A clinical comparison of sPESI to the original version has shown that it has similar prognostic accuracy and clinical utility but greater ease of use [105]. It appears to be the most usable for assessing risk for PE associated with dialysis access interventions.

In the original study [105], ROC curve analysis used to identify low-risk patients with PE for the sPESI determined that a score of only 1 point was the optimal cutoff between low- and high-risk groups. Patients with a score of 0 (i.e., no variables present) were categorized as low risk, and those with a score of 1 or more (any variable present) were categorized as high risk (see below).

Using Risk Factor Data

When dealing with a patient with a large clot load, one should be alert for signs that might suggest the occurrence of a pulmonary embolus such as the sudden onset of dyspnea, tachypnea, a sustained fall in oxygen saturation (less than 90 %), chest pain, syncope and/or hypotension, or shock [106–108]. In a review of 2,392 patients with acute PE [106], 108 (4.5 %) had massive PE, defined as a systolic arterial pressure <90 mmHg, and 2,284 (95.5 %) had non-massive PE with a systolic arterial pressure ≥ 90 mmHg; the symptoms listed in Table 26.1 were noted.

Given symptoms suggestive of a PE, a decision has to be made concerning the initiation of emergency treatment. In some instances this may require that the patient be transferred from an outpatient facility to a location where such treatment can be performed and time is often critical. Although most episodes of PE, even if significant, do not lead to sudden death, most patients who do succumb to pulmonary embolism do so within the first few hours of the event (Fig. 26.7). In fact, 15 % of all cases (all cause) of sudden death are attributable to PE. As a cause of sudden death, massive pulmonary embolism is second only to sudden cardiac death. In patients who survive the immediate effects of a PE, death can often be prevented with prompt diagnosis and therapy [106].

Faced with the sudden appearance of signs or symptoms compatible with the occurrence of a PE, superimposed upon a clinical situation in which such an adverse event is possible (large clot load), the availability of a risk index such as sPESI is helpful in making a decision to take the necessary steps to immediately initiate what could be lifesaving therapy. While both the PESI and sPESI have been validated with PE associated primarily with DVT, it seems only reasonable that similar results would be obtained with an embolus from another source.

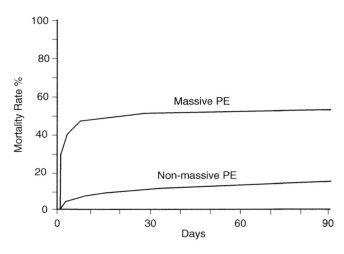

Fig. 26.7 Mortality rate from acute PE (Modified from Kucher et al. [106])

Table 26.2 Modified sPESI: a score of 1 or greater should be considered high risk

Variable	Modified PESI
Age >80 years	1
Heart failure	1
Chronic lung disease	1
Pulse ≥100	1
Systolic BP <100	1
Respiratory rate ≥30/min	1
Arterial O_2 saturation <90 %	1

We suggest a modification of sPESI to better fit the dialysis access circumstance (Table 26.2). The sPESI index combines cardiac and respiratory categories into a single variable. In the dialysis population because of the frequency with which each of these comorbidities is seen, the case can be made for keeping them separate. Since events such as a drop in blood pressure, tachycardia, and a drop in oxygen saturation is not infrequent, these index variables should be taken to mean a persistent change (>15 min) rather than a transient alteration. When dealing with a patient with the potential for a massive PE, the index would be applicable for determining the appropriate level of management (Fig. 26.8).

26.5.2 Diagnosis

In making the diagnosis of an acute PE, time is critical. The overall mortality in patients with PE who are untreated can be as high as 30 % [109] while the correct diagnosis and appropriate timely therapy can significantly lower mortality to 2.5–10 % [87, 110, 111]. Unfortunately, making an accurate clinical diagnosis is difficult since there are no symptoms or physical findings that are specific for the event. However, interventionalists should maintain a high index of suspicion, especially in the clinical setting of a thrombectomy being performed on an arteriovenous access with a large clot load (equal to or greater than LCV-50). If there is the sudden onset of suggestive symptoms, a presumptive diagnosis should be made and appropriate action taken. Symptoms that are suggestive in this setting are dyspnea, tachypnea, a sustained fall in oxygen saturation (less than 90 %), chest pain, syncope and/or sustained hypotension, or shock [106–108].

Since some of the suggestive symptoms are not uncommon in the dialysis patient, to arouse concern there should be a change from the patient's baseline and should be persistent. Hypotension in this instance should be <90 mmHg lasting for 15 min or more or a decrease in systolic blood pressure

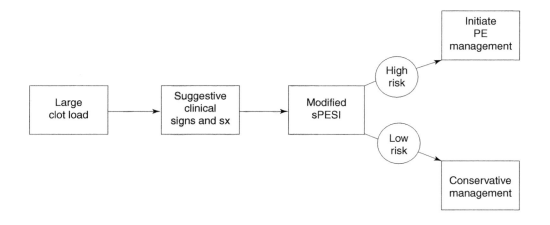

Fig. 26.8 Application of modified sPESI

≥40 mmHg from the patient's stable level [108]. PE is generally associated with hypoxemia, but up to 20 % of patients with PE have a normal oxygen saturation level [112]. Electrocardiographic signs of right ventricular strain, such as inversion of T waves in leads V1–V4, a QR pattern in lead V1, the classic S1Q3T3 type, and incomplete or complete right bundle-branch block, may be helpful if of new onset [113, 114].

In patients with suspected PE and cardiogenic shock, the decision to obtain diagnostic studies such as computed tomogram or a ventilation–perfusion scan can excessively delay the initiation of reperfusion therapy. In the presence of evidence of severe right ventricular dysfunction, reperfusion therapy should be initiated immediately without the time delay required in obtaining these studies.

Plasma D-Dimer

D-dimer is a degradation product of cross-linked fibrin. Levels are elevated in the plasma in the presence of an acute clot because of simultaneous activation of coagulation and fibrinolysis. Measurement of plasma D-dimer levels is often used as an aid in the diagnosis of suspected PE [115, 116]. However, utility is primarily in ruling out rather than confirming a PE [107] because there are a number of other conditions that can cause an elevation. Since one of these conditions is the presence of an acute clot, it is of no value as an aid to the diagnosis of a PE in a patient having a dialysis access thrombectomy. One would expect that these cases would always have an elevated plasma D-dimer level.

Radiological Tests

Pulmonary angiography is traditionally considered the gold standard of diagnosis of PE. However, it is infrequently performed because it is an invasive and expensive method and requires experienced radiologists/physicians to both perform the test and interpret the results [117]. As a result other tests are more likely to be used.

Ventilation–Perfusion Scintigraphy

Ventilation–perfusion scintigraphy (V/Q scan) has been widely used as an aid in the diagnosis of PE (Fig. 26.9). The basic principle of the test depends upon an intravenous injection of technetium-labelled macroaggregated albumin particles, which block a small fraction of pulmonary capillaries and thereby enable scintigraphic assessment of lung perfusion at the tissue level. Where there is occlusion of pulmonary arterial branches, the peripheral capillary bed will not receive particles, rendering the area "cold" on subsequent images. Perfusion scans are combined with ventilation studies, in which a radioactive-labelled tracer (generally a gas) is inhaled. The purpose of the additional ventilation scan is to increase specificity by the identification of hypoventilation as a non-embolic cause of hypoperfusion due to reactive vasoconstriction (perfusion–ventilation match). In the case of PE, ventilation is expected to be normal in hypoperfused segments (perfusion–ventilation mismatch) [118, 119].

Lung scan results are frequently classified according to criteria established in the North American PIOPED trial

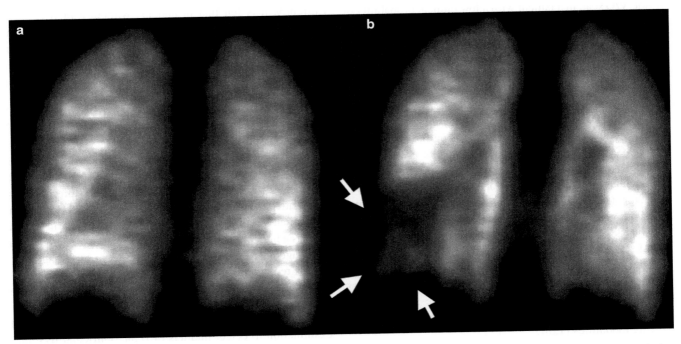

Fig. 26.9 V/Q Scan of lung with ventilation–perfusion mismatch. (**a**) Ventilation scan shows no pathologic change. (**b**) Defect on the perfusion scan (*arrows*) indication location of PE

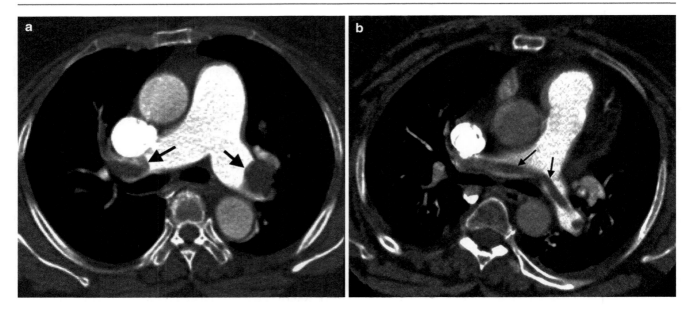

Fig. 26.10 CT pulmonary angiography. (**a**) Thrombus occluding right and left pulmonary arteries (*arrows*). (**b**) Saddle embolus (*arrows*)

[120] into four categories: normal or near-normal, low, intermediate (nondiagnostic), and high probability of PE. Although this classification has been questioned [121, 122], the validity of a normal perfusion lung scan has been evaluated in several studies which have indicated that it is a safe practice to withhold anticoagulant therapy in patients with a normal perfusion scan [123–125]. It is generally accepted that a normal perfusion scan is very safe for excluding PE. Although less well validated, the combination of a nondiagnostic V/Q scan in a patient with a low clinical probability of PE is an acceptable criterion for excluding PE. A high-probability ventilation–perfusion scan establishes the diagnosis of PE with a high degree of probability, but further tests may be considered in selected patients with a low clinical probability [107].

Computed Tomography (CT)

Contrast-enhanced multi-slice spiral CT pulmonary angiography (CTPA) has shown promising results [126, 127] in diagnosing PE (Fig. 26.10). There are two approaches to this technology, single detector (SD-CTPA) and multidetector (MD-CTPA). Two large clinical studies using SD-CTPA reported a sensitivity of 70 % and a specificity of 90 % [128, 129]. It was concluded that the overall sensitivity of spiral CT for PE was too low to endorse its use as the sole test to exclude PE. This was true even for patients with larger PE in segmental or larger pulmonary artery branches [128, 129]. It was felt, however, that these studies could replace angiography in combined strategies that include testing modalities [128].

Actually, MD-CTPA with high spatial and temporal resolution and quality of arterial opacification has become the

method of choice for imaging the pulmonary vasculature for suspected PE in routine clinical practice. It allows adequate visualization of the pulmonary arteries up to at least the segmental level [130–132]. In an early study, a sensitivity and specificity for PE above 90 % were reported in an early series [133]. In a later, larger series (PIOPED II), a sensitivity of 83 % and a specificity of 96 % were observed [126].

A SD-CTPA or MD-CTPA showing a thrombus up to the segmental level can be taken as adequate evidence of PE. Currently, it is felt that in patients without a high clinical probability, a negative SD-CTPA must be combined with other testing modalities to safely exclude PE, whereas MD-CTPA may be used as a stand-alone test [107].

26.5.3 Treatment of Pulmonary Embolization

General

In addition to general support measures which are critical to success (Table 26.3), there are two approaches to the initial treatment of PE, anticoagulation alone and thrombolysis with anticoagulation. The choice of therapy depends upon the patient's risk stratification [134]. For patients in whom there is a high clinical suspicion of PE, initial treatment with anticoagulants while awaiting the outcome of diagnostic tests is recommended as long as the patient is stable. In the absence of a contraindication, anticoagulation should not be delayed until diagnostic testing for PE has been completed. As quickly as possible, it is important to conduct a physical examination to detect findings of right ventricular dysfunction such as distended jugular veins, a systolic murmur of tricuspid regurgitation, or an accentuated P2. Clues on the

Table 26.3 Summary of management of high-risk pulmonary embolism [107]

Anticoagulation with unfractionated heparin should be initiated without delay
Systemic hypotension should be corrected to prevent progression of RV failure and death
Vasopressive drugs are recommended for hypotensive patients
Aggressive fluid challenge is not recommended
Oxygen should be administered in patients with hypoxemia
Thrombolytic therapy should be used in patients presenting with cardiogenic shock and/or persistent arterial hypotension
Surgical pulmonary embolectomy is a recommended therapeutic alternative if thrombolysis is absolutely contraindicated or has failed
Catheter embolectomy or fragmentation of proximal pulmonary arterial clots may be considered as an alternative to surgical treatment

ECG include right bundle-branch block, S1Q3T3, and T wave inversion in leads V1 through V4.

Poor prognostic indicators include patients who appear critically ill, with marked dyspnea, anxiety, and low oxygen saturation; elevated troponin, indicating right ventricular microinfarction; right ventricular dysfunction on echocardiography; and right ventricular enlargement on chest CT. Patients with any or a combination of these changes are at high risk for an adverse outcome and may derive benefit from immediate thrombolytic therapy, even if they initially maintain systemic arterial pressure [134]. Major contraindications to thrombolytic therapy include intracranial disease, uncontrolled hypertension at presentation, and recent major surgery or trauma [135].

Shock or systemic blood hypotension at presentation represents the most important clinical sign of poor prognosis in patients with acute PE [93, 94, 106]. The presence of shock in these patients defines a three- to sevenfold increase in mortality, with a majority of deaths occurring within 1 h of occurrence [95]. Thrombolytic therapy is recommended in these cases unless there are major contraindications related to bleeding risk. Thrombolysis in these patients should not be delayed; irreversible cardiogenic shock may ensue [134].

There is widespread agreement that thrombolytic therapy should be used to treat PE associated with hemodynamic compromise. Compared with anticoagulation alone, thrombolytic therapy has demonstrated acceleration of thrombus lysis as evidenced by more rapid resolution of perfusion scan abnormalities, decrement in angiographic thrombus, reduction in elevated pulmonary artery pressures, normalization of right ventricular dysfunction, and a trend toward improved clinical outcomes [134]. However, studies comparing anticoagulation and thrombolytic therapy have shown an increased incidence of bleeding in the latter group. In one study intracranial bleeding occurred in 3.0 % of patients who received thrombolytic therapy, compared with 0.3 % of the non-thrombolysis-treated patients [106].

When a lytic agent is deemed appropriate for treating PE, current evidence indicates that thrombolytic therapy should be infused into a peripheral vein rather than given directly into a pulmonary artery. Centrally administering the agent does not accelerate thrombolysis but does cause more frequent bleeding at the catheter insertion site [136]. An infusion of tPA at a dose of 100 mg should be administered over a 2-h period or less [134]. More prolonged infusions of thrombolytic agents (e.g., 12 h or more) are associated with higher rates of bleeding [137, 138]. Additionally, a 2-h infusion achieves more rapid clot lysis than 12- or 24-h infusions [138–140]. In patients with imminent or actual cardiac arrest, bolus infusion of thrombolytic therapy is indicated [134].

Before thrombolytic therapy is administered, IV heparin (unfractionated) should be administered in full therapeutic doses (e.g., bolus of 80 U/kg followed by 18 U/kg/h initially) [134]. During administration of thrombolytic therapy, it is acceptable to either continue or suspend heparin infusion.

Mechanical Thrombectomy Devices

The use of mechanical thrombectomy devices in the treatment of PE has been reported. Kuo et al. [141] reported a meta-analysis of 594 patients from 35 studies (six prospective, 29 retrospective) who were treated with catheter-directed mechanical therapy for massive PE. The pooled clinical success rate for this group of cases was 86.5 %. Pooled risks of minor and major procedural complications were 7.9 and 2.4 %, respectively. In 546 of 571 cases with data available (95 %), catheter-directed mechanical therapy was used as the first adjunct to anticoagulation without previous intravenous thrombolysis.

The purpose of the mechanical device is to fragment thrombus either in an effort to send particles more distally and expose a larger aggregate surface area of the thrombus to pharmacologic thrombolytic agents [142] or more often to aspirate the fragments with a catheter [143]. The goal is to reduce pulmonary arterial resistance enough to reduce pulmonary artery hypertension, alleviating right ventricular dilatation and dysfunction, and rapidly increase cardiac output. Hemodynamic improvement can be dramatic following successful thrombus fragmentation. Substantial improvement in pulmonary blood flow may result from what appears to be only modest angiographic change [107].

Unfortunately, these endovascular techniques have not been compared with other forms of therapy in prospective randomized controlled studies. The American College of Chest Physicians Clinical Practice Guidelines [134] recommends against use of interventional catheterization techniques for most patients. However, in selected, highly compromised patients who are unable to receive thrombolytic therapy because of bleeding risk, or whose critical status does not allow sufficient time for systemic thrombolytic therapy to be effective, interventional catheterization techniques may be considered as an alternative to surgical treatment [107, 134].

Surgical Embolectomy

Emergency surgical embolectomy with cardiopulmonary bypass has been used as a management strategy for cases with massive PE [144–146]. The American College of Chest Physicians Clinical Practice Guidelines [134] recommend that in selected highly compromised patients who are unable to receive thrombolytic therapy because of bleeding risk, or whose critical status does not allow sufficient time for systemic thrombolytic therapy to be effective, pulmonary embolectomy should be considered.

Practice guidelines for the diagnosis and management of pulmonary embolism published by the Japanese Circulation Society [108] take a stronger view on the role of surgery. Pointing out evidence that surgical treatment has been shown to improve the condition of patients with unstable hemodynamics due to massive PE [144, 147, 148], they recommend that a patient with an acute pulmonary embolus be closely monitored during medical therapy for evidence of deterioration and a need for surgical intervention.

If the patient develops circulatory failure or shock, prompt recanalization of the occluded pulmonary arteries is essential [106]. Surgical pulmonary thrombectomy under cardiopulmonary bypass should be considered for these patients. In patients without shock, conventional surgical pulmonary thrombectomy is indicated when (1) tachycardia persists in the absence of hypotension and medical treatment is not effective; (2) thrombus is observed (using some type of imaging modality) in the pulmonary arterial trunk or both right and left main pulmonary arteries, and heart failure and/or respiratory failure is rapidly progressive; (3) thrombolytic therapy is contraindicated; and (4) free thrombus is present in the right atrium and/or ventricle [149].

References

1. Deffebach ME, Charan NB, Lakshminarayan S, Butler J. The bronchial circulation. Small, but a vital attribute of the lung. Am Rev Respir Dis. 1987;135:463.
2. Wagenvoort C, Wagenvoort N. Pathology of pulmonary hypertension. 1st ed. New York: Wiley; 1977.
3. Virmani R, Roberts W. Pulmonary arteries in congenital heart disease: a structure-function analysis. Philadelphia: Davis; 1987. p. 77–130.
4. Mathes M, Holman E, Reichert F. A study of the bronchial, pulmonary, and lymphatic circulations of the lung under various pathologic conditions experimentally produced. J Thorac Surg. 1932;1:339.
5. Kauczor H, Schwickert H, Mayer E, et al. Spiral CT of bronchial arteries in chronic thromboembolism. J Comput Assist Tomogr. 1994;18:855.
6. Dalen J, Haffajee C, Alpert J, et al. Pulmonary embolism, pulmonary hemorrhage, and pulmonary infarction. N Engl J Med. 1977;296:1431.
7. Tsao MS, Schraufnagel D, Wang NS. Pathogenesis of pulmonary infarction. Am J Med. 1982;72:599.
8. Wagenvoort CA. Pathology of pulmonary thromboembolism. Chest. 1995;107:10S.
9. Schraufnagel DE, Tsao MS, Yao YT, Wang NS. Factors associated with pulmonary infarction. A discriminant analysis study. Am J Clin Pathol. 1985;84:15.
10. Alderson PO, Martin EC. Pulmonary embolism: diagnosis with multiple imaging modalities. Radiology. 1987;164:297.
11. Rosenberg RD, Aird WC. Vascular-bed–specific hemostasis and hypercoagulable states. N Engl J Med. 1999;340:1555.
12. Chapman HA, Allen CL, Stone OL. Abnormalities in pathways of alveolar fibrin turnover among patients with interstitial lung disease. Am Rev Respir Dis. 1986;133:437.
13. Bowen RM, Hoidal JR, Estensen RD. Urokinase-type plasminogen activator in alveolar macrophages and bronchoalveolar lavage fluid from normal and smoke-exposed hamsters and humans. J Lab Clin Med. 1985;106:667.
14. Chapman Jr HA, Stone OL, Vavrin Z. Degradation of fibrin and elastin by intact human alveolar macrophages in vitro. Characterization of a plasminogen activator and its role in matrix degradation. J Clin Invest. 1984;73:806.
15. Marshall BC, Brown BR, Rothstein MA, et al. Alveolar epithelial cells express both plasminogen activator and tissue factor. Potential role in repair of lung injury. Chest. 1991;99:25S.
16. Marshall BC, Sageser DS, Rao NV, et al. Alveolar epithelial cell plasminogen activator. Characterization and regulation. J Biol Chem. 1990;265:8198.
17. Dano K, Andreasen PA, Grondahl-Hansen J, et al. Plasminogen activators, tissue degradation, and cancer. Adv Cancer Res. 1985;44:139.
18. Rolle F, Pengloan J, Abazza M, et al. Identification of microemboli during haemodialysis using Doppler ultrasound. Nephrol Dial Transplant. 2000;15:1420.
19. Woltmann D, Fatica RA, Rubin JM, Weitzel W. Ultrasound detection of microembolic signals in hemodialysis accesses. Am J Kidney Dis. 2000;35:526.
20. Droste DW, Kuhne K, Schaefer RM, Ringelstein EB. Detection of microemboli in the subclavian vein of patients undergoing haemodialysis and haemodiafiltration using pulsed Doppler ultrasound. Nephrol Dial Transplant. 2002;17:462.
21. Forsberg U, Jonsson P, Stegmayr C, Stegmayr B. Microemboli, developed during haemodialysis, pass the lung barrier and may cause ischaemic lesions in organs such as the brain. Nephrol Dial Transplant. 2010;25:2691.
22. Trerotola SO, Lund GB, Scheel Jr PJ, et al. Thrombosed dialysis access grafts: percutaneous mechanical declotting without urokinase. Radiology. 1994;191:721.
23. Middlebrook MR, Amygdalos MA, Soulen MC, et al. Thrombosed hemodialysis grafts: percutaneous mechanical balloon declotting versus thrombolysis. Radiology. 1995;196:73.
24. Trerotola SO, Johnson WM, Winkler T, Dreesen RG. Percutaneous creation of arteriovenous hemodialysis grafts: work in progress. J Vasc Interv Radiol. 1995;6:675.
25. Beathard GA, Welch BR, Maidment HJ. Mechanical thrombolysis for the treatment of thrombosed hemodialysis access grafts. Radiology. 1996;200:711.
26. Smits HF, Van Rijk PP, Van Isselt JW, et al. Pulmonary embolism after thrombolysis of hemodialysis grafts. J Am Soc Nephrol. 1997;8:1458.
27. Winkler TA, Trerotola SO, Davidson DD, Milgrom ML. Study of thrombus from thrombosed hemodialysis access grafts. Radiology. 1995;197:461.
28. Swan TL, Smyth SH, Ruffenach SJ, et al. Pulmonary embolism following hemodialysis access thrombolysis/thrombectomy. J Vasc Interv Radiol. 1995;6:683.
29. Kinney TB, Valji K, Rose SC, et al. Pulmonary embolism from pulse-spray pharmacomechanical thrombolysis of clotted hemodialysis grafts: urokinase versus heparinized saline. J Vasc Interv Radiol. 2000;11:1143.

30. Petronis JD, Regan F, Briefel G, et al. Ventilation-perfusion scintigraphic evaluation of pulmonary clot burden after percutaneous thrombolysis of clotted hemodialysis access grafts. Am J Kidney Dis. 1999;34:207.

31. Yigla M, Nakhoul F, Sabag A, et al. Pulmonary hypertension in patients with end-stage renal disease. Chest. 2003;123:1577.

32. Dolmatch BL, Gray RJ, Horton KM. Will iatrogenic pulmonary embolization be our pulmonary embarrassment? Radiology. 1994; 191:615.

33. Clark AR, Burrowes KS, Tawhai MH. The impact of micro-embolism size on haemodynamic changes in the pulmonary micro-circulation. Respir Physiol Neurobiol. 2011;175:365.

34. Harp RJ, Stavropoulos SW, Wasserstein AG, Clark TW. Pulmonary hypertension among end-stage renal failure patients following hemodialysis access thrombectomy. Cardiovasc Intervent Radiol. 2005;28:17.

35. Hagen PT, Scholz DG, Edwards WD. Incidence and size of patent foramen ovale during the first 10 decades of life: an autopsy study of 965 normal hearts. Mayo Clin Proc. 1984;59:17.

36. Ward R, Jones D, Haponik EF. Paradoxical embolism. An under-recognized problem. Chest. 1995;108:549.

37. Meister SG, Grossman W, Dexter L, Dalen JE. Paradoxical embolism. Diagnosis during life. Am J Med. 1972;53:292.

38. Sharma GV, McIntyre KM, Sharma S, Sasahara AA. Clinical and hemodynamic correlates in pulmonary embolism. Clin Chest Med. 1984;5:421.

39. Briefel GR, Regan F, Petronis JD. Cerebral embolism after mechanical thrombolysis of a clotted hemodialysis access. Am J Kidney Dis. 1999;34:341.

40. Loscalzo J. Paradoxical embolism: clinical presentation, diagnostic strategies, and therapeutic options. Am Heart J. 1986;112:141.

41. Webster MW, Chancellor AM, Smith HJ, et al. Patent foramen ovale in young stroke patients. Lancet. 1988;2:11.

42. Overell JR, Bone I, Lees KR. Interatrial septal abnormalities and stroke: a meta-analysis of case–control studies. Neurology. 2000;55:1172.

43. Owens CA, Yaghmai B, Aletich V, et al. Fatal paradoxic embolism during percutaneous thrombolysis of a hemodialysis graft. AJR Am J Roentgenol. 1998;170:742.

44. Petrea RE, Koyfman F, Pikula A, et al. Acute stroke, catheter related venous thrombosis, and paradoxical cerebral embolism: report of two cases. J Neuroimaging. 2013;23:111–4.

45. Wu S, Ahmad I, Qayyum S, et al. Paradoxical embolism after declotting of hemodialysis fistulae/grafts in patients with patent foramen ovale. Clin J Am Soc Nephrol. 2011;6:1333.

46. Beathard GA, Litchfield T. Effectiveness and safety of dialysis vascular access procedures performed by interventional nephrologists. Kidney Int. 2004;66:1622.

47. Eichhorn V, Bender A, Reuter DA. Paradoxical air embolism from a central venous catheter. Br J Anaesth. 2009;102:717.

48. Kariya S, Tanigawa N, Komemushi A, et al. Asymptomatic paradoxical and symptomatic pulmonary air embolism during central venous catheter insertion. Jpn J Radiol. 2010;28:473.

49. Oyama N, Sakaguchi M, Kitagawa K. Air tract in the thrombus: paradoxical cerebral air embolism through a residual catheter track. J Stroke Cerebrovasc Dis. 2012;21:905.e11–3.

50. Rocha JL, Gonzalez-Roncero F, Lopez-Hidalgo R, et al. Inverse paradoxical embolism in a patient on chronic hemodialysis with aortic bacterial endocarditis. Am J Kidney Dis. 1999;34:338.

51. Haage P, Vorwerk D, Wildberger JE, et al. Percutaneous treatment of thrombosed primary arteriovenous hemodialysis access fistulae. Kidney Int. 2000;57:1169.

52. Dexter L, Smith GT. Quantitative studies of pulmonary embolism. Am J Med Sci. 1964;247:641.

53. Knisely WH, Wallace JM, Mahaley Jr MS, Satterwhite Jr WM. Evidence, including in vivo observations, suggesting mechanical blockage rather than reflex vasospasm as the cause of death in pulmonary embolization. Am Heart J. 1957;54:482.

54. Mc ER, Harder RA, Dale WA. Respiratory and cardiovascular phenomena associated with pulmonary embolism. Surg Gynecol Obstet. 1958;106:271.

55. McIntyre KM, Sasahara AA. The hemodynamic response to pulmonary embolism in patients without prior cardiopulmonary disease. Am J Cardiol. 1971;28:288.

56. Gorham LW. A study of pulmonary embolism. II. The mechanism of death; based on a clinicopathological investigation of 100 cases of massive and 285 cases of minor embolism of the pulmonary artery. Arch Intern Med. 1961;108:189.

57. Wu AS, Pezzullo JA, Cronan JJ, et al. CT pulmonary angiography: quantification of pulmonary embolus as a predictor of patient outcome–initial experience. Radiology. 2004;230:831.

58. Qanadli SD, El Hajjam M, Vieillard-Baron A, et al. New CT index to quantify arterial obstruction in pulmonary embolism: comparison with angiographic index and echocardiography. AJR Am J Roentgenol. 2001;176:1415.

59. Venkatesh SK, Wang SC. Central clot score at computed tomography as a predictor of 30-day mortality after acute pulmonary embolism. Ann Acad Med Singapore. 2010;39:442.

60. McIntyre KM, Sasahara AA. Determinants of right ventricular function and hemodynamics after pulmonary embolism. Chest. 1974;65:534.

61. Miller RL, Das S, Anandarangam T, et al. Association between right ventricular function and perfusion abnormalities in hemodynamically stable patients with acute pulmonary embolism. Chest. 1998;113:665.

62. Boldt J, Muller M, Uphus D, et al. Cardiorespiratory changes in patients undergoing pulmonary resection using different anesthetic management techniques. J Cardiothorac Vasc Anesth. 1996; 10:854.

63. Alpert JS, Godtfredsen J, Ockene IS, et al. Pulmonary hypertension secondary to minor pulmonary embolism. Chest. 1978;73:795.

64. Smulders YM. Pathophysiology and treatment of haemodynamic instability in acute pulmonary embolism: the pivotal role of pulmonary vasoconstriction. Cardiovasc Res. 2000;48:23.

65. Wiedemann HP, Matthay RA. Acute right heart failure. Crit Care Clin. 1985;1:631.

66. Lualdi JC, Goldhaber SZ. Right ventricular dysfunction after acute pulmonary embolism: pathophysiologic factors, detection, and therapeutic implications. Am Heart J. 1995;130:1276.

67. Parmley Jr LF, North RL, Ott BS. Hemodynamic alterations of acute pulmonary thromboembolism. Circ Res. 1962;11:450.

68. Kovacs GS, Hill JD, Aberg T, et al. Pathogenesis of arterial hypoxemia in pulmonary embolism. Arch Surg. 1966;93:813.

69. McIntyre KM, Sasahara AA. The ratio of pulmonary arterial pressure to pulmonary vascular obstruction: index of preembolic cardiopulmonary status. Chest. 1977;71:692.

70. Moser KM. Pulmonary embolism. Am Rev Respir Dis. 1977;115:829.

71. Milnor WR, Jose AD, McGaff CJ. Pulmonary vascular volume, resistance, and compliance in man. Circulation. 1960;22:130.

72. Moser KM, Guisan M, Bartimmo EE, et al. In vivo and post mortem dissolution rates of pulmonary emboli and venous thrombi in the dog. Circulation. 1973;48:170.

73. Tow DE, Wagner Jr HN. Recovery of pulmonary arterial blood flow in patients with pulmonary embolism. N Engl J Med. 1967;276:1053.

74. Nijkeuter M, Hovens MM, Davidson BL, Huisman MV. Resolution of thromboemboli in patients with acute pulmonary embolism: a systematic review. Chest. 2006;129:192.

75. Chait A, Summers D, Krasnow N, Wechsler BM. Observations on the fate of large pulmonary emboli. Am J Roentgenol Radium Ther Nucl Med. 1967;100:364.

76. Dalen JE, Banas Jr JS, Brooks HL, et al. Resolution rate of acute pulmonary embolism in man. N Engl J Med. 1969;280:1194.

77. Walker RH, Goodwin J, Jackson JA. Resolution of pulmonary embolism. Br Med J. 1970;4:135.

78. Winebright JW, Gerdes AJ, Nelp WB. Restoration of blood flow after pulmonary embolism. Arch Intern Med. 1970;125:241.

79. Paraskos JA, Adelstein SJ, Smith RE, et al. Late prognosis of acute pulmonary embolism. N Engl J Med. 1973;289:55.

80. Hall RJ, Sutton GC, Kerr IH. Long-term prognosis of treated acute massive pulmonary embolism. Br Heart J. 1977;39:1128.

81. Riedel M, Stanek V, Widimsky J, Prerovsky I. Longterm follow-up of patients with pulmonary thromboembolism. Late prognosis and evolution of hemodynamic and respiratory data. Chest. 1982;81:151.

82. Pacho R, Pruszczyk P, Chlebus M. Monitoring of thrombi regression in massive acute pulmonary embolism with repeated CT [abstract]. Radiology. 1996;201:304.

83. Otero-Candelera R, Rodriguez-Panadero F, Ramos A, et al. Evolution of pulmonary scintigraphy in the follow-up of pulmonary embolism. Effect of anticoagulant treatment and other associated factors. Arch Bronconeumol. 1997;33:129.

84. Palla A, Donnamaria V, Petruzzelli S, Giuntini C. Follow-up of pulmonary perfusion recovery after embolism. J Nucl Med Allied Sci. 1986;30:23.

85. Ribeiro A, Lindmarker P, Johnsson H, et al. Pulmonary embolism: a follow-up study of the relation between the degree of right ventricle overload and the extent of perfusion defects. J Intern Med. 1999;245:601.

86. Owen WR, Thomas WA, Castleman B, Bland EF. Unrecognized emboli to the lungs with subsequent cor pulmonale. N Engl J Med. 1953;249:919.

87. Dalen JE, Alpert JS. Natural history of pulmonary embolism. Prog Cardiovasc Dis. 1975;17:259.

88. Ribeiro A, Lindmarker P, Johnsson H, et al. Pulmonary embolism: one-year follow-up with echocardiography doppler and five-year survival analysis. Circulation. 1999;99:1325.

89. Pengo V, Lensing AW, Prins MH, et al. Incidence of chronic thromboembolic pulmonary hypertension after pulmonary embolism. N Engl J Med. 2004;350:2257.

90. Fedullo PF, Auger WR, Kerr KM, Rubin LJ. Chronic thromboembolic pulmonary hypertension. N Engl J Med. 2001;345:1465.

91. de Perrot M, McRae K, Shargall Y, et al. Pulmonary endarterectomy for chronic thromboembolic pulmonary hypertension: the Toronto experience. Can J Cardiol. 2011;27:692.

92. Heit JA, Silverstein MD, Mohr DN, et al. Predictors of survival after deep vein thrombosis and pulmonary embolism: a population-based, cohort study. Arch Intern Med. 1999;159:445.

93. White RH. The epidemiology of venous thromboembolism. Circulation. 2003;107:I4.

94. Goldhaber SZ, Visani L, De Rosa M. Acute pulmonary embolism: clinical outcomes in the International Cooperative Pulmonary Embolism Registry (ICOPER). Lancet. 1999;353:1386.

95. Wood KE. The presence of shock defines the threshold to initiate thrombolytic therapy in patients with pulmonary embolism. Intensive Care Med. 2002;28:1537.

96. Aujesky D, Roy PM, Le Manach CP, et al. Validation of a model to predict adverse outcomes in patients with pulmonary embolism. Eur Heart J. 2006;27:476.

97. Jimenez D, Yusen RD. Prognostic models for selecting patients with acute pulmonary embolism for initial outpatient therapy. Curr Opin Pulm Med. 2008;14:414.

98. Becattini C, Vedovati MC, Agnelli G. Prognostic value of troponins in acute pulmonary embolism: a meta-analysis. Circulation. 2007;116:427.

99. Klok FA, Mos IC, Huisman MV. Brain-type natriuretic peptide levels in the prediction of adverse outcome in patients with pulmonary embolism: a systematic review and meta-analysis. Am J Respir Crit Care Med. 2008;178:425.

100. Moores LK, Holley AB. Computed tomography pulmonary angiography and venography: diagnostic and prognostic properties. Semin Respir Crit Care Med. 2008;29:3.

101. Douketis JD, Leeuwenkamp O, Grobara P, et al. The incidence and prognostic significance of elevated cardiac troponins in patients with submassive pulmonary embolism. J Thromb Haemost. 2005;3:508.

102. Moores L, Aujesky D, Jimenez D, et al. Pulmonary Embolism Severity Index and troponin testing for the selection of low-risk patients with acute symptomatic pulmonary embolism. J Thromb Haemost. 2010;8:517.

103. Donze J, Le Gal G, Fine MJ, et al. Prospective validation of the Pulmonary Embolism Severity Index. A clinical prognostic model for pulmonary embolism. Thromb Haemost. 2008;100:943.

104. Choi WH, Kwon SU, Jwa YJ, et al. The pulmonary embolism severity index in predicting the prognosis of patients with pulmonary embolism. Korean J Intern Med. 2009;24:123.

105. Jimenez D, Aujesky D, Moores L, et al. Simplification of the pulmonary embolism severity index for prognostication in patients with acute symptomatic pulmonary embolism. Arch Intern Med. 2010;170:1383.

106. Kucher N, Rossi E, De Rosa M, Goldhaber SZ. Massive pulmonary embolism. Circulation. 2006;113:577.

107. Torbicki A, Perrier A, Konstantinides S, et al. Guidelines on the diagnosis and management of acute pulmonary embolism: the Task Force for the Diagnosis and Management of Acute Pulmonary Embolism of the European Society of Cardiology (ESC). Eur Heart J. 2008;29:2276.

108. JCS Joint Working Group. Guidelines for the diagnosis, treatment and prevention of pulmonary thromboembolism and deep vein thrombosis (JCS 2009). Circ J. 2011;75:1258.

109. Soudry G, Dibos PE. Gated myocardial perfusion scan leading to diagnosis of unsuspected massive pulmonary embolism. Ann Intern Med. 2000;132:845.

110. Carson JL, Kelley MA, Duff A, et al. The clinical course of pulmonary embolism. N Engl J Med. 1992;326:1240.

111. Barritt DW, Jordan SC. Anticoagulant drugs in the treatment of pulmonary embolism. A controlled trial. Lancet. 1960;1:1309.

112. Stein PD, Goldhaber SZ, Henry JW, Miller AC. Arterial blood gas analysis in the assessment of suspected acute pulmonary embolism. Chest. 1996;109:78.

113. Rodger M, Makropoulos D, Turek M, et al. Diagnostic value of the electrocardiogram in suspected pulmonary embolism. Am J Cardiol. 2000;86:807.

114. Geibel A, Zehender M, Kasper W, et al. Prognostic value of the ECG on admission in patients with acute major pulmonary embolism. Eur Respir J. 2005;25:843.

115. Stein PD, Hull RD, Patel KC, et al. D-dimer for the exclusion of acute venous thrombosis and pulmonary embolism: a systematic review. Ann Intern Med. 2004;140:589.

116. Di Nisio M, Squizzato A, Rutjes AW, et al. Diagnostic accuracy of D-dimer test for exclusion of venous thromboembolism: a systematic review. J Thromb Haemost. 2007;5:296.

117. He J, Wang F, Dai HJ, et al. Chinese multi-center study of lung scintigraphy and CT pulmonary angiography for the diagnosis of pulmonary embolism. Int J Cardiovasc Imaging. 2012;28:1799–805.

118. Alderson PO. Scintigraphic evaluation of pulmonary embolism. Eur J Nucl Med. 1987;13(Suppl):S6.

119. Miller RF, O'Doherty MJ. Pulmonary nuclear medicine. Eur J Nucl Med. 1992;19:355.

120. Value of the ventilation/perfusion scan in acute pulmonary embolism. Results of the Prospective Investigation of Pulmonary Embolism Diagnosis (PIOPED). JAMA. 1990;263:2753.

121. Gottschalk A, Sostman HD, Coleman RE, et al. Ventilation-perfusion scintigraphy in the PIOPED study. Part II. Evaluation of the scintigraphic criteria and interpretations. J Nucl Med. 1993;34:1119.

122. Sostman HD, Coleman RE, DeLong DM, et al. Evaluation of revised criteria for ventilation-perfusion scintigraphy in patients with suspected pulmonary embolism. Radiology. 1994;193:103.

123. Kruip MJ, Leclercq MG, van der Heul C, et al. Diagnostic strategies for excluding pulmonary embolism in clinical outcome studies. A systematic review. Ann Intern Med. 2003;138:941.

124. Ten Wolde M, Hagen PJ, Macgillavry MR, et al. Non-invasive diagnostic work-up of patients with clinically suspected pulmonary embolism; results of a management study. J Thromb Haemost. 2004;2:1110.

125. Anderson DR, Kahn SR, Rodger MA, et al. Computed tomographic pulmonary angiography vs ventilation-perfusion lung scanning in patients with suspected pulmonary embolism: a randomized controlled trial. JAMA. 2007;298:2743.

126. Stein PD, Fowler SE, Goodman LR, et al. Multidetector computed tomography for acute pulmonary embolism. N Engl J Med. 2006;354:2317.

127. Musset D, Parent F, Meyer G, et al. Diagnostic strategy for patients with suspected pulmonary embolism: a prospective multicentre outcome study. Lancet. 2002;360:1914.

128. Perrier A, Howarth N, Didier D, et al. Performance of helical computed tomography in unselected outpatients with suspected pulmonary embolism. Ann Intern Med. 2001;135:88.

129. Van Strijen MJ, De Monye W, Kieft GJ, et al. Accuracy of single-detector spiral CT in the diagnosis of pulmonary embolism: a prospective multicenter cohort study of consecutive patients with abnormal perfusion scintigraphy. J Thromb Haemost. 2005;3:17.

130. Ghaye B, Szapiro D, Mastora I, et al. Peripheral pulmonary arteries: how far in the lung does multi-detector row spiral CT allow analysis? Radiology. 2001;219:629.

131. Remy-Jardin M, Remy J, Wattinne L, Giraud F. Central pulmonary thromboembolism: diagnosis with spiral volumetric CT with the single-breath-hold technique–comparison with pulmonary angiography. Radiology. 1992;185:381.

132. Patel S, Kazerooni EA, Cascade PN. Pulmonary embolism: optimization of small pulmonary artery visualization at multi-detector row CT. Radiology. 2003;227:455.

133. Winer-Muram HT, Rydberg J, Johnson MS, et al. Suspected acute pulmonary embolism: evaluation with multi-detector row CT versus digital subtraction pulmonary arteriography. Radiology. 2004;233:806.

134. Kearon C, Kahn SR, Agnelli G, et al. Antithrombotic therapy for venous thromboembolic disease: American College of Chest Physicians Evidence-Based Clinical Practice Guidelines (8th Edition). Chest. 2008;133:454S.

135. Kanter DS, Mikkola KM, Patel SR, et al. Thrombolytic therapy for pulmonary embolism. Frequency of intracranial hemorrhage and associated risk factors. Chest. 1997;111:1241.

136. Verstraete M, Miller GA, Bounameaux H, et al. Intravenous and intrapulmonary recombinant tissue-type plasminogen activator in the treatment of acute massive pulmonary embolism. Circulation. 1988;77:353.

137. Urokinase-streptokinase embolism trial: phase 2 result. JAMA. 1974;229:1606.

138. Goldhaber SZ, Kessler CM, Heit J, et al. Randomised controlled trial of recombinant tissue plasminogen activator versus urokinase in the treatment of acute pulmonary embolism. Lancet. 1988;2: 293.

139. Meneveau N, Schiele F, Vuillemenot A, et al. Streptokinase vs alteplase in massive pulmonary embolism. A randomized trial assessing right heart haemodynamics and pulmonary vascular obstruction. Eur Heart J. 1997;18:1141.

140. Meyer G, Sors H, Charbonnier B, et al. Effects of intravenous urokinase versus alteplase on total pulmonary resistance in acute massive pulmonary embolism: a European multicenter double-blind trial. The European Cooperative Study Group for Pulmonary Embolism. J Am Coll Cardiol. 1992;19:239.

141. Kuo WT, Gould MK, Louie JD, et al. Catheter-directed therapy for the treatment of massive pulmonary embolism: systematic review and meta-analysis of modern techniques. J Vasc Interv Radiol. 2009;20:1431.

142. Chamsuddin A, Nazzal L, Kang B, et al. Catheter-directed thrombolysis with the Endowave system in the treatment of acute massive pulmonary embolism: a retrospective multicenter case series. J Vasc Interv Radiol. 2008;19:372.

143. Zeni Jr PT, Blank BG, Peeler DW. Use of rheolytic thrombectomy in treatment of acute massive pulmonary embolism. J Vasc Interv Radiol. 2003;14:1511.

144. Leacche M, Unic D, Goldhaber SZ, et al. Modern surgical treatment of massive pulmonary embolism: results in 47 consecutive patients after rapid diagnosis and aggressive surgical approach. J Thorac Cardiovasc Surg. 2005;129:1018.

145. Meneveau N, Seronde MF, Blonde MC, et al. Management of unsuccessful thrombolysis in acute massive pulmonary embolism. Chest. 2006;129:1043.

146. Sukhija R, Aronow WS, Lee J, et al. Association of right ventricular dysfunction with in-hospital mortality in patients with acute pulmonary embolism and reduction in mortality in patients with right ventricular dysfunction by pulmonary embolectomy. Am J Cardiol. 2005;95:695.

147. Yalamanchili K, Fleisher AG, Lehrman SG, et al. Open pulmonary embolectomy for treatment of major pulmonary embolism. Ann Thorac Surg. 2004;77:819.

148. Digonnet A, Moya-Plana A, Aubert S, et al. Acute pulmonary embolism: a current surgical approach. Interact Cardiovasc Thorac Surg. 2007;6:27.

149. Meyer G, Tamisier D, Sors H, et al. Pulmonary embolectomy: a 20-year experience at one center. Ann Thorac Surg. 1991;51: 232.

Stent Migration

Ramanath Dukkipati

27.1 Introduction

Central vein stenosis is common in hemodialysis patients. Risk factors include history of tunneled dialysis catheter placement. In hemodialysis patients in the USA, endovascular stent placement is increasingly being used to manage these lesions. In dialysis vascular access, only the Flair™ endovascular stent graft has been approved by the FDA, and their role in extending a graft cumulative survival has been debated. Some commonly used self-expanding stents are shown in Fig. 27.1. Stent placement is considered to be an adjuvant for angioplasty as it is used to limit elastic recoil of venous stenotic lesions after angioplasty, counteract extrinsic vein compression, and limit extravasation of blood in dissected vasculature and has been approved for vein-graft stenotic lesions in hemodialysis patients. Complications related to placement of stent include migration, fracture, thrombosis, infection, shortening, vessel rupture due to attempts at advancement of stent after partial or complete deployment, occlusion of side branches of a vessel, and instent stenosis.

The incidence of stent migration has been reported to be as low as 3 %. In one series migration of stent has occurred in 20 % of the cases.

27.2 What Causes Migration of a Stent?

Stents once placed are partially covered by endothelium and are thought to be more susceptible to move from its originally intended location prior to this endothelialization. The causes of migration of stent include (a) improper sizing of stent (too small a stent) relative to the diameter of vein lumen resulting in incomplete contact between the stent and the

R. Dukkipati, MD
Division of Nephrology, University of California,
Torrance, Los Angeles, CA, USA
e-mail: ramdukkipati@gmail.com

vessel lumen, (b) placement of stent in a vein close to a joint such as shoulder joint which mobilizes the stent leading to movement of stent into a larger diameter vein, (c) fracture of stent which can lead to migration from its intended native location to a proximal or central location, and (d) susceptibility of self-expanding stent to move and migrate with inspiration prior to its attachment to the vessel lumen. Lack of sharp flared filament ends in Wallstents and lack of fixation hooks in other types of stents (Gianturco stent) could play an additional role in migration of these stents centrally. There is also a concern that stent grafts may impair stent wall apposition in comparison to the uncovered bare metal stent. This may be a reason for more oversizing of the stent graft compared to a bare metal stent.

27.3 Case Reports

Migration of stents has been reported for virtually every kind of stent placed in the central venous system. Susceptibility of one type of stent for over the other to migrate has not been compared in a randomized clinical trial.

27.4 Complications Related to Stent Migration

Migration of the stent can result in potentially serious complications. Stents can migrate to right atrium, right ventricle, and pulmonary artery. This migration can lead to no symptoms at all or lead to complications such as tricuspid regurgitation, pulmonary infarction, acute myocardial infarction, and cardiogenic shock. Placement of a stent near the subclavian–innominate vein junction will cover the orifice of the ipsilateral internal jugular vein, and attempted central venous catheterization of the subclavian vein can dislodge the stent and embolize the stent into the right heart and pulmonary artery.

A.S. Yevzlin et al. (eds.), *Interventional Nephrology*,
DOI 10.1007/978-1-4614-8803-3_27, © Springer Science+Business Media New York 2014

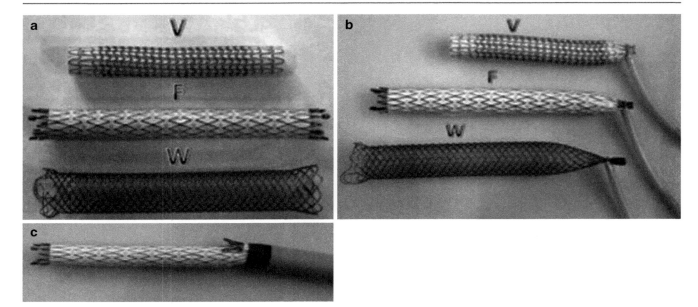

Fig. 27.1 (**a**) Three self-expanding covered endovascular stents (*V*) 6 50 mm Viabahn, (*F*) 6 60 mm Fluency, (*W*) 8 60 mm Wallflex. (**b**) 15 mm gooseneck snare crimping the edge of the stent. (**c**) Gooseneck snare applied to stent's edge and the Fluency stent enfolding within a 16 Fr sheath (Adapted with permission from Catheterization and Cardiovascular Interventions)

27.5 Management Options

Management strategies include (1) conservative approach of observation, (2) percutaneous removal of stent through a vascular sheath, (3) redeployment of stent in external iliac veins, and (4) surgical approach. Management should depend on the clinical circumstance, operator and institution experience, and best judgement.

One approach of retrieval of stents in the right heart could be the following. Place a long percutaneous (e.g., a 45 cm 16 French) sheath into the femoral vein. Insert an Amplatz gooseneck snare (e.g., a 15–25 mm size diameter) through the abovementioned sheath and snare the stent and draw the stent into the sheath. During retraction of the stent, care has to be taken so as to prevent the coned edge from snagging the tricuspid valves. Once this is accomplished, the sheath with the stent in the sheath can be removed. If excessive resistance is encountered, surgical solution should be considered.

A dual-snare approach is employed by some interventionalists. When the snared stent is withdrawn to the level of the mid-inferior vena cava, a second sheath (around 16 French – 35 cm) is placed in the contralateral vein (femoral or internal jugular vein). A second gooseneck snare is placed over the opposite end of the stent. The advantage here is that the second snare secures the stent into the sheath. The first snare is released once the second snare is placed on the opposite end of the stent.

In patients with a permanent inferior vena caval filter already in place, snaring of stent will not be possible. The

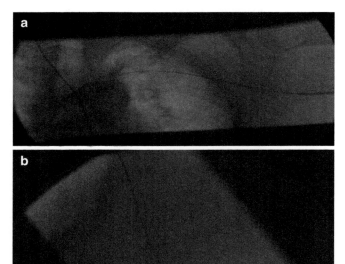

Fig. 27.2 (**a**) Fractured stent (8 mm×6 cm) in the proximal basilic vein. (**b**) Fractured stent (8 mm×6 cm) kept in place by placing an oversized stent (12 mm×4 cm) in the fractured stent

nitinol Smart stent is not readily amenable to crimping like a Wallstent with a gooseneck snare and therefore cannot be drawn into a sheath.

The flared ends are more compressible than the central part of the stents. Another approach for retrieval of embolized stent has been published. This involves inserting and inflating a slightly oversized balloon proximal to the embolized stent and guiding the stent migration from the right heart into the inferior or superior vena cava. Once the balloon and stent combination is closer to the sheath, the stent can be snared and then removed along with the sheath and the balloon. Alternatively a wire can be passed through the embolized stent, and if this can be guided into the femoral vein, then the stent can be surgically removed. There is risk of entanglement of the stent in the right heart with this approach.

There are published case reports of conservative approach with embolized uncovered stents. These patients had terminal illness or serious comorbidities which made surgical procedures to remove stents very high risk.

Surgical approach may be needed if percutaneous approaches fail.

In patients who have a stent fracture (Fig. 27.2a), an oversized stent (new stent larger in diameter than the fractured stent) can be placed in the fractured stent to keep the stent in place (Fig. 27.2b).

27.6 Strategies to Decrease Stent Migration

Oversizing of the stent by 1–2 mm helps the stent to come in complete contact with the vessel wall. A large stent is more likely to be lodged in the innominate vein than migrate into the right heart or pulmonary artery. Large-diameter self-expanding stents are now available which do not shorten as their diameter increases, but the milking action of the vein with respiration can still dislodge the stent in the absence of a mechanism to hold the stent to the vessel wall.

Foreign Body Retrieval

28

Karthik Ramani and Davinder Wadehra

28.1 Introduction

Widespread use of percutaneous techniques in the fields of cardiology, urology, interventional radiology, and interventional nephrology has resulted in an increased rate of dislodgement of foreign bodies. Several endovascular techniques have evolved over time to retrieve the same. Little literature and studies are present that describe the success and failure of different methods of retrieval.

Removal of foreign bodies via nonsurgical methods was initially described in the 1960s [1] and has grown to become a rare but important skill set to have in the armamentarium of an interventionist. This chapter will provide an overview of the nature of foreign bodies one can encounter and describe different techniques and approaches for endovascular removal of foreign bodies.

28.2 Types of Intravascular Foreign Bodies

Most intravascular foreign bodies are iatrogenic in etiology although vascular embolization with bullets and ureteric/bile duct calculi has been described. Our discussion is going to focus primarily on iatrogenic foreign bodies.

Various classifications exist of foreign bodies based on type, location, and description which are illustrated in Table 28.1 below [2–4].

The most common foreign bodies are fragments of catheters, guide wires, angioplasty balloons, and migrated endovascular stents. The final localization of foreign bodies depends on the characteristics of the embolized foreign body such as

the length, weight, stiffness, mobility, and geometry of the foreign body [2]. It also depends on the vessel characteristics such as vessel morphology, site of flow, and blood flow [2].

28.3 Localization of Foreign Body

It is imperative to identify the exact location of foreign body for intravascular foreign body retrieval. Fluoroscopy is excellent for identification and removal of radiopaque foreign bodies. Monoplane fluoroscopy is useful in most instances for removal, but biplane fluoroscopy may be required in some instances for proper topographical localization of foreign bodies in complex anatomical sites. Angiography with road map may be used to supplement fluoroscopy to assist in foreign body removal.

Radiolucent bodies may be difficult to identify, and alternative techniques need to be used for localization. Radiolucent foreign bodies in cardiac structures may be identified via transthoracic or transesophageal echocardiography. For certain intravascular foreign bodies especially coronary stents, intravascular ultrasound may be used [5].

28.4 Complications of Foreign Bodies

Complications of foreign bodies may happen immediately or later [6–13]. The minor and major complications are listed in Table 28.2 below. Fatal complications occur rarely; however, bacterial contamination in the absence of bacteremia has been reported in some studies to be as high as 25 %.

28.5 Indications/Contraindications for Foreign Body Removal

Not every foreign body requires removal, and decision to remove depends on careful assessment of the risk-benefit ratio of every individual case. With the evolution of newer

K. Ramani, MD (✉)
Division of Nephrology and Hypertension,
University of Cincinnati, Cincinnati, OH, USA
e-mail: drkarthikramani@gmail.com

D. Wadehra, MD
LMC Diabetes and Endocrinology,
2130 North Park Dr, Brampton, ON, Canada
e-mail: davinder.wadehra@gmail.com

A.S. Yevzlin et al. (eds.), *Interventional Nephrology*,
DOI 10.1007/978-1-4614-8803-3_28, © Springer Science+Business Media New York 2014

devices and better techniques, the risks for removal have reduced significantly.

If the patient has life-threatening complications such as described in Table 28.2, it warrants prompt removal [2, 3, 14–16]. Foreign bodies lost in the peripheral circulation may be left alone unless they have a propensity to embolize, thrombose, and cause infection or injury. If despite the use of available imaging modalities the foreign body cannot be localized, the search must be discontinued and the patient monitored closely. The decision to anticoagulate depends on the individual situation, and there has been no benefit to anti-

Table 28.1 Commonly encountered foreign bodies

1. Classified on TYPE
(a) Fragments of
Diagnostic catheters
Angioplasty/embolectomy balloons (deflated vs inflated fragments)
Guide wires/sheaths
Pacemaker electrodes
(b) Stents
(c) Embolization coils
(d) IVC filters
(e) Closure devices
2. Classified on LOCATION
(a) Foreign bodies in the venous circulation
Central veins
Peripheral veins
Special situations – within the HD access, right atrium/ventricle and pulmonary circulation
(b) Foreign bodies in the arterial circulation
Aorta
Coronary arteries
Peripheral arteries
3. Classified based on APPEARANCE
(a) Long and skinny
Segment of central venous catheter
Fragment of IVC filter/guide wire
Migrating stent
(b) Round and slippery
Embolization coils
Occlusion devices
Bullets/shotgun pellets
Pressure balls and beads

Table 28.2 Complications of foreign bodies

Major complications	Minor complications
1. Unstable arrhythmias	1. Pain
2. Rupture of large vessels/injury to cardiac structures	2. Thrombosis of peripheral vessels
3. Embolization to vital structures	3. Localized Infection
4. Sepsis/endocarditis	

Table 28.3 Indications for retrieval

Absolute indications	Relative indications
1. Active infection (sepsis)/endocarditis	1. Pain
2. High risk of embolization to vital structure.	2. Thrombosis
3. High risk of perforation/arrhythmia	3. Cross-talk interference between pacemaker and ICD electrode.
4. Foreign body entrapped in cardiac chamber/large vessel	

biotic administration in the absence of systemic signs of infection.

Percutaneous retrieval obviates the need for surgery and is safer and simpler to perform. The common indications are listed in Table 28.3 below. There are no absolute contraindications to removal other than the procedure that must be done in a setting to avoid life-threatening complications.

28.6 Equipment and Devices for Foreign Body Retrieval

Over the years devices and techniques have evolved for the retrieval of foreign bodies. The first reports described the use of Dormia/Dotter retrieval baskets and self-made wire snare as there were no other tools available at that time. Newer devices [16–21] include the use of wire loop snare, retrieval basket, grasping forceps, pincher devices, tip-deflecting wire, goose neck snare, and balloon catheters, to name a few. The choice of device depends on location, type of foreign body, and operator choice/preference. Every device has its pros and cons; the most commonly used device is the loop snares. In this section a brief description of the commonly used commercial devices will be given.

28.6.1 Baskets

The first basket used for foreign body retrieval was a stone retrieval basket designed for the ureteric system [21]. Since these early stone baskets were designed for stone retrieval, they were relatively traumatic and, hence, underwent evolution to be designed specifically for intravascular use. Their newer designs are atraumatic and flexible and can pass over a guide wire.

Description of Dotter Retrieval Basket
The Dotter basket is a flexible, onion shaped wire mesh that is constrained within a guiding sheath. It is available in different sizes and can be navigated past the foreign body and advanced with a slight rotatory to-and-fro motion, opened, and pulled back to trap the foreign body. After the foreign body is trapped, the guiding sheath is advanced to entrap the foreign body.

28.6.2 Foreign Body Retrieval Forceps

The design of the forceps [22] like other retrieval devices has evolved into a highly flexible and atraumatic over the guide wire design. The most obvious advantage that these devices have over the snare system is that the foreign body need not be grasped at the free end. For example, if the guide wire/catheter fragment has both ends embedded in the vascular endothelium, the retrieval forceps would provide a plausible means for extraction, in comparison to loop-snare systems which would need an alternative device to expose the free end to facilitate extraction.

Types of Retrieval Forceps [1]

1. Rat-tooth forceps – two diametrically opposing jaws that contain a single distal tooth.
2. Alligator forceps – similar to rat-tooth except for multiple teeth.
3. Three/four-pronged retrieval forceps – shaped like a cone with three/four wire legs. As the legs are closed, they draw the foreign body to the central axis assisting in removal.

   With forceps with a guiding wire, the forceps is advanced and positioned near the foreign body under fluoroscopic guidance. The handle of the device is used to open the forceps and positioned around the foreign body. The jaws are now closed, and the whole unit, i.e., the guiding catheter and the sheath, is withdrawn.
4. Snares – are the most commonly used device for intravascular foreign body extraction. It primarily consists of a radiopaque nitinol-coated loop which can be collapsed into the catheter shaft and assumes the shape of the vessel.

Historically, the snares really started to evolve from the 1970s when Randall and colleagues initially described a 0.018″ loop at right angles to the guide wire, thus facilitating greater coverage of the vessel. In the 1990s, Furui and group reported a loop-snare device constructed of a 7 F, 80–110 cm long triple-lumen multipurpose configuration at the end. A 0.035″ glide wire is passed through the most distal lumen, and the other two openings are present near the catheter tip. To create a loop, a 0.18″ glide wire is passed through one lumen and brought out through the other. The loop was crimped to produce a right-angled loop. These snares were problematic as they caused trauma to the vessel walls and the doubled over glide wire resulted in internal friction. To overcome these problems, a new right-angled nitinol-braided snare (Amplatz gooseneck snare) was made which was the precursor to snares used in practice nowadays.

The different types of nitinol snares are described below:

(a) *Amplatz gooseneck snare* (*ev3*) – Comes in a variety of loop sizes and is provided with either 4- or 6-French guiding catheters, although substitution with any of several soft, blunt-tipped guiding catheters is possible.[2] The Amplatz snare loop is at a right angle to the catheter; this facilitates the capture of foreign bodies, devices, or catheters. The loop of the snare itself contains gold tungsten coils to enhance visualization (nitinol is poorly radiopaque). It also contains a platinum-iridium radiopaque marker band. The snare comes in a kit and in a variety of sizes ranging from 5 to 35 mm. The snare size used should be chosen based upon the size of the vessel involved. The two that are most applicable to dialysis vascular access procedure are the 10 and the 15 mm. The components of the snare kit are the introducer, torquing device, and the snare. This device is available in a range of sizes, including an Amplatz GooseNeck Microsnare Kit.

(b) *En Snare* (*Merit Medical*) – Consists of interlaced nitinol loops which is incorporated with platinum strands.[3] It also contains a platinum-iridium radiopaque marker band to enhance fluoroscopic visibility. It has a 15-degree-angled tip, is kink resistant, and provides torque control. It comes in a variety of sizes ranging from the 4–8 mm mini snare system to 36–40 mm. The most commonly used diameter in dialysis access would be 6–10 mm standard snare system which comes 6-French catheter size and is 100 cm long. The components of the snare system consist of the introducer, torquing device, catheter, and the snare.

Advantages – The advantages of these snares over the previously described snares are:

1. Multiple preformed sizes for maximal cross-sectional coverage of any vessel
2. Lack of a sharp or potentially traumatic design
3. Ultra-high fluoroscopic visibility
4. Maximum flexibility of both the loop and guide wire
5. Preformed right-angled design without a transition zone between the loop and guiding catheter/cable

Disadvantage – The only disadvantage of a snare-type device is the ability to access the free end of the object to facilitate removal. In some case reports, it has been shown that use of a tip-deflecting device/angioplasty balloon in conjunction with the snare facilitates retrieval of the foreign body when the free end is not accessible.

Steps for Deployment of Snares [23]:

In general, the following principles can be used for deployment of snares:

1. Pass the wire beyond the target object.
2. Position the diagnostic catheter (straight/hockey stick) close to the target object.

---

[1] ASDIN 8th annual scientific meeting pre-course presentation on foreign body retrieval. www.asdin.org.

[2] See footnote 1.

[3] http://www.merit.com/products/default.aspx?code=ensnare.

3. Feed snare into diagnostic catheter and position beyond target object.
4. Pull back the diagnostic catheter and use a torquing motion to grab the object.
5. Advance the diagnostic catheter to close the lasso of the snare and tighten your grip.
6. Now, remove the unit as a whole through the sheath.

Specific situations to warrant removal of objects, i.e., coil and guide wire, will be discussed under the clinical case scenario section [15, 24–29].

28.7 Dialysis Access Specific: Case Scenarios

(a) 42-year-old female with immature left brachiocephalic fistula with large accessory vein mid body of fistula. Attempt to place embolization coil in accessory vein resulted in malposition of coil.

Steps to follow in using snare to retrieve a misplaced coil:
- Deploy the snare above the coil.
- Pull the snare back in a deployed configuration until it catches on the coil
- Use torquing device to manipulate the snare.
- Advance the snare catheter up to the snare and pin the coil as the snare is compressed.
- Advance the catheter rather than pulling back on snare once the snare has caught on the coil.
- Extract the entire unit maintaining pressure on the snare with forward pressure on the catheter.

(b) 36-year-old male with right internal jugular-tunneled dialysis catheter fragment lodged in superior vena cava.

Steps to follow in using snare to retrieve dislodged catheter fragment:

If *free end of catheter is accessible*, use snare technique.
- Position the snare beyond the free edge of the catheter fragment.
- Use torquing device to manipulate the snare.
- Advance the snare catheter up to the snare and pin the fragment as the snare is compressed.
- Advance the catheter rather than pulling back on snare once the snare has caught on the fragment.
- Extract the entire unit maintaining pressure on the snare with forward pressure on the catheter.

If *free end is NOT accessible, use one of the two methods described below.*

*Femoral approach – Use retrieval forceps from a femor*al approach using an appropriate sheath/introducer.
- Position the retrieval forceps at target site.

- Push the button on the handle to open the jaws of the forceps and engage the foreign body. Avoid traumatizing the vessel wall in the process.
- Close the jaw of the forceps by pulling the button of the handle assembly backward. Maintain pressure to assist in removal.
- Pull back the retrieval forceps into the sheath and remove as one unit.
- If multiple fragments have to be removed, rinse the forceps with heparinized saline between withdrawals.

Alternative approach – Fragment is engaged with a deflecting catheter/wire, and once the free end of the fragment is exposed, it is retrieved using a loop snare using the technique described before.

(c) 40-year-old female with left brachiocephalic fistula and straight FLAIR stent placed in cephalic arch which migrated

Approaches – retrieve stent and pull back or trap with another stent.

Reason for migration – poorly sized stent and insufficient wall contact

Steps to follow in using snare to retrieve a migrated stent:

Balloon + Snare approach[4]
- Pass the wire through the stent.
- Pass an appropriately sized angioplasty balloon and inflate the balloon.
- Deploy the snare and snare the balloon and stent together.
- Extract the entire unit maintaining pressure on the snare with forward pressure on the catheter.

Snare-only approach – If free end is accessible:
- Position the snare before/behind the free edge of the stent.
- Use a torquing device to manipulate the snare.
- Advance the snare catheter up to the snare and pin the edge as the snare is compressed.
- Advance the catheter rather than pulling back on snare once the snare has caught on the fragment.
- Extract the entire unit maintaining pressure on the snare with forward pressure on the catheter.

(d) 73 years male with dysfunctional right internal jugular-tunneled dialysis catheter.

Initial fluoroscopic image showed tip of catheter high up in the SVC.

Snares can also be utilized for repositioning of malpositioned catheters.

Steps to repositioning of catheter using a snare[5]:
- Position the snare beyond the free edge of the catheter, using a femoral approach.

---

[4] See footnote 1.
[5] See footnote 1.

- Use torquing device to manipulate the snare.
- Advance the snare catheter up to the snare and pin the edge as the snare is compressed.
- Withdraw the catheter rather than pulling back on snare once the snare has caught the free edge of the catheter. Avoid using excessive force while pulling as it may tear the catheter.
- Position the tip of the catheter using the snare under fluoroscopy guidance.

28.8 Coding

Please refer to the current ASDIN manual for coding to get the latest updates on coding.

The current recommendations for coding are 37203 for transcatheter percutaneous removal of foreign body and 75961 for radiological supervision and interpretation.

Conclusion

This chapter has provided an overview of indications, described different retrieval devices and modes of usage, and focused on access specific scenarios from personal experiences and extensive literature review.

Techniques for extraction of intravascular foreign bodies have undergone significant changes over the years. With the increase in number and complexity of endovascular procedures and given the low incidence of morbidity with an endovascular approach to foreign body retrieval compared to surgery, endovascular modes of retrieval have developed into an important part of the arsenal as an interventionist.

References

1. Thomas J, Sinclair-Smith B, Bloomfield D, Davachi A. Non-surgical retrieval of a broken segment of steel spring guide from right atrium and inferior vena cava. Circulation. 1964;30:106–8.
2. Uflacker R, Lima S, Melichar AC. Intravascular foreign bodies: percutaneous retrieval. Radiology. 1986;160:731–5.
3. Egglin TK, Dickey KW, Rosenblatt M, Pollak JS. Retrieval of intravascular foreign bodies: experience in 32 cases. AJR Am J Roentgenol. 1995;164:1259–64.
4. Thompson K. Non-surgical retrieval of devices and foreign bodies. Endovasc Today. 2010:29–32.
5. Miller SF, McCowan TC, Eidt JF, et al. Embolization of a prosthetic mitral valve leaflet: localization with intravascular US. J Vasc Interv Radiol. 1991;2:375–8.
6. Bernhardt LC, Wegner GP, Mendenhall JT. Intravenous catheter embolization of the pulmonary artery. Chest. 1970;57:329–32.
7. Richardson JD, Grover FL, Trinkle JK. Intravenous catheter emboli: experience with 20 cases and collective review. Am J Surg. 1974;128:722–7.
8. Doering RB, Stemmer EA, Connolly JE. Complications of indwelling venous catheters with particular reference to catheter embolus. Am J Surg. 1967;114:259–66.
9. Cantor WJ, Lazzam C, Cohen EA, et al. Failed coronary stent deployment. Am Heart J. 1998;136:1088–95.
10. Druskin MS, Siegel DD. Bacterial contamination of indwelling intravenous polyethylene catheter. JAMA. 1963;185:966–70.
11. Prahlow JA, Obryant TJ, Barnard JJ. Cardiac perforation due to Wallstent embolization: a fatal complication of the transjugular intrahepatic portosystemic shunt procedure. Radiology. 1997;205:170–2.
12. Kozman H, Wiseman AH, Cook JR. Long-term outcome following coronary stent embolization or misdeployment. Am J Cardiol. 2001;88:630–4.
13. Kammler J, Leisch F, Kerschner K, et al. Long-term follow-up in patients with last coronary stents during interventional procedures. Am J Cardiol. 2006;98:367–9.
14. Dotter CT, Roesch J, Bilbao MK. Transluminal extraction of catheter and guide fragments from the heart and great vessels: 29 collected cases. AJR Am J Roentgenol. 1971;111:467–72.
15. Curry JL. Recovery of detached intravascular catheter or guide wire fragments. A proposed method. AJR Am J Roentgenol. 1969;105:894–6.
16. Dondelinger RF, Lepoutre B, Kurdziel JC. Percutaneous vascular foreign body retrieval: experience of an 11-year period. Eur J Radiol. 1991;12:4–10.
17. Fischer RG, Ferreyro R. Evaluation of current techniques for nonsurgical removal of intravascular iatrogenic foreign bodies. AJR Am J Roentgenol. 1978;130:541–8.
18. Slonim SM, Dake MD, Razavi MK, et al. Management of misplaced or migrated endovascular stents. J Vasc Interv Radiol. 1999;10:851–9.
19. Yedlicka Jr JW, Carson JE, Hunter DW, et al. Nitinol gooseneck snare for removal of foreign bodies: experimental study and clinical evaluation. Radiology. 1991;178:691–3.
20. Cekirge S, Weiss JP, Foster RG, et al. Percutaneous retrieval of foreign bodies: experience with the nitinol goose neck snare. J Vasc Interv Radiol. 1993;4:805–10.
21. Lassers BW, Pickering D. Removal of an iatrogenic foreign body from the aorta by means of a ureteric stone catcher. Am Heart J. 1967;73(3):375–8.
22. Trerotola S. Textbook of vascular interventional radiology with clinical perspectives. 2nd Ed. Thieme Publishing Group, 2000. p. 612–20.
23. Beathard G. ASDIN Core Curriculum for Interventional Nephrology. 13th Ed. ASDIN (American Society of Diagnostic Interventional Nephrology). p. 53–5.
24. Gabelmann A, Krämer S, Görich J. Percutaneous retrieval of lost or misplaced intravascular objects. AJR Am J Roentgenol. 2001;176:1509–13.
25. Hartnell GG, Jordan SJ. Percutaneous removal of a misplaced Palmaz stent with a coaxial snare technique. J Vasc Interv Radiol. 1995;6:799–801.
26. Greenfield LJ, Crute SL. Retrieval of the Greenfield vena caval filter. Surgery. 1980;88:719–22.
27. Sanchez RB, Roberts AC, Valji K, et al. Wallstent misplacement during transjugular placement of an intrahepatic portosystemic shunt: retrieval with a loop snare. AJR Am J Roentgenol. 1992;159:129–30.
28. Gabelmann A, Krämer SC, Tomczak R, Görich J. Percutaneous technique for managing maldeployed or migrated stents. J Endovasc Ther. 2001;8:291–302.
29. Savage C, Ozkan OS, Walser EM, et al. Percutaneous retrieval of chronic intravascular foreign bodies. Cardiovasc Intervent Radiol. 2003;26:440–2.

Contrast and Medication Allergic Reactions

29

Adrian Sequeira, Zulqarnain Abro, and Kenneth Abreo

Every drug increases and complicates the patient's condition.

—*Robert Henderson, M.D.*

29.1 Clinical Vignette

Mr. Wilson is a 50-year-old male with end-stage renal disease (ESRD), hypertension, and diabetes mellitus type 2 (DM 2). He is referred from another nephrology practice for a clotted right upper extremity AV graft. This is the first time his graft has clotted. He has never had a contrast study before. He denies any history of an allergic reaction to medications. The thrombectomy procedure (declot) including potential complications is explained to him. The initial 30 minutes of the procedure are uneventful. The central vessels are noted to be patent using 15 cc of a radiocontrast agent. However while attempting to pass the Fogarty catheter through the arterial anastomosis, he starts coughing and informs you that he feels his "throat is swollen." The procedure is stopped and you note that his face and the area around his eyes are swollen!

29.2 Introduction

The clinical scenario described above is by no means an uncommon occurrence. It has been estimated that more than 50 million radiographic contrast medium (RCM) administrations are made worldwide each year [1, 2]. With more than ten million radiological procedures requiring RCMs within the USA [3], the probability of witnessing an allergic reaction to contrast agents is certainly high. It is therefore the dual intent of this chapter to expose interventional nephrologists to the clinical manifestations of allergic reactions to contrast agents and provide them with an understanding of its management.

29.3 Classification of Radiocontrast Agents

Tri-iodinated benzoic acid derivatives by nature, RCMs are either monomers or dimers. A monomer contains a single benzene ring with three iodine atoms, while a dimer contains two benzene rings with six iodine atoms. The iodine is responsible for providing radiographic contrast with the surrounding tissues. Depending on their ability to dissociate in solution (thereby producing an anion and a cation), they may be ionic or nonionic. Thus four classes of derivatives are present – ionic monomers, nonionic monomers, ionic dimers, and nonionic dimers. In interventional nephrology, the predominant RCMs used are nonionic monomers (e.g., ioxilan) and nonionic dimers (e.g., iodixanol). Lastly, based on their osmolality (Table 29.1), they are classified as:

1. High-osmolar contrast media (HOCM): These have osmolalities ranging from 1,200 to 2,400 mOsm/kg and are ionic monomers.
2. Low-osmolar contrast media (LOCM): These have osmolalities between 600 and 860 mOsm/kg and are either ionic (dimers) or nonionic (monomers).
3. Iso-osmolar contrast media (IOCM): These have an osmolality (290 mOsm/kg) close to the plasma osmolality and are nonionic dimers.

Table 29.1 Classification of contrast agents

Classification	Contrast agent
High-osmolar agents (ionic monomers)	Iothalamate meglumine (*Conray*)
Low-osmolar agents	
Ionic dimer	Ioxilan (*Oxilan*)
Nonionic monomer	Ioxaglate (*Hexabrix*)
Iso-osmolar agents (Nonionic dimer)	Iodixanol (*Visipaque*)

A. Sequeira (✉) • Z. Abro • K. Abreo, MD
Nephrology Section, Department of Medicine,
LSU Health Sciences Center, Shreveport, LA, USA
e-mail: adrian_sequeira@yahoo.com; kabreo@lsuhsc.edu

A.S. Yevzlin et al. (eds.), *Interventional Nephrology*,
DOI 10.1007/978-1-4614-8803-3_29, © Springer Science+Business Media New York 2014

29.4   Pharmacokinetics

The commonly used RCMs in the interventional suite are chemically nonreactive with very limited protein binding [4]. They are not metabolized and are primarily excreted unchanged in the urine by glomerular filtration [5]. Only 1–2 % is excreted via the gastrointestinal and biliary system. They have a half-life of 1–2 h in those with normal renal function [4]. In those with impaired renal function, 20–30 % of the agent is eliminated by the gastrointestinal and biliary system, and their elimination half-life is delayed into hours. These agents are completely dialyzable in 2–3 hemodialysis sessions [5].

29.5   Incidence

The incidence of reactions varies with the osmolality of the RCM, such that reactions tend to be fewer as the osmolality of the agent decreases. The incidence of mild allergic reactions to HOCM varies from 5 to 15 % [6, 7], whereas with LOCM it is between 1 and 3 % [6, 7]. Moderate reactions to HOCM have an incidence of 1–2 % in contrast to 0.2–0.4 % with LOCM [6, 8]. The incidence of severe reactions with HOCM is 0.2–0.06 % [6], while with LOCM it is 0.04 % [8]. Fatal reactions are thankfully rare and occur at the rate of 1/100,000 with both types of agents [9].

29.6   Classification of Allergic Reactions

Clinically, allergic reactions may be classified based on their severity (Table 29.2), organ system involvement, or timing of the reaction.

(a) Based on the severity of the reaction, they are classified as:
  1. Mild: These are self-limiting and no treatment is required.
  2. Moderate: These can potentially become life threatening and require treatment.
  3. Severe: These are life threatening and therefore need hospitalization.
  4. Fatal
(b) These reactions may also be described based on the organ-specific involvement (Table 29.3).
    An alternative, Ring and Messmer classification [10] involves four organ systems and is used to grade moderate to severe reactions (Table 29.4).
(c) Based on timing, allergic reactions are classified as:
  1. *Immediate reactions*: These occur within the first hour of RCM administration [2]. Immediate reactions comprise two-thirds of all reactions [11] and are classified as anaphylactoid or non-anaphylactoid (chemotoxic reaction) based on their pathogenic mechanisms [3].
  2. *Delayed reactions*: These occur 1 h to 7 days after RCM administration [4].

Table 29.2 Allergic reactions classified based on severity

Mild	Moderate	Severe
Dizziness	Bronchospasm (mild)	Convulsions
Headache	Head/chest/abdominal pain	Cyanosis
Nausea/vomiting	Hypo-/hypertension	Paralysis
Pain at injection site	Severe vomiting	Profound hypotension
Rash/pruritus	Tachy-/bradycardia	Unresponsiveness
Urticaria (limited)	Thrombophlebitis	Cardiopulmonary arrest
Warmth	Cutaneous reactions/ extensive urticaria	Pulmonary edema
Diaphoresis	Facial and laryngeal edema	Arrhythmias

Table 29.3 Allergic reactions classified based on organ involvement

Organ system	Signs and symptoms
Cardiovascular	Hypotension, hypertension, tachy- or bradycardia, cardiac arrest, arrhythmia, chest pain
Respiratory	Laryngeal edema, pulmonary edema, dyspnea, wheezing
Gastrointestinal	Vomiting, diarrhea, nausea, abdominal pain
Neurological	Convulsions, headache, confusion
Skin	Erythema, urticaria, angioedema, pruritus, maculopapular rash
Salivary gland	Parotitis
Kidney	Contrast-induced nephropathy

Table 29.4 Ring and Messmer classification of allergic reactions

Grade	Skin	Abdomen	Respiratory	Cardiovascular
1	Erythema Urticaria Angioedema			
2	Erythema Urticaria Angioedema	Nausea Cramping	Dyspnea	Tachycardia Hypotension Arrhythmia
3	Erythema Urticaria Angioedema	Vomiting Diarrhea	Bronchospasm Cyanosis Laryngeal edema	Shock
4	Erythema Urticaria Angioedema	Vomiting Diarrhea	Respiratory arrest	Cardiac arrest

29.7   Immediate Reactions

29.7.1   Anaphylactoid Reactions

Anaphylactoid reactions by pathogenesis are non-IgE mediated. They are idiosyncratic and unpredictable, occurring independent of the dose administered. They do not require any prior exposure. Majority of these reactions are believed to be secondary to the release of preformed mediators such

Table 29.5 Non-anaphylactoid reactions

Physiochemical properties	Manifestations
Ionicity [3, 5]	Arrhythmia
	Neurotoxicity
High osmolality [3, 5, 18, 19]	Renal injury
	Hypotension
	Tachycardia
	Sickling
	Flushing
	Hyperkalemia
	Pain, warmth sensation
	Pulmonary edema, heart failure
High viscosity [3]	Pain during injection
Iodine concentration [3, 20]	Hyperthyroidism
	Thyroid storm
	Suppression of I-131 uptake

Table 29.6 Risk factors for contrast media reactions

History of allergies: 2–3× increased risk [3, 8, 13, 21]
Pulmonary conditions: asthma (2–6× increased risk) [3, 8, 24, 25]
Heart disease [3, 26]
Hematological conditions: myeloma, sickle-cell anemia [8, 25]
Drugs : NSAIDS, β-blockers, interleukin-2 [8, 25]
History of previous contrast reactions: 3–5× increased risk [3, 13, 22, 23]
Endocrine conditions: thyroid disease, pheochromocytoma [3]
Renal insufficiency [3, 8]
Anxiety [3, 13, 25]

as histamine from basophils and eosinophils and tryptase from mast cells [12]. This release may occur by direct interaction with cell membrane receptors of mast cells and basophils; by the generation of anaphylatoxins (C3a, C5a); activation of cascade pathways such as the kinin, coagulation, and fibrinolytic systems; and complement activation by enzyme induction [13]. Mast cell activation and the subsequent liberation of various vasoactive mediators (histamine, leukotrienes) as well as collagen-degrading compounds (tryptase) can precipitate angina and myocardial infarction that has been named the *Kounis syndrome* [14]. In approximately 4 % of cases, the reactions may in fact be IgE mediated [15, 16]. In these patients, the reactions are severe and anti-RCM IgE antibodies have been demonstrated [13, 17].

29.7.2 Non-anaphylactoid Reactions

These reactions are related to the physiochemical properties of the RCM such as ionicity, osmolality, viscosity, and iodine concentration [3]. They are predictable and dose dependent. Table 29.5 provides an overview of such reactions.

29.7.3 Risk Factors

While these reactions are more common in women [21] and those between 20 and 50 years of age [8, 21], it is the coexisting comorbid conditions in the elderly that predispose them to severe reactions. Risk factors for death include the 4 Ws: white, women, wrinkled (elderly), and weakened (debilitating medical conditions) [8]. A history of a previous reaction increases the risk for a recurrent reaction by a factor of 5 for both ionic and nonionic media [22, 23], while a switch from an ionic to a nonionic RCM results in a 4-fold reduction in the incidence of repeat reactions [22]. Anxiety may contribute to vasovagal reactions which can mimic an allergic reaction [3]. Debilitated and medically unstable patients are

more prone to non-anaphylactoid reactions [7]. Table 29.6 provides a list of risk factors.

29.8 Delayed Reactions

These are T cell mediated and occur 1 h to 7 days after contrast injection. Majority however occur after a latent period of 3 h to 2–3 days [1, 27]. The incidence of delayed reactions is 2–3 % when followed for a week after contrast administration [1]. Since these reactions may occur a week later, other drugs that patients are on or have been initiated later on are usually blamed. These reactions are more frequent with iso-osmolar agents [28, 29]. Manifestations include dermatological, respiratory, or gastrointestinal though dermatological (maculopapular exanthema followed by urticaria and angioedema) manifestations are the most common [27]. Serious reactions occur with a frequency of 0.004–0.008 % [1] and include erythema multiforme, fixed drug eruptions, Stevens-Johnson syndrome, toxic epidermal necrolysis, and cutaneous vasculitis [1]. There is no evidence so far indicating that those with a history of delayed reaction are at risk for an immediate reaction [1, 21]. Rarely, patients may have features of both immediate and delayed reactions [1, 3].

29.8.1 Risk Factors

Risk factors for delayed reactions include women, adults in the third to fifth decades, those on interleukin-2 therapy, and those of Japanese descent [3, 6, 30]. The recurrence rate in those with a previous reaction varies between 13 and 27 % [30, 31]. In fact, on reexposure, a repeat reaction occurs earlier (within 1–2 days) and may be more severe than the initial reaction [1, 27]. Those with a history of allergy have a two-fold risk of such reactions [27]. Reactions appear to be common during the pollen season [27]. Comorbid conditions like diabetes and cardiac, renal, and liver disease also predispose to delayed reactions. Systemic lupus erythematosus patients, those on hydralazine, and bone marrow transplant recipients have been reported to have severe skin reactions [32]. It has been suggested that since this is a T cell-mediated reaction, patients with an active viral or autoimmune disease are at an increased risk for a reaction [1].

29.9 Clinical Vignette

29.9.1 Iodide Mumps

A 60-year-old African American woman with hypertension, DM 2, and ESRD on dialysis with a right internal jugular vein tunneled catheter was referred to the vascular access clinic for a workup for the placement of a vascular access. She has a history of a previous left internal jugular catheter as well as failed accesses in both upper arms. A CT with contrast was done to evaluate the vasculature of both lower extremities. Two hours after the procedure, she complained of painful swellings below her lower jaw. On examination, she was noted to have tender, swollen submandibular glands bilaterally (Fig. 29.1)!

First described by Sussman and Miller in 1956 [33], iodide mumps is characterized by painful swelling of the salivary glands after contrast administration. Onset varies from a few minutes to 5 days after contrast administration

[34]. Other clinical features include photophobia, dyspnea, lacrimal gland enlargement, thyroiditis, and facial nerve paralysis [34, 35]. Ultrasound demonstrates diffuse enlargement of the glands with prominent ducts and increased vascularity [36]. Renal failure is a risk factor. Normally 98 % of the contrast media is excreted unchanged in the urine, while 2 % is excreted from the liver and salivary, lacrimal, and sweat glands [33]. With renal failure, the elimination half-life increases from 60 min to 20–140 h [5]. Contrast media contain a small amount of inorganic iodide and a large amount of organically bound iodine. In renal failure, the retained iodine undergoes deiodination to nonorganic iodide which accumulates in the ducts of the salivary glands and induces inflammation [33, 34, 37]. Treatment consists of analgesics [33] and 2–3 sessions of hemodialysis to remove these agents completely [5, 33] (Fig. 29.2). In patients without renal failure, the reaction may spontaneously subside within a few days. Switching contrast media does not help, and premedication with steroids and antihistaminics does not prevent a recurrence [35]. This condition is not a contraindication for recurrent contrast administration as no serious reactions have been described [33, 35].

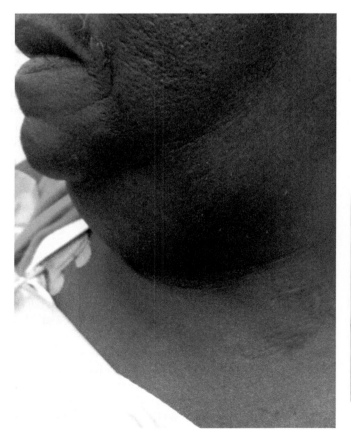

Fig. 29.1 Iodide mumps

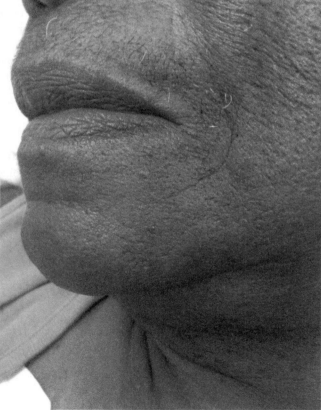

Fig. 29.2 Resolution post dialysis

29.10 Seafood Allergy and Contrast Media

There is a prevalent misconception amongst physicians that seafood allergy predisposes one to a disproportionately higher risk for contrast reactions. How this started is not entirely clear. However, the perception has been around at least since the 1970s. Witten et al. in 1973 and later *Shehadi* in 1975 reported on this association. They reported that 6–15 % of their study population with seafood allergy also had an allergic reaction to RCM. Interestingly, a similar percentage of people with allergies to other food products also had a reaction to RCMs [38, 39]. It is plausible that physicians of their own accord then concluded that iodine was the culprit in these allergic reactions [38]. Iodine is an essential trace mineral, and therefore it is unlikely that people are allergic to iodine itself. The iodine atom while too small to initiate an antigen-antibody reaction might act as a hapten [40]. In vitro animal studies have shown that iodine can induce the formation of iodinated protein antigens under certain conditions and this can generate an immune response [41]. While it is true that a history of allergy or atopy increases the risk of a reaction to RCM (2–3 times that of general population), seafood allergy does not disproportionately increase the risk. In fact, from *Shehadi's* study, 85 % of those with seafood allergy did not have an adverse reaction to RCM [39, 40]. People allergic to seafood have IgE directed either toward parvalbumin (fish protein) or tropomyosin (shellfish protein). Hence people who are allergic to shellfish (crustaceans and mollusks) can eat scaled fish. It is important to differentiate seafood allergy from seafood *intolerance*. The latter occurs after the ingestion of food rich in histamine together with drugs or alcohol that inhibits histaminases. The increased histamine concentration causes a pruritic skin rash, diarrhea, and bronchospasm [42]. Hence patients with seafood allergy should always be questioned about the nature of their reaction. There is also no relationship between contact dermatitis to iodine-containing antiseptics and anaphylactoid reactions to contrast media [40].

29.11 Prevention of Allergic Reactions

> Forewarned, forearmed; to be prepared is half the victory.
> —Miguel de Cervantes Saavedra

The risk of adverse reactions has decreased dramatically with the use of low-osmolar nonionic contrast media. However, adverse reactions can occur at any time even in patients who have no previous history. Hence the dictum in the suite should be "BE VIGILANT, BE PREPARED!" Certain precautionary steps can be taken to minimize this risk, beginning with a focused history. Inquire into the indication for the procedure. In those with a history of a severe reaction, the use of an alternative radiographic modality is justified. Assess risk factors and the manifestation as well as circumstances of any previous reaction. Keep in mind that the etiological differential for a reaction may include other drugs that may have been given during the procedure like antibiotics and narcotics or maybe secondary to the use of latex gloves [43]. A history of a severe reaction and non-cardiogenic pulmonary edema are contraindications to the use of RCMs [17, 44]. If the culprit RCM is known, then utilization of another class of RCMs or a structurally different RCM has been advocated [1, 12, 21]; for example, an iso-osmolar RCM may be used in place of LOCM. An important caveat to remember is that since many of the RCMs cross-react, this may not definitely prevent a reaction [1, 11, 45]. Note the medications the patient is on, as these may worsen some of the manifestations of an adverse reaction. For example, the duration and severity of anaphylactoid symptoms may be particularly prolonged and severe with prior use of β-blockers [3, 46]. Anxiety is a well-known contributor to an adverse reaction. Going over the procedural steps and informing the patient what he or she may encounter during the procedure goes a long way in alleviating anxiety [25]. Once the patient is in the suite, good IV access must be secured. All personnel involved in the procedure should be well versed with the manifestations of various adverse events. It is very important to identify the symptoms early. Mild reactions if not picked up early may progress to more severe reactions. In addition, if noted early, lower doses of resuscitative medications may be utilized to control symptoms and prevent untoward side effects [7]. Since most of the serious reactions occur in the first 20 min after contrast injection, it is important to observe a patient for at least 30 min after RCM administration in order to identify early symptoms of a reaction [47]. A well-stocked crash cart along with other functioning resuscitative equipment and up-to-date basic life support (BLS) and advanced cardiac life support (ACLS) certification of all the members of the interventional team is mandatory.

As the overall incidence of anaphylactoid reactions is low, the American College of Radiology (ACR) has advocated the use of antihistaminics and steroids in those with a history of moderate to severe reactions [12]. However, Bierry [48] argues that premedication should be administered to anyone with a history of a reaction irrespective of severity. The rationale being that in patients with a prior history of a mild to moderate reaction, a severe life-threatening reaction could occur on subsequent reexposure to RCM. The initial study in 1987, Lasser et al. showed that premedication decreases the risk of adverse reactions when used with HOCM [49]. Methylprednisolone was given in two doses, 32 mg PO at 12 h and at 2 h prior to the procedure. This study reported that steroids given as a single dose 2 h before a procedure did not offer any protection. In 1994, Lasser et al. reported that

Table 29.7 Premedication protocols [3]

1. Prednisone 50 mg PO at 13, 7, and 1 h prior to the study + diphenhydramine 50 mg IV/PO/IM 1 h prior to study
2. Methylprednisolone 32 mg PO at 12 and 2 h prior to study with or without diphenhydramine 50 mg 1 h prior to study
3. In an EMERGENCY or when unable to take PO: hydrocortisone 200 mg immediately IV and q 4 h with IM/IV diphenhydramine 50 mg 1 h prior to study. H2 blocker (1 h before study) optional. Use LOCM

Table 29.8 Steps to prevention an adverse reaction

1. Identify at risk individuals
2. Inquire as to the nature of the previous reaction, keeping in mind the differentials
3. Consider other non-contrast modalities that can be used instead of RCM
4. Stop β-blockers if possible prior to study
5. Premedicate with steroids and antihistaminics (H2 blocker optional)
6. Use a structurally different LOCM agent or switch from LOCM to IOCM
7. Use small amounts of RCM and lowest doses when possible
8. Minimize anxiety
9. Be prepared for breakthrough reactions which may be severe
10. Refer to an allergologist

using the 2-dose protocol of steroids also decreased the incidence of adverse reactions when LOCM was used [50]. The study also demonstrated that this protocol should be started at least 6 h prior to a procedure for any benefit. Golberger et al. used a three-dose protocol, prednisone 50 mg given 13, 7, and 1 h prior to a procedure along with 50 mg diphenhydramine (1 h before a procedure) and use of a LOCM in patients with a previous reaction to HOCM [51]. This protocol also decreased the number of total adverse reactions. However, not everyone is in favor of premedication sighting flaws in previous studies on premedication, extra costs and side effects from premedication, delay or postponing of the procedure till the patient has been premedicated, and possibly neglecting appropriate patient evaluation and treatment while premedicated [47, 52]. In addition, breakthrough reactions occur in 10 % of patients despite premedication [53]. These reactions tend to be similar to the original reaction in a majority of patients, but in 10 % of cases the reaction may increase in severity [53, 54]. If the previous reaction is mild, then in 70–90 % the breakthrough reactions are also mild [53, 54]. If the initial reaction is moderate or severe, then in 40–60 % the breakthrough reaction will be of similar severity [54]. Table 29.7 provides a list of the different premedication protocols. H2 blocker use is optional. There are a few things to be aware of on premedication. Steroids have to be given at least 6 h for it to be effective. Steroids have been shown to decrease the number of circulating basophils and eosinophils as well as levels of histamine. These effects are maximal after 4–8 h of administration [55]. In addition, steroids increase functional C1 esterase inhibitor level which inhibits activated factor XII (Hageman factor) thereby inhibiting the formation of bradykinin [56]. Steroids must be used cautiously in those with a history of psychosis and those with a history of acid peptic disease or diverticulitis within the past year [57]. Avoid them in patients with systemic infections [58]. Do not use H2 blockers in the absence of H1 blockers as this may cause coronary vasoconstriction from unopposed H1 stimulation in the presence of a histamine surge [7]. Always use the smallest volume of RCM during a procedure. Table 29.8 provides a brief protocol that can be followed in high-risk individuals. Steroids are of no benefit in chemotoxic reactions [59]. Drug rechallenges and test doses are not recommended as they can be fatal [60]. Patients

may be referred to an allergologist to evaluate if the reaction is in fact IgE mediated [15, 61].

In patients with a previous history of a delayed reaction, avoid the offending agent if known and use a structurally different RCM [4]. However, reactions can still occur because of cross-reactivity between RCMs [4]. It is advisable to refer the patient beforehand to an allergologist so that cross-reacting RCMs may be detected and avoided [1]. Watanbe et al. have recommended the use of IV steroids *after* an imaging study [62]. Romano et al., in 2002, used a combination of 100 mg PO of cyclosporine and 40 mg IM of methylprednisolone daily, 1 week prior to and 2 weeks after a contrast study. No antihistaminics were used [4]. Premedication with steroids and antihistaminics is beneficial in patients on IL-2 therapy [63].

29.12 Treatment of Reactions

If there is any early evidence that a reaction has started, it is imperative to stop the interventional procedure immediately and assess the symptoms. Talk to and reassure the patient. Check vitals and oxygen saturation and ensure oxygen flow. Rule out hypoglycemia. Record the symptoms of the reaction, the amount of RCM given, and the time to the reaction after administration of RCM. Once treatment has been initiated, note the response to treatment as well. Remember many of the treatment protocols require 6–10 L/min of oxygen by mask to be initiated. Epinephrine (1:1,000) is the initial drug of choice in most of the serious reactions. This must be given intramuscular (IM) in the lateral aspect of the thigh. Knowledge amongst radiologists and trainees is surprisingly poor with regard to appropriate management in such situations [64, 65]. In a telephone survey of radiologists from Canada and the USA, none were able to provide the ideal response to a case scenario of a severe allergic reaction, and less than 50 % provided an acceptable administration route,

Table 29.9 Reactions and their management

Clinical diagnosis	Management [7, 12, 21, 23, 25, 65]
Urticaria	
Transient, scattered	Observe (may progress to severe reaction)
	Mark areas involved
	Supportive care
Protracted, scattered	Diphenhydramine 25–50 mg IV/ IM, q 2–3 h
Severe	Diphenhydramine 25–50 mg IV/ IM, q 2–3 h
	Cimetidine 300 mg IV, q 6–8 h
	Adrenaline (1:1,000) 0.1–0.3 mL (0.1–0.3 mg) SQ/IM[a,b], q 6–8 h
	Admit
	Consult dermatologist and an allergologist
Facial or laryngeal edema	Oxygen by mask (6–10 L/min)
	Adrenaline (1:1,000) 0.1–0.3 mL SQ/IM[a,b]
	Airway suction
	Call code team if severe
	Admit
	If facial edema is mild without progression, then observe only
Nausea, vomiting	Diphenhydramine 25 mg IV/IM
Bronchospasm	
Mild	Oxygen by mask (6–10 L/min)
	β2-adrenergic agonist nebulization q 4 h
Severe	Oxygen by mask (6–10 L/min)
	β2-adrenergic agonist nebulization q 4 h
	Adrenaline (1:1,000) 0.1–0.3 mL IM[a,b], q 10–15 min
	Admit
Hypotension with bradycardia (vagal reaction)	Elevate patient's leg
	Oxygen by mask (6–10 L/min)
	IV fluids
	Atropine 0.6–1 mg IV (repeat to a maximum does of 3 mg, q 3–5 min)
Generalized anaphylactoid reaction (severe bronchospasm, hypotension, laryngospasm, angioedema)	Call code team
	Oxygen by mask (6–10 L/min)
	Airway suction
	Leg elevation
	IV fluids
	β2-adrenergic agonist nebulization
	Diphenhydramine 25–50 mg IV/IM
	Cimetidine 300 mg IV, q 6–8 h
	Hydrocortisone 500 mg IV
	Adrenaline (1:1,000) 0.5 mL IM[a,b]
	Admit
For patients on β-blockers, instead of adrenaline	Glucagon 1–5 mg IV and then infusion 5–15 µg/min
	or
	Isoproterenol (1:5,000 solution, 0.2 mg/mL) IV (diluted to 10 mL normal saline). Give 1 mL/min (20 µg) increments

[a]IM to be given in the lateral aspect of the thigh
[b]To give adrenaline IV (use 1:10,000 solution) 1 mL (0.1 mg) under EKG monitoring. Give slowly over 2–5 min, up to 3 mL/dose. Repeat in 5–30 min as needed

concentration, and dose of epinephrine, while 17 % provided an overdose [64]. Hence patients may not be receiving appropriate therapy. Therefore it is useful to have laminated placards of common reactions with drug doses and administration routes available for quick reference (Table 29.9). Patients on nonselective β-blockers may pose a special situation. Epinephrine has both α- and β-agonist properties. β-receptor sites need smaller doses of epinephrine than do the α-receptor regions. When given subcutaneously or slowly IV, the β-agonist property predominates while giving it rapidly IV, and in larger doses, its α-agonist property predominates [7]. Therefore, if the appropriate β-adrenergic response (bronchodilation) is not obtained, the physician may give more epinephrine thereby producing unwanted α-adrenergic effects. Hence it may be better to use isoproterenol (β1- and β2-agonist). Asthmatic patients who are on chronic β-agonist medications will require larger doses of β-agonist medications possibly secondary to desensitization [7]. Steroids generally have no role in an acute reaction except for reducing the severity of delayed symptoms.

Management of delayed reactions is symptomatic as the reactions are mostly mild and self-limiting. Localized reactions may need emollients and steroid creams. However, serious skin reactions will need systemic steroids and antihistaminics. Dermatological evaluation may be warranted.

Once treated, a record of the incident must be made in the patient's chart, and he/she must be informed about the RCM that caused the reaction. Some have suggested the patient wears a bracelet to warn other physicians of such a reaction [47].

29.13 Allergic Reactions to Drugs Used in Conscious Sedation

In interventional nephrology midazolam and fentanyl are used for conscious sedation. This combination is used because of its quick onset, short duration of action, and good potency in terms of pain relief and anxiolysis. While these drugs are safe, they do have adverse reactions that may mimic an allergic reaction.

29.13.1 Opioids

Opioids belong to four different classes [66]. These are:
1. Phenylpiperidines, e.g., fentanyl and meperidine (*Demerol*)
2. Phenanthrenes, e.g., morphine, hydromorphone (*Dilaudid*), codeine, hydrocodone (*Lortab, Vicodin*), and oxycodone (*Oxycontin*)
3. Diphenylheptanes, e.g., methadone and propoxyphene (*Darvon*)
4. Benzomorphans, e.g., pentazocine (mixed agonist/antagonist effect)

When a patient states that he/she is allergic to an opioid, they are usually referring to a pharmacologic action of the opioid that occurred unexpectedly. This occurs in more than 80 % of the cases and is not a true allergy [67]. True opioid allergy is rare [67]. Besides the parent compound, an allergy may also be related to the preservative used [68]. Immune-mediated reactions are IgE or T cell mediated and present similar to RCM reactions.

Patients with a true allergy to a particular opioid should be treated with a non-opioid analgesic or with a structurally different opioid *with close monitoring* (see above classification) [67]. It is believed that cross-reactivity between different classes is low. However, there is evidence that a patient maybe allergic to more than one class of derivatives [69]. Pentazocine is related to morphine, and from a practical perspective, it is useful to consider the first three classes only when considering a substitution [70].

Pseudoallergic reactions secondary to direct release of mediators (e.g., histamine) from mast cells are more common [71]. Codeine, meperidine, and morphine are the usual culprits [67, 72]. They characteristically affect skin mast cells and not those present in the lung. Hence only cutaneous reactions are noted rather than bronchospasm [73]. If respiratory symptoms do occur in an "anaphylactoid reaction," it should be considered an immune-mediated reaction [74]. These reactions are related to the potency of an opioid [75]. Potent derivatives (like fentanyl) are less likely to produce such a reaction as less amount of drug is present at the mast cell membrane [73].

There are a few treatment options in such cases. These include:

- Use of non-opioid analgesics
- Concurrent administration of an antihistaminic with a reduced dose or a slow rate of infusion of culprit opioid [72]
- Use of more potent opioid at a low dose and slow rate of infusion
  - The relative potency of IV opioids from high to low are:
    Fentanyl > hydromorphone > methadone > morphine > meperidine [76, 77].
  - The relative potency of PO opioids from high to low are:
    Hydromorphone > Oxycodone and methadone > hydrocodone and morphine > codeine [76, 77].

29.13.2 Midazolam

Severe allergic reactions (anaphylactic and anaphylactoid) can occur with midazolam, though these are rare [78, 79]. Some of the well-known adverse reactions like laryngospasm, respiratory depression, and respiratory arrest [78] can be mistaken for a severe reaction. Other adverse reactions

include chest wall rigidity and paradoxical agitation. Respiratory depression and respiratory arrest are precipitated when the drug is given rapidly as a bolus [80]. To avoid this, the drug should be given slowly IV over 2 min! [80, 81]. Flumazenil can reverse only some of the adverse effects like laryngospasm, sedation, and paradoxical agitation [81, 82]. In the elderly and those with hepatic and renal impairment, the duration of action of midazolam is prolonged from 1 to 4 h [81]. Consequently, re-sedation and respiratory depression may recur in spite of treatment with flumazenil as its half-life is shorter than that of midazolam [81]. Therefore patients must be monitored for at least 1 h after the last dose of midazolam [83]. Repeated doses of flumazenil may be needed to reverse sedation. Like RCMs, skin testing is required to prove a true allergic reaction.

29.14 Clinical Vignette

29.14.1 Contrast-Induced Nephropathy

A 74-year-old African American male with a past medical history of hyperlipidemia, hypertension, and CKD stage 3 with baseline serum creatinine of 1.5 mg/dL presents to the emergency department complaining of chest pain associated with shortness of breath for the past 3 h. The patient was noted to have new T-wave inversions in II, III, and AVF. Subsequent laboratory testing confirmed a myocardial infarction (troponin I −15.0 ng/mL). Therapy of acute coronary syndrome was initiated which included aspirin, clopidogrel, nitrates, and intravenous heparin. The patient was taken emergently for a left heart cardiac catheterization and received iodixanol contrast. A lesion of the right coronary artery was identified. One drug-eluting stent was placed, and a total of 250 mL iodixanol contrast was used during the entire procedure. After 48 h post cardiac catheterization, the creatinine increased to 2.0 mg/dL accompanied by a decrease in urine output.

What are this patient's risk factors for developing contrast-induced nephropathy (CIN), and what measures could potentially modify those risks significantly? This section reviews the recent literature on acute kidney injury that results from the administration of contrast media.

The administration of radiocontrast agents is a common cause of acute kidney injury (AKI). Contrast-induced nephropathy (CIN) remains the third leading cause of hospital-acquired acute renal failure, after surgery and hypotension, accounting for up to 10 % of all hospitalized patients [84]. This is very important information to know especially for interventional nephrologists, cardiologist, and radiologist who give contrast media on a routine basis when performing procedures. Patients who get these procedures often have advanced chronic kidney disease which places them at higher risk for CIN. Renal failure associated with contrast carries an increased risk of mortality related to complications such as sepsis, bleeding, and respiratory failure [84]. This grave risk of mortality calls for a heightened awareness of the diagnosis and prevention of CIN.

CIN is defined as a sudden decline in kidney function after contrast administration. Typically, the serum creatinine begins to increase by at least 0.5 mg/dL from baseline at 24–72 h after the administration of contrast, peaks at 3–5 days, and requires another 3–5 days to return to baseline [85]. Large doses and multiple injections of contrast media within 72 h increase the risk of developing CIN [85]. The major risk factors for development of acute renal failure after radiocontrast administration include diabetic nephropathy, preexisting renal dysfunction, severe congestive heart failure, volume depletion, hypotension, elderly age group, multiple myeloma, intra-arterial administration of contrast, large doses and multiple injections of contrast within 72 h, concomitant treatment with ACE inhibitors, NSAIDS, or exposure to other nephrotoxins [86]. Preexisting renal dysfunction is the most documented and most significant risk factor for the development of CIN [87].

CIN seems to be related to the agent's vasoactive properties. In animal models, contrast injections initially cause vasodilatation of the renal circulation, followed by potent and persistent vasoconstriction. The persistent vasoconstriction causes renal tubular injury and medullary ischemia. The exact cause of the injury is not well defined but involves several pathogenic factors. The proposed mechanism may include increased vasoconstriction, enhanced endothelin release with increase intracellular calcium levels, reduced production of vasodilator prostaglandins and nitric oxide (NO), increase in oxygen free radicals causing direct toxic injury to the renal tubular cells, contrast-induced diuresis, increased urinary viscosity, and tubular obstruction, all leading to medullary ischemia [88–91].

Clinical presentation of CIN is typically nonoliguric, but in severe cases one can see oliguria or anuria. The urine sediment is usually unremarkable, and the fractional excretion of sodium is usually <1 %, reflecting the prerenal component of injury. The injury can be mild, with transient reduction of renal dysfunction or severe enough to require hemodialysis. Strategies for the prevention of CIN include selection of contrast agents, volume of administration, pharmacologic therapy, hemodialysis or hemofiltration, and avoidance of concomitant nephrotoxins.

Selection of contrast agents will be discussed first in the prevention strategy. In one large study of 1,196 patients, it was shown that patients receiving diatrizoate (HOCM) were 3.3 times as likely to develop CIN as those receiving iohexol (LOCM) [92]. Subsequent meta-analysis of 31 trials also concluded that the use of LOCM rather than HOCM was beneficial to patients with preexisting renal failure [93]. Chalmers and Jackson [94] were first to suggest that there was a decreased incidence of CIN with iodixanol (IOCM). They looked at 124 consecutive patients with renal impairment (estimated Ccr <60 mL/min) undergoing renal angiography, peripheral angiography, or both (half of whom had diabetes) and found that

iodixanol was 50 % less nephrotoxic than iohexol (>10 % increase in serum creatinine levels in 15 % of the iodixanol group vs. 30 % in the iohexol group; $P<0.05$). This was confirmed by a double-blind randomized controlled study of 129 patients by Aspelin et al. in 2003 [95], which suggested that high-risk patients tend to develop less contrast nephropathy by using IOCM, as compared with an LOCM (odds were 11 times lower) [95]. The effect of using high-volume IOCM on renal function in chronic kidney disease patients has also been investigated. A retrospective cohort study that looked at 117 patients with a creatinine clearance <60 mL/min (not on dialysis) concluded that volume did not affect the incidence of CIN when iso-osmolar media were used [96]. The mean dose of contrast used was 84.3 ± 67 mL. The average dose of contrast used in interventional nephrology procedures is less than 50 mL. Kian and Asif et al. have shown that using <20 mL of LOCM during access salvage procedures and venography is associated with a low incidence (4 %) of CIN [97, 98]. The exact mechanism as to why IOCM are less nephrotoxic is not very well understood. It has been purposed that using IOCM causes less of a diuretic effect. HOCM enhance distal delivery of sodium, consequently increasing the workload of the renal medulla causing hypoxic injury in addition to volume depletion [99].

29.15 Minimizing Contrast-Induced Nephropathy

There are techniques proposed for minimizing the dose of CIN, one of which is digital subtraction angiography (DSA). This allows for one to see vascular structures more clearly. DSA achieves this by subtracting all the superimposed objects within the field to get a great image using low amounts of contrast. A second method of minimizing the dose of contrast media is by diluting the contrast agent with 50 % saline. Minimizing contrast use is particularly useful in patients with marginal renal function (CKD3–5) in whom contrast nephrotoxicity can result in the need for hemodialysis.

Several drug interventions have been tested in clinical trials for prophylaxis against the development of CIN. These will be discussed in the following section but have generated few significant positive results and are not widely used. At present, only IV hydration and avoidance of nephrotoxic agents are extensively used to decrease the incidence of contrast-induced renal dysfunction.

Adequate hydration is the most cost effective and simplest way of preserving kidney function. High-risk patients should be given an IV infusion of 0.9 % saline at a rate of 1 mL/kg/h. One must adjust the volume of infusion appropriate to the patient's current volume status and cardiovascular condition. This treatment should be started 6–12 h before the procedure and continued for up to 12–24 h after the radiographic examination has been completed [100]. A retrospective nested cohort study conducted in 518 patients with impaired renal function (serum creatinine levels >1.9 mg/dL) reported that the 76 patients who developed CIN (defined as an increase in serum creatinine levels >0.5 mg/dL over 48 h) had lower blood pressure before angiography and had less hydration before the procedure than 82 matched controls [101]. Similarly, results were seen in a smaller magnitude in an uncontrolled study of 25 patients with chronic renal insufficiency (serum creatinine levels >1.8 mg/dL), who received intraoperative hydration (550 mL/h of 0.9 % saline) and did not developed renal dysfunction [102].

Using IV bicarbonate as an alternative to normal saline has been studied in the prevention of CIN. A single-center randomized trial of 119 patients by Merten et al. [103] showed that the use of sodium bicarbonate hydration was superior to sodium chloride. Rates of CIN were significantly lower in the sodium bicarbonate group (1.7 %, $n=1$) when compared with the sodium chloride group (13.6 %, $n=8$) when both cohorts were administered 154 mEq/L of either solution IV (mean difference, 11.9 %; 95 % confidence interval (CI), 2.6–21.2 %; $P=0.02$). The study authors concluded that using bicarbonate ion is more efficacious than chloride and suggested that contrast-induced free-radical formation (which usually causes an acidic environment) was abrogated by the increased pH in the extracellular fluid induced by sodium bicarbonate. Repeat studies have failed to show any benefit in using sodium bicarbonate including a recent randomized prospective trial [104]. In this study 258 patients with renal insufficiency who were undergoing intravascular contrast procedures were randomized to receive intravenous volume supplementation with either (A) sodium chloride 0.9 % 1 mL/kg/h for at least 12 h prior and after the procedure or (B) sodium bicarbonate (166 mEq/L) 3 mL/kg for 1 h before and 1 mL/kg/h for 6 h after the procedure or (C) sodium bicarbonate (166 mEq/L) 3 mL/kg over 20 min before the procedure plus sodium bicarbonate orally (500 mg per 10 kg). The incidence of CIN was significantly lower in Group A (1 %) vs. Group B (9 %, $P=0.02$) and similar between Groups B and C (10 %, $P=0.9$). This study therefore concluded that volume supplementation with 24 h sodium chloride 0.9 % is superior to sodium bicarbonate for the prevention of CIN [104]. A meta-analysis evaluating the value of sodium bicarbonate as a prophylaxis for contrast-induced nephropathy also showed no significant benefit [105].

There is some evidence that reactive oxygen species play a role in the renal damage caused by radiocontrast agents [106]. N-acetylcysteine (NAC), an antioxidant, can act as a free-radical scavenger. NAC increases nitric oxide (NO) formation by increasing the expression of NO synthase and also increases the biologic effects of NO by combining with NO to form S-nitrosothiol which is a potent vasodilator [107]. NAC has been shown to reduce ischemic renal failure in animal models [108]. Tepel et al. [109] found that the incidence of contrast nephropathy after CT in patients with chronic renal insufficiency was greatly decreased with NAC. Patients were given

1,200 mg of N-acetylcysteine per day, orally in divided doses on the day before and the day of administration of the contrast agent. This prevented the expected decline in renal function in all patients with chronic renal insufficiency (mean serum creatinine levels, $2.4\pm1.3(\pm$ SD) mg/dL; creatinine clearance, <50 mL/min). However, the study was limited by its lack of power ($n=83$) and long-term follow-up. A meta-analysis of the use of NAC for the prevention of CIN was conducted by Kelly in 2008 which showed a very mild benefit [110]. The usefulness of using NAC in clinical practice is a matter of some debate. However, given the association of renal dysfunction associated with increased morbidity/mortality rates and inpatient hospital stays, the use of NAC seems reasonable in the high-risk groups. An oral dose of 600 mg twice daily the day before and the day of procedure is the most commonly used regimen, IV doses of 150 mg/kg over half an hour before the procedure followed by 50 mg/kg administered over 4 h can be used in critically ill patients or in those who are unable to take NAC orally [111]. Other agents have also been investigated such as mannitol, theophylline, furosemide, anaritide (the synthetic form of atrial natriuretic peptide), fenoldopam (dopamine agonist), and atorvastatin for prevention of CIN; however, none of these have shown any benefit.

Removal of contrast media by hemodialysis and hemofiltration after the procedure in patients with preexisting renal failure has also been investigated. These studies have shown no effect on CIN and proven to be unwarranted as a routine clinical practice [112, 113]. Vogt et al. [114] evaluated prophylactic hemodialysis to see if the contrast agent could be efficiently removed, thus reducing the concentration to which the kidneys were exposed, but this procedure showed no beneficial effect compared with using saline hydration alone. Table 29.10 summarizes the strategies for prevention of CIN.

Table 29.10 Steps to minimize radiocontrast-induced nephropathy (RCN)

Prior to procedure
1. Withdraw potential nephrotoxic agents (NSAIDS, diuretics)
2. Hydrate with normal saline (1 mL/kg/h for 6–12 h) or increase salt and fluid intake if not contraindicated
3. Use N-acetylcysteine (NAC) 600 mg PO bid
During procedure
1. Use low or iso-osmolar agents
2. Use low volume of radiocontrast (<20 mL)
(a) Dilute with normal saline when using LOCM (1:1 or 1:3 ratio)
(b) Use small puffs of contrast (1–3 mL)
(c) Utilize digital subtraction
Post procedure
1. Continue hydration for 12–24 h
2. Continue NAC
3. Avoid repeat contrast study within 72 h
4. Check serum creatinine in 2–3 days

Conclusion

The intent of this chapter is to provide a comprehensive review of allergic reactions to commonly used drugs in the interventional suite. As responsible physicians, one must be aware of common and life-threatening presentations and know how to manage them. An ounce of prevention is worth a pound of cure and this starts by knowing risk factors and taking a good history. Vigilance and early interpretation of symptoms during a procedure are required to provide timely care. Patients need to be informed of their reactions and such information must be noted in their charts as well. CIN is another inevitable complication that can occur. Adequate hydration and use of small doses of LOCM or use of IOCM may prevent this complication.

References

1. Christiansen C. Late-onset allergy-like reactions to X-ray contrast media. Curr Opin Allergy Clin Immunol. 2002;2:333–9.
2. Brockow K, Ring J. Anaphylaxis to radiographic contrast media. Curr Opin Allergy Clin Immunol. 2011;11:326–31.
3. Costa N. Understanding contrast media. J Infus Nurs. 2004;27(5):302–12.
4. Guent-Rodriguez RM, Romano A, Brabaud A, et al. Hypersensitivity reactions to iodinated contrast media. Curr Pharm Des. 2006;12:3359–72.
5. Widmark JM. Imaging- related medications: a class overview. Proc (Bayl Univ Med Cent). 2007;20(4):408–17.
6. Thomsen HS, Morcos SK. Radiographic contrast media. BJU Int. 2000;86 Suppl 1:1–10.
7. Bush WH, Swanson DP. Acute reactions to intravascular contrast media: types, risk factors, recognition and specific treatment. AJR Am J Roentgenol. 1991;157:1153–61.
8. Namasivayam S, Kalra MK, Torees WE, Small WC. Adverse reactions to intravenous iodinated contrast media: a primer for radiologists. Emerg Radiol. 2006;12:210–5.
9. Caro JJ, Trindade E, McGregor M. The risks of death and of severe nonfatal reactions with high vs low osmolality contrast media: a meta- analysis. Am J Roentgenol. 1991;156:825–32.
10. Idee JM, Pines E, Prigent P, Corot C. Allergy like reactions to iodinated contrast agents. A critical analysis. Fundam Clin Pharmacol. 2005;19:263–81.
11. Scherer K, Harr T, Bach S, Bircher AJ. The role of iodine in hypersensitivity reactions to radiocontrast media. Clin Exp Allergy. 2010;40:468–75.
12. American College of Radiology. ACR manual on contrast media: version 7. American College of Radiology, 2010.
13. Canter L. Anaphylactoid reactions to radiocontrast media. Allergy Asthma Proc. 2005;26:199–203.
14. Lopez PR, Peiris AN. Kounis syndrome. South Med J. 2010;103(11):1148–55.
15. Trcka J, Schmidt C, Seitz CS, et al. Anaphylaxis to iodinated contrast material: nonallergic hypersensitivity or IgE mediated allergy? AJR Am J Roentgenol. 2008;190:666–70.
16. Laroche D, Namour F, Lefrancois C. Anaphylactoid and anaphylactic reactions to iodinated contrast material. Allergy. 1999;54 suppl 58:13–6.
17. Lieberman PL, Seigle R. Reactions to radiocontrast material. Clin Rev Allergy Immunol. 1999;17:469–96.
18. Rao VM, Rao AK, Steiner RM. The effect of ionic and nonionic contrast media on the sickling phenomenon. Radiology. 1982;144(2):291–3.
19. Aronson JK. "Radiologic contrast media". Side effects of drugs annual 27. 1st ed. Amsterdam: Elsevier B.V; 2004.
20. Nygaard B, Nygaard T, Jensen LI, et al. Iohexol: effects on uptake of radioactive iodine in the thyroid and on thyroid function. Acad Radiol. 1998;5:409–14.
21. Meth MJ, Maibach HI. Current understanding of contrast media reactions and implications for clinical management. Drug Saf. 2006;29(2):133–41.
22. Katayma H, Yamaguchi K, Kozuka T, et al. Adverse reactions to ionic and nonionic media. Radiology. 1990;175:621–8.
23. Morcos SK, Thomsen HS. Adverse reactions to iodinated contrast media. Eur Radiol. 2001;11:1267–75.
24. Thomsen HS, Morocs SK. Management of acute adverse reactions to contrast media. Eur Radiol. 2004;14:476–81.
25. Singh J, Daftary A. Iodinated contrast media and their adverse reactions. J Nucl Med Technol. 2008;36:69–74.
26. Lang DM, Allpern MB, Visintainer PF, et al. Elevated risk of anaphylactoid reaction from radiographic contrast media is associated with both beta-blocker exposure and cardiovascular disorders. Arch Intern Med. 1993;153(17):2033–40.
27. Christiansen C, Pichler WJ, Skotland T. Delayed allergy- like reactions to x-ray contrast media: mechanistic considerations. Eur Radiol. 2000;10:1965–75.
28. Webb JAW, Stacul F, Thomsen HS, et al. Late adverse reactions to intravascular iodinated contrast media. Eur Radiol. 2003;13:181–4.
29. Sutton AGC, Finn P, Grech ED, et al. Early and late reactions after the use of iopamidol 340, ioxaglate 320 and iodixanol 320 in cardiac catheterization. Am Heart J. 2001;141:677–83.
30. Mikkonen R, Kontkanen T, Kivisaari L. Acute and late adverse reactions to low osmolal contrast media. Acta Radiol. 1995; 36:72–6.
31. Yoshikawa H. Late adverse reactions to nonionic contrast media. Radiology. 1992;183(3):737–40.
32. Baert AL. Adverse reactions, iodinated contrast media, delayed. Encyclopedia of diagnostic imaging, vol. 2. Berlin: Springer; 2008.
33. Bohora S, Harikrishnan S, Tharakan J. Iodide mumps. Int J Cardiol. 2008;130:82–3.
34. Christensen J. Iodide mumps after intravenous administration of a nonionic contrast medium. Acta Radiol. 1995;36:82–4.
35. Wyplosz B, Louet AL, Scotte F, et al. Recurrent iodide mumps after repeated administration of contrast media. Ann Intern Med. 2006;145(2):155–6.
36. Greco S, Centenaro R, Lavecchia G, et al. Iodide mumps: sonographic appearance. J Clin Ultrasound. 2010;38(8):438–9.
37. Moisey RS, McPherson S, Wright M, et al. Thyroiditis and iodide mumps following an angioplasty. Nephrol Dial Transplant. 2007; 22:1250–2.
38. Schabelman E, Witting M. The relationship of radiocontrast, iodine and seafood allergies: a medical myth exposed. J Emerg Med. 2010;39(5):701–7.
39. Shehadi WH. Adverse reactions to intravascularly administered contrast media. A comprehensive study based on a prospective survey. Am J Roentgenol Radium Ther Nucl Med. 1975;124:145–52.
40. Coakley FV, Panicek DM. Iodine allergy: an oyster without a pearl? AJR Am J Roentgenol. 1997;169:951–2.
41. Shionoya H, Sugihara Y, Okano K, et al. Studies on experimental iodine allergy: 2. Iodinated protein antigens and their generation from inorganic and organic iodine containing chemicals. J Toxicol Sci. 2004;29(2):137–45.
42. Boehm I. Letter to the editor. Seafood allergy and radiocontrast media: are physicians propagating a myth? Am J Med. 2008; 121(8):e19.

43. Lierberman P. Anaphylactic reactions during surgical and medical procedures. J Allergy Clin Immunol. 2002;110:S64–9.

44. Goldsmith SR, Steinberg P. Noncardiogenic pulmonary edema induced by nonionic low osmolality radiographic contrast media. J Allergy Clin Immunol. 1995;96:698–9.

45. Brockow K, Christiansen C, Kanny G, et al. Management of hypersensitivity reactions to iodinated contrast media. Allergy. 2005;60:150–8.

46. Hash RB. Intravascular radiographic contrast media: issues for family physicians. J Am Board Fam Pract. 1999;12(1):32–42.

47. Liccardi G, Lobefalo G, Di Floro E, et al. Strategies for the prevention of asthmatic, anaphylactic and anaphylactoid reactions during the administration of anesthetics and or contrast media. J Investig Allergol Clin Immunol. 2008;18(1):1–11.

48. Bierry G. Letter to the editor. Management of patients with history of adverse effects to contrast media when pulmonary artery CT angiography is required. Radiology. 2007;245(3):919.

49. Lasser EC, Berry CC, Talner LB. Pretreatment with corticosteroids to alleviate reactions to intravenous contrast material. N Engl J Med. 1987;317:845–9.

50. Lasser EC, Berry CC, Mishkin MM. Pretreatment with corticosteroids to prevent adverse reaction to nonionic contrast media. Am J Roentgenol. 1994;162(3):523–6.

51. Greenberger PA, Patterson R. The prevention of immediate generalized reactions to radiocontrast media in high risk patients. J Allergy Clin Immunol. 1991;87(4):867–72.

52. Dawson P. Adverse reactions to intravascular contrast agents. BMJ. 2006;333:663–4.

53. Freed KS, Leder RA, Alexander C, et al. Breakthrough adverse reactions to low osmolar contrast media after steroid premedication. Am J Roentgenol. 2001;176:1389–92.

54. Davenport MS, Cohan RH, Caoili EM, et al. Repeat contrast medium reactions in premedicated patients: frequency and severity. Radiology. 2009;253(2):372–9.

55. Dunsky EH, Zweiman B, Fischler E, et al. Early effects of corticosteroids on basophils, leukocyte histamine, and tissue histamine. J Allergy Clin Immunol. 1979;63(6):426–32.

56. Morcos SK. Acute serious and fatal reactions to contrast media: our current understanding. Br J Radiol. 2005;78:686–93.

57. Lasser EC. Pretreatment with corticosteroids to prevent reactions to IV contrast material: overview and implications. AJR Am J Roentgenol. 1988;150:257–9.

58. Dunnick NR, Cohan RH. Cost, corticosteroids and contrast media. AJR Am J Roentgenol. 1994;162:527–9.

59. Delaney A, Carter A, Fisher M. The prevention of anaphylactoid reactions to iodinated radiological contrast media: a systematic review. BMC Med Imaging. 2006;6:2.

60. Dawson P. Editorial. Adverse reactions to intravascular contrast agents. BMJ. 2008;333(30):663–4.

61. Caimmi S, Benyahia B, Suau D, et al. Clinical value of negative skin tests to iodinated contrast media. Clin Exp Allergy. 2010;40:805–10.

62. Watanabe H, Sueki H, Nakada T, et al. Multiple fixed drug eruption caused by iomeprol (Iomeron), a nonionic contrast medium. Dermatology. 1999;198:291–4.

63. Zukiwski AA, David CL, Coan J, et al. Increased incidence of hypersensitivity to iodine- containing radiographic contrast media after interleukin- 2 administration. Cancer. 1990;65: 1521–4.

64. Wang CL, Cohan RH, Ellis JH, et al. Frequency, outcome and appropriateness of treatment of nonionic iodinated contrast reactions. AJR Am J Roentgenol. 2008;191:409–15.

65. Lightfoot CB, Abraham RJ, Mammen T, et al. Survey of radiologists' knowledge regarding the management of severe contrast material- induced allergic reactions. Radiology. 2009;251(3): 691–6.

66. Trescot AM, Datta S, Lee M, et al. Opioid pharmacology. Pain Physician. 2008;11:S133–53.

67. Gilbar PJ, Ridge AM. Inappropriate labeling of patients as opioid allergic. J Oncol Pharm Pract. 2004;10:177–82.

68. Fakuda T, Dohi S. Anaphylactic reaction to fentanyl or preservative. Can Anaesth Soc J. 1986;33:826–7.

69. Baldo BA, Pham NH, Zhao Z. Chemistry of drug allergenicity. Curr Opin Allergy Clin Immunol. 2001;1:327–35.

70. Baumann TJ. Therapy consultation. Analgesic selection when the patient is allergic to codeine. Clin Pharm. 1991;10:658.

71. Weiss ME, Adkinson NF, Hirshman CA. Evaluation of allergic drug reactions in the perioperative period. Anesthesiology. 1989;71:483–6.

72. Harle DG, Baldo BA, Coroneos NJ, et al. Anaphylaxis following administration of papaveretum. Case report: implication for Ig E antibodies that react with morphine and codeine and identification of an allergic determinant. Anesthesiology. 1989;71: 489–94.

73. Erush SC. Narcotic allergy. P&T. 1996;21:250–2, 292.

74. Fisher MM, Harle DG, Baldo BA. Anaphylactoid reactions to narcotic analgesics. Clin Rev Allergy. 1991;9:309–18.

75. Blunk JA, Schmelz M, Zeck S, et al. Opioid induced mast cell activation and vascular responses is not mediated by μ-opioid receptors: an in vivo microdialysis study in human skin. Anesth Anal. 2004;98:364–70.

76. Chalverus C. Clinically important meperidine toxicities. J Pharm Care Pain Symptom Control. 2001;9:37–55.

77. Jou D, Shane R. Meeting the JHACO challenge for improving pain management: the Cedars-Sinai approach. J Pharm Care Pain Symptom Control. 2001;9:7–35.

78. Yakel DL, Whittaker SE, Elstad MR. Midazolam- induced angioedema and bronchoconstriction. Crit Care Med. 1992;20:307–8.

79. Fujita Y, Ishikawa H, Yokota K. Anaphylactoid reaction to midazolam. Anesth Analg. 1994;79:811–2.

80. Karch AM, Karch FE. Not so fast! IV push drugs can be dangerous when given too rapidly. AJN. 2003;103:71.

81. Nordt SP, Clark RF. Midazolam: a review of therapeutic uses and toxicity. J Emerg Med. 1997;15:357–65.

82. Davis DP, Hamilton RS, Webster TH. Reversal of midazolam-induced laryngospasm with flumazenil. Ann Emerg Med. 1998;32:263–5.

83. Chudnofsky CR. Safety and efficacy of flumazenil in reversing conscious sedation in the emergency department. Acad Emerg Med. 1997;4:944–9.

84. Tublin ME, Murphy ME, Tessler FN. Current concepts in contrast media-induced nephropathy. Am J Roentgenol. 1998;171: 933–9.

85. Asif A, Preston RA, Roth D. Radiocontrast –induced nephropathy. Am J Ther. 2003;10:137–47.

86. Oliveira DB. Prophylaxis against contrast-induced nephropathy. Lancet. 1999;353:1638–9.

87. Lindholt JS. Radiocontrast induced nephropathy. Eur J Vasc Endovasc Surg. 2003;25:296–304.

88. Brezis M, Rosen AS. Hypoxia of the renal medulla: its implications for disease. N Engl J Med. 1995;332:647–55.

89. Bakris GL, Lass N, Gaber AO, et al. Radiocontrast medium induced declines in renal function: a role for oxygen free radicals. Am J Physiol. 1990;258(1 Pt 2):F115–20.

90. Prasad PV, Priatna A, Spokes K, et al. Changes in intra-renal oxygenation as evaluated by BOLD MRI in a rat kidney model for radiocontrast nephropathy. J Magn Reson Imaging. 2000;13:744–7.

91. Weisberg LS, Kurnik PB, Kurnik BR. Radiocontrast-induced nephropathy in humans: role of renal vasoconstriction. Kidney Int. 1992;41:1408–15.

92. Rudnick MR, Goldfarb S, Wexler L, et al. Nephrotoxicity of ionic and nonionic contrast media in 1196 patients: a random-

ized trial. The Iohexol Cooperative Study. Kidney Int. 1995;47: 254–61.

93. Barrett BJ, Carlisle EJ. Meta-analysis of the relative nephrotoxicity of high- and low-osmolality iodinated contrast media. Radiology. 1993;188:171–8.

94. Chalmers N, Jackson RW. Comparison of iodixanol and iohexol in renal impairment. Br J Radiol. 1999;72:701–3.

95. Aspelin P, Aubry P, Fransson SG, et al. Nephrotoxic effects in high-risk patients undergoing angiography. N Engl J Med. 2003;348(6):491–8.

96. Tadros GM, Malik JA, Manske CL, et al. Iso-osmolar radio contrast iodixanol in patients with chronic kidney disease. J Invasive Cardiol. 2005;17:211–5.

97. Kian K, Wyatt C, Schon D, et al. Safety of low dose radiocontrast for interventional kidney disease AV fistula salvage in stage 4 chronic patients. Kidney Int. 2006;69:1444–9.

98. Asif A, Cherla G, Merrill D, et al. Venous mapping using venography and the risk of radiocontrast-induced nephropathy. Semin Dial. 2005;18(3):239–42.

99. Anto H, Chou SY, Porush J, et al. Infusion intravenous pyelography and renal function: effects of hypertonic mannitol in patients with chronic renal insufficiency. Arch Intern Med. 1981;141: 1652–6.

100. Gleeson TG, Bulugahapitiya S. Review of contrast induced nephropathy. Am J Radiol. 2004;183:1673–89.

101. Brown RS, Ransil B, Clark BA. Prehydration protects against contrast nephropathy in high risk patients undergoing cardiac catheterization. J Am Soc Nephrol. 1990;1:330A.

102. Eisenberg RL, Bank WO, Hedgock MW. Renal failure after major angiography can be avoided with hydration. Am J Roentgenol. 1985;136:859–63.

103. Merten GJ, Burgess WP, Gray LV, et al. Prevention of contrast-induced nephropathy with sodium bicarbonate: a randomized controlled trial. JAMA. 2004;291:2328–34.

104. Klima T, Christ A, Marana I, et al. Sodium chloride vs. sodium bicarbonate for the prevention of contrast medium-induced nephropathy: a randomized controlled trial. Eur Heart J. 2012; 33(16):2071–9.

105. Zoungas S, Ninomiya T, Huxley R, et al. Systematic review: sodium bicarbonate therapy for contrast induced acute kidney injury. Ann Intern Med. 2009;151:631–8.

106. Love L, Johnson M, Bresler M, et al. The persistent computed tomography nephrogram: its significance in the diagnosis of contrast-associated nephropathy. Br J Radiol. 1994;67:951–7.

107. Safirstein R, Andrade L, Vierira JM. Acetylcysteine and nephrotoxic effects of radiographic contrast agents: a new use for an old drug. (editorial). N Engl J Med. 2000;343:210–2.

108. DiMari J, Megyesi J, Udvarhelyi N, et al. N-acetylcysteine ameliorates ischemic renal failure. Am J Physiol. 1997;272:F292–8.

109. Tepel M, Van Der Giet M, Schwarzfeld C, et al. Prevention of radiographic-contrast-agent-induced reductions in renal function by acetylcysteine. N Engl J Med. 2000;343:180–4.

110. Kelly AM, Dwamena B, Cronin P, et al. Meta-analysis of N-acetylcysteine for prevention of CIN. Ann Intern Med. 2008;48:284–94.

111. Baker C, Wragg A, Kumar S, et al. A rapid protocol for the prevention of contrast-induced renal dysfunction: the RAPID study. J Am Coll Cardiol. 2003;41:2114–8.

112. Lehnert T, Keller E, Condolf K, et al. Effect of hemodialysis after contrast medium administration in patients with renal insufficiency. Nephrol Dial Transplant. 1998;13:358–62.

113. Younathan CM, Kaude JV, Cook MD, et al. Dialysis is not indicated immediately after administration of nonionic contrast agents in patients with end-stage renal disease treated by maintenance dialysis. Am J Roentgenol. 1994;163:969–71.

114. Vogt B, Ferrari P, Schonholzer C, et al. Prophylactic hemodialysis after radiocontrast media in patients with renal insufficiency is potentially harmful. Am J Med. 2001;111:692–8.

The Management of Serious Adverse Events Associated with Interventional Procedures

30

Gerald A. Beathard

30.1 Introduction

Interventional procedures have become the standard of practice for the management and salvage of dialysis access dysfunction. In addition, vascular access such as catheters and ports are frequently placed by interventionalists. These procedures are associated with the occurrence of complications. These events can be classified as (1) mechanical complications that are procedure related (PRC), (2) complications associated with sedation/analgesia (SARC), and (3) idiosyncratic or hypersensitivity-related complications (HRC) associated with the administration of radiocontrast and other drugs. It is critically important that the interventionalist managing dialysis access problems be in a position to deal with these adverse occurrences. This means two things – (1) being knowledgeable in complication recognition and management and (2) having the proper equipment and supplies readily at hand to do what needs to be done. For the interventional nephrologist, most of these procedures are performed in freestanding clinics, not attached to a hospital. There is the potential for the occurrence of a complication whose management will require facilities beyond the scope of this setting. It is important, therefore, that a policy be in place within these clinics to avoid these situations to the degree that avoidance is possible by identifying situations where there is a significant risk that the complication might occur. These cases should be referred to the hospital setting for care. It is also important to recognize that there are situations in which the appropriate management of the complication may only entail stabilization of the patient for transport to a hospital setting.

As the title suggests, this review is not intended to be totally inclusive. Fortunately, most adverse events are not of major consequence and their management is generally not complicated. Often it is simply intuitive, e.g., if it is bleeding, apply finger pressure. We will not devote time to these. Others are much more serious and are of such a nature that the patient's life or limb is at risk, specific action is required and action must be immediate. Often, the situation does not safely allow for invention, a definite, pre-rehearsed plan must be already in mind. These are the situations upon which we will concentrate our discussion. Additionally, most of discussion will be from the viewpoint of an interventional nephrologist practicing in a freestanding facility.

30.2 Procedure-Related Complications (PRC)

30.2.1 Introduction

Procedure-related complications (PRCs) can be divided into two categories. Firstly, there are PRCs that represent an adverse event that can be expected to occur with some degree of frequency. The rate at which it can be expected to occur varies with the individual procedure. The actual rate observed can be affected by external factors such as the manner in which the procedure is performed. One can, with the application of good practices, affect the frequency of the adverse event; nevertheless, a background occurrence rate is to be expected. However, the rate should not exceed a defined acceptable norm. An excessive complication rate suggests the need for critical evaluation of techniques and procedures. Secondly, there are PRCs that represent operator error. In general, these iatrogenic adverse events should not occur, yet they do. Some can have a disastrous result if not quickly recognized and managed appropriately. All interventionalists working with dialysis vascular access should be knowledgeable in preventing these occurrences but be prepared in the event that the unexpected actually occurs.

The bulk of the cases performed within a dialysis access center consist of only three categories and their variations – catheter-related procedures (placement, exchange, and removal), angioplasty, and thrombectomy. The latter two

G.A. Beathard, MD, PhD, FASN
Department of Internal Medicine,
University of Texas Medical Branch,
Galveston, TX, USA
e-mail: gbeathard@msn.com

A.S. Yevzlin et al. (eds.), *Interventional Nephrology*,
DOI 10.1007/978-1-4614-8803-3_30, © Springer Science+Business Media New York 2014

procedures are performed on both fistulas and grafts which expands the variety somewhat, but only slightly. Each of these types of procedure is associated with a set of PRCs. The list for catheter-related cases is relatively unique; however, there is considerable overlap between angioplasty and thrombectomy.

30.2.2 PRCS Related to Catheter Procedures

In general, the serious, potentially life-threatening PRCs related to dialysis catheter procedures are mechanical and related to catheter placement. The primary factors determining the development of a PRC during insertion are the experience of the operator [1–3] and the use of real-time imaging techniques [3–6]. Insertion of a catheter by a physician who has performed 50 or more catheterizations is half as likely to result in a mechanical complication as insertion by a physician who has performed fewer than 50 catheterizations [1]. The incidence of mechanical complications after three or more insertion attempts is six times the rate after one attempt [7]. Even in skilled hands, catheter insertion based only on topographic anatomy has been reported to be associated with an incidence of complications reaching 5.9 % [8, 9]. The use of ultrasound guidance during central venous catheterization has been shown to markedly reduce the number of cannulation-related complications [4, 10–16]. In a large, prospective, randomized study of 900 patients receiving internal jugular catheters [12], comparisons were made between patients in whom the procedure was performed using landmark-based techniques and those assigned to ultrasound guidance. The key benefits from use of ultrasound included reduction in needle puncture time, increased overall success rate (100 % versus 94 %), reduction in carotid puncture (1 % versus 11 %), reduction in carotid-associated hematomas (0.4 % versus 8.4 %), reduction in hemothorax (0 % versus 1.7 %), decreased pneumothorax (0 % versus 2.4 %), and reduction in catheter-related infection (10 % versus 16 %). For these reasons, the use of this modality is strongly recommended even for the most experienced operator, many would consider it mandatory.

The complications which we shall address are shown in Table 30.1. It should be noted that a great deal of the information in the literature concerning some of these issues is derived from experience with non-dialysis catheters. However, the principles still apply for our purposes.

Hemorrhage

Some bleeding following catheter insertion is not uncommon, but as a rule it should only be minimal. Even when there is considerable bleeding at the vein entry site during catheter insertion, it is rarely a problem after closure of the incision, although if the patient has a paroxysm of cough, it

Table 30.1 Major PRCs associated with dialysis catheter placement

Hemorrhage
Pneumothorax
Air embolization
Perforation of central vein
Perforation of heart
Cannulation of artery

can result in a hematoma. After the catheter placement has been completed, a persistent trickle of blood from the exit site may be problematic in patients with high venous pressure. In these cases this is generally "tunnel bleeding," or bleeding that is originating at the venotomy site and coming down the tunnel. This can be especially problematic if the patient is sent immediately to the dialysis facility.

Management of Tunnel Bleeding

The solution for tunnel bleeding is to occlude the tunnel. This can be done by placing a bolster dressing over the catheter tract, incorporating the catheter and occluding the tunnel (Fig. 30.1). This is performed by rolling a stack of 3 or 4 gauze 4×4 s into a tight roll which is then placed longitudinally over the catheter tunnel. It is then attached using 2-0 suture on an FSLX needle. This is a relatively large suture (strong) which allows for it to be tied very tightly. The letters FSL (the needle commonly used) and FSLX refer to needle sizes. Both of these are curved needles. Their shape is that of a 3/8 circle. The standard FSL needle is 30 mm in length and the FSLX is 40 mm. It is easier to get around the catheter without damaging it using this longer needle. Holding the gauze roll firmly in place, place two stitches around the bolster and catheter by passing the needle beneath the catheter and then double back and pass the needle in the opposite direction to come out on the starting side. This creates two sutures without cutting the material. The sutures can then be tied together as one. This should be tied very tightly using a surgeon's square knot in order to seal the tunnel. It will not affect catheter function. The suture should be removed after 24 h. This is easily accomplished by simply cutting it over the bolster. It should be noted that this suture is generally somewhat uncomfortable for the patient so it should not be left in place longer than necessary.

Pneumothorax

Pneumothorax (PT) is defined as the presence of air or gas within the pleural cavity, the potential space between the visceral and parietal pleura of the lung (Fig. 30.2). The clinical results are dependent on the degree of collapse of the lung on the affected side. If large, a PT can impair oxygenation and/or ventilation. If the PT is significant, it can cause a shift of the mediastinum and compromise hemodynamic stability.

Unless the subclavian vein is being cannulated (Fig. 30.3), PT as a complication for the placement of a dialysis catheter

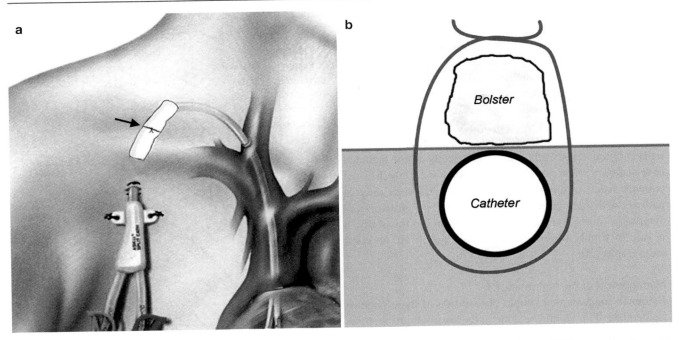

Fig. 30.1 Bolster dressing used to staunch tunnel bleeding. (**a**) Bolster in place over track of subcutaneous catheter. (**b**) Cross-sectional appearance of suture surrounding catheter and bolster

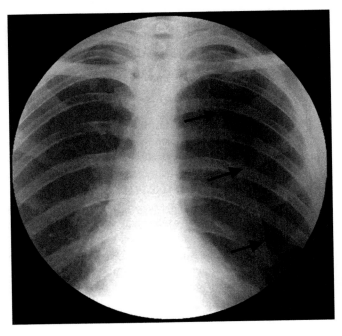

Fig. 30.2 Pneumothorax. *Arrows* indicate edge of collapsed lung on left. Notice the mediastinal shift

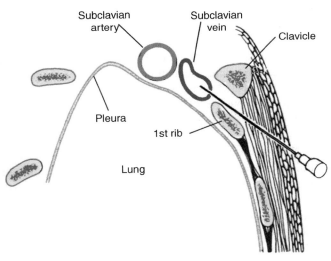

Fig. 30.3 Sagittal view of relationship between subclavian vessels and pleural dome

is not a common event [5], especially if ultrasound guidance is being used. In a report of 1,765 tunneled dialysis catheters placed in the internal jugular vein by nephrologists using ultrasound [17], there was only a single case of PT. A prospective study of 450 cases using ultrasound guidance and internal jugular placement encountered no cases [12]. However, when that rare case does occur, early recognition and appropriate management can be critical [18, 19]. PT can be divided into two categories – asymptomatic and symptomatic. The management of these is quite different.

Asymptomatic Pneumothorax

The symptoms produced by a PT are dependent primarily upon its size. If the volume of air that enters the pleural space is small, there may be no associated symptoms. The condition is recognized only radiographically (if at all). The hemodynamically stable patient with no symptoms is not likely to have pathology requiring treatment. Stated another way, patients requiring intervention will almost certainly have abnormal clinical parameters.

A multicenter, prospective, observational study was conducted that reported on more than 500 trauma patients with occult (no symptoms) PT identified on CT scan, with an initially normal chest radiograph. The study arms included observation versus chest tube thoracostomy. Only 6 % of patients failed observation. This failure was seen only in patients with radiographic evidence of PT progression and symptoms of respiratory distress. According to this study, it is safe to simply observe patients with occult PT on chest radiographs [20].

Management of Asymptomatic PT
Evidence suggests that simple observation of these patients is adequate. This should be done in the hospital setting, however. Oxygen administration at 3 L/min nasal cannula or higher flow in these cases can be used to treat possible hypoxemia (not generally present) and has been reported to be associated with a fourfold increase in the rate of pleural air absorption compared with room air alone [20].

Symptomatic Pneumothorax
If the volume of air in the pleural space is large, symptoms occur and immediate recognition and appropriate management are critical. In most instances, one is dealing with a tension pneumothorax (TPT). This is defined as the accumulation of air under pressure within the pleural space. This compresses the lung, displaces the mediastinum and its structures toward the opposite side, and eventually causes cardiopulmonary impairment [21]. With inspiration, air enters the pleural space, but with expiration it cannot exit. The situation tends to get progressively worse. Symptoms associated with this situation are variable but can be dramatic (Table 30.2).

The usual clinical picture is chest pain and respiratory distress (shortness of breath, feelings of smothering, tachypnea) which can develop suddenly. This is frequently associated with tachycardia. Hypotension and decreased oxygen saturation may also occur; their occurrence is the general rule in serious cases. If the route for air entry into the pleural space is still open and constitutes a one-way valve, rapid deterioration will occur if remedial action is not taken promptly.

Management of TPT
When the clinical situation is such that a TPT is suspected, the first step is to immediately evaluate the ABC mnemonic (Airway, Breathing, and Circulation). One must be prepared

Table 30.2 Symptoms and signs of tension pneumothorax (TPT) [22]

Universal findings	Common findings (50–75 % cases)
Chest pain	Tachycardia
Respiratory distress	Ipsilateral decreased air entry
Inconsistent findings (<25 % of cases)	Rare findings (about 10 % cases)
Low O$_2$ saturation	Cyanosis
Tracheal deviation	Decreasing level of consciousness
Hypotension	Ipsilateral chest hyperresonance

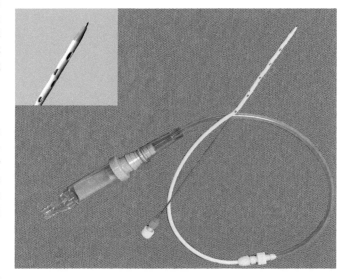

Fig. 30.4 Pneumothorax set (Arrow International), note tip of device (*inset*)

to support these functions. Administer oxygen, ventilate the patient, and establish an intravenous line if one is not already available (the dialysis catheter may serve). Immediate thoracostomy must be performed in any patient who presents with hemodynamic instability or hypoxia [18, 19]. Since immediate, effective treatment may be necessary to save the patient's life, it is essential that the interventional facility has the equipment and supply items necessary to manage a TPT until the patient can be transported to the hospital. Failure can result in rapid clinical deterioration and cardiac arrest. There are several ways that an effective thoracostomy can be accomplished:

Catheter Kit A device that is ideally suited for emergency use is the Pneumothorax Set (Arrow International, Pennsylvania) containing an 18-gauge over-the-needle catheter which is 8 Fr and 16 cm in length (Fig. 30.4). This kit contains the items necessary for insertion and attachment of the catheter to a Heimlich valve. This is a flutter valve consisting of a single piece of soft flexible rubber tubing enclosed in a hard transparent plastic case. When attached to the catheter, it permits only one-way passage (outward) of air.

The use of this device has been found to be very effective in the treatment of TPT [23]. The fact that it is simple and easily inserted is a significant advantage for those not accustomed to creating a thoracostomy. A meta-analysis of studies reported in the literature comparing treatment regimens indicated that this type of device is at least as safe and effective as a chest tube thoracostomy for management of primary spontaneous TPT [24]. The package insert with this device recommends placement in the second intercostal space at the midclavicular line: however, the author feels that placement in the fifth interspace at the anterior axillary line might be safer as explained below (Fig. 30.5).

Thoracic Vent Also available is the thoracic vent (Tru-Close®, Uresil, Skokie, IL). This is a minimally invasive self-contained device designed for the treatment of pneumothorax. It consists of a 13 Fr polyurethane catheter with a removable in-line trocar for insertion. This catheter is connected to a plastic chamber containing a one-way valve. A unique signal diaphragm reflects pressure changes in the pleural space and indicates initial entry of the trocar into the pleural space during insertion. This device is designed to be inserted under local anesthesia, generally in the second intercostal space in the midclavicular line on the affected side [25]. The thoracic vent has also been shown to be very effective in the treatment of TPT [25, 26].

Manual Aspiration In cases in which a commercially available treatment device is not available, the insertion of large-bore needle, sheath, or catheter may be lifesaving as an emergency measure. The insertion of one of these devices is most safely accomplished from a lateral approach at the fifth intercostal space (Fig. 30.5) and the anterior axillary line [27–30]. In a study involving manual aspiration [31], 102 cases of PT following interventional radiological procedures underwent percutaneous manual aspiration of a TPT. Air was aspirated from the pleural space using an 18- or 20-gauge intravenous catheter. After the pleural space was entered (indicated by aspiration of air), the needle was extracted leaving the catheter in place. The catheter was connected to a 3-way stopcock and a 60-mL syringe was used to aspirate air. Manual aspiration was continued until no more air could be aspirated. In 87 of the 102 patients (85.3 %), the pneumothorax had resolved completely on follow-up chest radiographs without chest tube placement. This success rate was subsequently confirmed in a larger series of 243 cases by the same investigators [32].

Standard Intravascular Sheath In the freestanding interventional facility, if a thoracostomy device is not immediately available, an intravascular sheath can be used to effectively treat a TPT. A sheath length of at least 4.5 cm is required [33]. To accomplish this, make a small incision

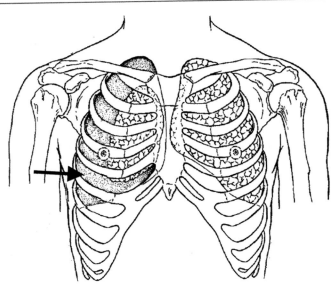

Fig. 30.5 Lateral site for insertion of thoracostomy needle, 5th interspace at the anterior axillary line axillary line (*arrow*)

Table 30.3 Risks of air embolization with catheter procedures

Open needle hub after cannulation
Open dilator after insertion
Open sheath after insertion
Catheter clamp open after insertion
Fractured catheter
Catheter removal in upright position (especially acute catheter)

under local anesthesia over the 5th intercostal space at the anterior axillary line on the affected side (Fig. 30.5). Insert an 18-gauge introducer needle with a syringe attached into the pleural space; entry is indicated by the aspiration of air. Pass the guidewire that comes with the sheath into the pleural space, remove the needle, and insert the sheath. As soon as the pleural space is entered, start backing the dilator out (do not completely remove yet) so as to not injure the lung with the dilator tip. Once the sheath is in, fix it in place with a stitch. Attach a large syringe to the side arm and begin aspirating air. This can be facilitated by attaching a three-way stopcock to the sheath side arm. After the bulk of the air has been aspirated, a finger condom or the finger of a rubber glove with its tip removed to serve as a makeshift one-way valve device can be attached to the side arm. The patient should then be transported to the hospital for observation.

Venous Air Embolism (VAE)

With dialysis catheter-related procedures, there are multiple opportunities for air to enter the systemic venous system and result in a VAE (Table 30.3). This is likely to occur any time there is an open passage for air to pass, and a pressure gradient exists that favors air passage in an inward direction.

In the use of intravenous devices, it is not unusual for a small amount of air to enter the circulation. This is dissipated in the lungs and very rarely produces symptoms. However, death may occur if a large bubble of air (VAE) becomes lodged in the heart or the right ventricular outflow tract stopping blood from flowing from the right ventricle to the lungs.

The two fundamental factors determining the morbidity and mortality of a VAE are the volume of air involved and the rate of its accumulation. It has been shown [34] that a pressure decrease of 5 cmH₂O across a 14-gauge needle (internal diameter of 0.072 in. or slightly less than 6 Fr) is capable of transmitting approximately 100 mL of air/s. This rate of entry will easily exceed lethal accumulation if not quickly stopped. Although the types of needles commonly used for vein cannulation when placing a dialysis catheter are smaller than this (18-gauge introducer needle internal diameter is about 0.035 in. or about 3 Fr), they can nevertheless transmit a significant amount of air very quickly. It should be borne in mind that dialysis catheters are much larger than this (15–16 Fr). Although classical teaching states that 5–8 mL/kg of air can be tolerated, the maximum safe amount in man is not really known. As little as 20 mL of air may show symptoms and 70–300 mL of air has been reported to be fatal [35–37]. With the entry of air into the heart, a paradoxical embolus is always a possibility. It has been observed that only 0.5 mL of air can be lethal when entered into the left side of the circulation [38, 39].

The reported frequency of air embolism associated with use of a central catheter has been reported to range from 0.1 [40] to 2 % [41], with a total mortality rate of 23 % when such an event occurs [42]. The risk of catheter-related air embolism is increased by a number of factors that reduce central venous pressure [41, 43], such as deep inspiration during insertion or removal, hypovolemia, and an upright position of the patient. There is a high incidence of sleep apnea in dialysis patients [44]; with sedation many of these patients will demonstrate loud snoring due to inspiration against a partially obstructed airway. This makes them especially susceptible to an air embolus during catheter insertion. An event that probably poses the greatest risk is the removal of a long-dwelling dialysis catheter with the patient in a sitting position because of a persistent patent catheter tract following removal that is frequent present [45–47]. This is especially true for acute catheters.

Clinical Manifestations

With catheter-related procedures in the interventional dialysis access facility, a VAE is usually small to medium. The clinical manifestations of these are variable and generally nonspecific, often asymptomatic. Signs and symptoms of larger VAEs are also nonspecific and may include the sudden onset of air hunger, dyspnea, cough, dizziness, chest pain, and a feeling of impending death [38, 48, 49]. Tachycardia,

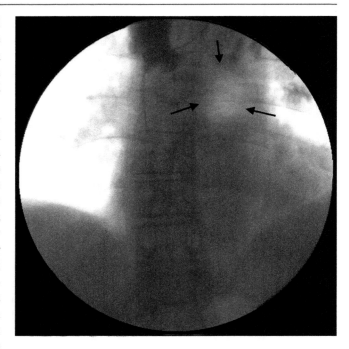

Fig. 30.6 Air embolus (*arrows*) in pulmonary artery

tachypnea, a drop in oxygen saturation, and hypotension are frequently present, and occasionally, a relatively specific drumlike or "mill wheel" heart murmur is heard [38, 48, 49]. A "gasp reflex" consisting of a short cough followed by brief expiration and several seconds of forced inspiration may be observed in some cases and has been described as typical of VAE [50]. This gasp reflex may actually increase the volume of air that embolizes by suddenly decreasing right atrial pressure. With a large volume of air, neurologic symptoms such as altered mental status, convulsions, and coma have been reported to occur in 42 % of patients [38]. Electrocardiographic changes may occur and can include tachyarrhythmias, variable degrees of atrioventricular block, right ventricular strain, and 3-T segment (lead V1–V3) changes [50].

The diagnosis of VAE in the course of a catheter-related procedure is facilitated by the fact that these cases are performed under fluoroscopic observation. In the typical case, chest radiographic findings of VAE consist of radiolucency (air) in the main pulmonary artery (Fig. 30.6) [49]. Air in the distal main pulmonary artery has been described as having a characteristic bell shape [49]. Air in the more distal pulmonary vessels is rarely detected on chest radiographs.

Pathophysiology

When a large volume of air embolizes, the air becomes lodged in the heart or the pulmonary artery, stopping blood from flowing from the right ventricle into the lungs. The major cause of death from massive VAE is due to circulatory obstruction and ultimately cardiac arrest resulting from air trapped in the right ventricular outflow tract [51]. The air that is transported to the lung through the pulmonary arteries can cause interference with gas exchange, cardiac arrhythmia, pulmonary hypertension, and right ventricular strain.

Large emboli may cause paradoxical (arterial) embolization by acutely increasing right atrial pressure, facilitating a right-to-left shunting through a patent foramen ovale or as small emboli passing across the pulmonary capillary bed [52]. This later situation is especially likely to occur in patients with chronic obstructive pulmonary disease who have greater intrapulmonary anatomical shunting than normal subjects [53]. Additionally, if the filter function of the pulmonary capillary network is overloaded due to excessive entry of air, the air can pass on into the left heart and the systemic arterial circulation [42, 54].

Management

It must be kept in mind that the optimum management for VAE is prevention. Care must be taken to avoid the occurrence of such an adverse event. Small VAE may require no treatment. However, the appearance of a small embolus should raise concern and result in an immediate evaluation of the situation to avoid a recurrence or worsening of the situation. A small VAE generally dissipates very quickly.

With a larger volume of air, treatment should be instituted. The first goal of management is identification of the source of air entry and prevention of further air embolization [55, 56]. Secondly (simultaneously), the patient should be placed on 100 % oxygen with a non-rebreather mask [57, 58]. In most cases this therapy alone is adequate. The air making up the embolus consists of 78 % nitrogen (room air). This nitrogen is not metabolized so with an air bubble in the circulation, it tends to dissipate very slowly. A non-rebreather mask delivers a high concentration of oxygen to the patient (60–100 %). This rids the blood of nitrogen, creating a large nitrogen gradient between the inside and outside of the air embolus. In this manner, nitrogen flows out of the air bubble and it shrinks. This generally happens very quickly.

In instances in which the VAE is very large, or in compromised patients, aggressive cardiopulmonary resuscitation may be required [46]. In the past, attempting to relieve the air lock in the right side of the heart either by placing the patient in the Durant position which is the left lateral decubitus position with the head down 30–45° [51] or simply placing the patient in the Trendelenburg position if the patient was hemodynamically unstable was advocated. However, this positioning to optimize hemodynamics has been questioned [59]. In fact, the concept of repositioning the patient at all during a suspected episode of VAE has been challenged by reports from animal studies [60]. There are no data in humans, however. Nevertheless, this maneuver should be regarded as being of little value.

Rapid initiation of cardiopulmonary resuscitation with defibrillation and chest compression has been shown to be effective for massive VAE that results in cardiac arrest [61]. Even without the need for cardiopulmonary resuscitation, closed-chest massage has been advocated to force air out of the pulmonary outflow tract into the smaller pulmonary vessels, thus improving forward blood flow. There is clinical evidence of the efficacy of this approach [62].

Paradoxical Air Embolization

As stated above it is possible for a paradoxical air embolus to occur [42, 54, 63]. Air entering the arterial circulation can have disastrous effects. When an air bubble travels along an artery, it moves through a system of blood vessels that gradually become increasingly smaller. At some point, the embolus will block a small artery and cut off the blood supply to a particular area of the body. The most common symptoms heralding the occurrence of a paradoxical embolus are neurologic [42]. In these instances hyperbaric oxygen therapy has been recommended [43, 64]. Even patients with very dense neurologic deficits may experience reversal of symptoms with this therapy [65].

Perforation of a Central Vein

With the use of a dialysis catheter, there is the possibility of iatrogenic perforation of a central vein or the heart. This problem can be divided into acute and delayed types. The acute event occurs at the time of catheter placement. The delayed version occurs after the passage of hours or days. Either one can have serious consequences.

Acute Perforation

Acute perforation of a central vein has been reported to occur with catheter insertion with an incidence of approximately 0.25–0.4 % [66], but underreporting is very likely. This complication is higher for catheters inserted on the left side than on the right. This risk of perforation is created by the angles that must be negotiated as a device is passed through the central vein on that side in order to reach the superior vena cava (SVC) [67]. The left internal jugular vein joins the brachiocephalic vein at almost a 90° angle, and a similar angle is found between the left brachiocephalic and the SVC. This is in addition to a sharp angulation as the vein drapes over the aorta or arch vessels in the midline. Additionally, the high incidence of central vein stenosis in the dialysis patient may very well contribute to the incidence of this complication in some cases [68].

Sequelae resulting from the perforation of a central vein are variable. Many interventionalists have had the experience of perforating a central vein and having no adverse effect. This may be due in part to the low pressure within the right atrium and SVC (2–6 mmHg and even lower if patient is hypovolemic) and the fact that the perforation was high in the SVC or in brachiocephalic (above the pericardial reflection). However, perforation can lead to bleeding either into

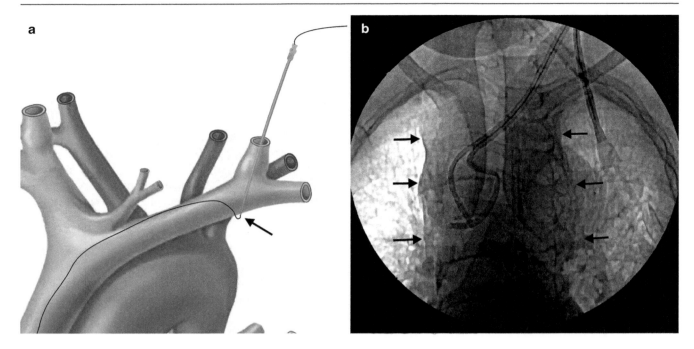

Fig. 30.7 Dialysis catheter placed blindly resulting in hemo-mediastinum. (**a**) Mechanism of adverse event (*arrow*). (**b**) Catheter in mediastinum, note widening of mediastinum (*arrows*)

the pleural space or into the mediastinum [68–73]. The upper half of the SVC is covered by mediastinal connective tissue. In this region perforation can result in hemo- or hydrothorax/mediastinum [66] (Fig. 30.7). Life-threatening cardiac tamponade may result if a catheter perforates the right heart or that part of the SVC that is within the pericardial space (below the pericardial reflection).

With large-bore hemodialysis catheters, injuries may cause voluminous bleeding leading to hemodynamic instability, hypovolemic shock, and even death [68, 70, 74, 75]. Serious damage to the central veins can result from failure to use the large-bore vein dilators properly when preparing a cannulation site for the insertion of the dialysis catheter. To be safe, the dilator must follow the course of the guidewire into and down the central vein. This path is not completely straight, even on the right side. Initially, it angles downward as one enters the vein and then turns caudally following the path of the central vein (much more circuitous than this on the left). Additionally, because of the close proximity of the patient's neck and head to the entry site, there is a tendency for the operator to angle the proximal end of the dilator outward. Because of these issues, the guidewire can become kinked and instead of the serving as a track to direct the passage of the device, it is advanced with it. If the tip of the dilator is pressing against the side of the vein, the advancing guidewire can act as a blade (Fig. 30.8), slicing the vein as it moves along its course [70].

Normally, when a large-bore dilator is used to dilate the vein entry site, some degree of force is required to pass the device through superficial structures and the vein wall into

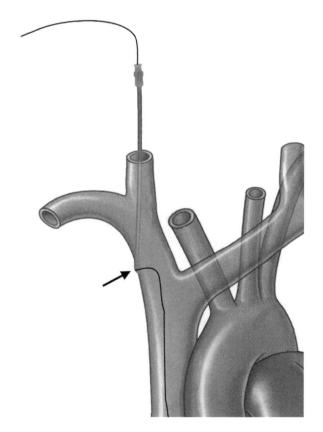

Fig. 30.8 Kinked guidewire. Guidewire is kinked and pressed against vein wall (*arrow*) becoming a blade

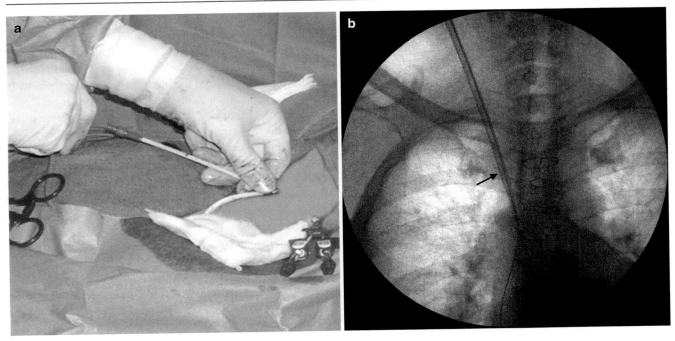

Fig. 30.9 Practices for safe passage of dilators for catheter insertion. (**a**) Assuring that guidewire is not advancing with dilator. (**b**) Direct fluoroscopic visualization

the lumen of the target vessel. If the guidewire is kinked, this force is being applied toward destruction of the vein. The result can be disastrous.

Actually, for a successful catheter insertion, it is necessary for the dilator to only be passed just far enough into the vein to dilate it. This requires only a few centimeters. If it is advanced considerable beyond this point, damage to the vein is more likely to occur and be much worse if it does occur.

In a retrospective review of 4,000 [76], 10 patients had a vascular perforation, an incidence of 0.25 %. Operator error was the primary cause of the problem; the injury was caused by kinking of the guidewire followed by forcing the vessel dilator or peel-away sheath into the central vein. The initial error, kinking of the guide wire, was the result of the operator's failure to firmly hold and stabilize the guidewire while advancing the vessel dilator. Of these ten cases, four were fatal.

This problem can be prevented by checking free passage of the guidewire in and out of the dilator repeatedly during insertion (Fig. 30.9). Additionally, direct observation under fluoroscopy will alert the operator to any untoward dilator-guidewire interaction. Careful attention to these two issues can prevent the occurrence of this problem.

Delayed Perforation

Some cases of vascular perforation (usually the SVC) are delayed and occur hours to days after catheter insertion [77–80], 3 days or more after the procedure in 41 % of patients [81]. Left-sided catheter placement and large-bore catheters are reported to be risk factors for delayed vascular

perforations [82, 83]. In a review of 2,992 catheters [84] (non-dialysis), an incidence of 0.17 % was observed with a mean time to onset of symptoms of 3.6 days following catheter insertion. The most common clinical symptoms and diagnostic findings were dyspnea, new or rapidly progressive pleural effusions, chest pain with radiation to the left or right shoulder, hypotension, coughing, fever, and mediastinal widening. It is of interest that delayed perforation is associated with a higher incidence of hydrothorax, in contrast to hemothorax, which is more commonly found when perforation occurs at the time of catheter insertion (acute) [85].

Delayed perforation of the SVC is almost exclusively a left-sided catheter placement problem. Because of the horizontal orientation of the left brachiocephalic vein and its 90° junction with the SVC, catheters introduced via the left jugular vein must turn an acute angle to enter the SVC. If the catheter is too short to extend well beyond this curve, its tip may impinge upon the lateral wall of the vein (Fig. 30.10). Catheter tip impingement is regularly observed in left-sided catheters with their tip positioned in the upper SVC [85–87]. It has been reported that a chest X-ray frequently shows a horizontal catheter with a gentle curve at the tip before clinical or radiographic recognition of perforation in many of these cases [88]. Continuous catheter motion can be observed on fluoroscopy during the respiratory and cardiac cycles. Associated with tenting of the vessel wall from the catheter tip, this results in continuous mechanical irritation and injury [89, 90]. This is in contrast to the catheter that runs parallel with the vessel wall if the tip is positioned in the lower SVC [85–87].

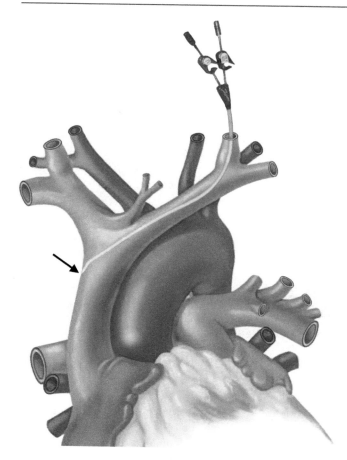

Fig. 30.10 Catheter tip impingement on wall of SVC (*arrow*) creating a risk for perforation

of the device involved and whether the perforation is into the pleural space or into the mediastinum. If it is only the needle, there are usually no ill effects and no treatment is required. One may not even recognize that it has occurred, unless the guidewire is passed into the pleural space. Even then, withdrawal is frequently not followed by adverse changes.

With a larger device such as a dilator, management will depend on the extent of the injury, general status of the patient and efficiency of the patient's clotting system [71]. It should be remembered that the removal of the offending device can result in massive hemorrhage requiring surgical intervention which cannot be accomplished in a freestanding facility. Passage into the mediastinum may result in a hematoma that may be self-limiting. Passage into the pleural space can result in a hemothorax (or a pneumothorax, if the device is open to the air). However, one can never be sure what will happen once the device is removed leaving a large defect in the vein. It is better to leave the device in place and transfer the patient to a hospital setting where it can be removed with surgical support available. Detailed diagnostic imaging procedures should be performed. Removal of the offending object can result in massive hemorrhage requiring an exploratory thoracotomy to repair the defect [74, 92] although there are reports of endovascular management of such an injury [71, 93]. In one case report [93], the perforation site was repaired using a stent graft. In this instance the stent graft was placed through a femoral approach prior to withdrawal of the catheter. If the event results in a large defect as can occur in the situation depicted in Fig. 30.8, it is almost uniformly fatal.

As with acute perforations, detailed diagnostic imaging procedures should be performed when delayed perforation is suspected. The management must be individualized depending upon the extent of the injury and general status of the patient. Although in some cases the catheter can be simply removed [94], an exploratory thoracotomy to repair the defect [74, 92] is frequently required for these vascular perforations.

Most cases of delayed vascular preformation involve the SVC. However, with the insertion of catheters in the lower extremity, delayed perforation can also occur following femoral vein catheter placement leading to severe hemorrhage and retroperitoneal hematoma formation [91].

Management of Central Vein Perforation

Since this is a complication that is generally related to operator error, the most effective step in management is to take precautions to avoid it. The use of ultrasound-guided cannulation is very important. Blind cannulation should be avoided. Good practices in the use of guidewires and dilators plus use of fluoroscopic observation (Fig. 30.9) will go a long way toward eliminating this as an acute problem. With newer materials being used for catheter manufacturing, delayed perforation is very uncommon, but still possible. The selection of an appropriate catheter length is also important in prevention.

Since the effects of central vein perforation are variable, the management will also be variable and largely dependent upon observation of changes in the individual patient. The sequelae of perforation are largely dependent upon the size

Cardiac Perforation

In addition to central vein perforation, there is a risk of cardiac perforation with the insertion of a catheter. This is the most deadly of the complication associated with central venous catheters. This event has been observed primarily with the insertion of catheters that are longer than necessary for a right internal jugular insertion and are somewhat rigid (but not always). In the dialysis patient, this relates primarily to the use of acute (non-tunneled) catheters. When this problem occurs, it results in cardiac tamponade and the consequences are frequently fatal [95] especially those involving the atrium [96]. The exception has been in cases in which the patient was in the surgical suite on the operating table at the time of occurrence [97].

This problem can occur early as a result of operator error during the insertion procedure or late as a result of vascular injury from the catheter tip eroding through the myocardium [98]. Cardiac tamponade has been reported 24 h or more catheter placement in 50 % of patients who have had the complication [99, 100]. This delay is generally thought to be related to the placement of a catheter that was too long, was not well secured, and was inadvertently advanced during the course of its use.

Delayed complications have a high mortality, frequently due to late identification of the problem. The mortality rate of cardiac tamponade in these situations has ranged from 44 to 77 % [99]. In a review of eight cases of cardiac perforation (non-dialysis catheters), it was noted that although right ventricular perforations detected early had a relatively benign course, those detected late and those that involved right atrial perforations required emergent surgical exploration and often have catastrophic consequences [96].

In a review of 23 cases of cardiac perforation (non-dialysis catheters), 22 patients developed cardiac tamponade. Seventeen patients developed cardiac tamponade during the process of catheter placement, and five were found at 2–14 h after the procedure. Pericardiocentesis and pericardial catheter drainage were performed in 20 patients and 11 were successful. Among the other 11 patients with tamponade, 7 had a successful thoracotomy and 4 died [101].

In another review of 25 cases of cardiac tamponade from central venous catheters [102], it was found that all patients developed unexplained hypotension from hours to 1 week after catheter placement. Pulmonary symptoms were common. Eight patients complained of chest tightness, 12 of shortness of breath, and 15 were noted to have air hunger up to 6 h prior to the occurrence of significant changes in vital signs. Fourteen patients (56 %) developed tachycardia and eight patients (32 %) were noted to be bradycardic. In 22 cases the catheters were "stiff" and 3 were Silastic. The site of catheter erosion could be determined for 80 %. Fifteen occurred in the right atrium, four in the right ventricle, and one at the intrapericardial junction of the superior vena cava and right atrium. Post-insertion chest radiographs were available for review in 22 cases. The tip of the catheter was in the right atrium in 15, the right ventricle in 2, at the junction of the superior vena cava and right atrium in 2, and at the junction of the right atrium and right ventricle in 3. One catheter followed a markedly abnormal course across the heart. All of the catheters were within the pericardial silhouette on chest radiograph. Eighty percent of the patients died, and 12 % remained in a persistent vegetative state as a direct result of the tamponade. Only 2 patients (8 %) survived without any neurologic residual.

In 1989, the FDA published a precautionary statement regarding the positioning of central venous catheters that states that "the catheter tip should not be placed in or allowed to migrate into the heart" [103, 104]. In 2006, the NKF/KDOQI practice guidelines recommend that acute catheters be placed with their tip in the SVC and that the position should be verified radiographically [105].

Unfortunately, the SVC-atrial junction cannot be accurately identified fluoroscopically, and the length of the SVC is quite variable. In an anatomical study based upon preserved adult cadavers, it was found that the median length of the SVC was 61 mm, but the range was 46–111 mm [66]. Of significance to cardiac tamponade from SVC perforation is the fact that the pericardial reflection onto the SVC is also variable. This same study found that the median intrapericardial part of the medial SVC was 32.5 mm with a range of 18–54 mm and the lateral SVC was 20.5 mm with a range of 8–44 mm [66]. Because of these individual anatomical variations, the exact catheter length that should be used cannot be stated with absolute certainty; however, the author feels that a good estimate of the location of the SVC-atrial junction can be obtained by moving down the lateral cardiac silhouette approximately one-third. To be safe, an acute dialysis catheter placed in the right internal jugular should not exceed 15–16 cm in length.

The catheter material and its stiffness are also risk factors for vascular damage [106–109]. The majority of vascular and cardiac perforations related to central venous catheters were reported at a time when catheter material was relatively stiff and more rigid than today [110]. Additionally, imaging guidance during insertion procedures was not generally used. The availability of softer catheter materials such as silicone and polyurethane has substantially decreased the likelihood of this complication [111]. Nevertheless, catheter-related vascular erosions with catheters constructed of polyurethane have been reported [83, 112]. This suggests that vascular damage and subsequent perforation can occur with any catheter if the distal tip is positioned against a vascular wall [113]. Any patient with a central venous catheter who develops unexplained hypotension, air hunger, shortness of breath, or chest tightness should have cardiac tamponade included in their differential diagnosis [102].

Arterial Perforation

Mechanical complications from catheter-related cervicothoracic arterial injury (CRCAI) due to the misplacement of large-caliber devices associated with central vein catheter placement have been reported to have an incidence of 0.1–0.8 % [114]. These complications include hematoma, which can potentially expand and obstruct the airway [115], hemothorax [116, 117], pseudoaneurysm [117], arteriovenous fistula [118], and stroke [114, 119].

The problem generated by perforation of an artery during the insertion of a dialysis catheter is largely dependent upon the point in the procedure in which the event occurs.

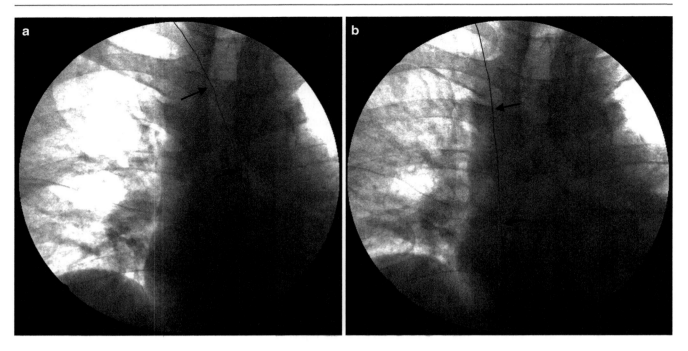

Fig. 30.11 Position of guidewires (*arrows*). (**a**) Guidewire in carotid, extending into aorta. (**b**) Guidewire in internal jugular extending into vena cava (guidewires enhanced for illustration)

In general, this event has to be initiated by insertion of the cannulation needle into the artery. In most instances this is immediately recognized because of the appearance of pulsatile red blood from the hub of the needle. The risk of this occurrence is markedly decreased, but not totally eliminated, by the use of ultrasound-guided cannulation [120].

Many interventionalists use a 21-gauge needle (Micropuncture® Introducer Set, Cook Medical, Bloomington, IN) for cannulation. Removing such a small needle from a carotid artery and applying external pressure to prevent hemorrhagic complications is a common management approach, and the event is inconsequential in most cases [1, 121, 122]. It is probable that this occurrence is frequently not reported in the medical record and is underreported in the literature. As a result, very few cases of major complications related to needles in carotid arteries or the aorta have been reported [114, 123, 124]. In these cases, inadvertent carotid puncture occurred with a larger-gauge needle and was treated by external compression for 3–15 min. Many of these patients had significant carotid atherosclerotic plaque and presented with an embolic stroke within the first 48 h post-procedure.

Even insertion of a guidewire is generally not a problem; it can be removed in most cases without any adverse sequelae as long as external pressure is applied for several minutes to prevent the formation of a hematoma. It is important to be able to recognize the characteristic appearance of a guidewire that has entered the carotid and is passing into the arch of the aorta (Fig. 30.11) so that the procedure can be stopped at this point before a larger device is introduced.

The nature of the situation changes once one has gone beyond the guidewire insertion point. With the insertion of a dilator, the defect created in the artery can be very problematic if not handled properly. The low internal jugular vein approach that is commonly used for the catheter insertion procedure can injure not only the carotid artery but also the subclavian or brachiocephalic vessels and even the aorta [125]. Subclavian approaches can also injure the aorta, common carotid, or brachiocephalic artery.

Two different approaches to these arterial injuries have been taken: (1) removal of the device, followed by the application of local pressure, and (2) immediate direct surgical or endovascular arterial repair. The first of these can be problematic. Although the usual target vein runs in parallel to the artery, if the arterial injury is remote from the intended access venous site, its location may preclude effective external pressure to tamponade the bleeding from the puncture.

In a retrospective study, two groups of patients with CRCAI were analyzed [120]. The first group consisted of 13 patients who were treated in the study institutions. Five of these underwent immediate catheter removal and compression, and all had severe complications. One case experienced a major stroke and died. The other four of the five cases required intervention either for massive bleeding or for a false aneurysm. The remaining eight patients were treated immediately for the arterial injury without complications by either an open repair (six) or through an endovascular approach (two). The second group of patients reviewed in this study consisted of 30 cases derived from the published medical literature used for comparison. Of these, 17 were treated by immediate catheter removal and direct external pressure. Eight (47 %) of these had major complications requiring further interventions and two died. The remaining 13 patients were treated by immediate surgical exploration, catheter removal and artery repair under direct vision, without any complications.

Under no circumstances should prolonged arterial cannulation be tolerated. Several cases have been described with thrombus found at the site of the arterial injury, especially after prolonged catheterization. Heparinization should be considered if immediate treatment is not possible [120].

Management

As is the case with the other categories of complications listed above, prevention is an extremely important aspect of the CRCAI issue. The use of ultrasound guidance with cannulation and paying attention to the course followed by guidewires as they are passed under direct fluoroscopic observation (Fig. 30.11) is very important. Blood flow (backflash) through a micropuncture needle also may be useful. Blood will rarely independently back up through a disconnected 21-gauge needle when it is within a vein. If backflow is observed, arterial entry should be considered. The color of the blood is also a helpful guide, unless the patient is very hypoxic (check the pulse oximeter), arterial blood will be bright red, unlike the darker color typical of venous blood. Careful attention to these points should eliminate most of these problems.

If the puncture injury is small (<7 Fr) the pull and pressure method is reasonable as long as the arterial site is in a location where effective pressure can be applied. Pressure should be applied for 20 min and the patient should be monitored (for a minimum of 1 h) for hematoma formation [120]. This may not be effective; however, once the device is removed, direct pressure is difficult to place on the arterial entry site because it is often distal to the skin puncture site. Additionally, the patient may become very uncomfortable with the pressure required to compress the artery. Unfortunately, adequate compression in the cervical area for larger defects is not possible without jeopardizing cerebral perfusion. In these cases, an enlarging hematoma after the removal of a misplaced dilator or catheter can occur. This can expand rapidly and result in airway compression requiring difficult emergent intubation [116, 126].

If the device causing the injury is 7 Fr or greater, then it should be left in place. Vascular surgery consultation should be sought and the patient transferred to the hospital. In the past, treatment was exclusively surgical; however, more recently, endovascular techniques, with the placement of a stent graft or a percutaneous arterial closure device, have been reported [127]. These options are ideal for arterial trauma sites in the proximal carotid and subclavian artery.

Arterial trauma below the sternoclavicular joint should not be repaired through a cervical approach. Clinical suspicion of these low injuries should prompt preoperative imaging to clarify the injury site and aid in the development of an appropriate treatment plan [120].

30.2.3 PRCS Related to Arteriovenous Access Procedures

When dealing with an arteriovenous access (synthetic grafts and arteriovenous fistulas) problems, there are two procedures that are commonly performed that can result in significant adverse events – angioplasty and thrombectomy. The most frequent procedure-related complication seen in association with angioplasty that dictates the need for intervention is venous rupture. The same is true for thrombectomy with the addition of arterial embolization. Although rare, symptomatic pulmonary embolism can also occur [128].

Venous Rupture

The most frequent PRC seen in association with angioplasty that requires intervention is venous rupture. Although some investigators have reported an alarmingly high incidence of vein rupture in association with angioplasty treatment of autologous fistulae [129, 130], in other reports the occurrence has been relatively low [17, 131–134], generally 2 % or less. In a series of 1,222 cases with dysfunctional hemodialysis grafts, angioplasty-induced vascular ruptures occurred in 24 (2.0 %) [133]. In another report of 1,796 angioplasty procedures, an overall complication rate (all types) of 2.4 % (44 cases) was seen. This series was composed of 73 % synthetic grafts (1,311 cases with a 1.8 % complication rate) and 27 % autologous fistulae (485 cases with a 4.1 % complication rate). Seventy percent of these complications (34 cases) were vein rupture of some degree [17].

Venous rupture appears to be more commonly associated with the treatment of fistulas than with grafts [129, 135]. In a series of 75 instances of vein rupture in 1,985 hemodialysis interventions [135], this problem occurred more often in fistulas (5.6 % of 693) as a group than in grafts (2.8 % of 1,292). Transposed fistulas were more problematic (10.7 % of 187) than non-transposed ones (3.8 % of 506). Actually, when only non-transposed fistulas were compared to grafts, there was no difference. The terminal arch of the cephalic vein (cephalic arch) is a venous site that is especially susceptible to rupture [129, 131, 136]. It has been reported that the incidence of venous rupture is higher in female patients than in males, one study finding a 2:1 ratio [135].

The clinical significance of this complication varies considerably, ranging from none to a loss of the access. The difference lies in the severity of the rupture and the success of the management. The presence of this complicating event is

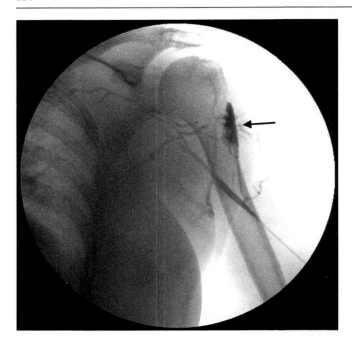

Fig. 30.12 Subclinical extravasation of contrast (*arrow*)

Table 30.4 Extravasation classification

Subclinical extravasation of contrast (SEC)
No associated hematoma[a]
Only evident on fluoroscopy
Grade 1 hematoma
Does not interfere with flow[a]
Size variable
Requires no therapy
Stable[a]
Grade 2 hematoma
Slows or stops flow[a]
Size variable
Therapy required
Stable[a]
Grade 3 hematoma (vein disruption)
Large extravasation or hematoma
Size variable, generally large
Continues to expand may be rapid[a]
Pulsatile[a]

[a]Denotes defining feature

Table 30.5 Managing extravasation

Subclinical extravasation of contrast
No treatment required
Grade 1 hematoma
Symptomatic management of symptoms
Grade 2 hematoma
Restore lumen with prolonged balloon dilatation (primary)
Endovascular stent (secondary)
Grade 3 hematoma (vein disruption)
Endovascular stent (primary)
Occlude access (secondary)

heralded by the extravasation of radiocontrast, blood, or both. As soon as the occurrence of a venous rupture has been recognized, the access should be manually occluded to arrest further extravasation until an evaluation of the situation has been completed [137].

Some of the clinical problems occur when the extravasation that occurs is associated with the formation of a hematoma. A classification system has been devised for extravasation (Table 30.4). This is based primarily upon clinical significance of the hematoma [138, 139].

Subclinical Extravasation of Contrast (SEC)

An SEC simply represents the extravasation of a small amount of radiocontrast at the site of the dilatation: there is no associated hematoma (Fig. 30.12, Table 30.4). These small extravasations are of no clinical significance. It is not unusual to observe a small ecchymosis over the treated site the day following therapy making it obvious that a small, subclinical extravasation of blood has occurred. Although there may be a slight degree of tenderness, an SEC is generally asymptomatic and only obvious on fluoroscopy.

Management

The SEC is of no consequence and may be totally missed except by the patient who may not mention it. Nothing need be done for these cases except to reassure the patient (Table 30.5).

Grade 1 Hematoma

A grade 1 hematoma is stable, e.g., not continuing to grow, and does not affect flow (Fig. 30.13, Table 30.4). It is of no

real consequence to the outcome of the procedure. This is true regardless of its size. In general, a hematoma that remains stable over 30 min to an hour period will continue to behave in this manner as long as the downstream vascular drainage is patent. This is the most common complication associated with venous angioplasty [17].

Management

Since the condition is stable and flow is not affected, no specific treatment is required for a grade 1 hematoma. The area may be moderately tender, and the patient may experience some mild pain, more intense symptoms are uncommon. The patient may benefit from symptomatic measures, however (Table 30.5).

Grade 2 Hematoma

If a hematoma is stable but affects flow, it is classified as a grade 2 hematoma (Fig. 30.14, Table 30.4). This is the only feature that distinguishes it from a grade 1. Most of these lesions stabilize very quickly after they form. If they do not, they may progress rapidly which signifies that it is actually a grade 3 hematoma in most instances.

Management

These cases require treatment in order to restore flow. Two mechanisms that can obstruct flow are in effect; firstly, the tear in the wall of the vessel may be displaced into the former lumen resulting in its obstruction, and secondly, the hematoma can compress the vessel obstructing its lumen. The goal of treatment is to press the vessel wall and the tear outward to open the lumen and restore flow (Table 30.5). This treatment requires that a guidewire be positioned across the lesion. If this is the case, the likelihood of salvage is in the range of 90 % or better. If the guidewire has been inadvertently removed, the chances of passing it across the site again are probably no better than 50 %.

As mentioned above, manual occlusion of the arterial inflow should be effected and maintained while the problem

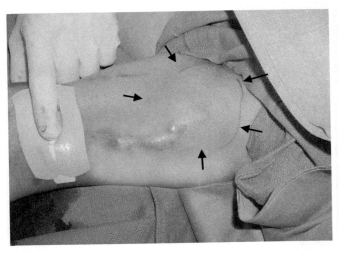

Fig. 30.13 Grade 1 hematoma (*arrows*), the condition is stable and flow is not affected

is assessed. Additionally, the occlusion should be continued during treatment. The angioplasty balloon that was used for the basic treatment should be positioned across the site of the rupture and inflated with a low pressure; only the amount necessary to fully expand the balloon should be applied. This should be maintained for a period of 4–5 min. After that time, the balloon should be deflated and gently removed. The site should then be checked using a puff of radiocontrast to determine if flow has been restored. If flow appears normal or relatively so and the hematoma is stable, nothing further needs to be done. Actually, attempts to do more can lead to additional problems. However, if flow continues to be significantly affected, balloon tamponade should be repeated. If the problem persists after this, insertion of an endovascular stent should be considered [140–143]. If this treatment is unsuccessful, the access may be lost if surgical revision is not possible.

Grade 3 Hematoma

The defining feature of a grade 3 hematoma is that it is unstable (Fig. 30.15, Table 30.4). It continues to enlarge. Hematoma formation generally occurs very rapidly after the angioplasty dilatation and in some instances may be painful (dampened by sedation/analgesia). The size attained by the hematoma, however, is quite variable. It depends on how quickly the condition is recognized and extravasation is controlled (with manual occlusion). The hematoma begins, expands rapidly, and is pulsatile. Arterial blood is being pumped directly into the tissue surrounding the area. Early recognition is critical; unfortunately the site may be covered by the drapes and not quickly recognized. Dilatation of the vein with angioplasty may elicit pain, but it should immediately resolve with balloon deflation. Pain and discomfort that continues should arouse suspicion of a venous rupture.

Management

When a grade 3 hematoma occurs, there is a definite risk of losing the access. There is also the risk of sizable blood loss,

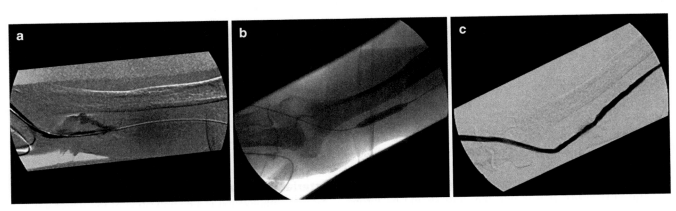

Fig. 30.14 Grade 2 hematoma. (**a**) Hematoma with no flow. (**b**) Balloon tamponade. (**c**) Restoration of flow

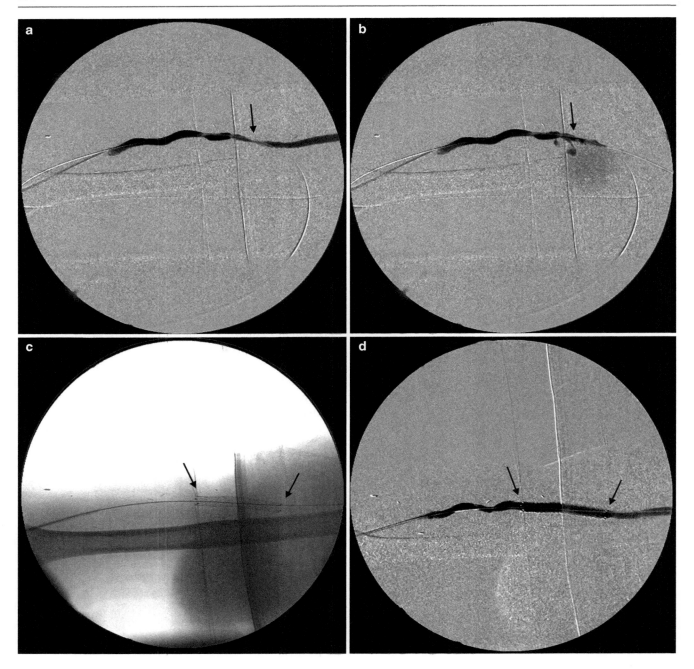

Fig. 30.15 Grade 3 hematoma. (**a**) Lesion prior to PTA (*arrow*), (**b**) vein rupture (*arrow*) which was unstable and did not respond to tamponade, (**c**) stent graft in place (*arrows*), (**d**) restoration of flow through stented area (*arrows*)

if not quickly controlled. The primary goal in the management of a grade 3 hematoma is to arrest its progression as quickly as possible. This is critical to limit the size of the hematoma and the volume of blood lost. As soon as the situation is recognized, the access should be manually occluded to arrest further extravasation [137]. Salvage using a stent graft (Table 30.5) should be attempted and is frequently successful [131, 144]. If it is not, the graft should be thrombosed. To accomplish this, simply inflate the angioplasty balloon to a low pressure within the access below the site of

rupture and leave it in position until the access is thrombosed. This generally necessitates an overnight admission for observation. Emergency surgery is not necessary; however, the patient will need a dialysis access for both the short and long term.

Arterial Embolization

Arterial embolization is a complication of thrombectomy that can occur regardless of whether a mechanical or surgical technique is used [128, 145]. The occluded graft contains two types

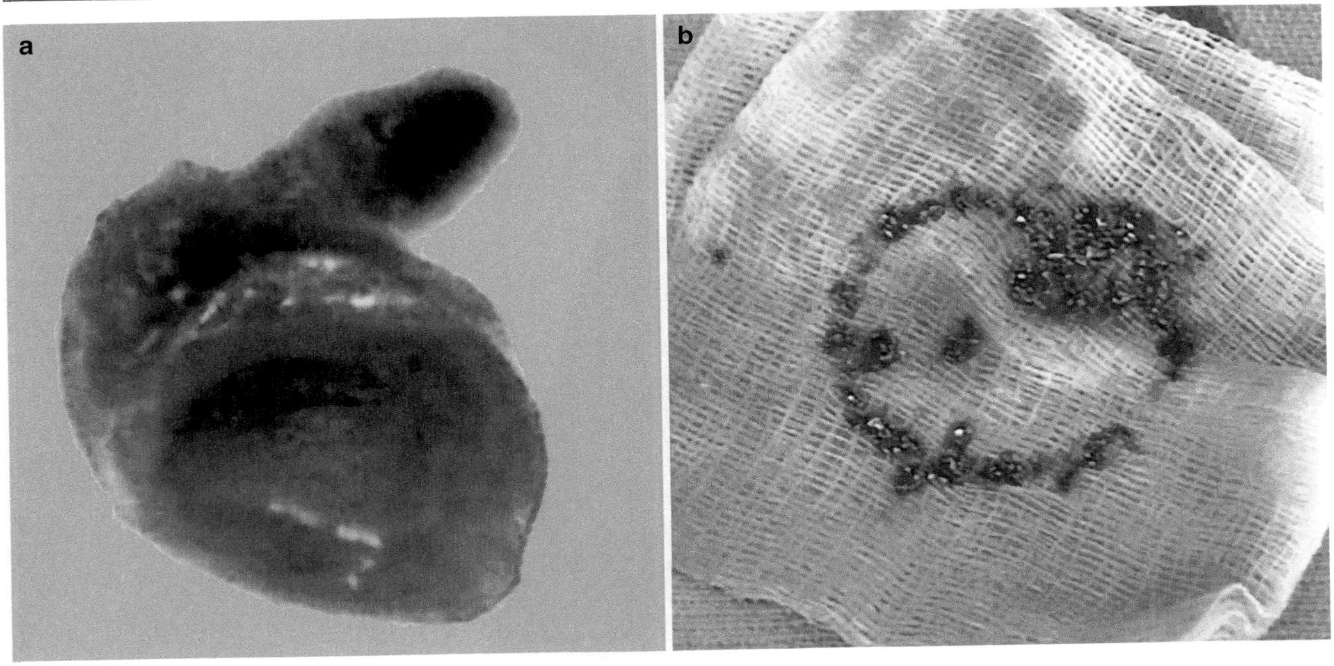

Fig. 30.16 Clot from thrombosed graft. (**a**) Arterial plug, (**b**) clot fragments that make up most of thrombus that is present

of thrombus, a firm arterial plug and a variable amount of soft thrombus (Fig. 30.16). Most of the clot present is of the latter type. This is poorly organized red thrombus that is friable and disintegrates easily. The arterial plug consists of a firm, laminated, organizing thrombus ranging from 5 mm to 3 cm in size [146]. It is found just downstream (antegrade) from the arterial anastomosis. This thrombus has a concave surface and forms a plug (Fig. 30.16) that is firmly attached to the wall of the graft at the point of maximum turbulence from the arterial inflow. It has been reported to be somewhat resistant to enzyme lysis [147, 148]. Any thrombotic material within the access has the potential for giving rise to an embolus; however, it is usually the arterial plug that is involved or at least a piece of it. With an upper arm access, the clot generally lodges in the brachial artery just above the bifurcation.

Arterial emboli are more commonly associated with the thrombectomy of a graft than with a fistula but can occur with either [17]. Although the reasons for this are not clear, it should be noted that the thrombus present in a fistula is mildly inflammatory and tends to become attached to the vessel wall. This decreases its ability to become detached and embolize.

Signs and Symptoms

The symptoms of embolization are those of hand ischemia. The hand and especially the fingers turn cold and take on a bluish discoloration that becomes mottled. These changes generally come on with the sudden onset of pain. In evaluating a patient's hand for a suspected embolus, it is important to compare it with the opposite hand. If both are cold and mottled, it is not likely that the hand in question reflects an acute

problem. The pulses at the wrist are generally absent or considerably diminished, a change that can be appreciated only if the patient was carefully evaluated prior to having the thrombectomy procedure. A Doppler signal is generally present over the arteries at the wrist even when the pulse is not palpable, although it is frequently diminished. If nothing is detected with Doppler examination, the urgency for immediate treatment to avoid tissue damage is even greater than usual.

Management

As is the case with all PRCs, the first aspect of management is avoidance. Although the occurrence of small asymptomatic and therefore inconsequential emboli may be unavoidable when doing a thrombectomy procedure, it is important to take measures to avoid the introduction of large clot fragments across the arterial anastomosis. Fluids (saline, radiocontrast, medications) are commonly introduced into the access during a thrombectomy procedure; care should be exerted to avoid doing it too rapidly and never doing it if the outflow is obstructed. The volume of a graft is actually rather small, injected fluid has to go somewhere. If the outflow is not open, it will generally go retrograde due to pressurization of the graft lumen. This risks refluxing thrombotic material across the arterial anastomosis. This is true even after the thrombectomy procedure is completed. One should never occlude the access and do a retrograde injection to visualize the anastomosis and adjacent artery. Even if the graft looks clean angiographically, clot fragments may still be present. Additionally, care must be used in passing devices across the arterial anastomosis during the thrombectomy procedure. It is possible to push material into the artery resulting in a problem.

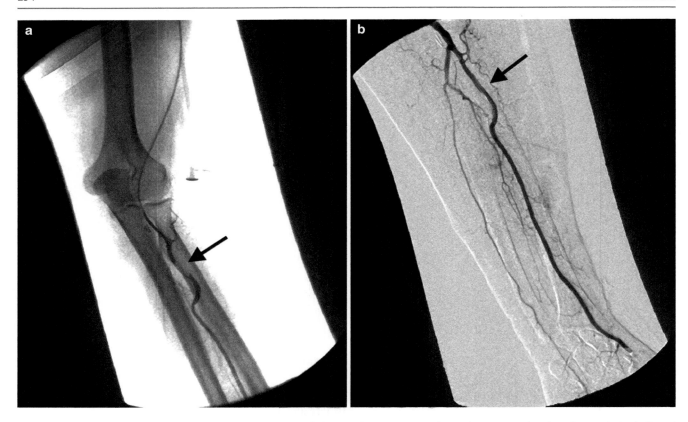

Fig. 30.17 Arterial embolus. (**a**) Embolus (*arrow*) occluding radial artery. (**b**) Appearance after embolectomy (site of previous embolus indicated by *arrow*)

Table 30.6 Treatment modalities for arterial emboli

Percutaneous – mechanical
Balloon catheter embolectomy
Catheter thromboaspiration
Back-bleeding
Percutaneous – pharmacological
Thrombolysis
Surgical embolectomy

Table 30.7 Balloon catheter embolectomy

Document the presence and location of the embolus
Pass a guidewire (a hydrophilic guidewire has a potential advantage) past the blockage
Insert a balloon catheter, angioplasty or occlusion balloon, beyond the embolus
Inflate and pull back to retrieve the clot into the access
Document the final appearance of the vessel angiographically

Symptomatic emboli (Fig. 30.17) must be treated in a timely fashion in order to prevent permanent sequelae. Treatment should be directed at restoring flow to the ischemic hand as quickly as possible in order to relieve the patient's pain and preserve hand function by avoiding secondary muscle ischemia and necrosis. Outcomes and prognosis largely depend on a rapid diagnosis and initiation of appropriate and effective therapy [149]. There are several approaches to the therapy of symptomatic peripheral artery emboli (Table 30.6). These can be divided into percutaneous and surgical. Further, the percutaneous approach can be subdivided into mechanical and pharmacological.

Percutaneous Mechanical Three percutaneous mechanical techniques for the treatment of an arterial embolus in this situation have been described.

Balloon Catheter Embolectomy As usually performed [137, 144], this technique involves the passage of a guidewire beyond the embolus once it has be identified and localized angiographically. Then a balloon, either an occlusion balloon (Boston Scientific, Natick, MA, USA) or an angioplasty balloon, is passed over the guidewire to a level below the embolus, inflated and withdrawn to extract the clot (Table 30.7).

Catheter Thromboaspiration The percutaneous aspiration thrombectomy technique uses a large-bore catheter connected to a syringe to aspirate clot from vessels. With this technique [150, 151], after the embolus is identified and localized angiographically, a 7 or 8 French catheter is passed down to a point that it is in contact with the embolus. Suction is then applied with a large syringe to secure the clot to the end of the catheter. The catheter is then withdrawn along with the clot as continuous suction is applied (Table 30.8).

Table 30.8 Catheter thromboaspiration

Document the presence and location of the embolus angiographically
Pass a guidewire beyond the clot fragment and insert a 7 or 8 F catheter
Position the catheter just above the embolus and in contact with it
Apply strong manual aspiration pressure using a 50 mL Luer-Lok syringe attached to the catheter as it is slowly withdrawn
Check the aspirate to see if the clot has been removed
Repeated the angiogram with a small volume of radiocontrast to document the result

Table 30.9 Back-bleeding

Document the presence and location of the embolus angiographically
Occlude the distal brachial artery central to the anastomosis using a balloon – Fogarty catheter or an angioplasty balloon
Instructed the patient to exercise their hand vigorously for approximately 1 min
This increases blood flow to the hand through collaterals and enhances the backflow up the artery pushing the clot back into the access
After the occluding balloon has been deflated, perform an arteriogram to document the result

Back-Bleeding The back-bleeding technique [152] is dependent upon the fact that, except in the face of severe peripheral artery disease, when the distal brachial artery is occluded, there is enough blood flow to the distal extremity through other vessels to still provide adequate perfusion. Success of this procedure is dependent upon the presence of this persistent perfusion causing blood to flow retrograde in the distal artery. This pushes the clot upward and into the graft relieving the obstruction. For this to work the access must be open and flowing. Firstly, the artery above the anastomosis is occluded with a balloon catheter. The patient is then instructed to exercise their hand for 1 min. A repeat angiogram is performed to check the result (Table 30.9).

Percutaneous Pharmacological This technique is generally referred to as regional intra-arterial infusion [149]. Firstly, the occluded arterial segment is selectively catheterized with the catheter tip positioned just proximal to the embolus. A lytic agent is then infused directly onto the clot. Tissue plasminogen activator (t-PA) is the agent generally used which is a very effective fibrinolytic agent and has the additional advantage of an extremely short half-life (5.0 ± 1.8 min).

This technique is usually reserved as a backup in the event of failure of one or more of the other percutaneous techniques and generally requires that the patient be referred to the hospital. Patients with evidence of severe ischemia should not be treated with this technique because catheter-based thrombolytic therapy often takes several hours and threatened ischemic changes may become irreversible over the course of treatment. These patients should be treated surgically on an emergent basis [149]. Additionally, the arterial plug is frequently the clot that results in an embolus, and it is somewhat resistant to fibrinolysis [147, 148]. Absolute and relative contraindications to thrombolytic therapy should be observed when this technique is considered [149, 153]. A significant number of patients will be found to fall within this category [154]. If these cases cannot be managed with mechanical means, surgical management is indicated.

Surgical Embolectomy A surgical thrombectomy generally consists of opening the exposed artery and extracting the clot using an embolectomy balloon. This procedure is facilitated considerably by localizing the exact site of the embolus angiographically prior to beginning. Clot resistance plus the fact that thrombolysis is not rapid has led some to feel that prompt surgical treatment may have an advantage. This is especially true in cases of severe ischemia requiring emergent reperfusion [149].

Pulmonary Embolization

There are reports of patients experiencing acute cardiopulmonary distress and even dyspnea and chest pain, soon after dislodgement of the arterial plug in the thrombectomy procedure. This temporal relationship strongly suggests that dislodgement of the arterial plug, and subsequent embolization of thrombotic material to the pulmonary arteries, is the cause of these clinical symptoms [128, 155–158]. There is no doubt that during a thrombectomy procedure, there is some degree of embolization to the lungs of the patient. Even during dialysis, there is microembolization to the lungs [159–161].

Clinical studies have demonstrated that the entire contents of a thrombosed hemodialysis graft can be safely embolized to the pulmonary circulation [162–165]. Although the majority of patients tolerate iatrogenic pulmonary emboli, the long-term consequence of these "silent" emboli has raised concern [166]. A high incidence (40–52 %) of pulmonary hypertension as detected by Doppler echocardiography has been reported in patients receiving chronic hemodialysis therapy via an arteriovenous access [167, 168]. A relationship between this and both microembolization associated with dialysis [160] and embolization from recurrent access thrombectomy [168] has been suggested.

Several different investigators have utilized ventilation and perfusion lung scans to evaluate post-thrombectomy pulmonary embolization [163, 169–171]. Some have shown no problems [170]. However, in other series abnormal perfusion scans following percutaneous thrombectomy of hemodialysis grafts have been high even though patients remained asymptomatic [163, 171]. This is thought to be related to the fact that the quantity of thrombus present in a thrombosed access is generally small [146]. However, death from acute pulmonary embolism in this setting has been reported [169]. Patients with severe cardiopulmonary disease are at high risk for complications during a percutaneous thrombectomy

Table 30.10 Modified sPESI Index

Age >80 years
Heart failure
Chronic lung disease
Pulse ≥100
Systolic BP ≤100 mmHg
Respiratory rate ≥30/min
Arterial oxygen saturation <90 %

procedure. The clinical significance of pulmonary emboliza-tion is not entirely based upon the volume of thrombus [166]. Even smaller emboli can result in the release of vasoactive substances that cause constriction of the pulmonary arteri-oles and an acute elevation of pulmonary arterial pressure. Patients with preexisting heart failure may not be able to tol-erate this additional increase in pulmonary arterial pressure. Patients with a large clot load associated with large dilated, aneurysmal fistulas are at much greater risk of serious effects from embolized thrombus.

A probe-patent foramen ovale has been reported to be present in 27–35 % of the general population at autopsy [172, 173], meaning that a probe can be passed across the opening although its flap-valve like architecture is such that it normally prevents the passage of blood. These individuals do not have right-to-left shunts normally; however, in dialy-sis patients with severe pulmonary hypertension, shunting from right to left can occur. These individuals are at risk of developing paradoxical emboli [174, 175]. A fatality due to a paradoxical embolism that occurred during a hemodialysis graft thrombectomy procedure has been reported [176].

Management

As is always the case, the first principle of management is to take steps to minimize the risk. There are cases of access thrombosis in which the clot load is quite large. It is advis-able, for safety sake, that before doing an endovascular thrombectomy, the case be evaluated for the size of the thrombotic material that is present. If the clot load appears to be large, as in a dilated aneurysmal fistula (mega-fistula), the procedure should not be performed in a freestanding facility. If it is to be done (many actually need surgical revision or replacement), it should be performed in the hospital setting.

Faced with the sudden appearance of signs or symptoms compatible with the occurrence of a PE, superimposed upon a clinical situation in which such an adverse event is possible (large clot load), a determination should be made as to whether the patient is at high risk for an adverse outcome. In order to accomplish this task, the use of a risk scale has been recommended [177]. If any of the variables listed in Table 30.10 (sPESI) are present, the patient should be evacu-ated immediately to the hospital for emergency care. Since events such as a drop in blood pressure, tachycardia, and a

drop in oxygen saturation are not infrequent, these index variables should be taken to mean a persistent change (>15 min) rather than a transient alteration.

30.3 Sedation/Analgesia-Related Complications (SARC)

30.3.1 Introduction

Most of the endovascular procedures performed for dialy-sis vascular access maintenance are painful and require the use of sedation/analgesia in order to minimize discomfort and relieve anxiety. This requirement takes on even greater significance in dealing with hemodialysis patients in that maintenance of their vascular access is a procedure-inten-sive endeavor generally necessitating repeated visits to an interventional facility [178]. An unpleasant episode or one associated with pain and discomfort adds greatly to the anxi-ety and stress associated with subsequent episodes of access dysfunction.

"Sedation and analgesia" describes a specific sedated state that allows a patient to tolerate unpleasant procedures while maintaining adequate cardiorespiratory functions and the ability to respond purposely to verbal command and/or tactile stimulation. With appropriate sedation/analgesia, the patient retains the ability to maintain their airway independently and continuously and to respond appropriately to physical stimu-lation and verbal command. Although this is quite different from anesthesia, it definitively creates an increased level of risk to the patient and complications can occur.

30.3.2 Agents Used

Sedation/analgesia is most effectively accomplished through the use of intravenously administered medications. These include benzodiazepines and opioids, alone or in combina-tion [179]. In the typical dialysis access interventional facil-ity operated by an interventional nephrologist, the most common agents used are midazolam (benzodiazepine) and fentanyl (opioid).

Midazolam (Versed)

Although it is not an analgesic, midazolam is ideal as a sin-gle agent to provide the degree of sedation required for per-forming short minor surgical procedures [180]. When it is used appropriately, patients generally have no significant indications of pain or discomfort during the procedure or memory of pain afterwards. The onset of action with mid-azolam is rapid, 1–2 min, and the duration of action is short, in the range of 30 min. With procedures of long duration, multiple doses can be given successfully.

Table 30.11 Adverse effects of midazolam

Hiccups
Nausea, vomiting
Coughing
Hyperactive and agitated
Hypoventilation (decrease in tidal volume)
Decreased respiratory rate
Apnea
Hypotension
Tachycardia

Table 30.12 Adverse effects of fentanyl

Muscle rigidity
Bradycardia
Hypotension
Nausea, vomiting
Depresses brain stem ventilation
Reduction in respiratory rate
Decreased sensitivity to CO_2 stimulation
Apnea

It is important that the dose of midazolam administered be titrated to the effect desired because of individual patient differences. Titrated doses in the range of 0.05–0.15 mg/kg fall into the sedation range; doses in the range of 0.1–0.4 mg/kg generally induce sleep (anesthesia) [181]. For a 70 kg person, this would be 3.5–10.5 mg for sedation. In reviewing the sedation/analgesia records of 12,896 hemodialysis patients undergoing dialysis access maintenance procedures, it was found that when midazolam was administered for sedation as the sole agent, the mean dosage used was 3.4 ± 1.5 mg. This dosage is in line with that reported for other procedures of a like nature [182, 183]. However, the dosage used should be individualized based on the patient's response in achieving the desired clinical effect. It is very helpful to look back at previous procedures if available to see how much S/A medication the patient received and use this as a guide to how much they will need (tolerate).

The major adverse effects associated with midazolam administration are related to pulmonary and cardiovascular events [184–189] (Table 30.11) and are dose dependent [181, 190].

Reversal Agent

Flumazenil (Romazicon) is a specific benzodiazepine antagonist. Used intravenously, it has been shown to reverse sedation and ventilatory depression produced by benzodiazepines in healthy human volunteers [191]. Its onset of action is rapid, and usually, effects are seen within 1–2 min (much faster if given centrally). The peak effect is seen at 6–10 min. Since benzodiazepine effects are dose dependent and appear to correspond to the proportion of receptors that bind agonist drug, a titrated dose of flumazenil may initially reverse hypnosis and, upon continued titration, reverse sedation as well [192, 193].

For the reversal of the sedative effects of midazolam administered for sedation/analgesia, the recommended initial dose of flumazenil is 200 µg (2 mL) administered intravenously over 15 s. If the desired level of consciousness is not obtained after waiting an additional 45 s, a second dose of 200 µg (2 mL) can be injected and repeated at 60-s intervals where necessary to a maximum total dose of 1 mg (10 mL).

Fentanyl (Sublimaze)

Fentanyl is the opioid most commonly used for sedation/analgesia because of its short duration of action [194]. It is approximately 600 times more lipid soluble and 100 times more potent than morphine, with 100 µg of fentanyl being approximately equivalent to 10 mg of morphine and 75 mg of meperidine in analgesic activity [195]. Because of its lipid solubility, fentanyl is able to quickly cross from the blood into the brain. As a result, the onset of action of fentanyl is almost immediate when the medicine is given intravenously. However, the maximal analgesic and respiratory depressant effect may not be noted for several minutes. The usual duration of action of analgesic effect is 30–60 min after a single intravenous dose of up to 100 µg [196]. In elderly patients and patients with liver disease the half-life of fentanyl is prolonged; therefore, these patients should have a reduced dosage [195].

The dosage of fentanyl should also be individualized. Some of the factors to be considered in determining the dose are age, body weight, physical status, comorbidities, use of other medicines, and the procedure involved. The initial dose should be reduced in the elderly and in debilitated patients. The effect of the initial dose should be taken into account in determining supplemental doses.

When used to induce sedation/analgesia for dialysis vascular access interventional procedures, 50–100 µg should be administered intravenously initially. This may be repeated at 2- to 3-min intervals until the desired effect is achieved. A reduced dose as low as 25–50 µg is recommended in elderly and poor-risk patients. The dose may need to be adjusted if given with a benzodiazepine [197].

In the presence of renal impairment, fentanyl is considered to be one of the safest drugs available because it does not deliver a high active metabolite load or have a significantly prolonged clearance [195]. Nevertheless, it can have adverse effects [198–201] (Table 30.12). All adverse effects of fentanyl are dose related. The major adverse reaction is altered respiration. Like all opioids, analgesia is accompanied by marked respiratory depression, but with fentanyl its onset is more rapid [198]. The duration of the respiratory depressant effect of fentanyl may be longer than the analgesic effect [202, 203]. There is a direct depression of brain stem ventilation and a dose-dependent reduction in respiratory rate [201]. Sensitivity to CO_2 stimulation is also decreased and may persist longer than depression of respiratory rate. This diminished sensitivity frequently slows the respiratory rate.

Reversal Agent

Naloxone (Narcan) is a pure opioid antagonist preventing or reversing the effects of opioids, including respiratory depression, sedation, and hypotension, by direct competition at mu, kappa, and sigma opioid receptor binding sites. In patients with respiratory depression, an increase in respiratory rate is generally seen within 1 or 2 min. Sedative effects are reversed and blood pressure, if depressed, returns to normal [198]. Naloxone will reduce the systemic side effects of opioids in a dose-dependent manner. Higher doses will reverse analgesia; lower doses will reverse opioid-related side effects without antagonizing analgesia [204].

Naloxone should be administered parenterally. After intravenous administration, naloxone is rapidly distributed throughout the body. It is highly lipophilic and readily crosses into the brain. Onset of action after IV dosing is within 2 min. When treating a patient demonstrating the adverse effects of fentanyl, an initial dose of 0.4–2.0 mg of naloxone may be administered intravenously. If the desired degree of reversal of respiratory function is not obtained, the dose may be repeated at 2–3 min intervals. If no response is observed after 10 mg has been administered, the diagnosis of narcotic overdose should be questioned.

It has been recommended that patients who receive naloxone be continuously observed for a minimum of 2 h after the last dose [205]. Antagonism of opioid effects by naloxone may be accompanied by an "overshoot" phenomenon. If this occurs, the respiratory rate depressed by opioids transiently becomes higher than that before the period of depression. Rebound release of catecholamines may cause hypertension, tachycardia, and ventricular arrhythmias. Pulmonary edema has been reported in these cases [198].

In case in which both midazolam and fentanyl have been used, reversal of only the benzodiazepine by the administration of flumazenil alone is often effective [206].

30.3.3 Precautions

The physician who administers sedation/analgesia must be experienced in the use of the necessary drugs and in the ability to recognize and deal with the complications that might ensue. Expertise in airway management is essential. The use of a carefully designed patient safety protocol is important [177]. There are safety issues that are important pre- and post-procedure as well as intra-procedure.

Pre-procedure

A focused medical history and physical examination to detect issues that might make the patient more prone to a SARC or make the patient's management more difficult should such an adverse event arise are essential [207]. In addition, the risks of sedation/analgesia relate directly to the patient's overall clinical status. Two systems have been proposed – a Numerical Clinical Scoring (NCS) system [139, 208] and the American Society of Anesthesiologists Physical Status (ASA-PS) Classification system. The NCS system is similar to the Aldrete Scoring System that has been used in anesthesiology for more than 30 years and has been validated [138]. It is more detailed and specific to the dialysis patients, however.

Intra-procedure

Supplemental oxygen should be administered for all cases in which sedation/analgesia is used. In general, nasal oxygen at 2 L/min is appropriate. Vascular access for administration of medications is mandatory and should be maintained throughout the procedure and until the patient is no longer at risk for cardiorespiratory depression [178]. Dialysis access procedures are somewhat unique in that as a general rule, they cannot be done unless vascular access is established for the purposes of the treatment. This access can then be used for the purposes of administering medications; a dedicated intravenous line is not necessary in these cases.

The use of sedation/analgesia creates a mandatory requirement for careful patient monitoring. The availability of a nurse to monitor the patient's status reduces the risk of adverse events and should be considered mandatory [178]. Patients can experience cardiovascular decompensation or cerebral hypoxia as a result of over sedation or as a consequence of a hypersensitivity reaction to drugs (e.g., radiocontrast) that are administered during the procedure. The timely detection and treatment of these complications is dependent upon careful patient monitoring. Level of consciousness, ventilation, oxygenation, blood pressure, pulse rate, and pain levels should be monitored and recorded contemporaneously.

It is important that the dosages of medications administered for sedation/analgesia be titrated to the effect desired because of individual patient differences. Reduced doses should be used in patients that are elderly, small, debilitated, and hypovolemic, have COPD, or have sleep apnea.

No sedation/analgesia should ever be administered unless the pharmacological antagonist for the drug(s) used is readily and immediately available [178]. This should be taken to mean that the drug is setting out and available for immediate access, not in a locked cabinet. When there is a need for reversal of sedation/analgesia, it is because there is an emergent problem. Delay can lead to anoxia and the risk of neurological injury.

The immediate availability of a "crash cart" with equipment for establishing a patent airway, including intubation, and providing positive pressure ventilation with supplemental oxygen should also be considered mandatory whenever sedation/analgesia is administered [178]. Suction and a defibrillator in good working order should be on the cart. A full battery of resuscitation medications should also be considered essential for this piece of emergency equipment.

Post-procedure

After a procedure requiring sedation/analgesia is completed, the patient should be sent to a recovery area where continuous monitoring and resuscitative equipment are available. Patients need to recover fully to their pre-sedation level of consciousness and exhibit stable vital signs and intact protective reflexes prior to discharge.

30.3.4 SARCs

Examination of the side effects of the drugs used makes it apparent that the SARCs that can be anticipated to occur include hypotension, a drop in oxygen saturation below 90 %, and apnea [139, 208]. Because of the nature of the dialysis population involved, for these events to be significant, they should be more than transitory.

When the above described precautions are taken, the incidence of a SARC is relatively low. In a review of 12,869 cases [179], PRCs were observed in 2.9 % of the cases. However, there were only 17 cases (0.12 % of cohort, 4.6 % of the complications observed) in which complications were noted that were felt to be directly attributable to the medications used for sedation/analgesia. These consisted of a drop in blood pressure in 7 patients, an oxygen saturation of less than 90 % in 7, 1 episode of transient apnea, and 2 cases in which the NCS score was adverse post-procedure. Two deaths were observed but were temporally removed from the procedure and not felt to have occurred as a direct result of the procedure.

Hypotension

While criteria for judging the gravity of a fall in blood pressure have been suggested based upon the level of therapy required [139, 208], there are no guidelines based upon the degree of hypotension experienced by the patient. This is especially true for the dialysis patient. Actually, it is somewhat difficult to determine if a fall in blood pressure represents a definite SARC. It is not unusual for the dialysis patient to be hypertensive as a result of omitting the medication in preparation for the procedure or as a result of anxiety. The administration of sedation/analgesia often has an ameliorative effect. Some patients have chronic hypotension making the detection of a SARC difficult. However, if the systolic blood pressure falls below 100 mmHg and is more than transient in a patient not previously hypotensive, a complication related to the sedation/analgesia should be suspected. When this represents a definite SARC, it is frequently also accompanied by a fall in oxygen saturation.

Management

Because of the gravity of the situation that exists when a fall in blood pressure of the magnitude described occurs and because there are other reasons in this patient population for the development of hypotension, the best course of action is to administer the reversal agent flumazenil. This should effectively remove sedation from consideration as a cause for the problem very quickly.

In many instances the patient who is experiencing an adverse event related to sedation/analgesia has been given both a benzodiazepine and an opioid. It has been shown that in cases such as this where the problem is respiratory depression, the reversal of only the benzodiazepine by the administration of flumazenil alone is often sufficiently effective [206].

Drop in Oxygen Saturation

Nasal oxygen at 2 L/min should be administered routinely to all patients receiving sedation/analgesia. It is important to be able to interpret the information provided by the pulse oximeter. In order to do this, it is of value to understand how the device works and how it correlates with blood oxygen levels (paO_2). The color of blood varies depending on the amount of oxygen that it contains. The pulse oximeter shines two beams of light through the finger to which it is attached, one beam is red light (which is visible), and the other is infrared light (which is invisible). These two beams of light allow the pulse oximeter to detect the color of the arterial blood and from this, the oxygen saturation. However, there are other things in the finger which will absorb light, so in order to determine the color of the arterial blood, the pulse oximeter looks for the slight change in the overall color caused by a beat of the heart pushing arterial blood into the finger. This change in color is very small so pulse oximeters work best when there is a good strong pulse in the finger that the probe is on. If the signal is too low, it will not be able to work.

Oxygen saturation (SaO_2) measured in this way represents the percentage of all the available heme-binding sites saturated with oxygen in arterial blood. Technically what is being measured is the "fractional" oxygen saturation, that is, the amount of oxygen the hemoglobin is carrying as a percentage of the maximum possible that could be carried by that much hemoglobin could carry. Correlation coefficients between pulse oximetry and direct blood oxygen saturation measurement range from 0.77 to 0.99 when oxygen saturation is greater than 60 % [209].

Table 30.13 Correlations and significance of SaO$_2$ values [210]

	SaO$_2$ (%)	PaO$_2$ (mmHg)
Normal (range)	97 (95–100)	98 (80–100)
Slight hypoxemia	<95	<80
Mild hypoxemia	90–94	60–79
Moderate hypoxemia	75–89	40–59
Severe hypoxemia	<75	<40

Table 30.14 Primary algorithm

A – Airway
B – Breathing
C – Circulation
D – Drugs

Table 30.15 Secondary algorithm

A. Airway
B – Breathing
C – Circulation
D – Differential diagnosis

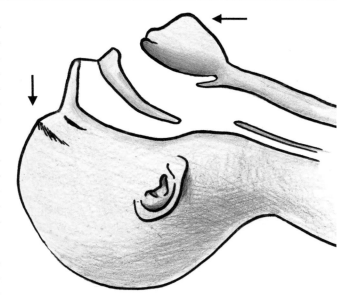

Fig. 30.18 Positioning to open airway (*arrows*) with head back and chin up

The normal range for SaO$_2$ is 95–100 %. It is useful to remember that an SaO$_2$ of 90 % correlates with a paO$_2$ of 60 mmHg. The 90-60-30 mnemonic may be helpful – 90 %=60 mmHg, 60 %=30 mmHg. Table 30.13 shows other correlations and a hypoxia classification indicating its significance.

SaO$_2$ by itself does not tell the whole story concerning the patient's respiration; at a minimum it is also necessary to record the respiratory rate and observe the patient's respiratory activity. A patient receiving oxygen with an acceptable SaO$_2$ who has gasping respiration at a normal rate is in trouble. It may take a few moments for the SaO$_2$ to fall, delaying problem recognition, if that is the only variable being monitored.

Management: Primary Algorithm

In assessing a situation where there is a drop in SaO$_2$, it is useful to use an ABCD mnemonic as shown in Tables 30.14 and 30.15. Primary and secondary algorithms are needed. The primary algorithm (Table 30.14) represents the first level of response to the adverse event. This should be a stepwise approach directed toward observing a rise in the patient's SaO$_2$. Once it has returned to normal levels, the event is over and further action is not required except to prevent a recurrence. The secondary algorithm is used in the event of failure of the first level of actions.

Airway

The first step is to check the airway. In most instances the patient has been positioned with a pillow under their head at the beginning of the procedure. As a first step, this should be removed. Additionally, repositioning the head to open the airway by getting the chin up is important (Fig. 30.18).

Breathing

The first step here is to be sure that the patient is actually breathing and not apneic. The patient should be stimulated verbally to take a deep breath. If this is not effective, they should be stimulated physically (pat face, pinch their neck or shoulder). Check to be sure that oxygen is actually on and increase the delivery rate to 4 L/min. Many patients are mouth breathers, especially when asleep. If this is the case, move the nasal prongs to the mouth to assure that they are actually inhaling the oxygen. Sleep apnea can cause partial obstruction to the airway. This will be made evident by loud snoring. This can generally be relieved by inserting a "nasal trumpet" (nasopharyngeal airway) into the mouth (Fig. 30.19). When the patient becomes more awake, they will spit it out. While taking these steps to relieve the problem, continue to watch the pulse oximeter reading for evidence of improvement.

Circulation

It is important to be sure that the fall in SaO$_2$ is not a manifestation of cardiopulmonary arrest. Check the EKG and assess the pattern, observe the pulse wave on the pulse oximeter and obtain the patient's blood pressure.

Drugs

The first step here is to assure that you have open access to the active circulation. One must remember that an access that is not flowing cannot be used to deliver medications. There must be access to a site that is actually circulating via a sheath or catheter. In most instances, the problem will be resolved before arriving at this step so reversal will not be needed. However, preparations for the administration of reversal agents should be made in the event that the above

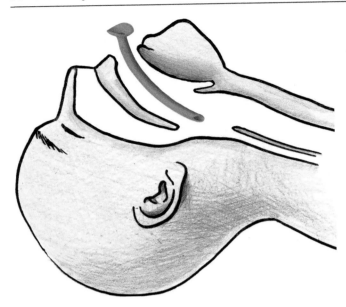

Fig. 30.19 Nasal trumpet inserted into patient's moth to relieve obstruction

listed actions do not result in an amelioration of the situation. If the patient has been given both a benzodiazepine and an opioid, the reversal of only the benzodiazepine by the administration of flumazenil alone is often effective [206].

Management: Secondary Algorithm

If the SaO_2 fails to respond by returning to a level that is at least above 90 %, the Secondary ABCD Algorithm (Table 30.15) should be instituted immediately. At this point, the failure of a response to the basic measures covered in the primary algorithm establishes that one is not dealing with a simple case of respiratory depression.

Airway

This is the time to check to be sure that the equipment required for the establishment of an airway from the crash cart is at hand and ready to use in the event that the fall in SaO_2 is a prelude to apnea. There are alternative devices available for establishing an airway. These are blind insertion airway devices, i.e., do not require the use of a laryngoscope.

The Combitube, also known as the double-lumen airway (Fig. 30.20), is designed for use in emergency situations and difficult airways. It can be placed without the need for visualization into the oropharynx and usually enters the esophagus when being inserted (as it should). It has a low volume inflatable distal cuff which occludes the esophagus and a much larger proximal cuff designed to occlude the pharynx [211–213]. Another blind insertion device is the laryngeal mask airway. It consists of a silicone mask (see inset, Fig. 30.20) that covers the larynx and is surrounded by an

inflatable cuff. This cuff forms a low-pressure seal around the laryngeal inlet permitting positive pressure ventilation.

Breathing

If the patient is breathing, the nasal cannula should be removed and replaced with a non-rebreather mask connected to the oxygen. This device is capable of delivering 60–100 % oxygen. Efforts should also be made to continue to stimulate patient verbally and physically.

Circulation

Continue to monitor the heart. Observe the EKG pattern for arrhythmia or any change in rate or pattern. Observe pulse wave for presence, rate, and amplitude. Check the blood pressure.

Differential Diagnosis

At this point the situation is not consistent with a simple overly aggressive sedation/analgesia situation. It is time to consider other diagnoses. One should consider a pulmonary event such as pulmonary embolization, air embolus, or pneumothorax; a cardiac event such as a myocardial infarction; or a hypersensitivity reaction to radiocontrast or one of the medications that have been used.

30.4 Hypersensitivity Drug Reactions (HDR)

30.4.1 Introduction

With the administration of any drug there is a risk of an adverse reaction, generally referred to simply as a drug reaction. The two primary types of adverse drug reactions have been referred to as type A and type B reactions [214]. In a type A adverse drug reaction, the effect observed is simply an extension of the pharmacological effect of the drug. With a type B adverse drug reaction, the effects observed are different than the pharmacological effect of the drug. Among these are the idiosyncratic drug reactions, commonly referred to as hypersensitivity drug reactions (HDR). These reactions occur rarely and unpredictably among any given population; the proposed mechanism for most HDRs is immune-mediated toxicity.

The most frequently observed HDRs are in response to antibiotics, especially penicillin and those that are cross-reactive. However, unless prophylactic antibiotics are being used, the most frequent drug associated with such a reaction in the dialysis access interventional facility is radiocontrast media (RCM). Relative to many available drugs, the radiocontrast products used today are exceptionally safe. Nevertheless, adverse and even fatal reactions can occur [215]. For this reason adverse reactions to RCM must be of

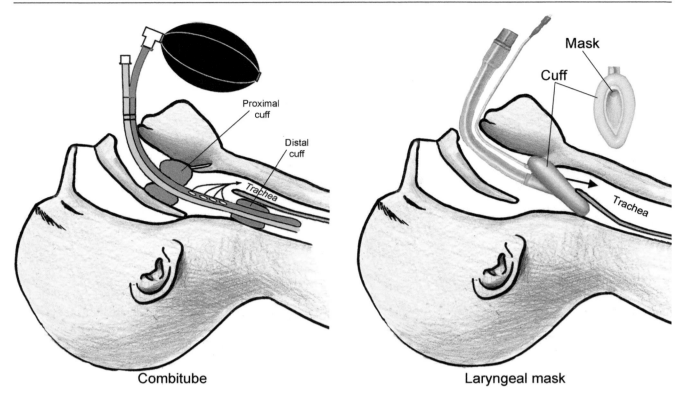

Fig. 30.20 Blind insertion airway devices

concern for all interventionalists working in these facilities because of the frequency with which iodinated radiocontrast materials are used.

30.4.2 Types of Radiocontrast Media (RCM)

All RCMs in current use are chemical modifications of a 2,4,6-tri-iodinated benzene ring with different side chains in the 1, 3, and 5 positions and different numbers of benzene rings. They are classified on the basis of their physical and chemical characteristics including osmolality, ionization in solution, and chemical structure. Currently, four classes of RCM are commercially available: ionic monomers, nonionic monomers, ionic dimers, and nonionic dimers [216, 217]. The oldest of the RCMs are the ionic monomers. In addition to ionizing in solution, these agents have relatively high osmolarity in solution (1,400 plus). Therefore, they are sometimes referred to as high-osmolar RCM or more commonly, ionic RCM.

Today, the RCMs most often used by interventional nephrologists are the nonionic monomers which have a lower osmolarity (500–900). These agents are sometimes referred to as low-osmolar radiocontrast media or more frequently simply as nonionic RCM. Iohexol, iopamidol, ioversol, iopromide, and ioxilan are examples of commonly used nonionic agents. A major issue that has contributed to the shift in RCM usage from ionic to nonionic is the significantly decreased incidence of HDR observed with the latter group of agents. Mild HDRs have been reported to occur in 3.8–12.7 % of patients receiving ionic agents in contrast to 0.7–3.1 % of patients receiving nonionic [218–220], while severe HDRs have been reported to occur with a frequency of 0.1–0.4 % versus 0.02–0.04 % for the two types of RCM, respectively [218–221].

A clinical study on adverse drug reactions to high-osmolar ionic RCM and low-osmolar nonionic RCM was performed prospectively [218] in which ionic RCM was administered in 169,284 cases (50.1 %) and nonionic in 168,363 cases (49.9 %). The overall prevalence of hypersensitivity reactions was 12.66 % in the ionic group and 3.13 % in the nonionic group. Severe anaphylactic reactions occurred in 0.22 % of the ionic and 0.04 % of the nonionic RCM examinations. One death occurred in each group, but a causal relationship to the contrast medium could not be established.

30.4.3 Reactions to RCM

The reactions that occur in response to the administration of RCM can be classified as chemotoxic and idiosyncratic or hypersensitivity [222]. Chemotoxic reactions result from the physiochemical properties of the RCM agent, the dose and the speed of the injection. All hemodynamic disturbances and localized symptoms affecting the distribution of vessels perfused by the RCM agent are included in this category. These include sensation of heat, vasovagal reactions, seizures, arrhythmias, and organ (such as renal) toxicity [223, 224]. We shall not discuss these further.

Hypersensitivity reactions to RCM are largely independent of dose and infusion rate [225]. In fact, they can occur in response to the administration of minute amounts. These reactions can be further subdivided into immediate (≤1 h) and delayed (>1 h) [226, 227]. Various types of exanthema resembling other drug-induced, non-immediate hypersensitivities, developing from 1 h to several days after administration account for the majority of RCM-induced delayed HDRs. This category includes mild to moderate cutaneous eruptions, urticaria/angioedema, and various uncommon reactions, including erythema multiforme minor, fixed drug eruption, Stevens-Johnson syndrome, flexural exanthema, and vasculitis [228, 229]. Such exanthemas have been reported to affect 1–3 % of RCM-exposed patients [230–232]. Unlike the immediate reactions, there appears to be a higher incidence of delayed reactions associated with dimeric nonionic RCM than to other types of RCM [233]. We shall not discuss these further, but instead will concentrate on the immediate group.

30.4.4 Signs and Symptoms of Immediate Hypersensitivity Reactions

Immediate hypersensitivity reactions to RCM are generally classified under the general heading of anaphylactic (referring to anaphylaxis) reactions. Anaphylaxis is classically defined as a condition caused by an IgE-mediated reaction. Anaphylactoid reactions are defined as those reactions that produce the same clinical picture as anaphylaxis but are not IgE mediated. The HDRs secondary to RCM fall into this category [234–236] although there is evidence that in some instances, they may also be IgE mediated [227, 237–240]. Anaphylactic (IgE-dependent) and anaphylactoid (IgE-independent) reactions differ mechanistically, but their clinical presentations are identical as is their acute management.

The onset of an immediate hypersensitivity reaction associated with RCM is generally very rapid, with about 70 % of all types occurring within 5 min [218, 241] and 96 % of severe or fatal reactions within 20 min after injection [242]. Signs and symptoms include flushing, pruritus, urticaria, angioedema bronchospasm and wheezing, laryngeal edema and stridor, decreased oxygen saturation, hypotension, and loss of consciousness [243]. When hypotension occurs, it may be associated with a loss of consciousness (anaphylactic

Table 30.16 Classification of hypersensitivity reactions to RCM

Categories of reactions	Signs/symptoms
Mild	Nausea, vomiting
Self-limited without evidence of progression	Pruritus, urticaria
	Edema – periorbital, face
Moderate	Generalized or diffuse erythema
More pronounced	Tachycardia/bradycardia
Moderate systemic signs/symptoms	Hypotension (SBP <90 mmHg)
	Dyspnea
	Bronchospasm, wheezing
	Laryngeal edema, stridor
Severe	Hypoxia (SpO$_2$ ≤90 %)
Signs/symptoms life threatening	Laryngeal edema
	Loss of consciousness
	Convulsions
	Profound hypotension
	Clinically manifest arrhythmias
	Cardiopulmonary arrest

Modified from American College of Radiology Committee on Drugs and Contrast Media [246]

shock) [218]. Tachycardia is the rule in anaphylaxis [244]. However, RCM can result in a vasovagal reaction (chemotoxic reaction) associated with bradycardia. Most fatalities when they occur are secondary to respiratory compromise and cardiovascular collapse [245]. The more rapidly anaphylaxis occurs after exposure, the more likely the reaction is to be severe and potentially life threatening [244].

Systemic immediate hypersensitivity reactions to RCM are often thought of in terms of three distinct clinical entities, urticaria, angioedema, and anaphylaxis; however, in actuality the responses observed represent a continuum of signs and symptoms ranging from mild to severe [244]. The clinical picture is best thought of as simply an anaphylactic reaction of varying degrees of severity. The grading system has been proposed by the American College of Radiology consisting of three levels – mild, moderate, and severe (Table 30.16).

In a study that reviewed 1,125 systemic hypersensitivity reactions (all causes) [215], the distribution of cases between the categories of severity was mild, 545; moderate, 441; severe, 139. Even when there are mild symptoms initially, the potential for progression to a severe and even irreversible outcome must be recognized [244]. It should be recognized that with each grade, there is also a spectrum of severity; the overall complex represents a continuum which ranges from the very mild to the extremely severe. Early recognition of an anaphylactic reaction is critical. Any delay in the recognition of the initial signs and symptoms can result in a fatal outcome either because of airway obstruction or vascular collapse. One study which examined fatal cases of anaphylaxis found that the median time to respiratory or cardiac arrest in cases that were iatrogenic was 5 min [245].

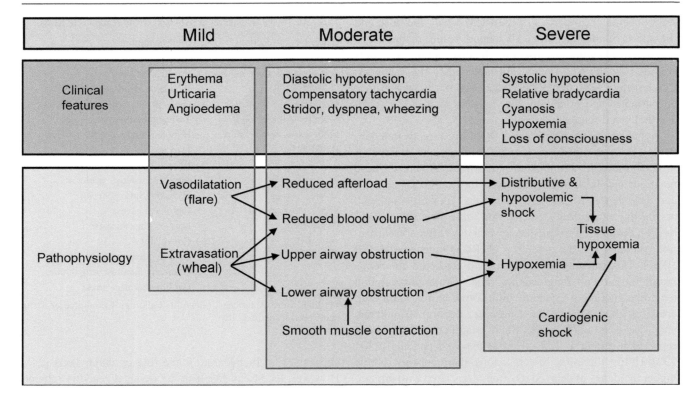

Fig. 30.21 Pathophysiology of anaphylaxis (Adapted from Brown [247])

30.4.5 Pathogenesis

With the onset of an anaphylactic reaction, a mast cell-leukocyte cytokine cascade is initiated, generating a number of mediators which in turn result in a variety of minor, but characteristic, skin, and mucosal symptoms as outlined in Table 30.16. Most pathophysiological effects can be ascribed to vasodilation, fluid extravasation, and smooth muscle contraction, leading to major clinical manifestations (Fig. 30.21) [247]. As the process progresses, fluid extravasation causes upper airway obstruction and, in combination with vasodilation, causes a mixed distributive-hypovolemic shock pattern; circulating blood volume can decrease by as much as 35 % within 10 min as a result of extravasation. As with severe asthma, lower airway obstruction in anaphylaxis can result from fluid extravasation (mucosal edema) and mucous plugging as well as smooth muscle contraction (bronchospasm) [248].

The major mediator culprit involved in this process is histamine. This agent exerts its actions by combining with specific cellular histamine receptors located on various target tissues. There are four histamine receptors that have been discovered in humans. These are designated H1 through H4; however, the pathophysiologic effects of histamine in anaphylaxis have been shown to be mediated only through H1 and H2 receptors, individually and in combination [249, 250]. H1 receptors are found on smooth muscle, endothelium, and central nervous system tissue. Their activation results in clinical features that include bronchoconstriction, bronchial smooth muscle contraction, vasodilation, separation of endothelial cells (responsible for urticaria), pain, and pruritus. H2 receptors are located on parietal cells and vascular smooth muscle cells; they are primarily involved in vasodilation but also stimulate gastric acid secretion.

Anaphylaxis is characterized by increased vascular permeability. This can be profound and can occur very rapidly. Urticaria and angioedema are a reflection of this increased permeability and are the most common manifestations of anaphylaxis occurring in 65–85 % of cases [218, 251, 252]. The absence of cutaneous symptoms should put the diagnosis of a hypersensitivity reaction in question [244]. However, with rapidly progressing anaphylaxis, hemodynamic collapse might occur rapidly with little or no cutaneous manifestations [244]. The two characteristic skin manifestations of this symptom complex should be discussed individually since their recognition is an important indicator for the presence of an anaphylactic reaction.

Urticaria

Urticaria (also referred to as hives) is a skin eruption notable for the presence of wheals (the typical lesion of urticaria). These are smooth, slightly elevated areas on the body surface, which may be either redder or paler than the surrounding skin (Fig. 30.22). Urticaria is generally associated with

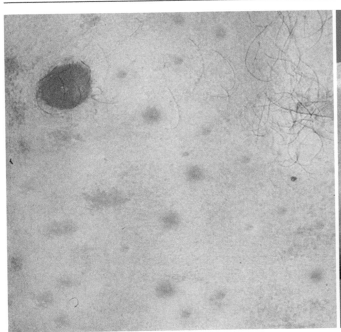
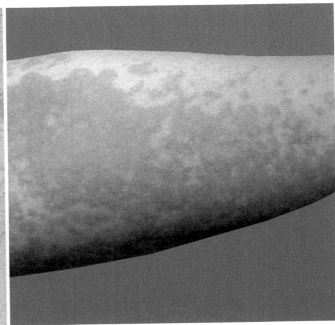

Fig. 30.22 Urticaria showing the typical wheals

pruritus which may precede its appearance by several minutes. Recognition of this problem may be confounded by the presence of preexisting pruritus in the dialysis patient. However, once the typical skin wheals appear, the diagnosis should be clear. In cases with only pruritus and no wheals, the diagnosis of urticaria should be doubted.

Angioedema

Unlike urticaria in which edema (wheals) occurs in the upper dermis, with angioedema, there is swelling of the dermis, subcutaneous tissue, mucosa, and submucosal tissues. The skin of the face, normally around the mouth (Fig. 30.23), the tongue, and the mucosa of the mouth and throat, become edematous over a period of minutes to several hours. This can occur simultaneous with the development of urticaria. This event, like most of the other types of reactions associated with HDR, can vary considerably in its severity and thus its symptoms. However, even though initially mild, it can progress and become a life-threatening problem. In severe cases, stridor of the airway occurs due to laryngeal edema, with gasping or wheezy inspiratory breath sounds and decreasing oxygen levels. Tracheal intubation is required in these situations to prevent respiratory arrest and risk of death.

30.4.6 Risk Factors

Significant predisposing risk factors (Fig. 30.24) for an HDR reaction to RCM include prior adverse reaction to contrast medium (four to six times greater risk), asthma (eight times

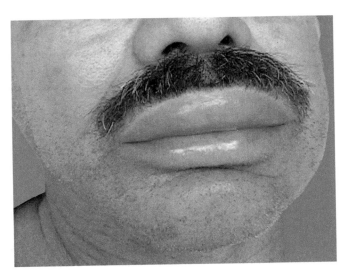

Fig. 30.23 Angioedema with marked swelling of lips

greater risk), and history of atopy (five times) [218]. A study of 34,371 patients reported a significant increase in risk for asthma patients with or without atopy (odds ratio of 8.74) [254]. Notably, allergy specific to seafood does not impose increased risk of an adverse reaction, because virtually no reactions to contrast media are truly allergic in nature nor are they related to the media's iodine content. Additionally, very few seafood allergies are in response to the iodine contained within the foods [255].

Additional risk factors for RCM reactions include cardiac disease, dehydration, hematologic conditions predisposing

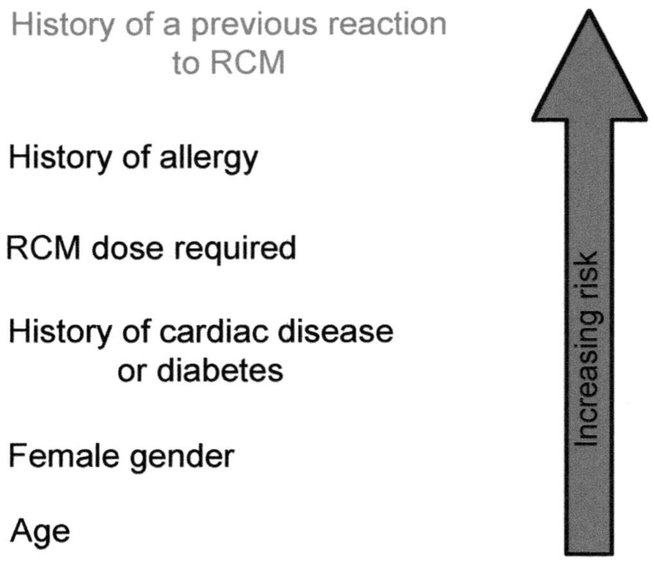

History of a previous reaction
to RCM

History of allergy

RCM dose required

History of cardiac disease
or diabetes

Female gender

Age

Fig. 30.24 Scale of priority for major risk factors for anaphylaxis upon administration of RCM (Modified from Liccardi et al. [253])

Table 30.17 Differential diagnosis for anaphylaxis

Cardiac arrhythmia
Bronchial asthma
Cardiogenic shock
Hemorrhage
Overdosage of sedation/analgesia drug
Pericardial tamponade
Pulmonary embolus
Pulmonary edema
Sepsis
Tension pneumothorax
Vasovagal reaction
Venous air embolism

to thrombosis, renal disease, and anxiety [243]. The use of beta-blocker therapy is a statistically significant risk factor for anaphylactoid reaction, with an odds ratio of 2.67 [254]. In addition, patients receiving beta-blockers have been reported to require hospitalization more often for their reactions [254]. This is thought to be most likely due to a reduced response to treatment.

Women more frequently exhibit adverse reactions than do men. In 5,264 consecutive patients receiving contrast-enhanced CT scans, 70 % of the 73 patients who experienced adverse reactions were women. Twenty-one of twenty-two severe anaphylactoid reactions occurred in women [256]. Studies examining the overall incidence of anaphylaxis and anaphylactoid events have similarly shown an increased occurrence in women [255].

No consistent pattern of adverse reaction risk has emerged related to the type of exam being conducted. Arterial and venous administrations appear to yield the same risks [255].

30.4.7 Treatment

Although it is not a frequent occurrence, an anaphylactic reaction to RCM can be life threatening. Preparedness, prompt recognition, and appropriate and aggressive treatment are integral to parts of successful management of anaphylaxis.

Preparedness

It is important that each facility that performs studies involving the administration of RCM be prepared to manage a patient who might develop a severe HDR. This should include the immediately availability of a completely equipped and supplied "crash cart." This needs to contain supplies and equipment necessary for the establishment of an airway, the administration of oxygen, and for cardiopulmonary resuscitation. Injectable medications should include epinephrine in both 1:1,000 and 1:10,000 dilutions, atropine, diphenhydramine, methylprednisolone, cimetidine, and 0.9 % normal saline. It is also important that regular cardiopulmonary resuscitation (CPR) drills be held.

Prompt Recognition

Early recognition of signs and maintaining a high level of suspicion of the possibility of a generalized reaction during the use of RCM is essential to prevent worsening of the reaction or a fatal outcome. Unfortunately, in many instances in the interventional facility, the recognition of an HDR to RCM may be somewhat hampered by the fact that the patient may have received sedation/analgesia medications. However, if shortly after injecting RCM the patient develops symptoms of pruritus, prolonged vomiting, a fall in oxygen saturation, or hypotension, the possibility of an anaphylactic reaction should be considered in the differential diagnosis (Table 30.17). This should be followed by an anaphylaxis-directed evaluation of the patient. The skin should be examined for the development of urticaria and the face for angioedema. Examine the exposed skin and remove the sterile drape to examine further. Both the upper and lower airways should be evaluated for evidence of stridor, cough, or wheezing. If necessary for evaluation, sedation/analgesia should be reversed.

Management

Appropriate and effective management of an anaphylactic reaction is dependent upon knowledge of the pharmacological agents that should be used and how they are to be applied.

Therapeutic Agents

Due to its central role in the pathogenesis, logic would suggest that antihistamines, agents with H1 and H2 activity, would play a major role in the treatment of an anaphylactic reaction. However, the mast cell-leukocyte cytokine cascade that is activated in this process has redundant and amplifying effects involving multiple mediators. Although histamine is the major culprit, a huge range of inflammatory mediators have been implicated in anaphylaxis. Additionally, studies have indicated that histamine levels peak early then return rapidly to normal despite the persistence of severe physiological compromise [257]. In fact, antagonists directed against histamine that initiated the process have not been found to be of primary therapeutic value. In the acute management of anaphylaxis, the emphasis is on physiological antagonism using epinephrine [247].

Epinephrin

Epinephrine is the most important drug for treating any moderate-to-severe anaphylactic reaction, although there has been no standard recommendation for dose or route. This agent is a direct-acting sympathomimetic agent with various properties that help to reverse the pathophysiological effects of anaphylaxis. The alpha-adrenergic actions of epinephrine work to increase peripheral vascular resistance and reverse peripheral vasodilation while also decreasing angioedema and urticaria. Its beta-1 adrenergic effects have positive chronotropic and inotropic effects on the heart, while the beta-2 adrenergic effects cause bronchodilation and reduction of inflammatory mediator release from mast cells and basophils [258]. In combination, these effects help to reverse the anaphylactic process and, in turn, improve the cutaneous, respiratory, and cardiovascular effects of the condition.

Epinephrine can be given intramuscularly or intravenously, either as a slow injection or an intravenous drip. Due to poor absorption resulting from vasoconstriction, it should not be given subcutaneously for anaphylaxis. Studies in human volunteers without anaphylaxis indicate that injection should be into the muscle of the lateral thigh because absorption here appears more reliable than the deltoid muscle [259, 260]. Direct intravenous administration of epinephrine is facilitated by the fact that during a dialysis access procedure one generally has access to the central circulation. However, great care must be used in administering it by this route. In one study looking at fatal cases of anaphylaxis, it was found that epinephrine was the cause of death in a significant number [248]. If the intravenous route is used, epinephrine must be diluted (1:10,000) and given slowly, and administration must be closely monitored for evidence of toxicity such as tachycardia or hypertension [261]. Fortunately, in the interventional facility continuous hemodynamic monitoring is a standard practice.

If epinephrine is administered as a continuous infusion, a solution of 1 mg to each 100 cc of intravenous fluid (either D5W or 0.9 % normal saline) should be prepared. This gives a concentration of 0.01 mg/cc (1:100,000). The infusion rate should be started at 30–100 mL/h. This can be titrated up or down according to the patients response in order to achieve the lowest effective infusion rate. Due to the short elimination half-life of epinephrine, a steady state is reached in 5–10 min following a change in infusion rate. Epinephrine toxicity is characterized by tachycardia, tremor, and pallor with a normal or elevated blood pressure. If toxicity becomes too severe, the infusion should be stopped briefly before continuing at a lower rate. As the anaphylactic reaction resolves, signs of epinephrine toxicity are more likely. With resolution, the infusion rate should be slowly decreased over a period of 30–45 min.

Antihistamine

Antihistamine falls into the category of a secondary drug in the treatment of anaphylaxis. There are no published trials that systematically examine their utility during anaphylaxis. H1 blockade appears to be useful for mild allergic reactions confined to the skin [262, 263]. There is some evidence in the literature that combined H1 (diphenhydramine) + H2 (cimetidine or ranitidine) blockade is more beneficial than H1 blockade alone for the skin reactions [264, 265]. It is recommended that an H1 blocker be used routinely in the management of all anaphylactic reactions to help counter histamine-mediated vasodilatation that may be continuing. This may not contribute in a major way, but has the virtue of safety. There is some evidence to suggest that an H1 blocker may shorten the duration of the reaction. The usual H1 drug that is used is diphenhydramine 25 or 50 mg given intravenously. Cimetidine, an H2 blocker, can also be administered intravenously at a dose of 300 mg.

Corticosteroids

Although generally used, there are no clinical trials of corticosteroids in the treatment of anaphylaxis, and they do not appear to totally prevent anaphylactic reactions [266, 267]. Current recommendations to consider these agents for patients with anaphylaxis-associated bronchospasm are based primarily upon an extrapolation from their known utility for the treatment of asthma [268]. Corticosteroids are slow-acting drugs and may take up to 4–6 h to have an effect even if given intravenously. They may, however, help in the emergency treatment of an acute attack, and they also have a role in preventing or shortening protracted reactions [268]. Methylprednisolone is the agent generally used. It can be administered intravenously at a dose of 125 mg.

Other Medications

In some cases other medications may be required. Atropine may be necessary if bradycardia occurs (vasovagal type reaction), and in the case of severe hypotension not responsive to fluids, vasopressor agents may be required [247]. These drugs should not be given prominence above fluid resuscitation, however.

Management Strategies

If an evaluation of the patient suggests the presence of anaphylaxis, treatment should be initiated immediately. It should be remembered that anaphylaxis occurs as part of a continuum. Symptoms not immediately life threatening can progress rapidly unless treated promptly.

The first step is to immediately stop the administration of the offending RCM. Subsequent treatment depends upon the severity of the reaction [269]. Sedation/analgesia should be reversed, if this has not already been done, so that breathing and level of consciousness can be more accurately assessed.

The specific treatment administered should be gauged to the grade of the anaphylactic reaction but should consist of some combination of epinephrine, H-1 blocker (diphenhydramine), H-2 blocker (cimetidine) steroid (methylprednisolone), oxygen, and fluid administration.

Mild Anaphylactic Reaction

These reactions tend to be localized and self-limiting. The major features within this classification are those of urticaria and mild angioedema. Some of the level of concern that should be generated by the recognition that an HDR is occurring relates to the rapidity with which it develops. Mild symptoms (pruritus, a few scattered urticarias, and no angioedema) that begin several minutes after the first infusion of RCM (often it is after the procedure has been completed) are often self-limited. These typically resolve fully in an hour or two. No treatment may be required in this situation; however, if the patient is complaining of pruritus, diphenhydramine (25–50 mg parentally or orally) can be administered for symptom control.

Symptoms that begin immediately after RCM infusion should always be treated, regardless of severity, as these reactions tend to persist or worsen. In this instance, diphenhydramine (50 mg intravenously) should be given immediately, and the patient should be observed carefully for any evidence of progression of symptoms. No additional RCM should be administered, even if the symptoms resolve, due to the high risk of recurrent and progressive symptoms.

H1 blockade appears to be useful for mild allergic reactions confined to the skin [262, 263], and there is some evidence in the literature that combined H1 (diphenhydramine)+H2 (cimetidine or ranitidine) blockade is more beneficial than H1 blockade alone [264, 265]. In instances in which the urticaria is severe or in which more than very mild angioedema is apparent, the administration of epinephrine should be considered. Epinephrine 1:1,000 can be given intramuscularly (lateral thigh muscle) at a dose of 0.1–0.3 mL or 1–3 mL of 1:10,000 administered intravenously very slowly with careful monitoring.

Moderate Anaphylactic Reaction

This is characterized by the appearance of systemic signs and symptoms. The major feature is worsening facial edema. The onset of respiratory problems indicates that the situation has deteriorated. This may be seen either as a progression from a picture that was initiated by the onset of urticaria or mild angioedema or it may be the first indication that an adverse event is occurring. This development should be taken as an indication for the immediate initiation of the algorithm outlined in Fig. 30.25 starting with the administration of epinephrine. In the interventional suite during a case in which one has access to the central circulation and the ability to closely monitor cardiovascular functions, epinephrine should be given intravenously (very slowly with monitoring). This should be given in dose of 3–5 mL of 1:10,000. Alternative an intravenous infusion (1:100,000) as described above can be started.

Severe Anaphylactic Reaction

This degree of severity is indicated by the development of life-threatening signs and symptoms – hypoxia, persistent hypotension, loss of consciousness, convulsions, and cardiopulmonary arrest. It should be noted that in a patient who has been sedated, some of these signs of worsening severity can escape notice. For this reason, sedation/analgesia should be reversed very early in the progress of the event. The algorithm outline in Fig. 30.25 should be followed. Only the intravenous route for epinephrine should be used in cases characterized by cardiovascular collapse [270, 271].

If the patient is breathing, a non-rebreather mask set to 100 % oxygen should be applied. It may be necessary to either intubate the patient or use a blind insertion airway device such as a Combitube or laryngeal mask airway. Blood pressure should be supported with fluid administration. This should start with a 200 mL bolus of 0.9 % normal saline as is used to treat hypotension that occurs during dialysis. Care must be exerted to not volume overload the patient. In the case of severe hypotension not responsive to fluids, vasopressor agents may be required.

Biphasic Reactions

Biphasic reactions, defined as a recurrence of anaphylactic symptoms after initial resolution, can occur anywhere from 1 to 72 h after the first onset of symptoms [272–275]. Approximately 5–20 % of patients with anaphylaxis experience a biphasic reaction often requiring oxygen, vasopressors, intubation, and repeat epinephrine administration [276]. Although no validated clinical predictors of biphasic reactions have been documented, some studies suggest that biphasic reactions are more likely to occur in patients who had delayed administration of epinephrine, who needed more than one dose of epinephrine or who initially presented with more severe symptoms [272–275]. Because of this phenomenon, a patient who has significant symptoms of an anaphylactic reaction should be admitted to the hospital for observation even if they responded well to treatment and the situation appears to be resolved.

Prevention

Despite the fact that the increased use of nonionic RCM has been associated with a decrease in the incidence of hypersensitivity reactions, prophylactic drug regimens

Fig. 30.25 Algorithm for treatment of anaphylaxis with systemic signs and symptoms

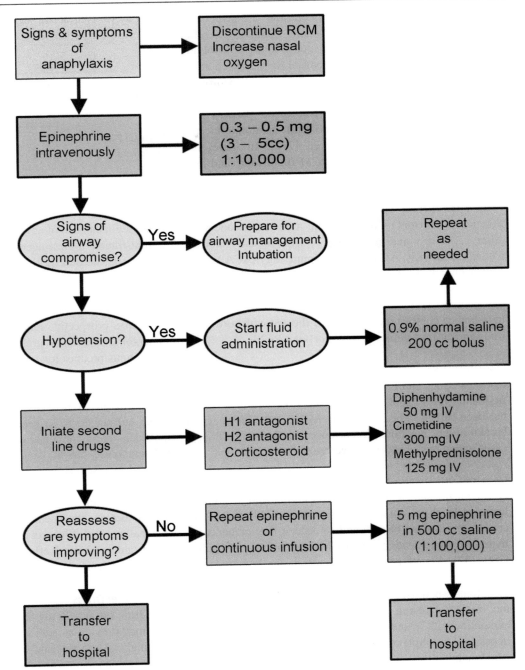

(premedication) that aim to decrease the incidence of breakthrough (recurrent) reactions are still widely used in clinical practice. Two basic questions that arise in relation to the use of premedication are whether it is warranted and whether or not pretreatment actually is effective.

Is It Warranted?

The question as to whether or not premedication will actually prevent breakthrough RCM-mediated HDR is actually somewhat controversial [277–279]. Many feel that sufficient data supporting the use of premedication in patients with a history of allergic reactions are lacking. However, most of the reported studies have included both patients with and those without a history of allergic reactions. It is possible if more restrictive investigation were conducted, more favorable results might be obtained. Additionally, some studies have involved ionic RCM which may not be meaningful in today's environment. Some have suggested that routine prophylaxis should be abandoned [277] and there are studies involving large numbers of cases using an ionic agent that have concluded that major reactions do not recur with any significant frequency even in the absence of premedication [280, 281].

Clinical studies to evaluate this question are difficult to design because a serious anaphylactic complication after administration of RCM is rare. In a meta-analysis involving more than 10,000 patients who received RCM, no reports of death, cardiopulmonary resuscitation, irreversible neurological deficit, or prolonged hospital stay were found [277]. In another series including more than 6,700 patients who received a nonionic-iodinated contrast medium, no life-threatening reaction was observed [282]. In more than 337,000 patients who received RCM (both ionic and non-ionic), 2 deaths occurred, but a causal relationship to the contrast medium could not be established [218].

In spite of these concerns, both the Joint Task Force on Practice Parameters representing the American Academy of Allergy, Asthma, and Immunology (AAAAI); the American College of Allergy, Asthma, and Immunology (ACAAI); the Joint Council of Allergy, Asthma, and Immunology [283]; and the American College of Radiology [284] recommend that patients with a known history of allergic-like reactions to iodinated contrast media be premedicated with corticosteroids and antihistamines before receiving RCM.

Does It Work?

Corticosteroids and H1- and H2-antihistamines are the most frequently used agents and premedication with these drugs has been shown to be effective in reducing the incidence of breakthrough reactions (recurrences) [227, 285–288] in cases with a prior history of a reaction.

Case for Corticosteroids

Although the mechanism by which corticosteroid prophylaxis works is not completely understood [289], the use of corticosteroids has been found to reduce the incidence of hypersensitivity reactions to RCM in a number of studies [290–292]. A meta-analysis of reports in the literature suggested that these agents prevented primarily respiratory symptoms when used as premedication [277]. Nevertheless, the value of using corticosteroid prophylaxis remains contentious [293], and the current opinion as to whether corticosteroid prophylaxis should be used with nonionic agents is not unanimous. For one thing prophylaxis does not totally prevent reactions, anaphylaxis has been reported in patients despite pretreatment with corticosteroids [294].

Not all physicians use these agents. In one survey of prophylaxis procedures in adult patients [295] receiving RCM, it was found that 91 % of respondents gave corticosteroids in high-risk patients. However, other surveys have reported that a significant percentage of responders did not use corticosteroid [296, 297].

Case for Antihistamines

The major clinical features of anaphylaxis are initiated by histamine release. Intuitively, antihistamines should be beneficial

Table 30.18 Pretreatment regimen for high-risk patients receiving RCM

Agent	Dose	Timing relative to procedure
Regimen 1		
Prednisone	50 mg orally	13, 7, and 1 h before
Diphenhydramine	50 mg orally (or parenterally)	1 h before
Regimen 2		
Prednisolone	32 mg orally	12 and 2 h before procedure

as prophylaxis. A number of studies have described a decreased incidence of adverse RCM reactions following the administration of these agents, either alone or in combination with corticosteroids [291, 298, 299]. Several reports have found that the combined use of anti-H1 and anti-H2 agents may give better protection against anaphylactic reactions than the administration of these drugs separately [249, 250, 300–303]. In a prospective randomized trial [304], 800 patients undergoing intravenous urography were pretreated with either intravenous prednisolone, an H1-antagonist (P/H1 group), a combination of H1 and H2 antagonists (H1/H2 group), or 0.9 % saline (control group). There was a significant difference in frequency between the control group and the H1/H2 group but not the P/H1 group. The authors suggested from their data that a combined application of histamine H1- and H2-antagonists might be useful in prophylaxis of RCM-induced adverse reactions. However, other reports have found that the addition of an H2 antagonist to regimens containing H1 antihistamines and corticosteroids did not further reduce the number of subsequent adverse reactions [290, 291, 305]. A meta-analysis of reports in the literature suggested that H1 antihistamine showed efficacy primarily against cutaneous symptoms when used as premedication [277].

Use of Other Drugs

Ephedrine sulfate, 25 mg orally, given 1 h before the procedure may provide an additional protective benefit; however, potential risks in patients with underlying heart disease or hypertension must be considered. For this reason, ephedrine is not commonly used.

Prevention Drug Regimens

The approach to the prevention of the recurrence of a hypersensitivity reaction to RCM involves the application of two principles, the use of a nonionic RCM and the administration of pharmacological agents. Although the optimal approach has not been determined [279, 290, 291, 304, 306–308], there are two regimens that have been applied (Table 30.18). The most widely accepted regimen (referred to herein as Regimen 1) is that recommended by the American College of Radiology which combines multiple doses of corticosteroids and a single dose of H1 antihistamine with the use of a nonionic RCM [279, 308, 309]. Regimen 2 involves only corticosteroid given at two times in advance of the procedure.

Effectiveness of Regimens

There is a considerable body of literature relating to pretreatment of patients with prior HDRs; however, most of it is based upon studies performed at a time when ionic RCM was used. This does not invalidate this work, but it does suggest that with the use of nonionic RCM the beneficial results might be better than those reported. In a study of 657 procedures using ionic RCM performed in 563 patients with a history of an HDR [306], it was reported that premedication using Regimen 1 (Table 30.18) reduced the rate of breakthrough reactions from a historical level of 17–60 %, down to 9 %. No deaths occurred, and only three episodes of transient hypotension developed, one of which required treatment with epinephrine. In this study, pretreatment was effective regardless of the severity of the patient's previous reaction (severe reactions may have been excluded from study).

In a prospective double-blind study utilizing Regimen 2 (Table 30.18) [292], two groups were studied. One group received the medication and the other did not and served as a control. A total of 1,155 patients and control subjects successfully completed the protocol. Corticosteroid pretreatment conferred protection for overall reactions (1.7 % versus 4.9 %, $p = .005$) and mild reactions (0.2 % versus 1.9 %, $p = .004$). Subjects receiving corticosteroids also had fewer moderate and severe reactions, but the total numbers involved were small, and the differences were not significant.

Who Should Be Premedicated

A number of risk factors for HDE have been identified; however, the only one significant enough to actually justify pretreatment is a definite prior reaction to RCM. Even if the patient alleges that they are "allergic to X-ray dye," one cannot be sure. An accurate history should be elicited to determine if the suspected event is actually credible for a hypersensitivity reaction to RCM. The administration of test doses of RCM should not be done. Fatalities have resulted from the administration of amounts as small as 1–2 mL as a test dose [310]. Additionally, severe and fatal reactions to RCM have occurred in patients who tolerated a test dose [280, 310–312]. It should also be noted that a patient can have a reaction to the very first dose, never having had a previous exposure (nonimmunologic and not IgE mediated) [229].

Breakthrough Reaction

Recurrent HDEs in spite of premedication are referred to as breakthrough reactions. Despite different protocols and administration routes, severe breakthrough reactions may still develop in patients who receive corticosteroid premedication [285]. In a study involving HDR to nonionic RCM, the estimated recurrence rate of RCM reaction after corticosteroid administration was estimated to be almost 10 % [285]. The severity of the breakthrough reaction is usually similar to the severity of the index reaction, and most RCM injections (especially nonionic) administered to premedicated patients do not result in a breakthrough reaction. Patients who experience a mild initial reaction have an extremely low risk of experiencing a severe breakthrough reaction. If one occurs, it is generally mild also [280, 288]. However, patients who experience a moderate or severe initial or breakthrough reaction are at high risk of experiencing another moderate or severe reaction should a breakthrough reaction occur [288]. Patients with this type of history should be referred to the hospital for their procedure.

In one study [285], breakthrough reactions were identified in approximately 10 % of patients who were premedicated with corticosteroids. Of these breakthrough reactions, 24 % were severe or life threatening. The severity of the breakthrough reaction was generally similar to that of the initial reaction; the breakthrough reaction was more severe 11 % of the time.

In another study [288], 140,775 injections of nonionic RCM resulted in 0.7 % hypersensitivity reactions. Their distribution was 928 mild, 99 moderate, and 17 severe. Of these, 18 % (190 cases) were breakthrough reactions (152 mild, 35 moderate, and 3 severe) that occurred in 175 patients. There were 122 female patients and 53 male patients. The severity of the initial reaction associated with 128 of the 190 breakthrough reactions was known. The breakthrough reaction was less severe in 15 (12 %), equally severe in 103 (81 %), and more severe in 10 (8 %) cases.

Emergent Procedures

In some instances, a patient with a prior history of a reaction to RCM is referred to the interventional facility for a dialysis access procedure without being premedicated. In these instances the question as to what should be done always arises. In many facilities it is common practice, if the prior reaction was mild (or questionable), for the patient to be given methylprednisolone, 125 mg and diphenhydramine, 50 mg intravenously immediately prior to the injection of RCM. The data upon which this practice is based is not clear.

There are only a few studies providing data relevant to this issue. Looking at cutaneous changes (pruritus and urticaria) associated with an HDR, there are two studies worthy of note. In a prospective controlled study, Small et al. [313] administered an antihistamine (chlorpheniramine) 15 min before the procedure in which RCM (type not specified) was administered. Cases were divided into 3 groups – medication (78), placebo (saline) (71), no treatment (71). Reactions were significantly decreased in the treatment group versus the two control groups (1/78 versus 15/142). Odds ratio was 0.25 (95 % confidence limits – 0.09–0.73). In another prospective controlled study, Wicke et al. [314] administered antihistamine (clemastine) to patients receiving RCM (ionic high osmolar). Cases were divided into two groups – treatment (92) and control (116). Only two reactions were observed in the study, both were within the control group. Odds ratio was 0.17 (95 % confidence limits – 0.01–2.71).

In a prospective controlled study, Chevrot et al. [315] administered corticosteroid (Betamethasone 8 mg IV) at the time of the procedure in which RCM was used (most were ionic high osmolar). No reactions were seen in the treated group (0/109) and one reaction (hypotension) was observed in the control group (1/112). Odds ratio was 0.14 (95 % confidence limits – 0.00–7.01).

Additionally there are small observational studies such as one involving ten cases with a prior history of an anaphylactic reaction [316]. In these cases, hydrocortisone 200 mg (equivalent to 40 mg of methylprednisolone) was administered intravenously immediately and every 4 h until the procedure was completed in addition to diphenhydramine, 50 mg intravenously, 1 h before the procedure. No reactions occurred in these patients.

It is difficult to know what a small study signifies and the prospective controlled studies can be faulted for having so few breakthrough reactions in their control groups giving odds ratios in a rather low range with very wide confidence limits. This is especially true in consideration of the fact previously mentioned that not all cases of a prior reaction will have a repeat reaction even in the absence of premedication [280, 281]. Nevertheless, these data do suggest the value of administration of premedication at the time of the procedure in which RCM is to be administered in cases in which the index reaction was mild.

Recommendations

All procedures should be performed using nonionic low-molecular-weight RCM in order to minimize the risk of an HDR. Cases with a history of a prior reaction to RCM should be considered to be at an increased risk for another reaction and should be premedicated. These repeat reactions will generally be of the same severity as the initial reaction or less, but one cannot depend upon this. If a patient has a history of a moderate-to-severe anaphylactic reaction, they should not be managed at a freestanding facility; they should be referred to the hospital setting with its full range of supportive measures. Regimen 1, Table 30.18 should be followed if time permits. Even though the evidence is not strong, patients with a history of a previous mild reaction to RCM who require an emergent procedure should receive pretreatment with 125 mg of methylprednisolone (or its equivalent) and diphenhydramine, 50 mg, intravenously immediately before the administration of RCM.

References

1. Sznajder JI, Zveibil FR, Bitterman H, et al. Central vein catheterization. Failure and complication rates by three percutaneous approaches. Arch Intern Med. 1986;146:259.
2. Fares 2nd LG, Block PH, Feldman SD. Improved house staff results with subclavian cannulation. Am Surg. 1986;52:108.
3. McGee DC, Gould MK. Preventing complications of central venous catheterization. N Engl J Med. 2003;348:1123.
4. Trerotola SO, Johnson MS, Harris VJ, et al. Outcome of tunneled hemodialysis catheters placed via the right internal jugular vein by interventional radiologists. Radiology. 1997;203:489.
5. Peris A, Zagli G, Bonizzoli M, et al. Implantation of 3951 long-term central venous catheters: performances, risk analysis, and patient comfort after ultrasound-guidance introduction. Anesth Analg. 2010;111:1194.
6. Rabindranath KS, Kumar E, Shail R, Vaux E. Use of real-time ultrasound guidance for the placement of hemodialysis catheters: a systematic review and meta-analysis of randomized controlled trials. Am J Kidney Dis. 2011;58:964.
7. Mansfield PF, Hohn DC, Fornage BD, et al. Complications and failures of subclavian-vein catheterization. N Engl J Med. 1994;331:1735.
8. Bour ES, Weaver AS, Yang HC, Gifford RR. Experience with the double lumen silastic catheter for hemoaccess. Surg Gynecol Obstet. 1990;171:33.
9. McDowell DE, Moss AH, Vasilakis C, et al. Percutaneously placed dual-lumen silicone catheters for long-term hemodialysis. Am Surg. 1993;59:569.
10. Randolph AG, Cook DJ, Gonzales CA, Pribble CG. Ultrasound guidance for placement of central venous catheters: a meta-analysis of the literature. Crit Care Med. 1996;24:2053.
11. Oguzkurt L, Tercan F, Kara G, et al. US-guided placement of temporary internal jugular vein catheters: immediate technical success and complications in normal and high-risk patients. Eur J Radiol. 2005;55:125.
12. Karakitsos D, Labropoulos N, De Groot E, et al. Real-time ultrasound-guided catheterisation of the internal jugular vein: a prospective comparison with the landmark technique in critical care patients. Crit Care. 2006;10:R162.
13. Lin BS, Huang TP, Tang GJ, et al. Ultrasound-guided cannulation of the internal jugular vein for dialysis vascular access in uremic patients. Nephron. 1998;78:423.
14. Lin BS, Kong CW, Tarng DC, et al. Anatomical variation of the internal jugular vein and its impact on temporary haemodialysis vascular access: an ultrasonographic survey in uraemic patients. Nephrol Dial Transplant. 1998;13:134.
15. Canaud B, Desmeules S, Klouche K, et al. Vascular access for dialysis in the intensive care unit. Best Pract Res Clin Anaesthesiol. 2004;18:159.
16. Tordor J, Haage P, Konner K, et al. EBPG on vascular access. Nephrol Dial Transplant. 2007;22 Suppl 2:103.
17. Beathard GA, Litchfield T. Effectiveness and safety of dialysis vascular access procedures performed by interventional nephrologists. Kidney Int. 2004;66:1622.
18. American College of Surgeons, Committee on Trauma. Advanced trauma life support course manual. Chicago: American College of Surgeons; 2004.
19. McPherson JJ, Feigin DS, Bellamy RF. Prevalence of tension pneumothorax in fatally wounded combat casualties. J Trauma. 2006;60:573.
20. Moore FO, Goslar PW, Coimbra R, et al. Blunt traumatic occult pneumothorax: is observation safe? – results of a prospective. AAST multicenter study. J Trauma. 2011;70:1019.
21. Kaufmann C. Initial assessment and management. New York: McGraw-Hill Medical; 2008.

22. Leigh-Smith S, Harris T. Tension pneumothorax – time for a re-think? Emerg Med J. 2005;22:8.

23. Choi SH, Lee SW, Hong YS, et al. Can spontaneous pneumothorax patients be treated by ambulatory care management? Eur J Cardiothorac Surg. 2007;31:491.

24. Zehtabchi S, Rios CL. Management of emergency department patients with primary spontaneous pneumothorax: needle aspiration or tube thoracostomy? Ann Emerg Med. 2008;51:91.

25. Samelson SL, Goldberg EM, Ferguson MK. The thoracic vent. Clinical experience with a new device for treating simple pneumothorax. Chest. 1991;100:880.

26. Martin T, Fontana G, Olak J, Ferguson M. Use of pleural catheter for the management of simple pneumothorax. Chest. 1996;110:1169.

27. Rawlins R, Brown KM, Carr CS, Cameron CR. Life threatening haemorrhage after anterior needle aspiration of pneumothoraces. A role for lateral needle aspiration in emergency decompression of spontaneous pneumothorax. Emerg Med J. 2003;20:383.

28. Heng K, Bystrzycki A, Fitzgerald M, et al. Complications of intercostal catheter insertion using EMST techniques for chest trauma. ANZ J Surg. 2004;74:420.

29. Jenkins C, Sudheer PS. Needle thoracocentesis fails to diagnose a large pneumothorax. Anaesthesia. 2000;55:925.

30. Biffl WL. Needle thoracostomy: a cautionary note. Acad Emerg Med. 2004;11:795.

31. Yamagami T, Kato T, Hirota T, et al. Usefulness and limitation of manual aspiration immediately after pneumothorax complicating interventional radiological procedures with the transthoracic approach. Cardiovasc Intervent Radiol. 2006;29:1027.

32. Yamagami T, Terayama K, Yoshimatsu R, et al. Role of manual aspiration in treating pneumothorax after computed tomography-guided lung biopsy. Acta Radiol. 2009;50:1126.

33. Ball CG, Wyrzykowski AD, Kirkpatrick AW, et al. Thoracic needle decompression for tension pneumothorax: clinical correlation with catheter length. Can J Surg. 2010;53:184.

34. Flanagan JP, Gradisar IA, Gross RJ, Kelly TR. Air embolus – a lethal complication of subclavian venipuncture. N Engl J Med. 1969;281:488.

35. Kashuk JL, Penn I. Air embolism after central venous catheterization. Surg Gynecol Obstet. 1984;159:249.

36. Yeakel AE. Lethal air embolism from plastic blood-storage container. JAMA. 1968;204:267.

37. Martland H. Air embolism: fatal air embolism due to powder insufflators used in gynecologic treatments. Am J Surg. 1945;68:164.

38. Orebaugh SL. Venous air embolism: clinical and experimental considerations. Crit Care Med. 1992;20:1169.

39. Olmedilla L, Garutti I, Perez-Pena J, et al. Fatal paradoxical air embolism during liver transplantation. Br J Anaesth. 2000; 84:112.

40. Scott WL. Complications associated with central venous catheters. A survey. Chest. 1988;94:1221.

41. Vesely TM. Air embolism during insertion of central venous catheters. J Vasc Interv Radiol. 2001;12:1291.

42. Heckmann JG, Lang CJ, Kindler K, et al. Neurologic manifestations of cerebral air embolism as a complication of central venous catheterization. Crit Care Med. 2000;28:1621.

43. Muth CM, Shank ES. Gas embolism. N Engl J Med. 2000;342:476.

44. Nicholl DD, Ahmed SB, Loewen AH, et al. Declining kidney function increases the prevalence of sleep apnea and nocturnal hypoxia. Chest. 2012;141:1422–30.

45. Eichhorn V, Bender A, Reuter DA. Paradoxical air embolism from a central venous catheter. Br J Anaesth. 2009;102:717.

46. Mirski MA, Lele AV, Fitzsimmons L, Toung TJ. Diagnosis and treatment of vascular air embolism. Anesthesiology. 2007;106:164.

47. Capozzoli G, Schenk C, Vezzali N. Cerebral air embolism after central dialysis line removal: the role of the fibrin sheath as portal (mechanism) of air entry. J Vasc Access. 2012;13:516–9.

48. King MB, Harmon KR. Unusual forms of pulmonary embolism. Clin Chest Med. 1994;15:561.

49. Kizer KW, Goodman PC. Radiographic manifestations of venous air embolism. Radiology. 1982;144:35.

50. Palmon SC, Moore LE, Lundberg J, Toung T. Venous air embolism: a review. J Clin Anesth. 1997;9:251.

51. Durant TM, Long J, Oppenheimer MJ. Pulmonary (venous) air embolism. Am Heart J. 1947;33:269.

52. Gottdiener JS, Papademetriou V, Notargiacomo A, et al. Incidence and cardiac effects of systemic venous air embolism. Echocardiographic evidence of arterial embolization via noncardiac shunt. Arch Intern Med. 1988;148:795.

53. Miller WC, Heard JG, Unger KM. Enlarged pulmonary arteriovenous vessels in COPD. Another possible mechanism of hypoxemia. Chest. 1984;86:704.

54. Ploner F, Saltuari L, Marosi MJ, et al. Cerebral air emboli with use of central venous catheter in mobile patient. Lancet. 1991;338:1331.

55. Papadopoulos G, Kuhly P, Brock M, et al. Venous and paradoxical air embolism in the sitting position, a prospective study with transoesophageal echocardiography. Acta Neurochir (Wien). 1994;126: 140.

56. Beck DH, McQuillan PJ. Fatal carbon dioxide embolism and severe haemorrhage during laparoscopic salpingectomy. Br J Anaesth. 1994;72:243.

57. Losasso TJ, Muzzi DA, Dietz NM, Cucchiara RF. Fifty percent nitrous oxide does not increase the risk of venous air embolism in neurosurgical patients operated upon in the sitting position. Anesthesiology. 1992;77:21.

58. Van Liew HD, Conkin J, Burkard ME. The oxygen window and decompression bubbles: estimates and significance. Aviat Space Environ Med. 1993;64:859.

59. Mehlhorn U, Burke EJ, Butler BD, et al. Body position does not affect the hemodynamic response to venous air embolism in dogs. Anesth Analg. 1994;79:734.

60. Geissler HJ, Allen SJ, Mehlhorn U, et al. Effect of body repositioning after venous air embolism. An echocardiographic study. Anesthesiology. 1997;86:710.

61. Ericsson JA, Gottlieb JD, Sweet RB. Closed-chest cardiac massage in the treatment of venous Air embolism. N Engl J Med. 1964;270: 1353.

62. Yeh PA, Chen HP, Tsai YC, et al. Successful management of air embolism-induced ventricular fibrillation in orthotopic liver transplantation. Acta Anaesthesiol Taiwan. 2005;43:243.

63. Han SS, Kim SS, Hong HP, et al. Massive paradoxical air embolism in brain occurring after central venous catheterization: a case report. J Korean Med Sci. 2010;25:1536.

64. Finsterer J, Stollberger C, Bastovansky A. Cardiac and cerebral air embolism from endoscopic retrograde cholangio-pancreatography. Eur J Gastroenterol Hepatol. 2010;22:1157.

65. Le Guen M, Trebbia G, Sage E, et al. Intraoperative cerebral air embolism during lung transplantation: treatment with early hyperbaric oxygen therapy. J Cardiothorac Vasc Anesth. 2012;26: 1077–9.

66. Bayer O, Schummer C, Richter K, et al. Implication of the anatomy of the pericardial reflection on positioning of central venous catheters. J Cardiothorac Vasc Anesth. 2006;20:777.

67. Salik E, Daftary A, Tal MG. Three-dimensional anatomy of the left central veins: implications for dialysis catheter placement. J Vasc Interv Radiol. 2007;18:361.

68. Schummer W, Schummer C, Fritz H. Perforation of the superior vena cava due to unrecognized stenosis. Case report of a lethal complication of central venous catheterization. Anaesthesist. 2001; 50:772.

69. Wicky S, Meuwly JY, Doenz F, et al. Life-threatening vascular complications after central venous catheter placement. Eur Radiol. 2002;12:901.

70. Jankovic Z, Boon A, Prasad R. Fatal haemothorax following large-bore percutaneous cannulation before liver transplantation. Br J Anaesth. 2005;95:472.

71. Wadelek J, Drobinski D, Szewczyk P, et al. Perforation of the internal jugular vein during cannulation for haemodialysis. Anestezjol Intens Ter. 2009;41:110.

72. Jost K, Leithauser M, Grosse-Thie C, et al. Perforation of the superior vena cava – a rare complication of central venous catheters. Onkologie. 2008;31:262.

73. Ko SF, Ng SH, Fang FM, et al. Left brachiocephalic vein perforation: computed tomographic features and treatment considerations. Am J Emerg Med. 2007;25:1051.

74. Wang CY, Liu K, Chia YY, Chen CH. Bedside ultrasonic detection of massive hemothorax due to superior vena cava perforation after hemodialysis catheter insertion. Acta Anaesthesiol Taiwan. 2009;47:95.

75. Elwali A, Drissi M, Bensghir M, et al. Fatal evolution of a left brachio-cephalic vein perforation by a catheter for hemodialysis. Nephrol Ther. 2011;7:562.

76. Robinson JF, Robinson WA, Cohn A, et al. Perforation of the great vessels during central venous line placement. Arch Intern Med. 1995;155:1225.

77. Edwards H, King TC. Cardiac tamponade from central venous catheters. Arch Surg. 1982;117:965.

78. Maschke SP, Rogove HJ. Cardiac tamponade associated with a multilumen central venous catheter. Crit Care Med. 1984;12:611.

79. Reilly JJ, Cosimi B, Russell PS. Delayed perforation of the innominate vein during hyperalimentation. Arch Surg. 1977; 112:96.

80. Ying-Chih L, Tung-Min Y. Delayed great-vessel perforation related to an indwelling haemodialysis catheter over the left internal jugular vein. Nephrology (Carlton). 2010;15:780.

81. Ishibashi H, Ohta K, Ochiai T, et al. Delayed hydrothorax induced by a pericutaneous central venous catheter; report of a case. Kyobu Geka. 2002;55:213.

82. Mukau L, Talamini MA, Sitzmann JV. Risk factors for central venous catheter-related vascular erosions. JPEN J Parenter Enteral Nutr. 1991;15:513.

83. Duntley P, Siever J, Korwes ML, et al. Vascular erosion by central venous catheters. Clinical features and outcome. Chest. 1992; 101:1633.

84. Walshe C, Phelan D, Bourke J, Buggy D. Vascular erosion by central venous catheters used for total parenteral nutrition. Intensive Care Med. 2007;33:534.

85. Iberti TJ, Katz LB, Reiner MA, et al. Hydrothorax as a late complication of central venous indwelling catheters. Surgery. 1983;94:842.

86. Schummer W, Schummer C, Gerold M. The placement of central venous catheters is a technically challenging procedure with various risks and well-known complications. Nutr Clin Pract. 2003;18:102.

87. Schummer W, Herrmann S, Schummer C, et al. Intra-atrial ECG is not a reliable method for positioning left internal jugular vein catheters. Br J Anaesth. 2003;91:481.

88. Tocino IM, Watanabe A. Impending catheter perforation of superior vena cava: radiographic recognition. AJR Am J Roentgenol. 1986;146:487.

89. Barton BR, Hermann G, Weil 3rd R. Cardiothoracic emergencies associated with subclavian hemodialysis catheters. JAMA. 1983;250:2660.

90. Leech RC, Watts AD, Heaton ND, Potter DR. Intraoperative cardiac tamponade after central venous cannulation in an infant during orthotopic liver transplantation. Anesth Analg. 1999;89:342.

91. Sirvent AE, Enriquez R, Millan I, et al. Severe hemorrhage because of delayed iliac vein rupture after dialysis catheter placement: is it preventable? Hemodial Int. 2012;16:315–9.

92. Florescu MC, Mousa A, Salifu M, Friedman EA. Accidental extravascular insertion of a subclavian hemodialysis catheter is signaled by nonvisualization of catheter tip. Hemodial Int. 2005; 9:341.

93. Azizzadeh A, Pham MT, Estrera AL, et al. Endovascular repair of an iatrogenic superior vena caval injury: a case report. J Vasc Surg. 2007;46:569.

94. Jaurrieta-Mas E, Rafecas A, Pallares R, et al. Successful diagnosis and treatment of cardiac perforation due to subclavian catheter during total parenteral nutrition. JPEN J Parenter Enteral Nutr. 1982;6:157.

95. Jay AW, Aldridge HE. Perforation of the heart or vena cava by central venous catheters inserted for monitoring or infusion therapy. Can Med Assoc J. 1986;135:1143.

96. Aliyev F, Celiker C, Turkoglu C, et al. Perforations of right heart chambers associated with electrophysiology catheters and temporary transvenous pacing leads. Turk Kardiyol Dern Ars. 2011;39:16.

97. Auxiliadora-Martins M, Apinages Dos Santos E, Adans Wenzinger D, et al. Perforation of the right ventricle induced by pulmonary artery catheter at induction of anesthesia for the surgery for liver transplantation: a case report and reviewed of literature. Case Rep Med. 2009;2009:650982.

98. Czepizak CA, O'Callaghan JM, Venus B. Evaluation of formulas for optimal positioning of central venous catheters. Chest. 1995;107:1662.

99. Greenall MJ, Blewitt RW, McMahon MJ. Cardiac tamponade and central venous catheters. Br Med J. 1975;2:595.

100. Giacoia GP. Cardiac tamponade and hydrothorax as complications of central venous parenteral nutrition in infants. JPEN J Parenter Enteral Nutr. 1991;15:110.

101. Shen X, Fang Z, Hu X, et al. Cardiac perforation and tamponade in percutaneous cardiac intervention. Zhong Nan Da Xue Xue Bao Yi Xue Ban. 2011;36:74.

102. Collier PE, Blocker SH, Graff DM, Doyle P. Cardiac tamponade from central venous catheters. Am J Surg. 1998;176:212.

103. Food and Drug Administration Task Force. Precautions necessary with central venous catheters. FDA Drug Bull. 1989:15–16.

104. Scott WL. Central venous catheters. An overview of Food and Drug Administration activities. Surg Oncol Clin N Am. 1995;4:377.

105. NKF-DOQI clinical practice guidelines for vascular access. Guideline 2: selection and placement of hemodialysis access, http://www.kidney.org/professionals/KDOQI/guideline_upHD_PD_VA/index.htm. Accessed 10 Dec 2013.

106. Bersten AD, Williams DR, Phillips GD. Central venous catheter stiffness and its relation to vascular perforation. Anaesth Intensive Care. 1988;16:342.

107. Gravenstein N, Blackshear RH. In vitro evaluation of relative perforating potential of central venous catheters: comparison of materials, selected models, number of lumens, and angles of incidence to simulated membrane. J Clin Monit. 1991;7:1.

108. Kearns PJ, Coleman S, Wehner JH. Complications of long arm-catheters: a randomized trial of central vs peripheral tip location. JPEN J Parenter Enteral Nutr. 1996;20:20.

109. Brandt RL, Foley WJ, Fink GH, Regan WJ. Mechanism of perforation of the heart with production of hydropericdium by a venous catheter and its prevention. Am J Surg. 1970;119:311.

110. Aldridge HE, Jay AW. Central venous catheters and heart perforation. CMAJ. 1986;135:1082.

111. Demers H, Siebold G, Schielke D, et al. Soft right atrial catheter for temporary or permanent vascular access. Nephrol Dial Transplant. 1989;18:130.

112. Tan PL, Chan C. Bilateral pleural effusions following central venous cannulation. J Postgrad Med. 2007;53:117.

113. Vesely TM. Central venous catheter tip position: a continuing controversy. J Vasc Interv Radiol. 2003;14:527.

114. Reuber M, Dunkley LA, Turton EP, et al. Stroke after internal jugular venous cannulation. Acta Neurol Scand. 2002; 105:235.
115. Shah PM, Babu SC, Goyal A, et al. Arterial misplacement of large-caliber cannulas during jugular vein catheterization: case for surgical management. J Am Coll Surg. 2004;198:939.
116. Eckhardt WF, Iaconetti J, Kwon JS, et al. Inadvertent carotid artery cannulation during pulmonary artery catheter insertion. J Cardiothorac Vasc Anesth. 1996;10:283.
117. Nicholson T, Ettles D, Robinson G. Managing inadvertent arterial catheterization during central venous access procedures. Cardiovasc Intervent Radiol. 2004;27:21.
118. Kulvatunyou N, Heard SO, Bankey PE. A subclavian artery injury, secondary to internal jugular vein cannulation, is a predictable right-sided phenomenon. Anesth Analg. 2002;95:564.
119. Mainland PA, Tam WH, Law B, Ngan Kee W. Stroke following central venous cannulation. Lancet. 1997;349:921.
120. Guilbert MC, Elkouri S, Bracco D, et al. Arterial trauma during central venous catheter insertion: case series, review and proposed algorithm. J Vasc Surg. 2008;48:918.
121. Slama M, Novara A, Safavian A, et al. Improvement of internal jugular vein cannulation using an ultrasound-guided technique. Intensive Care Med. 1997;23:916.
122. Ellison N, Jobes DR, Schwartz AJ. Percutaneous jugular cannulation. Ann Thorac Surg. 1979;28:204.
123. Heath KJ, Woulfe J, Lownie S, et al. A devastating complication of inadvertent carotid artery puncture. Anesthesiology. 1998; 89:1273.
124. Zaida N, Khan M, Naqvi H, Kamal R. Cerebral infarct following central venous cannulation. Anaesthesia. 1998;53:186.
125. Powell H, Beechey AP. Internal jugular catheterisation. Case report of a potentially fatal hazard. Anaesthesia. 1990;45:458.
126. Golden LR. Incidence and management of large-bore introducer sheath puncture of the carotid artery. J Cardiothorac Vasc Anesth. 1995;9:425.
127. Pikwer A, Acosta S, Kolbel T, et al. Management of inadvertent arterial catheterisation associated with central venous procedures. Eur J Vasc Endovasc Surg. 2009;38:707.
128. Vesely TM. Complications related to percutaneous thrombectomy of hemodialysis grafts. J Vasc Access. 2002;3:49.
129. Turmel-Rodrigues L, Pengloan J, Baudin S, et al. Treatment of stenosis and thrombosis in haemodialysis fistulas and grafts by interventional radiology. Nephrol Dial Transplant. 2000;15:2029.
130. Turmel-Rodrigues L, editor. Diagnosis and endovascular treatment for autologous fistula-related stenosis. New York: Lippincott Williams & Wilkins; 2002.
131. Raynaud AC, Angel CY, Sapoval MR, et al. Treatment of hemodialysis access rupture during PTA with Wallstent implantation. J Vasc Interv Radiol. 1998;9:437.
132. Beathard GA. The treatment of vascular access graft dysfunction: a nephrologist's view and experience. Adv Ren Replace Ther. 1994;1:131.
133. Pappas JN, Vesely TM. Vascular rupture during angioplasty of hemodialysis raft-related stenoses. J Vasc Access. 2002;3:120.
134. Beathard GA. Percutaneous transvenous angioplasty in the treatment of vascular access stenosis. Kidney Int. 1992;42:1390.
135. Kornfield ZN, Kwak A, Soulen MC, et al. Incidence and management of percutaneous transluminal angioplasty-induced venous rupture in the "fistula first" era. J Vasc Interv Radiol. 2009;20:744.
136. Rajan DK, Clark TW, Patel NK, et al. Prevalence and treatment of cephalic arch stenosis in dysfunctional autogenous hemodialysis fistulas. J Vasc Interv Radiol. 2003;14:567.
137. Beathard GA. Management of complications of endovascular dialysis access procedures. Semin Dial. 2003;16:309.
138. Beathard GA. Angioplasty for arteriovenous grafts and fistulae. Semin Nephrol. 2002;22:202.
139. Beathard GA, Urbanes A, Litchfield T. The classification of procedure-related complications – a fresh approach. Semin Dial. 2006;19:527.
140. Bittl JA. Venous rupture during percutaneous treatment of hemodialysis fistulas and grafts. Catheter Cardiovasc Interv. 2009;74:1097.
141. Funaki B, Szymski GX, Leef JA, et al. Wallstent deployment to salvage dialysis graft thrombolysis complicated by venous rupture: early and intermediate results. AJR Am J Roentgenol. 1997;169:1435.
142. Rundback JH, Leonardo RF, Poplausky MR, Rozenblit G. Venous rupture complicating hemodialysis access angioplasty: percutaneous treatment and outcomes in seven patients. AJR Am J Roentgenol. 1998;171:1081.
143. Rajan DK, Clark TW. Patency of Wallstents placed at the venous anastomosis of dialysis grafts for salvage of angioplasty-induced rupture. Cardiovasc Intervent Radiol. 2003;26:242.
144. Sofocleous CT, Schur I, Koh E, et al. Percutaneous treatment of complications occurring during hemodialysis graft recanalization. Eur J Radiol. 2003;47:237.
145. Trerotola SO, Johnson MS, Shah H, et al. Incidence and management of arterial emboli from hemodialysis graft surgical thrombectomy. J Vasc Interv Radiol. 1997;8:557.
146. Winkler TA, Trerotola SO, Davidson DD, Milgrom ML. Study of thrombus from thrombosed hemodialysis access grafts. Radiology. 1995;197:461.
147. Valji K, Bookstein JJ, Roberts AC, et al. Pulse-spray pharmacomechanical thrombolysis of thrombosed hemodialysis access grafts: long-term experience and comparison of original and current techniques. AJR Am J Roentgenol. 1995;164:1495.
148. Kumpe DA, Cohen MA. Angioplasty/thrombolytic treatment of failing and failed hemodialysis access sites: comparison with surgical treatment. Prog Cardiovasc Dis. 1992;34:263.
149. Rajan DK, Patel NH, Valji K, et al. Quality improvement guidelines for percutaneous management of acute limb ischemia. J Vasc Interv Radiol. 2005;16:585.
150. Sniderman KW, Bodner L, Saddekni S, et al. Percutaneous embolectomy by transcatheter aspiration. Work in progress. Radiology. 1984;150:357.
151. Turmel-Rodrigues LA, Beyssen B, Raynaud A, Sapoval M. Thromboaspiration to treat inadvertent arterial emboli during dialysis graft declotting. J Vasc Interv Radiol. 1998;9:849.
152. Trerotola SO, Johnson MS, Shah H, Namyslowski J. Backbleeding technique for treatment of arterial emboli resulting from dialysis graft thrombolysis. J Vasc Interv Radiol. 1998;9:141.
153. Working Party on Thrombolysis in the Management of Limb Ischemia. Thrombolysis in the management of lower limb peripheral arterial occlusion – a consensus document. Am J Cardiol. 1998;81:207.
154. The STILE Investigators. Results of a prospective randomized trial evaluating surgery versus thrombolysis for ischemia of the lower extremity. The STILE trial. Ann Surg. 1994;220:251.
155. Dolmatch BL, Casteneda F, McNamara TO, et al. Synthetic dialysis shunts: thrombolysis with the Cragg thrombolytic brush catheter. Radiology. 1999;213:180.
156. Vorwerk D, Schurmann K, Muller-Leisse C, et al. Hydrodynamic thrombectomy of haemodialysis grafts and fistulae: results of 51 procedures. Nephrol Dial Transplant. 1996;11:1058.
157. Sofocleous CT, Cooper SG, Schur I, et al. Retrospective comparison of the Amplatz thrombectomy device with modified pulse-spray pharmacomechanical thrombolysis in the treatment of thrombosed hemodialysis access grafts. Radiology. 1999;213:561.
158. Barth KH, Gosnell MR, Palestrant AM, et al. Hydrodynamic thrombectomy system versus pulse-spray thrombolysis for thrombosed hemodialysis grafts: a multicenter prospective randomized comparison. Radiology. 2000;217:678.

159. Bischel MD, Scoles BG, Mohler JG. Evidence for pulmonary microembolization during hemodialysis. Chest. 1975; 67:335.

160. Droste DW, Kuhne K, Schaefer RM, Ringelstein EB. Detection of microemboli in the subclavian vein of patients undergoing haemodialysis and haemodiafiltration using pulsed Doppler ultrasound. Nephrol Dial Transplant. 2002;17:462.

161. Rolle F, Pengloan J, Abazza M, et al. Identification of microemboli during haemodialysis using Doppler ultrasound. Nephrol Dial Transplant. 2000;15:1420.

162. Trerotola SO, Lund GB, Scheel Jr PJ, et al. Thrombosed dialysis access grafts: percutaneous mechanical declotting without urokinase. Radiology. 1994;191:721.

163. Beathard GA, Welch BR, Maidment HJ. Mechanical thrombolysis for the treatment of thrombosed hemodialysis access grafts. Radiology. 1996;200:711.

164. Middlebrook MR, Amygdalos MA, Soulen MC, et al. Thrombosed hemodialysis grafts: percutaneous mechanical balloon declotting versus thrombolysis. Radiology. 1995;196:73.

165. Soulen MC, Zaetta JM, Amygdalos MA, et al. Mechanical declotting of thrombosed dialysis grafts: experience in 86 cases. J Vasc Interv Radiol. 1997;8:563.

166. Dolmatch BL, Gray RJ, Horton KM. Will iatrogenic pulmonary embolization be our pulmonary embarrassment? Radiology. 1994;191:615.

167. Yigla M, Nakhoul F, Sabag A, et al. Pulmonary hypertension in patients with end-stage renal disease. Chest. 2003;123:1577.

168. Harp RJ, Stavropoulos SW, Wasserstein AG, Clark TW. Pulmonary hypertension among end-stage renal failure patients following hemodialysis access thrombectomy. Cardiovasc Intervent Radiol. 2005;28:17.

169. Swan TL, Smyth SH, Ruffenach SJ, et al. Pulmonary embolism following hemodialysis access thrombolysis/thrombectomy. J Vasc Interv Radiol. 1995;6:683.

170. Petronis JD, Regan F, Briefel G, et al. Ventilation-perfusion scintigraphic evaluation of pulmonary clot burden after percutaneous thrombolysis of clotted hemodialysis access grafts. Am J Kidney Dis. 1999;34:207.

171. Kinney TB, Valji K, Rose SC, et al. Pulmonary embolism from pulse-spray pharmacomechanical thrombolysis of clotted hemodialysis grafts: urokinase versus heparinized saline. J Vasc Interv Radiol. 2000;11:1143.

172. Hagen PT, Scholz DG, Edwards WD. Incidence and size of patent foramen ovale during the first 10 decades of life: an autopsy study of 965 normal hearts. Mayo Clin Proc. 1984;59:17.

173. Ward R, Jones D, Haponik EF. Paradoxical embolism. An under-recognized problem. Chest. 1995;108:549.

174. Briefel GR, Regan F, Petronis JD. Cerebral embolism after mechanical thrombolysis of a clotted hemodialysis access. Am J Kidney Dis. 1999;34:341.

175. Yu AS, Levy E. Paradoxical cerebral air embolism from a hemodialysis catheter. Am J Kidney Dis. 1997;29:453.

176. Owens CA, Yaghmai B, Aletich V, et al. Fatal paradoxic embolism during percutaneous thrombolysis of a hemodialysis graft. AJR Am J Roentgenol. 1998;170:742.

177. Jimenez D, Aujesky D, Moores L, et al. Simplification of the pulmonary embolism severity index for prognostication in patients with acute symptomatic pulmonary embolism. Arch Intern Med. 2010;170:1383.

178. American Society of Anesthesiologists Task Force on Sedation and Analgesia by Non-Anesthesiologists. Practice guidelines for sedation and analgesia by non-anesthesiologists. Anesthesiology. 2002;96:1004.

179. Beathard GA, Urbanes A, Litchfield T, Weinstein A. The risk of sedation/analgesia in hemodialysis patients undergoing interventional procedures. Semin Dial. 2011;24:97.

180. Vinik HR, Reves JG, Greenblatt DJ, et al. The pharmacokinetics of midazolam in chronic renal failure patients. Anesthesiology. 1983;59:390.

181. Reves JG, Fragen RJ, Vinik HR, Greenblatt DJ. Midazolam: pharmacology and uses. Anesthesiology. 1985;62:310.

182. Bergese SD, Patrick Bender S, McSweeney TD, et al. A comparative study of dexmedetomidine with midazolam and midazolam alone for sedation during elective awake fiberoptic intubation. J Clin Anesth. 2010;22:35.

183. Koshy G, Nair S, Norkus EP, et al. Propofol versus midazolam and meperidine for conscious sedation in GI endoscopy. Am J Gastroenterol. 2000;95:1476.

184. Brunton L, Lazo J, Parker K, editors. Goodman and Gilman's the pharmacological basis of therapeutics. 11th ed. New York: McGraw-Hill; 2006.

185. Forster A, Gardaz JP, Suter PM, Gemperle M. Respiratory depression by midazolam and diazepam. Anesthesiology. 1980;53:494.

186. Forster A, Gardaz JP, Suter PM, Gemperle M. I.V. midazolam as an induction agent for anaesthesia: a study in volunteers. Br J Anaesth. 1980;52:907.

187. Reves JG, Samuelson PN, Lewis S. Midazolam maleate induction in patients with ischaemic heart disease: haemodynamic observations. Can Anaesth Soc J. 1979;26:402.

188. Al-Khudhairi D, Whitwam JG, Chakrabarti MK, et al. Haemodynamic effects of midazolam and thiopentone during induction of anaesthesia for coronary artery surgery. Br J Anaesth. 1982;54:831.

189. Samuelson PN, Reves JG, Kouchoukos NT, et al. Hemodynamic responses to anesthetic induction with midazolam or diazepam in patients with ischemic heart disease. Anesth Analg. 1981; 60:802.

190. Bailey PL, Pace NL, Ashburn MA, et al. Frequent hypoxemia and apnea after sedation with midazolam and fentanyl. Anesthesiology. 1990;73:826.

191. Jensen S, Kirkegaard L, et al. Randomized clinical investigation of Ro 15-1788, a benzodiazepine antagonist, in reversing the central effects of flunitrazepam. Eur J Anaesth. 1987;4:113–118.

192. Klotz U, Ziegler G, Ludwig L, Reimann IW. Pharmacodynamic interaction between midazolam and a specific benzodiazepine antagonist in humans. J Clin Pharmacol. 1985;25:400.

193. Amrein R, Leishman B, Bentzinger C, Roncari G. Flumazenil in benzodiazepine antagonism. Actions and clinical use in intoxications and anaesthesiology. Med Toxicol Adverse Drug Exp. 1987;2:411.

194. Herz A, Akil H, Simon EJ, editors. Opioids I and II. Handbook of experimental pharmacology. Berlin: Springer; 1993.

195. Haberer JP, Schoeffler P, Couderc E, Duvaldestin P. Fentanyl pharmacokinetics in anaesthetized patients with cirrhosis. Br J Anaesth. 1982;54:1267.

196. Fassoulaki A, Theodoraki K, Melemeni A. Pharmacology of sedation agents and reversal agents. Digestion. 2010;82:80.

197. Kanto J, Sjovall S, Vuori A. Effect of different kinds of premedication on the induction properties of midazolam. Br J Anaesth. 1982;54:507.

198. Gutstein H, Akil H. Opiod analgesics. 11th ed. New York: McGraw-Hill; 2006.

199. Turski L, Havemann U, Schwarz M, Kuschinsky K. Disinhibition of nigral GABA output neurons mediates muscular rigidity elicited by striatal opioid receptor stimulation. Life Sci. 1982;31:2327.

200. Havemann U, Turski L, Kuschinsky K. Role of opioid receptors in the substantia nigra in morphine-induced muscular rigidity. Life Sci. 1982;31:2319.

201. Arunasalam K, Davenport HT, Painter S, Jones JG. Ventilatory response to morphine in young and old subjects. Anaesthesia. 1983;38:529.

202. Holmes CM. Supplementation of general anaesthesia with narcotic analgesics. Br J Anaesth. 1976;48:907.

203. Becker LD, Paulson BA, Miller RD, et al. Biphasic respiratory depression after fentanyldroperidol or fentanyl alone used to supplement nitrous oxide anesthesia. Anesthesiology. 1976;44:291.

204. Gan TJ, Ginsberg B, Glass PS, et al. Opioid-sparing effects of a low-dose infusion of naloxone in patient-administered morphine sulfate. Anesthesiology. 1997;87:1075.

205. Hall RC, Zisook S. Paradoxical reactions to benzodiazepines. Br J Clin Pharmacol. 1981;11 Suppl 1:99S.

206. Gross JB, Blouin RT, Zandsberg S, et al. Effect of flumazenil on ventilatory drive during sedation with midazolam and alfentanil. Anesthesiology. 1996;85:713.

207. Gupta S, Sharma R, Jain D. Airway assessment: predictors of difficult airway. Indian J Anaesth. 2005;49:257.

208. Vesely TM, Beathard G, Ash S, et al. A position statement from the American Society of Diagnostic and Interventional Nephrology. Semin Dial. 2007;20:359.

209. Bowes 3rd WA, Corke BC, Hulka J. Pulse oximetry: a review of the theory, accuracy, and clinical applications. Obstet Gynecol. 1989;74:541.

210. Williams AJ. ABC of oxygen: assessing and interpreting arterial blood gases and acid–base balance. BMJ. 1998;317:1213.

211. Bishop MJ, Kharasch ED. Is the Combitube a useful emergency airway device for anesthesiologists? Anesth Analg. 1998;86:1141.

212. Mercer MH, Gabbott DA. Insertion of the Combitube airway with the cervical spine immobilised in a rigid cervical collar. Anaesthesia. 1998;53:971.

213. Mercer MH, Gabbott DA. The influence of neck position on ventilation using the Combitube airway. Anaesthesia. 1998;53:146.

214. Rawlins M, Thompson J. Pathogenesis of adverse drug reactions. Oxford: Oxford University Press; 1977.

215. Brown SG. Clinical features and severity grading of anaphylaxis. J Allergy Clin Immunol. 2004;114:371.

216. Grainger R. Intravascular radiological iodinated contrast media. Oxford: Churchill Livingston; 2001.

217. Trcka J, Schmidt C, Seitz CS, et al. Anaphylaxis to iodinated contrast material: nonallergic hypersensitivity or IgE-mediated allergy? AJR Am J Roentgenol. 2008;190:666.

218. Katayama H, Yamaguchi K, Kozuka T, et al. Adverse reactions to ionic and nonionic contrast media. A report from the Japanese Committee on the Safety of Contrast Media. Radiology. 1990; 175:621.

219. Wolf GL, Arenson RL, Cross AP. A prospective trial of ionic vs nonionic contrast agents in routine clinical practice: comparison of adverse effects. AJR Am J Roentgenol. 1989;152:939.

220. Palmer FJ. The RACR survey of intravenous contrast media reactions. Final report. Australas Radiol. 1988;32:426.

221. Caro JJ, Trindade E, McGregor M. The risks of death and of severe nonfatal reactions with high- vs low-osmolality contrast media: a meta-analysis. AJR Am J Roentgenol. 1991;156:825.

222. Ansell G, Tweedie MC, West CR, et al. The current status of reactions to intravenous contrast media. Investigative Radiology. 1980;15(6 Suppl):S32.

223. Sandow BA, Donnal JF. Myelography complications and current practice patterns. AJR Am J Roentgenol. 2005;185:768.

224. Borish L, Matloff SM, Findlay SR. Radiographic contrast media-induced noncardiogenic pulmonary edema: case report and review of the literature. J Allergy Clin Immunol. 1984;74:104.

225. Federle MP, Willis LL, Swanson DP. Ionic versus nonionic contrast media: a prospective study of the effect of rapid bolus injection on nausea and anaphylactoid reactions. J Comput Assist Tomogr. 1998;22:341.

226. Brockow K. Contrast media hypersensitivity – scope of the problem. Toxicology. 2005;209:189.

227. Brockow K, Christiansen C, Kanny G, et al. Management of hypersensitivity reactions to iodinated contrast media. Allergy. 2005;60:150.

228. Hasdenteufel F, Waton J, Cordebar V, et al. Delayed hypersensitivity reactions caused by iodixanol: an assessment of cross-reactivity in 22 patients. J Allergy Clin Immunol. 2011;128:1356.

229. Brockow K. Immediate and delayed reactions to radiocontrast media: is there an allergic mechanism? Immunol Allergy Clin North Am. 2009;29:453.

230. Munechika H, Yasuda R, Michihiro K. Delayed adverse reaction of monomeric contrast media: comparison of plain CT and enhanced CT. Acad Radiol. 1998;5 Suppl 1:S157.

231. Yasuda R, Munechika H. Delayed adverse reactions to nonionic monomeric contrast-enhanced media. Invest Radiol. 1998;33:1.

232. Hosoya T, Yamaguchi K, Akutsu T, et al. Delayed adverse reactions to iodinated contrast media and their risk factors. Radiat Med. 2000;18:39.

233. Sutton AG, Finn P, Grech ED, et al. Early and late reactions after the use of iopamidol 340, ioxaglate 320, and iodixanol 320 in cardiac catheterization. Am Heart J. 2001;141:677.

234. Szebeni J. Complement activation-related pseudoallergy: a new class of drug-induced acute immune toxicity. Toxicology. 2005;216:106.

235. Greenberger PA. Contrast media reactions. J Allergy Clin Immunol. 1984;74:600.

236. Hong SJ, Wong JT, Bloch KJ. Reactions to radiocontrast media. Allergy Asthma Proc. 2002;23:347.

237. Laroche D, Aimone-Gastin I, Dubois F, et al. Mechanisms of severe, immediate reactions to iodinated contrast material. Radiology. 1998;209:183.

238. Mita H, Tadokoro K, Akiyama K. Detection of IgE antibody to a radiocontrast medium. Allergy. 1998;53:1133.

239. Wakkers-Garritsen BG, Houwerzijl J, Nater JP, Wakkers PJ. IgE-mediated adverse reactivity to a radiographic contrast medium. Ann Allergy. 1976;36:122.

240. Kanny G, Maria Y, Mentre B, Moneret-Vautrin DA. Case report: recurrent anaphylactic shock to radiographic contrast media, evidence supporting an exceptional IgE-mediated reaction. Allerg Immunol (Paris). 1993;25:425.

241. Brockow K, Romano A, Aberer W, et al. Skin testing in patients with hypersensitivity reactions to iodinated contrast media – a European multicenter study. Allergy. 2009;64:234.

242. Idee JM, Pines E, Prigent P, Corot C. Allergy-like reactions to iodinated contrast agents. A critical analysis. Fundam Clin Pharmacol. 2005;19:263.

243. Hagan JB. Anaphylactoid and adverse reactions to radiocontrast agents. Immunol Allergy Clin North Am. 2004;24:507.

244. (No authors listed). The diagnosis and management of anaphylaxis: an updated practice parameter. J Allergy Clin Immunol. 2005;115:S483.

245. Pumphrey RS. Lessons for management of anaphylaxis from a study of fatal reactions. Clin Exp Allergy. 2000;30:1144.

246. American College of Radiology Committee on Drugs and Contrast Media. ACR manual on contrast media. 6th ed. Reston: American College of Radiology; 2008.

247. Brown SG. Anaphylaxis: clinical concepts and research priorities. Emerg Med Australas. 2006;18:155.

248. Pumphrey RS, Roberts IS. Postmortem findings after fatal anaphylactic reactions. J Clin Pathol. 2000;53:273.

249. Lieberman P. The use of antihistamines in the prevention and treatment of anaphylaxis and anaphylactoid reactions. J Allergy Clin Immunol. 1990;86:684.

250. Wimbery S, Lieberman P. Histamine and antihistamines in anaphylaxis. Clin Allergy Immunol. 2002;17:287.

251. Kalimo K, Jansen CT, Kormano M. Allergological risk factors as predictors of radiographic contrast media hypersensitivity. Ann Allergy. 1980;45:253.

252. Witten J, Hirsch F, Hartman G. Acute reactions to urographic contrast medium. Am J Roentgenol. 1973;119:832.

253. Liccardi G, Lobefalo G, Di Florio E, et al. Strategies for the prevention of asthmatic, anaphylactic and anaphylactoid reactions during the administration of anesthetics and/or contrast media. J Investig Allergol Clin Immunol. 2008;18:1.

254. Lang DM, Alpern MB, Visintainer PF, Smith ST. Elevated risk of anaphylactoid reaction from radiographic contrast media is associated with both beta-blocker exposure and cardiovascular disorders. Arch Intern Med. 1993;153:2033.

255. Lieberman PL, Seigle RL. Reactions to radiocontrast material. Anaphylactoid events in radiology. Clin Rev Allergy Immunol. 1999;17:469.

256. Lang DM, Alpern MB, Visintainer PF, Smith ST. Gender risk for anaphylactoid reaction to radiographic contrast media. J Allergy Clin Immunol. 1995;95:813.

257. Smith PL, Kagey-Sobotka A, Bleecker ER, et al. Physiologic manifestations of human anaphylaxis. J Clin Invest. 1980;66:1072.

258. Davis JH, Foster TR, Tonelli M, Butcher SE. Role of metal ions in the tetraloop-receptor complex as analyzed by NMR. RNA. 2007;13:76.

259. Simons FE, Roberts JR, Gu X, Simons KJ. Epinephrine absorption in children with a history of anaphylaxis. J Allergy Clin Immunol. 1998;101:33.

260. Simons FE, Gu X, Simons KJ. Epinephrine absorption in adults: intramuscular versus subcutaneous injection. J Allergy Clin Immunol. 2001;108:871.

261. Brown SG. Cardiovascular aspects of anaphylaxis: implications for treatment and diagnosis. Curr Opin Allergy Clin Immunol. 2005;5:359.

262. Berchtold E, Maibach R, Muller U. Reduction of side effects from rush-immunotherapy with honey bee venom by pretreatment with terfenadine. Clin Exp Allergy. 1992;22:59.

263. Brockow K, Kiehn M, Riethmuller C, et al. Efficacy of antihistamine pretreatment in the prevention of adverse reactions to hymenoptera immunotherapy: a prospective, randomized, placebo-controlled trial. J Allergy Clin Immunol. 1997;100:458.

264. Lin RY, Curry A, Pesola GR, et al. Improved outcomes in patients with acute allergic syndromes who are treated with combined H1 and H2 antagonists. Ann Emerg Med. 2000;36:462.

265. Runge JW, Martinez JC, Caravati EM, et al. Histamine antagonists in the treatment of acute allergic reactions. Ann Emerg Med. 1992;21:237.

266. Brown SG. Parallel infusion of hydrocortisone with/without chlorpheniramine bolus injection to prevent acute adverse reactions to antivenom for snakebites. Med J Aust. 2004;180:428; author reply 428.

267. Gawarammana IB, Kularatne SA, Dissanayake WP, et al. Parallel infusion of hydrocortisone +/− chlorpheniramine bolus injection to prevent acute adverse reactions to antivenom for snakebites. Med J Aust. 2004;180:20.

268. Chamberlain D. Emergency medical treatment of anaphylactic reactions. Project Team of the Resuscitation Council (UK). J Accid Emerg Med. 1999;16:243.

269. Cochran ST. Anaphylactoid reactions to radiocontrast media. Curr Allergy Asthma Rep. 2005;5:28.

270. Fisher MM. Clinical observations on the pathophysiology and treatment of anaphylactic cardiovascular collapse. Anaesth Intensive Care. 1986;14:17.

271. Brown SG, Blackman KE, Stenlake V, Heddle RJ. Insect sting anaphylaxis; prospective evaluation of treatment with intravenous adrenaline and volume resuscitation. Emerg Med J. 2004;21:149.

272. Sampson HA, Mendelson L, Rosen JP. Fatal and near-fatal anaphylactic reactions to food in children and adolescents. N Engl J Med. 1992;327:380.

273. Lee JM, Greenes DS. Biphasic anaphylactic reactions in pediatrics. Pediatrics. 2000;106:762.

274. Stark BJ, Sullivan TJ. Biphasic and protracted anaphylaxis. J Allergy Clin Immunol. 1986;78:76.

275. Douglas DM, Sukenick E, Andrade WP, Brown JS. Biphasic systemic anaphylaxis: an inpatient and outpatient study. J Allergy Clin Immunol. 1994;93:977.

276. Mink SN, Simons FE, Simons KJ, et al. Constant infusion of epinephrine, but not bolus treatment, improves haemodynamic recovery in anaphylactic shock in dogs. Clin Exp Allergy. 2004;34:1776.

277. Tramer MR, von Elm E, Loubeyre P, Hauser C. Pharmacological prevention of serious anaphylactic reactions due to iodinated contrast media: systematic review. BMJ. 2006;333:675.

278. Kopp AF, Mortele KJ, Cho YD, et al. Prevalence of acute reactions to iopromide: postmarketing surveillance study of 74,717 patients. Acta Radiol. 2008;49:902.

279. Greenberger PA, Patterson R. The prevention of immediate generalized reactions to radiocontrast media in high-risk patients. J Allergy Clin Immunol. 1991;87:867.

280. Witten DM, Hirsch FD, Hartman GW. Acute reactions to urographic contrast medium: incidence, clinical characteristics and relationship to history of hypersensitivity states. Am J Roentgenol Radium Ther Nucl Med. 1973;119:832.

281. Shehadi WH. Adverse reactions to intravascularly administered contrast media. A comprehensive study based on a prospective survey. Am J Roentgenol Radium Ther Nucl Med. 1975;124:145.

282. Munechika H, Hiramatsu Y, Kudo S, et al. A prospective survey of delayed adverse reactions to iohexol in urography and computed tomography. Eur Radiol. 2003;13:185.

283. Lieberman P, Nicklas RA, Oppenheimer J, et al. The diagnosis and management of anaphylaxis practice parameter: 2010 update. J Allergy Clin Immunol. 2010;126:477.

284. American College of Radiology. ACR practice guideline for the use of intravascular contrast media. Reston: American College of Radiology; 2007. p. 73–8.

285. Freed KS, Leder RA, Alexander C, et al. Breakthrough adverse reactions to low-osmolar contrast media after steroid premedication. AJR Am J Roentgenol. 2001;176:1389.

286. Mohan JC, Reddy KS, Bhatia ML. Anaphylactoid reaction to angiographic contrast media: recurrence despite pretreatment with corticosteroids. Cathet Cardiovasc Diagn. 1984;10:465.

287. Raut CP, Hunt KK, Akins JS, et al. Incidence of anaphylactoid reactions to isosulfan blue dye during breast carcinoma lymphatic mapping in patients treated with preoperative prophylaxis: results of a surgical prospective clinical practice protocol. Cancer. 2005;104:692.

288. Davenport MS, Cohan RH, Caoili EM, Ellis JH. Repeat contrast medium reactions in premedicated patients: frequency and severity. Radiology. 2009;253:372.

289. Lasser EC, Lang JH, Lyon SG, et al. Glucocorticoid-induced elevations of C1-esterase inhibitor: a mechanism for protection against lethal dose range contrast challenge in rabbits. Invest Radiol. 1981;16:20.

290. Marshall Jr GD, Lieberman PL. Comparison of three pretreatment protocols to prevent anaphylactoid reactions to radiocontrast media. Ann Allergy. 1991;67:70.

291. Greenberger PA, Patterson R, Tapio CM. Prophylaxis against repeated radiocontrast media reactions in 857 cases. Adverse experience with cimetidine and safety of beta-adrenergic antagonists. Arch Intern Med. 1985;145:2197.

292. Lasser EC, Berry CC, Mishkin MM, et al. Pretreatment with corticosteroids to prevent adverse reactions to nonionic contrast media. AJR Am J Roentgenol. 1994;162:523.

293. Dawson P, Sidhu PS. Is there a role for corticosteroid prophylaxis in patients at increased risk of adverse reactions to intravascular contrast agents? Clin Radiol. 1993;48:225.

294. Worthley DL, Gillis D, Kette F, Smith W. Radiocontrast anaphylaxis with failure of premedication. Intern Med J. 2005;35:58.

295. Morcos SK, Thomsen HS, Webb JA. Prevention of generalized reactions to contrast media: a consensus report and guidelines. Eur Radiol. 2001;11:1720.

296. Seymour R, Halpin SF, Hardman JA, et al. Corticosteroid prophylaxis for patients with increased risk of adverse reactions to intravascular contrast agents: a survey of current practice in the UK. Clin Radiol. 1994;49:791.

297. Cohan RH, Ellis JH, Dunnick NR. Use of low-osmolar agents and premedication to reduce the frequency of adverse reactions to radiographic contrast media: a survey of the Society of Uroradiology. Radiology. 1995;194:357.

298. Barrett BJ, Parfrey PS, McDonald JR, et al. Nonionic low-osmolality versus ionic high-osmolality contrast material for intravenous use in patients perceived to be at high risk: randomized trial. Radiology. 1992;183:105.

299. Bertrand PR, Soyer PM, Rouleau PJ, et al. Comparative randomized double-blind study of hydroxyzine versus placebo as premedication before injection of iodinated contrast media. Radiology. 1992;184:383.

300. Tryba M, Zevounou F, Zenz M. Prevention of anaphylactoid reactions using intramuscular promethazine and cimetidine. Studies of a histamine infusion model. Anaesthesist. 1984;33:218.

301. Lorenz W, Doenicke A. H1 and H2 blockade: a prophylactic principle in anesthesia and surgery against histamine-release responses of any degree of severity: part 1. N Engl Reg Allergy Proc. 1985;6:37.

302. Lorenz W, Ennis M, Doenicke A, Dick W. Perioperative uses of histamine antagonists. J Clin Anesth. 1990;2:345.

303. Kimura K, Adachi M, Kubo K. H1- and H2-receptor antagonists prevent histamine release in allergic patients after the administration of midazolam-ketamine. A randomized controlled study. Inflamm Res. 1999;48:128.

304. Ring J, Rothenberger KH, Clauss W. Prevention of anaphylactoid reactions after radiographic contrast media infusion by combined histamine H1- and H2-receptor antagonists: results of a prospective controlled trial. Int Arch Allergy Appl Immunol. 1985;78:9.

305. Moneret-Vautrin DA, Laxenaire MC, Mouton C, et al. Change in skin reactivity in anaphylaxis to muscle relaxants and hypnotics after administration of anti H1, anti H2 and tritoqualine. Ann Fr Anesth Reanim. 1985;4:225.

306. Greenberger PA, Patterson R, Radin RC. Two pretreatment regimens for high-risk patients receiving radiographic contrast media. J Allergy Clin Immunol. 1984;74:540.

307. Lasser EC, Berry CC, Talner LB, et al. Pretreatment with corticosteroids to alleviate reactions to intravenous contrast material. N Engl J Med. 1987;317:845.

308. Greenberger PA, Patterson R. Adverse reactions to radiocontrast media. Prog Cardiovasc Dis. 1988;31:239.

309. American College of Radiology Committee on Drugs and Contrast Media. ACR manual on contrast media. 5th ed. Reston: American College of Radiology; 2004.

310. Fischer HW, Doust VL. An evaluation of pretesting in the problem of serious and fatal reactions to excretory urography. Radiology. 1972;103:497.

311. Yamaguchi K, Katayama H, Takashima T, et al. Prediction of severe adverse reactions to ionic and nonionic contrast media in Japan: evaluation of pretesting. A report from the Japanese Committee on the Safety of Contrast Media. Radiology. 1991;178:363.

312. Yamaguchi K, Katayama H, Kozuka T, et al. Pretesting as a predictor of severe adverse reactions to contrast media. Invest Radiol. 1990;25 Suppl 1:S22.

313. Small P, Satin R, Palayew MJ, Hyams B. Prophylactic antihistamines in the management of radiographic contrast reactions. Clin Allergy. 1982;12:289.

314. Wicke L, Seidl G, Kotscher E, et al. Side effects of roentgen contrast media injections with and without antihistaminics. Wien Med Wochenschr. 1975;725:698.

315. Chevrot A, Chevrot L, Sarrat P, Wallays C. Betamethasone in the prevention of allergic complications caused by intravenous iodine contrast media. Ann Radiol (Paris). 1988;31:193.

316. Greenberger PA, Halwig JM, Patterson R, Wallemark CB. Emergency administration of radiocontrast media in high-risk patients. J Allergy Clin Immunol. 1986;77:630.

Preoperative Evaluation of a Patient for Peritoneal Dialysis Catheter

Mary Buffington and Kenneth Abreo

31.1 Introduction

The goal of preoperative evaluation is to recognize patients at high risk for complications during the perioperative period. Risk factors for complications such as advanced age, diabetes, chronic renal failure, or end-stage renal disease could lead to complications. Because placement of a PD catheter will usually occur within 2 weeks of needing dialysis, patients undergoing this procedure will have advanced renal failure. Preoperative evaluation of a patient who is referred for peritoneal dialysis catheter placement should identify factors that indicate a contraindication for the peritoneoscopic or fluoroscopic procedure or identify medical factors that could lead to complications following the procedure. History taking should elicit information about prior surgeries and medical conditions that could lead to anatomic barriers to placement of the catheter or factors that could lead to complications following the surgery. Physical exam should search for physical signs of abdominal masses and abdominal wall weakness or hernias and also signs of bleeding irregularities or infection. Preoperative physical exam should include planning the exit site for the catheter. Additionally, guidelines are reviewed for additional preparatory measures such as placement of Foley catheter or bowel preparation.

31.2 Risk Assessment

The American College of Cardiology/American Heart Association guidelines on perioperative cardiovascular evaluation and care for noncardiac surgery classify surgical procedures as low risk, intermediate risk, and vascular surgery (Table 31.1). Two of the primary factors for the risk level are duration of surgery and fluid shifts caused by blood loss and third spacing that can cause myocardial ischemia and respiratory depression. Low-risk surgery has less than 1 % risk of cardiovascular complications even in high-risk patients. Examples of low-risk surgery are endoscopic procedures, superficial procedures, cataract surgery, breast surgery, and ambulatory surgery [1]. Of the low-risk procedures, superficial and ophthalmologic procedures represent the lowest risk and are rarely associated with excess morbidity and mortality [2].

Percutaneous PD catheter placement falls under the category of a low-risk procedure because it is a minimally invasive procedure performed under moderate (conscious) sedation and local anesthesia. Typically, the peritoneal dialysis catheter will be placed as the patient approaches renal replacement therapy, preferably at least 2 weeks prior to starting peritoneal dialysis in order to minimize dialysate leakage [3, 4]. The percutaneous placement of the catheter involves a superficial 3–4 cm incision lateral to the umbilicus with dissection to the rectus sheath, cannulation and dilation of the rectus muscle, then insertion of the catheter into the pelvis through a sheath with or without a guidewire, and then tunneling the exterior part of the catheter laterally through subcutaneous tissue to the exit site. Complications of this procedure are relatively minor [5–16] (Table 31.2). Bowel and bladder perforations are the most serious complications and these are rarely reported.

The patient should fast prior to the procedure in order to minimize the risk of aspiration during the period of sedation and should not have solid food for 6 h prior or liquid for 2 h prior to the procedure [17]. PD catheter placement can be performed safely as an outpatient surgical procedure [18]. In

M. Buffington, MD, JD • K. Abreo, MD (✉)
Nephrology Section,
Department of Medicine,
Louisiana State University Health Sciences Center,
1501 Kings Highway, Shreveport, LA 71130, USA
e-mail: mbuffi@lsuhsc.edu; kabreo@lsuhsc.edu

A.S. Yevzlin et al. (eds.), *Interventional Nephrology*,
DOI 10.1007/978-1-4614-8803-3_31, © Springer Science+Business Media New York 2014

Table 31.1 Cardiac risk
stratification for noncardiac
surgical procedures [1]

Risk stratification	Reported cardiac risk	Procedure examples
Vascular	More than 5 %	Aortic, other major vascular surgery, peripheral vascular surgery
Intermediate	1–5 %	Intraperitoneal and intrathoracic surgery, carotid endarterectomy, head and neck surgery, orthopedic surgery, prostate surgery
Low	Less than 1 %	Endoscopic procedures, superficial procedures, cataract surgery, breast surgery, ambulatory surgery

Table 31.2 Summary of perioperative complications of peritoneal dialysis catheter placement

Source	No. of catheters	Infection	Drainage problem	Bleeding	Leak	Perforation
Fluoroscopy guided						
Moon et al. [5]	134	2.2 %	1.5 %	1/134	3 %	0
Zaman et al. [6]	36	0	2.9 %	1/36	3 %	0
Vaux et al. [7]	209	8 %	5 %	NR	5 %	0
Maya [8]	32	0		0	0	GI 3 %
Jacobs et al. [9]	45	7 %	13.3 %	3/45	9 %	GI 4.4 %
Reddy et al. [10]	64	0	NR	4/64	1/64	0
Henderson et al. [11]	283	4 %	21 %	NR	6 %	
Perakis et al. [12]	86	12.7 %	23.2 %	5/86	23 %	0
Ozener et al. [13]	133	3 %	11.2 %	5/133	8.3 %	0
Peritoneoscope guided						
Goh et al. [14]	91	1 in 93.7 pt months	17.6 %	NR	NR	NR
Gadallah et al. [15]	76	2.6 %	Early 7.9 %	NR	Early 1.3 %	GI 1.3 %
Asif et al. [16]	82	0	0	4/82	0	0

NR not reported

that circumstance, a caregiver should accompany the patient if the procedure is done on an outpatient basis since the patient should not drive for 24 h [17, 19]. All medications should be taken on the morning of the procedure except for medications for diabetes and anticoagulation as will be discussed below.

Non-anesthesiologists frequently administer moderate sedation safely. A benzodiazepine is administered for anxiolysis and an opioid achieves pain control. Under moderate sedation, the patient has purposeful response to verbal or tactile stimulation with the ability to maintain the airway. Spontaneous ventilation and cardiovascular function are preserved [17]. Sedation is a continuum ranging from minimal to deep or general anesthesia. Should the patient's degree of sedation exceed the desired level, the benzodiazepine and opioid are reversible using flumazenil (Romazicon) and naloxone (Narcan), respectively.

Interventional radiology literature shows that the most common adverse events occurring in procedures under moderate sedation are hypoxia and hypotension. Arepally et al. evaluated the safety of moderate sedation in a prospective study of 594 patients over a 5-month period [20]. Adverse events were classified as respiratory, sedative, or major adverse events. Rates of these events were 4.7, 4.2, and 2 %, respectively. Procedures involving the biliary tract had an increased rate of adverse events, with 50 % of adverse events

occurring in those procedures. Respiratory adverse events were defined as excessive respiratory depression requiring Ambu bag use, jaw thrust, or oral airway placement. Sedation events consisted of hypoxia (oxygen saturation less than 90 %), unresponsiveness to verbal or tactile stimuli, agitation, or requirement of reversal with flumazenil or naloxone. Major adverse events were defined as hypotension (systolic blood pressure less than 80 mmHg), cardiac arrest, intubation, or cardiopulmonary resuscitation. Thus, hypotension was the only major adverse event that occurred in the study. In this study, no cardiac arrest occurred nor intubation was required. Catheter insertions had no respiratory complications. Another recent prospective study of 72 radiologic procedures involving the biliary system or abscess drainage showed hypotension in 6.9 % and hypoxia in 19.4 % [21].

Patients with significant underlying medical comorbidities may be at increased risk for complications of sedation [19]. The American Society of Anesthesiologists physical status classification describes the patient's baseline condition, with class I being a healthy patient with no comorbidities and class V being a moribund patient that is not expected to live without the operation (Table 31.3). Classifying your patient under this system helps identify patients who may be more likely to have an adverse reaction to sedation; however, in the Arepally study, this correlation was not established statistically [20, 22]. Patients at risk for sedation-related

Table 31.3 The American Society of Anesthesiologists physical status classification

Class	Baseline health characteristics
I	Normal healthy patient
II	Patient with mild systemic disease
III	Patient with severe systemic disease that is not incapacitating
IV	Incapacitating systemic disease that is a constant threat to life
V	Moribund patient who is not expected to survive for 24 h with or without the operation

complications include patients with airway obstruction or anatomic barriers to intubation if the patient is oversedated. Also, patients with impaired level of consciousness at baseline or inability to protect the airway or prevent aspiration will have a higher risk of adverse events. Patients with increased intracranial pressure and renal, cardiac, pulmonary, or hepatic disease could be more likely to have adverse reactions when undergoing sedation [19]. Classifying patients with renal failure is challenging and anesthesiologists have a greater variability for ASA grades given to these patients [23]. However, when the renal failure is stable and the patient is not incapacitated, the classification score should be class II or III depending on existence of other comorbidities.

As such, percutaneous PD catheter placement has a low risk of cardiovascular complications under this analysis. In low-risk procedures, preoperative cardiac testing is generally not warranted unless the patient is having active cardiac issues, such as unstable coronary syndromes, decompensated heart failure, significant arrhythmia, or severe valvular disease [24]. Unstable coronary syndrome is defined as unstable or severe angina or recent myocardial infarction within 30 days. Decompensated heart failure is worsening or new-onset heart failure or NYHA functional class IV heart failure. Significant arrhythmias include third degree AV block, atrial fibrillation with rapid ventricular rate, and symptomatic bradycardia. Severe valvular disease is severe aortic stenosis or symptomatic mitral stenosis [25].

Risks for postoperative pulmonary complications following PD catheter insertion are limited because the patient is not intubated and undergoes moderate sedation throughout the procedure. The patient must be able to remain in a supine position comfortably for at least 2 h. Preoperative risk assessment for pulmonary complications involves identification of risk factors and aggressive risk factor modification [26]. Risk factors for pulmonary complications are COPD, age, tobacco use, pulmonary hypertension, and obstructive sleep apnea. Nutritional factors such as low albumin and elevated BUN also contribute to increased risk for pulmonary complications. Risk modification strategies are smoking cessation 6–8 weeks prior to surgery and perioperative corticosteroids

and bronchodilators in appropriate cases. A chest radiograph is not necessary unless the physical examination reveals an abnormality that may prevent the patient from remaining supine during the procedure [27].

Obstructive sleep apnea (OSA) is the periodic, partial or complete obstruction of the upper airway during sleep. The American Society of Anesthesiologists has published guidelines for the perioperative management of patients with OSA [28]. Characteristics associated with OSA are increased body mass index (BMI), hypertension, larger neck circumference, history of snoring or respiratory pauses, and lower oxygen saturation. A patient's perioperative risk depends on the severity of OSA and the invasiveness of the surgical procedure. For superficial procedures, the use of local anesthesia or peripheral nerve blocks with or without moderate sedation is recommended [28]. Procedures typically performed on an outpatient basis in non-OSA patients may also be safely performed on an outpatient basis in patients who are at increased perioperative risk from OSA when local or regional anesthesia is administered. Patients with OSA should be monitored longer than their non-OSA counterparts before discharge from the facility [28].

31.3 History and Physical Exam

The history should elicit information about underlying conditions that could lead to complications during or after the procedure. The history should determine whether the patient had a prior reaction to sedation, difficulty with maintaining the airway, or has obstructive sleep apnea (OSA). Medications and allergies should be carefully evaluated to determine possible drug interactions or anticoagulation. A patient with an allergy to iodine-based contrast should be given steroids prior to the procedure to prevent an allergic reaction to the small amount of intraperitoneal contrast given during the procedure. Patients with minor reaction to contrast material, such as emesis, nausea, or hives, should receive methylprednisolone 32 mg orally 12 h before the procedure and 2 h before the procedure [29]. Another study showed that patients with a previous reaction to contrast material should be premedicated with prednisone 50 mg orally 13, 7, and 1 h before the procedure along with diphenhydramine 50 mg orally [30]. Low-osmolality contrast material used in selective cases may limit the occurrence of reactions to the contrast [30, 31].

The physician should elicit prior tobacco, alcohol, and illegal drug use. Previous abdominal surgeries or prior PD catheter placement or peritonitis should raise the question of whether the patient has anatomic barriers to percutaneous placement. Peritoneal adhesions have been reported in up to 90 % of patients following major abdominal surgery and 55–100 % of women undergoing pelvic surgery [32]. One prospective study found a history of previous abdominal surgery in 42.9 % of 217 PD catheter implantations [33]. Of those patients with prior surgery, 26.9 % had intraperitoneal adhesions and only 2.8 % of patients without prior abdominal surgery had intraperitoneal adhesions. Those patients with an extensive history of abdominal surgeries should be referred for laparoscopic placement of the catheter. Gastrointestinal pathology, fever, and infection would also raise questions about the suitability of catheter placement at that time, requiring postponement of the procedure when these issues are resolved.

A careful history should be directed toward potential cardiovascular, pulmonary, hematological conditions that could affect the perioperative condition of the patient. Regarding cardiovascular conditions, the physician should ask about chest pain, dyspnea, presyncope, recent or prior myocardial infarction, or percutaneous procedures involving cardiac stents. Recent pacemakers or defibrillators should be discussed. A history of congestive heart failure or valvular heart disease would be pertinent as to whether the patient needs preoperative cardiac evaluation. In addition, significant arrhythmias, such as symptomatic bradycardia or atrial fibrillation with uncontrolled ventricular rate, are active cardiac conditions that might require evaluation prior to the procedure; thus, questions regarding dyspnea, dizziness, light-headedness, or palpitations are important [25].

Episodes of ecchymoses, purpura, epistaxis, gingival bleeding, GI bleeding, or excessive bleeding after cuts should be elicited in the history to determine if uremic bleeding is occurring [34]. Careful review of medications for anticoagulants is extremely important.

31.4 Physical Exam

Vital signs will indicate acute conditions such as infection, hypotension, or hypertension. Hypertension is common in patients with renal failure. In the preoperative context, stage 1 or 2 hypertension under the JNC VI classification (systolic blood pressure below 180 mmHg and diastolic blood pressure below 110 mmHg) is not an independent risk factor for cardiovascular complications [25, 35, 36]. One study of patients presenting with elevated diastolic blood pressure of 110 mmHg evaluated preoperative reduction in blood pressure with intranasal nifedipine versus postponement of the surgery to treat elevated blood pressure. The subjects had a history of well-controlled hypertension and few comorbidities, and surgery was postponed in the control group. There was no statistically significant difference in the postoperative complications between the two groups [37]. In a retrospective study, hypertension was associated with negative surgical outcome in surgeries lasting longer the 220 min [38]. For stage 3 hypertension, the potential

benefit of postponing the procedure to optimize blood pressure control should be balanced against the negative consequences of delaying the procedure. Short-acting medications can bring the blood pressure within range in a matter of hours and allow the patient to have the PD catheter placed [25]. Suitable short-acting medications are clonidine and captopril. Alternatively, giving a missed dose of the patient's home medication can bring the blood pressure into an acceptable range.

An arrhythmia could manifest as tachycardia or irregular heart rate. Tachypnea can indicate pulmonary disease. Physical exam directed toward the airway can indicate if intubation would be difficult should the degree of sedation deepen. Indications for difficult intubations include obesity, short neck, limited neck extension, decreased hyoid-mental distance, neck mass, and dysmorphic facial features. The patient with small mouth, arched palate, macroglossia, nonvisible uvula, micrognathia, and retrognathia can be difficult to intubate [17]. Cardiac examination should evaluate for heart murmurs, S3 gallop, arrhythmia, and jugular venous distension. Pulmonary disease can manifest as wheezing or decreased breath sounds.

The physical exam should focus on the presence of abdominal hernias or abdominal wall weakness [39]. Preexisting hernias could be inguinal, incisional, umbilical, epigastric, Spigelian, or diaphragmatic [40]. These hernias can be repaired laparoscopically at the same time as catheter placement if they are identified and referral to surgery is made in a timely manner. This avoids delaying catheter placement following hernia repair [41–43].

Careful attention should be paid to hepatosplenomegaly, an enlarged bladder, and a pelvic mass such as that caused by uterine fibroids or polycystic kidneys that could make placement of the PD catheter difficult. Edema of the extremities could mean congestive heart failure, renal or hepatic failure, or deep vein thrombosis. Neurologically, the ability to swallow and protect the airway should be tested, and decreased ability to understand the procedure should be determined so that precautions can be taken to protect the patient during the procedure [44].

31.5 Plan the Location of Exit Site

Planning of the exit site must occur prior to the insertion procedure. Physical examination of the abdomen will guide determination of the optimal site for the catheter to exit [39]. With the patient clothed and laying supine, the physician can locate the point at which the deep cuff will be inserted into the rectus muscle by placing the upper edge of the coil of the catheter tip on the cephalad border of the pubic symphysis with the deep cuff 2–4 cm lateral to the umbilicus [6–8] (Fig. 31.1). The area under the deep cuff is the location of the

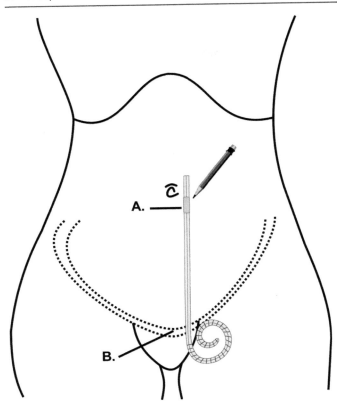

Fig. 31.1 Location of incision at point *A*. Locate coil of catheter at point *B*

incision [45]. Then the patient should sit and stand to confirm that neither the belt line nor the skin folds will interfere with catheter placement. Patients with a belt line above the umbilicus should have a catheter with a preformed bend in the inter-cuff segment with exit site directed downward. With a belt line below the umbilicus, the patient should have a catheter with straight inter-cuff segment with exit site directed laterally but not in upward direction. Preprinted stencils aid in location of exit site and especially with correct arc of straight inter-cuff segment catheters [46]. Extended catheters can be placed in obese patients with excessive skin folds and patients with ostomies, urinary or fecal incontinence, and chronic intertrigo [47]. In these cases, the exit site should be either in the upper abdomen or at a presternal location approximately 3 cm lateral to the midline [48].

31.5.1 Laboratory Testing

Catheter insertion usually occurs when the patient is approaching the need for dialysis; thus, laboratory testing will likely reflect abnormalities associated with advanced chronic kidney disease. Hyperkalemia is not uncommon in patients with severe renal dysfunction. Postoperative hyperkalemia is one of the most common complications following

surgery. In one study, hyperkalemia occurred in 19 % of surgical procedures [49]. Hyperkalemia can result in paresthesias and weakness with decreased deep tendon reflexes that can advance to a flaccid paralysis. Hyperkalemia can cause myocardial instability with or without changes on electrocardiograph (EKG). These changes result from reduced myocardial conduction velocity and accelerated repolarization manifesting on EKG as peaked T waves, prolonged PR interval, decreased P-wave amplitude, widening QRS complex, and ultimately sine-wave configuration [50]. Clinically, the patient can experience ventricular fibrillation and asystole. These effects result from a serum potassium level of 6.5 mmol/L or greater; however, a patient can have a normal EKG with even higher potassium levels. The onset of effects of hyperkalemia is unpredictable; thus, treatment should not be arbitrarily associated with a particular potassium level or EKG reading. Preoperative hyperkalemia should be treated with hemodialysis or medically with calcium gluconate, insulin and dextrose, kayexalate, albuterol, and sodium bicarbonate [50].

Coagulation tests such as protime (PT) time, international normalized ratio (INR), and partial thromboplastin time (PTT) may detect disorders involving coagulation factors that the patient may have that could lead to excessive bleeding during and after the procedure. Complete blood count will show the degree of anemia present. Also, an elevated white blood cell (wbc) count will indicate the presence of an infection, and a low wbc count would predispose the patient to infection. The presence of thrombocytopenia with platelet count less than 50,000/μL would be cause for concern in undergoing this procedure as discussed below.

Bleeding time is not routinely ordered in preoperative evaluation of chronic kidney disease patients. Uremia causes platelet dysfunction that leads to increased clinical evidence of bleeding such as ecchymosis, gingival bleeding, epistaxis, and purpura. Additionally, major GI bleeding or subdural hemorrhage can occur [34]. Bleeding time accurately correlates with uremia and platelet dysfunction [51, 52]. However, there is not a significant association between patients with abnormal bleeding time and other indicators of bleeding risk on the occurrence of clinically significant perioperative bleeding [53, 54]. As such, screening for preoperative bleeding time is not a reliable test to evaluate the risk of perioperative bleeding.

31.5.2 Hemostasis and Management of Anticoagulation

Bleeding is rarely a significant problem after catheter implantation and usually occurs at the exit site (Table 31.2). Blood may be present initially in the effluent drained, owing to the trauma of insertion, but the drainage should return to normal within a few days. Manual pressure or additional suturing can stop persistent bleeding, but hematomas can form subcutaneously following the procedure. Bleeding can occur when the epigastric vessels are perforated. Using ultrasound to visualize these vessels significantly reduces the risk of this complication [8].

The CBC and coagulation parameters will help identify patients at risk of bleeding. Often, patients with a platelet count less than 50,000/μL are transfused with platelets to prevent bleeding complications, although this practice is based on observational data [55, 56]. Patients with an elevated PT, INR, or PTT should have the cause of the abnormality identified and addressed. Those patients that are uremic and at risk of resulting platelet dysfunction should receive dDAVP.

A candidate for PD catheter may be on anticoagulant therapy, and the decision to continue or hold anticoagulation for the procedure is significant. The American College of Chest Physicians issued clinical practice guidelines to address this question [57, 58]. The decision to hold anticoagulation for a surgical procedure involves a balance between the risk of thromboembolism following withholding of the therapy and the risk of bleeding that the procedure itself presents. Perioperative bleeding not only causes complications like hematomas that can affect the function of the catheter and healing but also can cause a delay in resumption of anticoagulation after the procedure, which could increase the risk of thromboembolism.

The extent of perioperative bleeding inherent in a surgical procedure must be determined by the degree of invasiveness and duration. Surgical procedures associated with high bleeding risk are coronary artery bypass, heart valve replacement, aortic aneurysm repair, orthopedic surgery, and prostate and bladder surgery [57–59]. The guidelines also note procedures that seem to have a low risk of bleeding but should be cautiously undertaken with full anticoagulation on board. These procedures include resection of colon polyps, biopsy of the prostate or kidney, and pacemaker or defibrillator implantation. Caution regarding endoscopic resection of colon polyps in an anticoagulated patient is due to the risk that the polyp stalk can continue to bleed following removal. The kidney and prostate will have endogenous urokinase activity that can increase local anticoagulant activity and could increase the risk of bleeding following the procedure. Pacemaker or defibrillator implantation also has a low risk of bleeding but should be undertaken with caution when the patient is anticoagulated because the pacemaker pocket is prone to hematoma formation.

Minor procedures that do not require the interruption of vitamin K antagonists (VKA) are minor dental procedures such as a tooth extraction or root canal, superficial skin excisions, and cataract removal. Coagulant material can be directly applied to maintain hemostasis in dental surgeries.

Cataract surgery does not involve a highly vascular area that has a significant risk of bleeding. Superficial skin surgeries do have an increased risk of bleeding when patients are on anticoagulation, but most bleeding complications are manageable. Thus, the most significant risk of comorbidity in that context is from thromboembolism due to withholding anticoagulation [60, 61].

As discussed above, percutaneous PD catheter placement is a low-risk surgery in the context of perioperative cardiovascular complications. In the context of anticoagulant management in the ACCP guidelines, this procedure has a risk of bleeding associated with the incision and dissection to the rectus muscle and the risk of perforating the epigastric vessels. The duration is usually less than 1 h and the most invasive part of the surgery is the 3–4 cm incision made superficially lateral to the umbilicus. Mital et al. did a retrospective analysis of a prospective database to determine bleeding complications of surgical placement of PD catheters using the open surgical technique [62]. This study involved 292 catheters placed in 263 patients over an 11-year period of time. Six patients had episodes of major bleeding within 2 weeks of the procedure for a complication rate of 2 %. Three of the six patients with bleeding were anticoagulated with preoperative warfarin or postoperative heparin. Two of the six had no coagulation parameters drawn prior to surgery. The study concluded that the rate of bleeding complications related to catheter insertion was low and was associated with anticoagulation. The study concluded that coagulation parameters should be drawn prior to the procedure and abnormalities corrected. Anticoagulation before and immediately after the procedure should be avoided. Also, dDAVP should be given for bleeding after surgery.

Anticoagulation can be divided broadly into vitamin K antagonists (VKA) and antiplatelet agents. The most common reasons to be on vitamin K antagonists such as warfarin are heart valvular abnormality, atrial fibrillation, and venous thromboembolism (VTE). The risk that a patient may have a perioperative thromboembolism is stratified into high, moderate, or low risk based on risk factors identified in medical literature (Table 31.4). According to the ACCP guidelines on perioperative management of antithrombotic therapy, patients with a mechanical heart valve have a high risk of thromboembolism in the absence of VKA if they have a prosthetic mitral valve, have older aortic valve prosthesis, or have a recent transient ischemic attack or stroke. The risk is moderate with bileaflet aortic valve prosthesis along with another risk factor such as atrial fibrillation, age >75 years, congestive heart failure, diabetes, or prior stroke. The risk for thromboembolism when anticoagulation is held is low with a bileaflet aortic valve without atrial fibrillation or other risk factors.

A patient on VKA for prior venous thromboembolism is at a high risk of a thrombotic event in the absence of VKA if

Table 31.4 Risk stratification for perioperative thromboembolism [58]

Indication for VKA	High risk	Moderate risk	Low risk
Mechanical heart valve	Mitral valve prosthesis, stroke or TIA within 6 months, older design of prosthetic aortic valve	Bileaflet aortic valve plus atrial fibrillation, prior stroke/TIA, HTN, DM, CHF, or age >75 years old	Bileaflet aortic valve without atrial fibrillation or other risk factors for stroke
Atrial fibrillation	$CHADS_2$ score of 5 or 6, stroke/TIA within 3 months, rheumatic valvular heart disease	$CHADS_2$ score of 3 or 4	$CHADS_2$ score of 0–2 without history of prior stroke/TIA
Venous thromboembolism	VTE within 3 months, severe thrombophilia (protein C or S deficiency, antithrombin, antiphospholipid antibodies)	VTE within 3–12 months, recurrent VTE, cancer treated within 6 months or palliative care, less severe thrombophilic conditions	Single VTE occurring more than 12 months before without other risk factors

a VTE event has occurred within the past 3 months or with severe thrombophilia. Severe thrombophilia includes protein C or S deficiency, antithrombin, or antiphospholipid antibodies. Moderate risk exists with VTE event within 3–12 months, recurrent VTE, cancer that was treated in the last 6 months or with palliative care, or less severe thrombophilia such as with heterozygous factor V Leiden or factor II mutation. A patient with a single VTE event occurring more than 12 months ago with no other risk factors has a low risk for perioperative thromboembolism in the absence of VKA therapy.

A number of scoring systems using risk factor assessment have evaluated the risk of thromboembolism in the setting of atrial fibrillation, but none directly apply in the perioperative setting [63, 64]. The ACCP practice guideline uses the $CHADS_2$ scoring system to determine the risk of thromboembolism in the absence of anticoagulation (Table 31.5). This system gives a score for risk factors: *Cardiac* failure, *Hypertension, Age* (75 years of age or older), *Diabetes*, and *Stroke*. Each factor has a value of one point in the score except for stroke, which is two points. Hence, the acronym $CHADS_2$ provides a scoring system to evaluate risk of embolism without anticoagulation. A patient with atrial fibrillation is at high risk of VTE in the absence of VKA with $CHADS_2$ score of 5 or 6, stroke within 3 months, or rheumatic valvular disease. Moderate risk for VTE exists with $CHADS_2$ score of 3 or 4. Low risk exists with $CHADS_2$ score of less than 3 without previous TIA or stroke [57].

For patients on VKA at high risk for thromboembolism in the absence of anticoagulation, VKA should be held 5 days before surgery, and therapeutic dose of bridging anticoagulation either with low-molecular-weight heparin (LMWH) or heparin should be started when the INR is <2. If the INR is not <1.5 at the time of the procedure, then low-dose vitamin K can be given. The last dose of LMWH should be on the morning of the day before surgery. Unfractionated heparin administered IV should be held at least 4 h before the procedure [57, 58]. With a moderate risk of thromboembolism, VKA should be held 5 days before the procedure. The clinician can choose between alternative bridging therapies. The bridging therapy can be therapeutic-dose LMWH or unfractionated

Table 31.5 $CHADS_2$ scoring system

Risk factor	Point value
Congestive heart failure	1
Hypertension	1
Age >75	1
Diabetes mellitus	1
Stroke	2

heparin, intermediate-dose bridging regime, or low-dose bridging therapy [58]. Low-dose bridging therapy is LMWH at DVT prophylaxis dose or unfractionated heparin 5,000 IU twice a day. The intermediate regimen is a dose between low and therapeutic therapy, such as enoxaparin 40 mg bid. Those patients at low risk for thromboembolism can have bridging with low-dose LMWH or no bridging depending on the clinical judgment of the physician; however, the most recent ACCP guidelines recommend no bridging therapy in low-risk patients. The bridging therapy should be restarted within 12–24 h after the procedure when hemostasis has been achieved. Resumption of bridging therapy after surgeries with high risk of major bleeding can occur beyond 24 h afterward when hemostasis has been accomplished.

Dabigatran (Pradaxa), a direct thrombin inhibitor, is an alternative to warfarin to anticoagulate in the context of non-valvular atrial fibrillation [65, 66]. This medication should be discontinued prior to a surgical procedure on the same basis as VKA. Dabigatran is renally eliminated, and it should be stopped 1–2 days prior to surgery in patients with a creatinine clearance greater than 50 mL/min. In patients with a creatinine clearance less than 50 mL/min, dabigatran should be stopped 3–5 days prior to the procedure. Bridging therapy should be initiated within 12–24 h of the last dose, depending on renal function. This medication does not have a specific reversal agent at this time, but it may be dialyzable. Also, coagulation factors such as factor VIIa, II, IX, or X may be effective in limiting bleeding.

Antiplatelet therapy may be initiated for a number of reasons ranging from primary prevention of myocardial infarction or stroke to prevention of thromboembolism in a coronary artery stent, prevention of recurrence of recent stroke, or myocardial infarction. Patients at high risk for perioperative cardiovascular events in the absence of antiplatelet therapy should continue aspirin and clopidogrel (Plavix) therapy uninterrupted. High risk includes patients with a bare-metal stent placed in coronary artery within 6 weeks, drug-eluting coronary stent within 12 months of surgery, and myocardial infarction within 3 months of surgery [59]. In patients undergoing coronary artery bypass graft surgery, aspirin therapy should be continued, but clopidogrel should be stopped 5–10 days prior to surgery. Patients undergoing percutaneous coronary intervention (PCI) should continue aspirin and clopidogrel or load clopidogrel if the patient is not taking it. Patients who are at high risk for perioperative cardiac events undergoing noncardiac surgery should continue aspirin through surgery, but clopidogrel should be stopped 5–10 days prior to surgery. Patients who are not at high risk for cardiovascular events should stop antiplatelet therapy prior to surgery. Those at low risk for perioperative cardiovascular events include patients taking antiplatelet drugs for primary prevention of myocardial infarction or stroke. For patients receiving antiplatelet drugs alone that are stopped prior to surgery, bridging anticoagulation with LMWH or unfractionated heparin is not initiated. Antiplatelet medications should be restarted within 24 h of surgery. Plavix can be restarted at 75 mg daily dose or with a loading dose.

One prospective study of 52 PD catheter insertions, removals, or replacements with patients on aspirin therapy evaluated the risk of bleeding [67]. Twenty-nine of the procedures occurred in patients receiving aspirin, 26 on aspirin 100 mg daily, and 3 on aspirin 325 mg daily. The remaining 23 procedures were in patients not taking aspirin or other anticoagulant and served as the control group. All procedures were performed using the open surgical technique. Postoperative bleeding was defined as wound hematoma or persistent oozing from the incision or exit site. Minor bleeding was bleeding that did not require surgical intervention or transfusion. Major bleeding occurred when a transfusion of packed red blood cells was required. Minor bleeding occurred in five patients (17.2 %) in the aspirin group and three patients (13 %) in the control group. Major bleeding occurred in one patient in the control group, and this procedure involved replacement of a PD catheter with synchronous repair of an umbilical hernia. Six of the nine bleeding events occurred after a catheter removal, which involved dissection of the deep cuff out of the rectus. The study concluded that PD catheter-related procedures can be performed safely on low-dose aspirin therapy.

31.5.3 Prophylactic Antibiotics

Although the catheter placement procedure is performed under sterile conditions in an outpatient procedure room or surgery suite, an increased risk of infection exists because a foreign body, the catheter, remains in the peritoneum after the surgery. Postoperative peritonitis could injure and diminish the function of the peritoneal membrane and subsequently lead to decreased effectiveness of peritoneal dialysis for the patient [68].

The use of preoperative prophylactic antibiotics significantly reduces the risk for peritonitis developing in the postoperative period [69]. Guidelines recommend the use of prophylactic antibiotics either with vancomycin 1 g IV or with a first- or second-generation cephalosporin to reduce the risk of insertion-related peritonitis and exit site infections [4, 39, 70]. The antibiotic should be selected for individual patients with that choice based upon local patterns of antibiotic resistance and frequently occurring organisms [3].

A study by Bennett-Jones et al. was one of the first prospective studies to show that administering gentamicin 1.5 mg/kg IV at the beginning of surgery could reduce the incidence of exit site infections and peritonitis within 28 days following the procedure [71]. Subsequently, a small prospective study compared 25 patients receiving single-dose cefazolin 500 mg IV and gentamicin 80 mg IV to a control group of 25 patients who did not receive preoperative antibiotics. This study found no significant reduction in exit site infections or peritonitis by giving preoperative antibiotics [72]. Golper et al. conducted a prospective analysis of peritonitis in 1939 patients across 68 PD units comprising the Network 9 data set that found giving antibiotics prior to PD catheter placement lowered the rate of peritonitis by 39 % [73]. Thirty-eight patients were included in a prospective study of preoperative antibiotics by Wikdahl et al. [68]. The patients were divided into group I ($n=18$) that received cefuroxime 1.5 g IV and cefuroxime 250 mg intraperitoneally in the first liter of dialysate following implantation of the catheter and group II ($n=20$) that did not receive antibiotics. No patients in group I developed peritonitis in the 10 days following catheter placement; however, in group II six patients developed microbial growth in dialysate and four patients developed peritonitis. Preoperative antibiotics significantly reduced the risk of peritonitis ($p=0.021$).

Vancomycin is an effective choice to prevent peritonitis but should be used cautiously to limit development of resistant organisms. A prospective study comparing vancomycin and cefazolin found that vancomycin reduced the risk of postoperative peritonitis [74]. This study spanning 6 years included 221 patients with 254 catheter placements. Patients in group I ($n=86$) received vancomycin 1 g intravenously (IV) 12 h before the catheter placement procedure. Group II ($n=85$) received cefazolin 1 g IV 3 h before the procedure. Patients in group III ($n=83$) did not receive antibiotic prophylaxis. There were no significant differences between the three groups regarding demographic factors, history of prior catheter placements, or history of prior abdominal surgery. The study demonstrated a significant reduction in the incidence of postoperative peritonitis in the patients receiving vancomycin compared to group II or III. Results of this study showed that 1 % of patients ($n = 1$) in group I developed peritonitis within the 14-day monitoring period. Six patients in group II (7 %) and ten patients in group III (12 %) developed peritonitis within 14 days of the procedure ($p = 0.02$) [74]. The odds ratio of developing post-procedure peritonitis was 11.64 (confidence interval 1.456–93.14) in the control group, which received no antibiotics. The group receiving cefazolin had an odds ratio of 6.45 (confidence interval 0.76–54.8) for developing peritonitis. The vancomycin group had an odds ratio of 1.0 (with $p = 0.001$).

A first-generation cephalosporin is most frequently used as preoperative antibiotic prophylaxis, but in light of the above study, vancomycin is also a good choice [6, 8–11, 14]. Each program should consider the use of vancomycin in light of their patient population and organisms isolated in peritonitis balanced against the risk of vancomycin usage causing the development of resistant organisms [39, 70, 75].

Screening for nasal colonization of methicillin-resistant staphylococcus aureus (MRSA) allows identification of carriers and their treatment in order to reduce the rate of exit site infections [76, 77]. Some studies of PD catheter placements described testing for nasal carriage of MRSA prior to the procedure [7, 11]. Post-procedure application of mupirocin (Bactroban) ointment in nares twice a day for 5 days reduces the rate of exit site infection. There is no data regarding whether treating nasal MRSA carriage prior to catheter placement reduced subsequent exit site infections [70].

31.6 Other Preparation for Catheter Placement

Informed consent for the procedure and the use of moderate sedation should be obtained from the patient after the risks of the procedure have been explained fully to the patient and all questions have been answered. It is important that the patient empty the bladder just before the procedure to minimize the size of the bladder in the pelvis. Some physicians prefer to insert a Foley catheter into the bladder the morning of the procedure to prevent urinary retention from incomplete voiding and assist with early detection of inadvertent placement of the PD catheter into the bladder. However, this is considered optional. Most studies of PD catheter placement have patients empty the bladder rather than place a Foley catheter [7, 11, 14].

Bowel cleansing with a laxative or bowel prep will help prevent peritonitis in the unlikely event of a bowel perforation [39, 75]. The patient should shower the morning of the procedure and scrub the abdomen with soap or detergent. Chlorhexidine is the most commonly used agent in catheter placement reports [6, 7, 14]. Abdominal hair should be clipped if present [75].

Conclusion

Preoperative evaluation for placement of PD catheter involves detailed history and physical examination to determine risk factors for perioperative complications or conditions that could lead to failure to successfully place the catheter. Risk factors that could lead to complications of the procedure should be explored. Physical examination should focus on anatomic barriers to placement of the catheter and planning of the exit site. Laboratory testing should identify potential complications such as hyperkalemia and bleeding tendencies. Preparatory measures such as prophylactic antibiotics, bowel preparation, and bladder evacuation have also been reviewed.

Conflict of Interest The authors have no conflicts of interest.

References

1. Fleisher LA, et al. ACC/AHA 2007 guidelines on perioperative cardiovascular evaluation and care for noncardiac surgery: executive summary: a report of the American college of Cardiology/American Heart association Task Force on Practice Guidelines (Writing Committee to Revise the 2002 Guidelines on Perioperative Cardiovascular Evaluation for Noncardiac Surgery) Developed in Collaboration with the American Society of Echocardiography, American Society of Nuclear Cardiology, Heart Rhythm Society, Society of Cardiovascular Anesthesiologists, Society for Cardiovascular Angiography and Interventions, Society for Vascular Medicine and Biology, and Society for Vascular Surgery. J Am Coll Cardiol. 2007;50(17):1707–32.
2. American College of Cardiology Foundation/American Heart Association Task Force on Practice, G, et al. ACCF/AHA focused update on perioperative beta blockade incorporated into the ACC/AHA 2007 guidelines on perioperative cardiovascular evaluation and care for noncardiac surgery. J Am Coll Cardiol. 2009;54(22):e13–118.
3. Figueiredo A, et al. Clinical practice guidelines for peritoneal access. Perit Dial Int. 2010;30(4):424–9.
4. Dombros N, et al. European best practice guidelines for peritoneal dialysis. 3 Peritoneal access. Nephrol Dial Transplant. 2005;20 Suppl 9:ix8–12.
5. Moon JY, et al. Fluoroscopically guided peritoneal dialysis catheter placement: long-term results from a single center. Perit Dial Int. 2008;28(2):163–9.
6. Zaman F, et al. Fluoroscopy-assisted placement of peritoneal dialysis catheters by nephrologists. Semin Dial. 2005;18(3):247–51.
7. Vaux EC, et al. Percutaneous fluoroscopically guided placement of peritoneal dialysis catheters–a 10-year experience. Semin Dial. 2008;21(5):459–65.
8. Maya ID. Ultrasound/fluoroscopy-assisted placement of peritoneal dialysis catheters. Semin Dial. 2007;20(6):611–5.
9. Jacobs IG, et al. Radiologic placement of peritoneal dialysis catheters: preliminary experience. Radiology. 1992;182(1):251–5.
10. Reddy C, Dybbro PE, Guest S. Fluoroscopically guided percutaneous peritoneal dialysis catheter placement: single center experience and review of the literature. Ren Fail. 2010;32(3):294–9.
11. Henderson S, Brown E, Levy J. Safety and efficacy of percutaneous insertion of peritoneal dialysis catheters under sedation and local anaesthetic. Nephrol Dial Transplant. 2009;24(11):3499–504.
12. Perakis KE, et al. Long-term complication rates and survival of peritoneal dialysis catheters: the role of percutaneous versus surgical placement. Semin Dial. 2009;22(5):569–75.

13. Ozener C, Bihorac A, Akoglu E. Technical survival of CAPD catheters: comparison between percutaneous and conventional surgical placement techniques. Nephrol Dial Transplant. 2001;16(9):1893–9.

14. Goh BL, et al. Does peritoneal dialysis catheter insertion by interventional nephrologists enhance peritoneal dialysis penetration? Semin Dial. 2008;21(6):561–6.

15. Gadallah MF, et al. Peritoneoscopic versus surgical placement of peritoneal dialysis catheters: a prospective randomized study on outcome. Am J Kidney Dis. 1999;33(1):118–22.

16. Asif A, et al. Modification of the peritoneoscopic technique of peritoneal dialysis catheter insertion: experience of an interventional nephrology program. Semin Dial. 2004;17(2):171–3.

17. American Society of Anesthesiologists Task Force on, S. and N.-A. Analgesia by, practice guidelines for sedation and analgesia by non-anesthesiologists. Anesthesiology. 2002;96(4):1004–17.

18. Maya ID. Ambulatory setting for peritoneal dialysis catheter placement. Semin Dial. 2008;21(5):457–8.

19. Patatas K, Koukkoulli A. The use of sedation in the radiology department. Clin Radiol. 2009;64(7):655–63.

20. Arepally A, et al. Safety of conscious sedation in interventional radiology. Cardiovasc Intervent Radiol. 2001;24(3):185–90.

21. Kim TH. Safety and effectiveness of moderate sedation for radiologic non-vascular intervention. Korean J Radiol. 2006;7(2):125–30.

22. Wolters U, et al. ASA classification and perioperative variables as predictors of postoperative outcome. Br J Anaesth. 1996;77(2):217–22.

23. Cuvillon P, et al. American Society of Anesthesiologists' physical status system: a multicentre francophone study to analyse reasons for classification disagreement. Eur J Anaesthesiol. 2011;28(10):742–7.

24. Freeman WK, Gibbons RJ. Perioperative cardiovascular assessment of patients undergoing noncardiac surgery. Mayo Clin Proc. 2009;84(1):79–90.

25. Fleisher LA, et al. ACC/AHA 2007 guidelines on perioperative cardiovascular evaluation and care for noncardiac surgery: a report of the American College of Cardiology/American heart Association Task Force on Practice Guidelines (Writing Committee to Revise the 2002 Guidelines on Perioperative Cardiovascular Evaluation for Noncardiac Surgery) developed in collaboration with the American Society of Echocardiography, American Society of Nuclear Cardiology, Heart Rhythm Society, Society of Cardiovascular Anesthesiologists, Society for Cardiovascular Angiography and Interventions, Society for Vascular Medicine and Biology, and Society for Vascular Surgery. J Am Coll Cardiol. 2007;50(17):e159–241.

26. Bapoje SR, et al. Preoperative evaluation of the patient with pulmonary disease. Chest. 2007;132(5):1637–45.

27. Qaseem A, et al. Risk assessment for and strategies to reduce perioperative pulmonary complications for patients undergoing noncardiothoracic surgery: a guideline from the American College of Physicians. Ann Intern Med. 2006;144(8):575–80.

28. Gross JB, et al. Practice guidelines for the perioperative management of patients with obstructive sleep apnea: a report by the American Society of Anesthesiologists Task Force on Perioperative Management of patients with obstructive sleep apnea. Anesthesiology. 2006;104(5):1081–93; quiz 1117–8.

29. Lasser EC, et al. Pretreatment with corticosteroids to alleviate reactions to intravenous contrast material. N Engl J Med. 1987;317(14):845–9.

30. Greenberger PA, Patterson R. The prevention of immediate generalized reactions to radiocontrast media in high-risk patients. J Allergy Clin Immunol. 1991;87(4):867–72.

31. Bettmann MA, et al. Adverse events with radiographic contrast agents: results of the SCVIR Contrast Agent Registry. Radiology. 1997;203(3):611–20.

32. Liakakos T, et al. Peritoneal adhesions: etiology, pathophysiology, and clinical significance. Recent advances in prevention and management. Dig Surg. 2001;18(4):260–73.

33. Keshvari A, et al. The effects of previous abdominal operations and intraperitoneal adhesions on the outcome of peritoneal dialysis catheters. Perit Dial Int. 2010;30(1):41–5.

34. Remuzzi G. Bleeding in renal failure. Lancet. 1988;1(8596):1205–8.

35. The sixth report of the Joint National Committee on prevention, detection, evaluation, and treatment of high blood pressure. Arch Intern Med. 1997;157(21):2413–46.

36. Howell SJ, Sear JW, Foex P. Hypertension, hypertensive heart disease and perioperative cardiac risk. Br J Anaesth. 2004;92(4):570–83.

37. Weksler N, et al. The dilemma of immediate preoperative hypertension: to treat and operate, or to postpone surgery? J Clin Anesth. 2003;15(3):179–83.

38. Reich DL, et al. Intraoperative tachycardia and hypertension are independently associated with adverse outcome in noncardiac surgery of long duration. Anesth Analg. 2002;95(2):273–7, table of contents.

39. Flanigan M, Gokal R. Peritoneal catheters and exit-site practices toward optimum peritoneal access: a review of current developments. Perit Dial Int. 2005;25(2):132–9.

40. Nicholson ML, et al. Combined abdominal hernia repair and continuous ambulatory peritoneal dialysis (CAPD) catheter insertion. Perit Dial Int. 1989;9(4):307–8.

41. Crabtree JH. Hernia repair without delay in initiating or continuing peritoneal dialysis. Perit Dial Int. 2006;26(2):178–82.

42. Garcia-Urena MA, et al. Prevalence and management of hernias in peritoneal dialysis patients. Perit Dial Int. 2006;26(2):198–202.

43. Juhari Y, Nicholson ML. Combined laparoscopic peritoneal dialysis catheter insertion and epigastric hernia repair to avoid delaying dialysis. Ann R Coll Surg Engl. 2010;92(8):715.

44. Laine C, Williams SV, Wilson JF. In the clinic. Preoperative evaluation. Ann Intern Med. 2009;151(1):ITC1–15, quiz ITC16.

45. Crabtree JH. Selected best demonstrated practices in peritoneal dialysis access. Kidney Int Suppl. 2006;103:S27–37.

46. Crabtree JH, Burchette RJ, Siddiqi NA. Optimal peritoneal dialysis catheter type and exit site location: an anthropometric analysis. ASAIO J. 2005;51(6):743–7.

47. Sreenarasimhaiah VP, et al. Percutaneous technique of presternal peritoneal dialysis catheter placement. Semin Dial. 2004;17(5):407–10.

48. Crabtree JH, Burchette RJ. Comparative analysis of two-piece extended peritoneal dialysis catheters with remote exit-site locations and conventional abdominal catheters. Perit Dial Int. 2010;30(1):46–55.

49. Pinson CW, et al. Surgery in long-term dialysis patients. Experience with more than 300 cases. Am J Surg. 1986;151(5):567–71.

50. Ahmed J, Weisberg LS. Hyperkalemia in dialysis patients. Semin Dial. 2001;14(5):348–56.

51. Steiner RW, Coggins C, Carvalho AC. Bleeding time in uremia: a useful test to assess clinical bleeding. Am J Hematol. 1979;7(2):107–17.

52. Liu YK, et al. Thigh bleeding time as a valid indicator of hemostatic competency during surgical treatment of patients with advanced renal disease. Surg Gynecol Obstet. 1991;172(4):269–74.

53. Gewirtz AS, Miller ML, Keys TF. The clinical usefulness of the preoperative bleeding time. Arch Pathol Lab Med. 1996;120(4):353–6.

54. Lind SE. The bleeding time does not predict surgical bleeding. Blood. 1991;77(12):2547–52.

55. Strauss RG. Pretransfusion trigger platelet counts and dose for prophylactic platelet transfusions. Curr Opin Hematol. 2005;12(6):499–502.

56. O'Connor SD, et al. Coagulation concepts update. AJR Am J Roentgenol. 2009;193(6):1656–64.

57. Douketis JD, et al. The perioperative management of antithrombotic therapy: American College of Chest Physicians Evidence-Based Clinical Practice Guidelines (8th edition). Chest. 2008;133 (6 Suppl):299S–339S.

58. Douketis JD, et al. Perioperative management of antithrombotic therapy: antithrombotic therapy and prevention of thrombosis, 9th ed: American College of Chest Physicians Evidence-Based Clinical Practice Guidelines. Chest. 2012;141(2 Suppl):e326S–50S.

59. Douketis JD. Perioperative management of patients who are receiving warfarin therapy: an evidence-based and practical approach. Blood. 2011;117(19):5044–9.

60. Lewis KG, Dufresne Jr RG. A meta-analysis of complications attributed to anticoagulation among patients following cutaneous surgery. Dermatol Surg. 2008;34(2):160–4; discussion 164–5.

61. Syed S, et al. A prospective assessment of bleeding and international normalized ratio in warfarin-anticoagulated patients having cutaneous surgery. J Am Acad Dermatol. 2004;51(6):955–7.

62. Mital S, Fried LF, Piraino B. Bleeding complications associated with peritoneal dialysis catheter insertion. Perit Dial Int. 2004; 24(5):478–80.

63. Lip GY, et al. Refining clinical risk stratification for predicting stroke and thromboembolism in atrial fibrillation using a novel risk factor-based approach: the euro heart survey on atrial fibrillation. Chest. 2010;137(2):263–72.

64. Olesen JB, et al. Validation of risk stratification schemes for predicting stroke and thromboembolism in patients with atrial fibrillation: nationwide cohort study. BMJ. 2011;342:d124.

65. United States Food and Drug Administration. Prescribing Information for Pradaxa (dabigatran etexilate mesylate) capsules for oral use. Physicians Desk Reference, 2013. www.accessdata. fda.gov/drugsatfda_docs/label/2013/022512s011lbl.pdf.

66. Connolly SJ, et al. Dabigatran versus warfarin in patients with atrial fibrillation. N Engl J Med. 2009;361(12):1139–51.

67. Shpitz B, et al. Should aspirin therapy be withheld before insertion and/or removal of a permanent peritoneal dialysis catheter? Am Surg. 2002;68(9):762–4.

68. Wikdahl AM, et al. One-dose cefuroxime i.v. and i.p. reduces microbial growth in PD patients after catheter insertion. Nephrol Dial Transplant. 1997;12(1):157–60.

69. Strippoli GF, et al. Antimicrobial agents to prevent peritonitis in peritoneal dialysis: a systematic review of randomized controlled trials. Am J Kidney Dis. 2004;44(4):591–603.

70. Piraino B, et al. Peritoneal dialysis-related infections recommendations: 2005 update. Perit Dial Int. 2005;25(2):107–31.

71. Bennett-Jones DN, et al. Prophylactic gentamicin in the prevention of early exit-site infections and peritonitis in CAPD. In: Khanna R et al., editors. Advances in continuous ambulatory peritoneal dialysis. 8th annual CAPD conference. Toronto: Peritoneal Dialysis Bulletin, Inc; 1988. p. 147–50.

72. Lye WC, Lee EJ, Tan CC. Prophylactic antibiotics in the insertion of Tenckhoff catheters. Scand J Urol Nephrol. 1992;26(2): 177–80.

73. Golper TA, et al. Risk factors for peritonitis in long-term peritoneal dialysis: the network 9 peritonitis and catheter survival studies. Academic Subcommittee of the Steering Committee of the Network 9 Peritonitis and Catheter Survival Studies. Am J Kidney Dis. 1996;28(3):428–36.

74. Gadallah MF, et al. Role of preoperative antibiotic prophylaxis in preventing postoperative peritonitis in newly placed peritoneal dialysis catheters. Am J Kidney Dis. 2000;36(5):1014–9.

75. Gokal R, et al. Peritoneal catheters and exit-site practices: toward optimum peritoneal access. Perit Dial Int. 1993;13(1): 29–39.

76. Bonifati C, et al. Antimicrobial agents and catheter-related interventions to prevent peritonitis in peritoneal dialysis: using evidence in the context of clinical practice. Int J Artif Organs. 2006; 29(1):41–9.

77. Nasal mupirocin prevents Staphylococcus aureus exit-site infection during peritoneal dialysis. Mupirocin Study Group. J Am Soc Nephrol. 1996;7(11):2403–8.

Operative Considerations for Peritoneal Dialysis Catheter

32

Stephen R. Ash, Rajeev Narayan, Anil K. Agarwal, and John H. Crabtree

32.1 Introduction

Tunneled PD catheters are the most successful long-term transcutaneous access devices ever used in medical practice. While flow and infection problems complicate central venous catheters for hemodialysis in weeks to months, PD catheters can provide successful dialysis access for years with few problems in dialysate flow or infection. However, successful hydraulic function of a peritoneal catheter is a complex relationship between a simply shaped catheter and a natural, unique, and complex intraperitoneal space, which means that the hydraulic function is less predictable than hemodialysis catheters. The type of catheter chosen, the method of placing the catheter, the experience of the operating physician, and the intraperitoneal anatomy all affect the success of PD catheters. This chapter reviews the types of catheters available currently and recently, proper location of catheter components, preoperative evaluation of the patient including ultrasound of the abdominal wall and peritoneum, overview of methods of placement, embedding of PD catheters and exteriorization, catheter repositioning, repair of pericatheter leaks and hernias, and catheter removal.

S.R. Ash, MD, FACP (✉)
Indiana University Health Arnett, Lafayette, Indiana, USA

HemoCleanse, Inc. and Ash Access Technology, Inc.,
3601 Sagamore Parkway North, Suite B, Lafayette,
Indiana 47905, USA
e-mail: sash@hemocleanse.com

R. Narayan, MD
Clinical and Interventional Nephrology,
San Antonio Kidney Disease Center,
San Antonio, TX, USA

A.K. Agarwal, MD, FACP, FASN, FNKF
Division of Nephrology, The Ohio State University,
395 W 12th Avenue, Ground Floor,
Columbus, OH 43210, USA

J.H. Crabtree,
Department of Surgery, Kaiser Permanente,
Bellflower, CA, USA

32.2 Types of Current Chronic Peritoneal Catheters and Comparative Advantages

Chronic PD catheters used today are all constructed of silicone. The intraperitoneal portion contains numerous 0.5–1-mm side holes. All chronic PD catheters have one or two Dacron® (polyester) cuffs that lie in the rectus muscle or subcutaneous space, which promote a local inflammatory response. This inflammation results in a fibrous plug attached to the Dacron that fixes the catheter in position, prevents pericatheter fluid leaks, and prevents bacterial migration around the catheter. Although there are numerous designs for PD catheters, the method of placement and experience of the physician have more effect on the functional success and complications of the catheter than the catheter design [1].

On first view, there appears to be a bewildering variety of chronic peritoneal catheters currently on the market (Fig. 32.1). However, each portion of the catheter has only a few basic design options.

There are three designs of the intraperitoneal portion: (Fig. 32.1a)

- Straight Tenckhoff, with an 8-cm portion containing 1-mm side holes
- Curled Tenckhoff, with a coiled 16-cm portion containing 1-mm side holes
- Straight Tenckhoff, with perpendicular silicone discs (Toronto Western™ or Oreopoulos-Zellerman catheter)

There are two basic shapes of the subcutaneous portion between the muscle wall and the skin exit site: (Fig. 32.1b)

- Straight or a gently curved straight catheter
- A permanent 150° bend or arc (Swan Neck™)

There are four positions and designs for Dacron® (polyester) cuffs:

- Single cuff around the catheter, usually placed in the rectus muscle but sometimes on the anterior surface of the rectus sheath (depending on the procedure used to implant the catheter)

A.S. Yevzlin et al. (eds.), *Interventional Nephrology*,
DOI 10.1007/978-1-4614-8803-3_32, © Springer Science+Business Media New York 2014

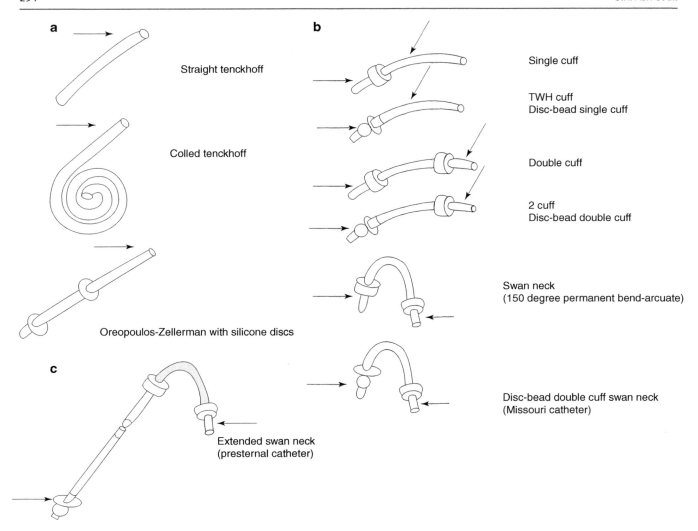

Fig. 32.1 Currently available peritoneal catheters; intraperitoneal and extraperitoneal designs; all are made from silicone with Dacron® cuffs. Arrows indicate usual position of parietal peritoneum and skin surface

relative to the catheter. (**a**) intraperitoneal portions, (**b**) subcutaneous portions, (**c**) swan neck presternal catheter extension

- Dual cuffs around the catheter, one in the rectus muscle and the other in subcutaneous tissue
- Disc-bead deep cuff, with parietal peritoneum and posterior rectus sheath sewn between a Dacron® disc (20 mm) and a silicone bead (12 mm), usually in combination with a subcutaneous cuff (Oreopoulos-Zellerman™ and Missouri™ catheters, Fig. 32.1b)
- Subcutaneous extension to a double cuff swan neck portion (presternal catheter)

The outer diameter of adult PD catheters is 5 mm, yielding a catheter size of about 15 French. There are two different internal diameters for adult PD catheters:

- 2.6 mm, the standard Tenckhoff catheter size (also Swan Neck™ catheter, Missouri™ Swan Neck™ catheter, and Oreopoulos-Zellerman™ catheter)
- 3.5 mm, the Flex-Neck® catheter, which provides faster flow rates and makes the catheter body less rigid

The various intraperitoneal designs have all been created to diminish the incidence of outflow obstruction due to omental attachment to the catheter. The shape of the curled Tenckhoff catheter and the discs of the Toronto Western™ catheter hold visceral peritoneal surfaces away from the side holes of the catheter. The optimal location for the standard deep cuff is within the rectus muscle. Fixation of the deep cuff within the muscle generally avoids problems associated with the deep cuff migration, including pericatheter leaks, pericatheter hernias, and exit-site erosion. However, outward migration still may occur over time, since the deep cuff can extrude from the muscle over time. The goal of more complicated deep cuff designs is to prevent this outward migration of the deep cuff and the catheter. The disc-bead deep cuff is fixed in position by the apposition of the bead against the parietal peritoneum and the disc against the posterior rectus sheath.

Variations in the subcutaneous catheter shapes are designed to provide a lateral or downward direction of the exit site. This direction minimizes the risk of exit infection. An upward directed exit site collects debris and fluid, increasing the risk of exit-site infection. The larger internal diameter of the Flex-Neck® catheters provides lower hydraulic resistance and more rapid dialysate flow during inflow and the early phase of outflow. In the latter part of outflow, the resistance to flow is determined mostly by the spaces formed by peritoneal surfaces as they approach the catheter, rather than the inside of the catheter, so the catheters do not increase blood flow at this part of outflow. All catheters with a larger internal diameter of the tubing have a thinner wall and therefore crimp somewhat more easily than the catheters with a smaller ID. Some extra training and caution are necessary for physicians to make sure that they do not bend the catheter too acutely in the subcutaneous space during placement, and patients should be advised to not repeatedly fold and crimp the external tubing of the catheter when bandaging the exit site.

Silicone rubber seems to be an ideal material for creation of PD catheters, but other materials could work well. Polyurethane catheters such as the Cruz "pail-handle" catheter have been marketed, but they did not provide a lower incidence of persisting peritonitis or omental attachment leading to outflow failure. Polyurethane catheters had a weaker bond to the Dacron® cuff, and loosening of this bond created pericatheter leaks and peritonitis quite frequently. Degradation of the tubing of polyurethane PD catheters also occurred in a number of patients, with catheter fracturing [2, 3]. These complications have not been seen in polyurethane central venous catheters, or in silicone catheters, so perhaps they were due to a peculiar interaction of polyurethane with fat, fatty acids, or surfactants in the abdominal subcutaneous tissue. More advanced copolymers such as polycarbonate-polyurethane are now used very successfully in central venous catheters, but these copolymers have not been used for construction of PD catheters.

The "presternal" PD catheter is designed to provide an exit site over the chest or the upper abdomen rather than in the mid-abdomen. It is an appropriate alternative when an abdominal catheter exit site is not suitable or desirable, such as obese patients, those with abdominal ostomies, incontinent patients with diapers, and those who desire to take a deep tub bath without risk of exit-site contamination [4]. The device consists of a standard peritoneal catheter placed in the usual manner with the deep cuff within the abdominal wall. From the primary incision, a second catheter with two cuffs is tunneled to the upper abdomen or chest. The two catheters are then joined by a titanium connector. Presternal catheter systems are available for both Missouri and standard Tenckhoff catheters [5]. Figure 32.1c shows the general configuration and position of the components of the presternal catheter. The presternal catheter exit-site location should be planned preoperatively. The exit site should avoid the open collar area, bra line, and fleshy part of the breast. The subcutaneous tract should be parasternal in location and not cross the midline in the event that the patient should subsequently require a midline sternotomy for cardiovascular surgery. The usual alignment of the Swan Neck presternal segment is such that the exit limb is oriented medially with the exit site at least 2.5–3 cm off of the midline.

Long-term outcomes for the presternal catheter have been excellent, especially considering that the patients are often obese. In non-randomized studies, the 2-year survival of presternal Missouri catheters was about 90 %, while the survival of abdominal Missouri catheters was about 75 % (though results were not significantly different and catheters removed for persistent peritonitis without signs of tunnel infection were not included) [6].

Another peritoneal catheter variation is the "self-locating" catheter, a modification of Tenckhoff catheter with a 12-g cylinder of Tungsten at the tip to ensure non-displacement of the catheter tip from the pouch of Douglas. The study from 16 Italian centers included 746 patients receiving a self-locating catheter compared to 216 patients receiving a traditional Tenckhoff catheter [7]. The results showed significantly better outcomes of the self-locating catheter including cuff extrusion, infection, peritonitis, early leakage, and obstruction that were statistically less frequent. This catheter is not available in the USA but is placed frequently in Italy and in Europe.

32.3 Proper Location of Catheter Components

There is general agreement on the proper location of the components of chronic peritoneal catheters (Figs. 32.2 and 32.3):

- The intraperitoneal portion should be between the parietal and visceral peritoneum and directed towards the pelvis to the right or left of the bladder.
- The deep cuff should be within the rectus muscle, at the medial or lateral border of the rectus sheath.
- The subcutaneous cuff should be approximately 2 cm from the skin exit site.

Placing the deep cuff within the rectus muscle promotes tissue ingrowth and therefore minimizes pericatheter hernias, leaks, catheter extrusion, and exit-site erosion [8]. At the parietal peritoneal surface, the squamous epithelium reflects along the surface of the catheter to reach the deep cuff. If the deep cuff is outside the muscle wall, the peritoneal extension creates a potential hernia. At the skin surface, the stratified squamous epithelium follows the surface of the catheter until it reaches the superficial cuff. If the exit-site tunnel is longer than 3 cm, the squamous epithelium does not reach the superficial cuff, and granulation tissue remains, producing a serous fluid that weeps into the tunnel to create an exit site that is continually wet and crusted. This increases the potential for exit-site infection.

Some peritoneal catheters have components that provide greater fixation of the deep cuff within the musculature such as the Missouri™, Toronto Western™, and the previously available Advantage™ and column-disc catheters. With all of these catheters, outward migration of the catheter is impossible, even if there is poor tissue ingrowth into the deep

cuff or disc. With exception of the Advantage catheter (no longer available), all of these catheters with parietal peritoneal fixation have been placed surgically.

In placement of peritoneal catheters, it is best to choose a deep cuff location that is free of major blood vessels (Fig. 32.4). The superficial epigastric arteries course from the femoral artery and ligament towards the umbilicus, anterior to the rectus sheath. The inferior epigastric arteries lie behind the rectus muscles, roughly in the middle of the rectus sheath. Considering the position of these arteries, the safest locations for placing the deep cuff are in the medial or lateral borders of the rectus muscle. For procedures using a cannula or needle insertion, it is best to aim directly at the perceived lateral border. This can be located in physical exam by finding the anterior superior iliac spine and the midline and determining the midpoint of the line between these two points. In patients without much subcutaneous fat, the lateral border of the rectus can be felt when the patient tightens their muscles. The medial border is located 1–2 cm from midline, below the umbilicus. The exact location of the medial and lateral border of the rectus muscle can be determined more precisely using ultrasound (as shown below). The intraperitoneal portion of the catheter should be placed adjacent to the parietal peritoneum.

32.4 Preoperative Evaluation and Ultrasound Imaging of the Abdominal Wall

When a peritoneal catheter placement is planned, the following information needs to be obtained:
- Previous abdominal surgeries and location of scars.
- Prior PD catheter placements, locations, operative findings, and reasons for catheter failure.

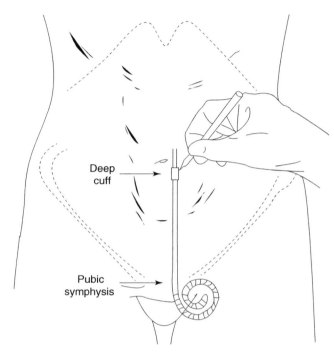

Fig. 32.2 Determining approximate location of deep cuff of PD catheter to assure that the coil of the catheter is behind the inguinal ligament. Deep cuff may be placed at the lateral border or medial border of the rectus muscle

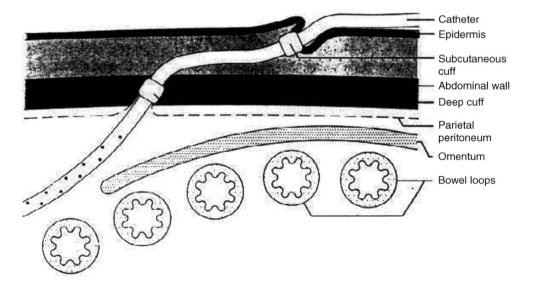

Fig. 32.3 Proper relationship of peritoneal cuffs to abdominal musculature, parietal and visceral peritoneum, and skin exit site for straight Tenckhoff catheter

Fig. 32.4 Major blood vessels and landmarks of the anterior abdominal wall. *Open squares* represent the preferred and safest points for location of the deep cuff of a chronic peritoneal catheter, within the medial or lateral border of the rectus muscle. *Solid squares* indicate the external landmarks used during blind insertion of a needle or cannula at the start of peritoneoscopic or blind catheter placement: ½ the distance between the anterior superior iliac spine for the lateral border of the rectus and 1–2 cm from midline below the umbilicus for the medial border of the rectus

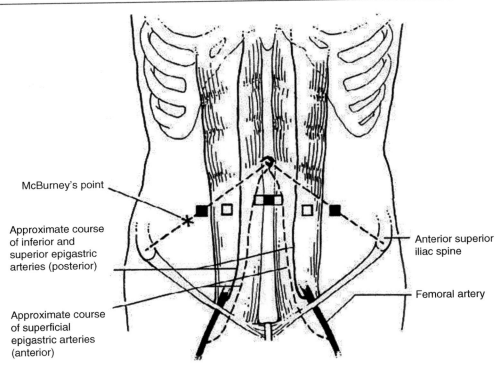

McBurney's point

Approximate course of inferior and superior epigastric arteries (posterior)

Approximate course of superficial epigastric arteries (anterior)

Anterior superior iliac spine

Femoral artery

- Presence of ventral hernias and whether bowels are present within the hernia (by physical exam, ultrasound, or x-ray evaluation). If bowels are present within the hernia, then it is imperative to have the hernia repaired before initiation of PD therapy.
- Bowel function, including constipation or diarrhea (if constipated, give laxatives for 2–3 days before the procedure).
- Bleeding risk, including low platelet count, use of antiplatelet drugs (aspirin or Plavix), anticoagulants (warfarin or newer agents), and intrinsic coagulopathies (factor V abnormalities, lupus anticoagulant, and cardiolipin antibodies).
- Blood tests relating to bleeding risks (placement of a PD catheter in a patient on Coumadin can be done safely if INR is below 2 and if platelet count is over 50,000).
- Allergy to antibiotics and sensitivity or allergy to sedatives or analgesics.
  Instructions to patient should include the following:
- Do not eat any solid food for 8 h before the procedure.
- Do not drink any liquids 2 h before the procedure (3 hours for diabetic patients).
- Urinate before coming to the facility and again after coming to the facility.
- Let the staff know if you have been constipated lately.
- If you are taking antiplatelet and anticoagulant drugs such as Coumadin, consult with your doctor to determine when they should be stopped before the procedure. Usually these medications are stopped 5 days before the catheter placement, but your physician may choose instead a

different time, a reduced dose, or substitution of another short-term anticoagulant such as Lovenox™ depending upon the need for anticoagulation. Your physician may also order a blood test to determine the function of your blood clotting system.

When the patient arrives at the center for catheter placement, the above information is reviewed, and a careful physical examination is performed. By physical examination, hernias can be confirmed, and the lateral and medial border of the rectus and the location of the anterior superior iliac spine (the deep cuff is generally placed cranial to this level) can be identified. The presence of panniculus can be determined, and an estimation of subcutaneous fat thickness at various potential locations of the deep cuff. With a catheter or a template, the planned location of the tip of the catheter can be determined, as well as the planned exit site (choosing an exit site above or below the belt line) as in Fig. 32.2.

PD catheters are often placed without a prior ultrasound evaluation of the anterior abdominal wall. However, many physicians have found that using ultrasound examination improves the ease and success of the placement procedure and occasionally prevents immediate failure of the procedure or catheter. Using a medium frequency probe such as used in placing IJ catheters, accurate information can be gained on:

- The exact location of the medial and lateral border of the rectus muscle, noted by thinning of the rectus sheath at these locations.
- The absence of bulky or firm adhesions between the visceral and parietal peritoneal surfaces (by observing free motion of the visceral peritoneum against the parietal

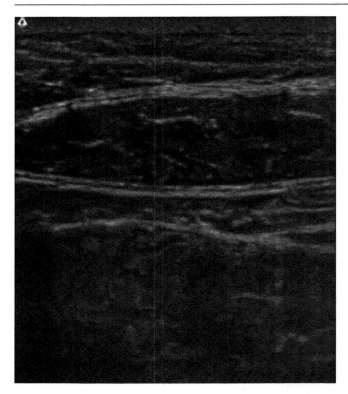

Fig. 32.5 Ultrasound of abdominal wall near the lateral border of the rectus. Tissue layers from top to bottom are: subcutaneous fat, anterior rectus sheath, rectus muscle, posterior rectus sheath, parietal peritoneum and mesenteric fat

peritoneum and, a clear single or double line of the peritoneum beneath the rectus sheath). Though this method is not perfect, it at least demonstrates dense adhesions and whether adhesions are more prominent on one side of the abdomen or the other.

- The location of the inferior epigastric artery within the rectus muscle (through finding a round, echo-free space which expands with heartbeats but does not compress under pressure from the probe). The epigastric artery is usually near the middle of the rectus muscle and lying against the posterior rectus sheath but has considerable variation. Smaller arteries can be identified by Doppler ultrasound. If the inferior epigastric artery is not found by either method of ultrasound, then it is small and unlikely to cause any bleeding problems during placement of the catheter.
- The thickness of the subcutaneous fat layer between the rectus muscle and the skin and a comparison of the fat layer thickness at levels. In general, the length of the skin incision over the deep cuff location should be the same as the depth of the fat layer.

To properly perform the ultrasound examination, the patient must lie flat in the supine position, as they will on the procedure table. Figure 32.5 is an example of an ultrasound of the lateral border of the rectus muscle in a normal patient.

During the ultrasound examination, there are sometimes surprises, such as subcutaneous veins which enlarge with SVC occlusion, connect through the rectus, and create a plexus in the pre-peritoneal space of the abdominal wall. A subcutaneous plexus of veins is shown in Fig. 32.6, a non-contrast CT of the anterior abdominal wall in a patient with asymptomatic SVC occlusion. Doppler ultrasound detected the SQ vessels and pre-peritoneal plexus of veins allowing placement of a catheter in an area free of both.

32.5   Placement Technique Overview

Throughout the history of PD, there has been a steady evolution of techniques of catheter placement. The goal of catheter placement techniques is to obtain:

- Proper placement of all of the components of the catheter (the catheter tip adjacent to the parietal peritoneum, deep cuff in rectus musculature, and subcutaneous cuff 2 cm below the exit site)
- A tight seal between the catheter cuffs and muscle and subcutaneous tissue
- A small exit site of size just large enough to permit passage of the catheter and without sutures
- Adequate hydraulic function for PD (manual or automated) and avoid:
  - Patient discomfort during or after the procedure
  - Pericatheter leaks
  - Trauma to tissues and organs surrounding the catheter
  - Bleeding from muscle, peritoneum, or subcutaneous tissues
  - Infection

The earliest tunneled and cuffed peritoneal catheters were placed blindly, using the Tenckhoff trocar, essentially a percutaneous technique. Surgical or dissective placement evolved soon after, and techniques evolved balancing the need for exposure of the peritoneum with making a small incision in the rectus muscle. Peritoneoscopic techniques using a 2.2-mm needlescope and an expandable guide for placing the deep cuff evolved in the 1980s, with the great advantage of visualizing the peritoneal space, avoiding adhesions, and placing the tip of the catheter next to the parietal peritoneum. Percutaneous placement blind technique with guidewire and split sheath followed the development of these techniques for placing tunneled IJ dialysis catheters. More recently the use of a fluoroscopy and a long guidewire to assist blind placement has been shown to improve results. Laparoscopic techniques for catheter placement have become popular among some surgeons and provide vision of adhesions and choice of the best catheter location. Especially if omentopexy is performed and a long downward tunnel in the rectus muscle is created during the procedure, results are excellent.

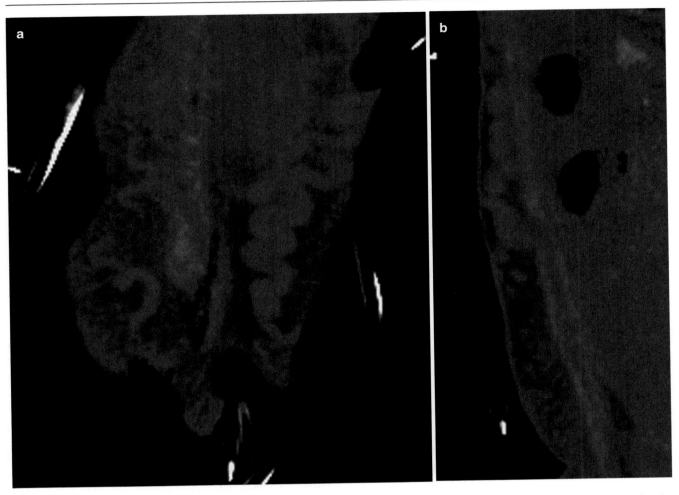

Fig. 32.6 Non-contrast CT of patient with subcutaneous plexus of veins developing after superior vena cava occlusion, shown penetrating the rectus muscle sheath. (**a**) coronal plane, anterior to rectus muscles. (**b**) sagittal plane

The advantages of percutaneous methods include the minimal trauma of the technique, ability to avoid general anesthesia, potential to avoid pericatheter leaks (allowing an earlier start of PD), and lower incidence of infections. Peritoneoscopic methods allow visualization of the parietal peritoneum and placement of the catheter against this surface, visualization and avoidance of adhesions, and choice of the longest and clearest space for placing the catheter. Surgical methods have the advantage that they are easily implemented by surgeons and exercising care in suturing the peritoneum and rectus sheath can result in very low leak rates. Some catheters such as the Missouri and Oreopoulos-Zellerman catheters can only be placed surgically. Laparoscopic techniques have the advantage of excellent intraperitoneal vision and the ability to perform omentopexy, tunneling of the catheter within the rectus sheath or pre-peritoneal space, and other procedures during catheter placement. Overall, the type of technique chosen determines outcome less than do the skill and experience of the physician. An excellent review of peritoneal catheter placement techniques is found in the 1998 "Best Practices" publication of ISPD [11].

32.5.1 Blind Placement by Tenckhoff Trocar

When Tenckhoff first described the twin cuffed PD catheter, he also described a device that could place this catheter into the peritoneum and position the cuffs in approximately the right position. The Tenckhoff trocar is still used in many centers for placement of Tenckhoff and similar catheters, especially in practices outside of the USA. After inserting the device tip through the rectus muscle, the stylet is removed, the PD catheter is advanced through the trocar, and the halves of trocar are removed around the catheter, leaving the deep cuff just outside the outer rectus sheath (Fig. 32.7). The cuff could then be advanced into the musculature with hemostats. Placement of the PD catheter by Tenckhoff trocar resulted in a 2–43 % risk of pericatheter leak, especially if PD was

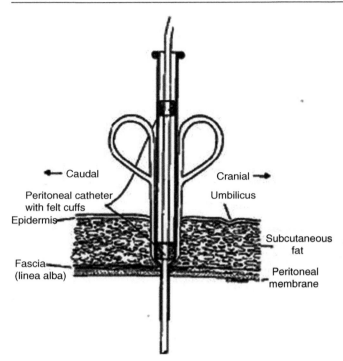

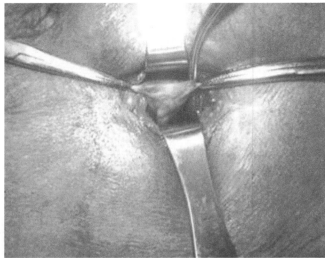

Fig. 32.8 Dissective implantation approach. Parietal peritoneum is being lifted through the rectus sheath incision

Fig. 32.7 The Tenckhoff trocar, as shown after removal of the trocar portion and with the catheter inserted. Removing the outer tube allowed the body of the cannula to split into two pieces, and each was then removed separately, leaving the cuff just outside the linea alba

initiated soon after placement of the catheter. There was a 5–50 % risk of outflow failure with this blind technique [1].

32.5.2 Dissection (Surgical)

Surgical dissection is still the most commonly used method for placement of chronic PD catheters, and some catheters require surgical placement (Toronto Western and Missouri catheters) [9, 10]. As reviewed by Dr. Crabtree, placement by dissection begins with either extensive local anesthesia or light general anesthesia. There are two general approaches: the lateral and the paramedian. The skin, subcutaneous tissue, and anterior rectus sheath over the desired entry site are dissected, resulting in creation of the primary incision. After blunt dissection through the rectus muscle, the posterior rectus sheath is identified and a 1–2-cm incision made. The peritoneum is identified, lifted, and opened with a 1–2-cm incision as in Fig. 32.8. The space between the parietal and visceral peritoneum is identified. If the omentum is prominent in this location, the surgeon can perform a local, partial *omentectomy* by pulling out 7–10 cm of omentum and resecting it, though this is done mostly in placement of peritoneal catheters in children. The catheter is prepared by wetting and injecting with saline and squeezing all air bubbles out of the cuffs under saline to promote better tissue ingrowth. It is washed with sterile normal saline, 20 mL of which is injected

through it to remove particulates. It is then advanced through the incision into the peritoneal cavity by feel using a stylet or a large, curved, blunt clamp. With an internal stylet, the Tenckhoff is inserted into the peritoneum while the stylet is retracted. A curled Tenckhoff then uncoils and advances within the peritoneal space. The proper location of the catheter tip should be just beneath the left or right inguinal ligament, between the anterior abdominal wall and the mass of omentum and bowel loops. In this location, there is less chance of functional outflow obstruction from bowel loops and omentum. After proper positioning of the catheter tip, the peritoneum is closed tightly around the catheter below the level of the deep cuff using a running lock stitch. The abdominal musculature and posterior and anterior rectus sheath are closed around the cuff with sutures.

The skin exit site is then selected. The location can be estimated by laying the outer part of the catheter over the skin, accommodating for a bend to direct the exit towards the patient's feet. If the catheter does not have a preformed arcuate bend, create a gentle bend in the subcutaneous tract to direct the exit site laterally or downward. A sharply arcuate subcutaneous course creates tension between the two cuffs and tends to displace the intra-abdominal portion from the pelvis. A straight course between the cuffs also creates tension between the cuffs. The skin exit site should be approximately 2 cm distant from the location of the superficial cuff. This distance is necessary to allow proper epithelialization of the tract down towards the superficial cuff.

A tunneling tool is then passed subcutaneously from the primary incision to the skin exit site from below. The skin is nicked over the tool to create the exit site, and the catheter is pulled through the tunnel by attachment to the tunneling tool. The tunnel is widened through the primary incision with hemostats lightly attached to the catheter to facilitate passage of the superficial cuff through the tunnel to its proper position near the exit site.

A limitation of the dissective approach is that there is limited visualization of the peritoneal space, and the catheter tip is advanced into the peritoneum mostly by "feel" as the catheter is advanced. A local omentectomy may be performed through the incision to the peritoneum, but the technique is limited by the size of the peritoneal opening.

32.5.3 Laparoscopic Placement, with Omentopexy and Long Rectus Tunnel Options

As stated by Dr. John Crabtree [5], with the revolutionary introduction of laparoscopic cholecystectomy into surgical practice, surgeons have endeavored to apply the laparoscope to virtually every abdominal procedure. However, laparoscopic techniques used by surgeons to establish PD access are still evolving. Currently, there is no standardized methodology for laparoscopic PD catheter implantation. The process is partially impeded by the attempted use of ordinary laparoscopic equipment that is familiar to surgeons but is not suitably adapted to catheter insertion. As a consequence, reported outcomes have been extremely variable and frequently demonstrate no clear advantage to implantation of catheters by standard open dissection.

The strength of laparoscopy is that it allows an opportunity to visibly address problems that adversely affect catheter outcome, namely, catheter tip migration, omental entrapment, and peritoneal adhesions [11–13]. Identifying and preemptively correcting these problems at the time of the implantation procedure are potential advantages of surgical laparoscopy over other catheter insertion techniques.

One of the impediments for using laparoscopy as a means of implanting PD catheters has been the necessity for general anesthesia. The instruments used during laparoscopy are large, at least 5-mm diameter, as shown in Fig. 32.9. Insufflation of CO_2 gas to create the pneumoperitoneum produces pain and requires general anesthesia. In addition, insufflation of CO_2 can produce metabolic acidosis and cardiac arrhythmias. Recently, the use of alternative insufflation gases (nitrous oxide, helium) that are painless and metabolically inert has permitted safe laparoscopy under local anesthesia [13, 14]. Air is also painless when infused into the peritoneum, and this is used in the peritoneoscopic technique described below. For infusion of all gases, care must be taken to assure that the gas enters the peritoneal space and not into blood vessels or solid tissues.

Laparoscopic dialysis catheter implantation is accomplished using a 2-port technique as shown in Fig. 32.9. The peritoneal catheter is inserted through a port at the previously designated paramedian site while continuously monitoring the implant procedure with a laparoscope from a second port location. Any patient that is a candidate for catheter insertion by open dissection is a candidate for laparoscopic implantation. A history of previous abdominal surgery and the location of surgical scars only dictates the manner in which the gas insufflation needle (Veress needle) and the initial camera port are inserted. Under local anesthesia, with the patient protruding and tensing the abdominal wall to create a rigid platform, the Veress needle is safely inserted using the closed method through a pararectus incision on the side opposite of the planned catheter insertion site. Under general anesthesia, closed insertion of the Veress needle can be achieved at the lateral border of the rectus sheath below the costal margin in either of the upper abdominal quadrants. Alternatively, and in the event of midline scars or multiple previous abdominal surgeries, the initial port is placed by opening the peritoneum under direct vision.

After insertion of the camera port and creation of a satisfactory pneumoperitoneum, laparoscopic exploration of the peritoneal cavity is performed. The laparoscope permits evaluation for undiagnosed abdominal wall hernias, redundant omentum, and adhesions that create compartmentalization or obscure the planned catheter insertion site. Rectus sheath tunneling is important for maintaining pelvic orientation of the catheter to prevent catheter tip migration, as shown in Fig. 32.10 [15–17]. In addition, the tangential passage of the catheter through the abdominal wall reduces the risk of pericannular leak or hernia. The PD catheter, straightened over a stylet, is advanced through the port under laparoscopic control. The stylet is partially withdrawn as the catheter is advanced. The catheter tip is positioned in the retrovesical space. To make sure that the deep cuff has passed through the anterior rectus sheath, the catheter is advanced until the cuff is visible in the peritoneal cavity. Once the port and stylet are removed, the catheter is gently withdrawn until the deep cuff is just below the anterior rectus sheath. Subcutaneous tunneling of the catheter to the selected exit site will be discussed in a separate section to follow. After establishing careful wound hemostasis, the subcutaneous tissue and skin are sutured in separate layers.

Redundant, thin, filmy omentum that extends into the pelvis that lies in juxtaposition to the catheter tip increases the risk of omental entrapment. The performance of an omental tacking-up procedure (omentopexy) as shown in Fig. 32.9 eliminates this complication [18, 19]. The procedure is performed only when the omentum is found to extend into the pelvis. Employing selective criteria for omentopexy eliminates the performance of unnecessary procedures and minimizes cost. Omentopexy requires insertion of an additional port through which grasping forceps are used to pull the omentum into the upper abdomen. Here it is fixed to the abdominal wall or the falciform ligament with a suture or tacking device. Laparoscopic resection of the omentum has been performed but requires more instrumentation and procedure time without increasing the benefit provided by

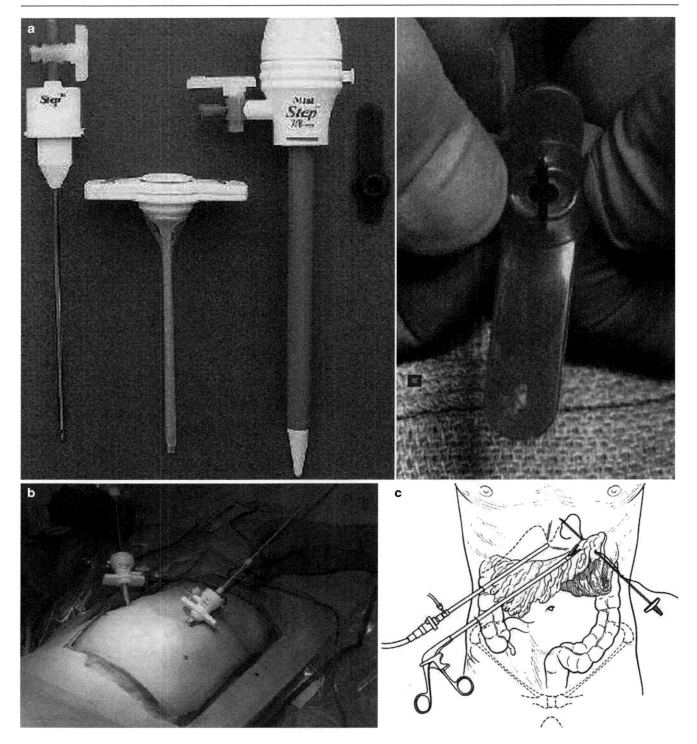

Fig. 32.9 (a) Laparoscopic atraumatic port system includes, from left to right, Veress-type needle for pneumoperitoneum, radially expandable plastic sleeve, 7/8-mm dilator-cannula assembly with attachable valve.

(b) close-up of valve. (c) operative field during laparoscopic placement of PD catheter. (d) diagram of omentopexy procedure. (Courtesy Dr. John Crabtree)

omentopexy. Alternatively, teasing the omentum out through one of the port incision sites has permitted partial omental resection. Although the procedure is shorter than laparoscopic resection and requires no extra instrumentation, partial omentectomy is still followed with an incidence of flow obstruction as high as 10 % [15, 20–22].

Adhesions from previous abdominal surgery may involve the parietal peritoneum at the planned site for catheter

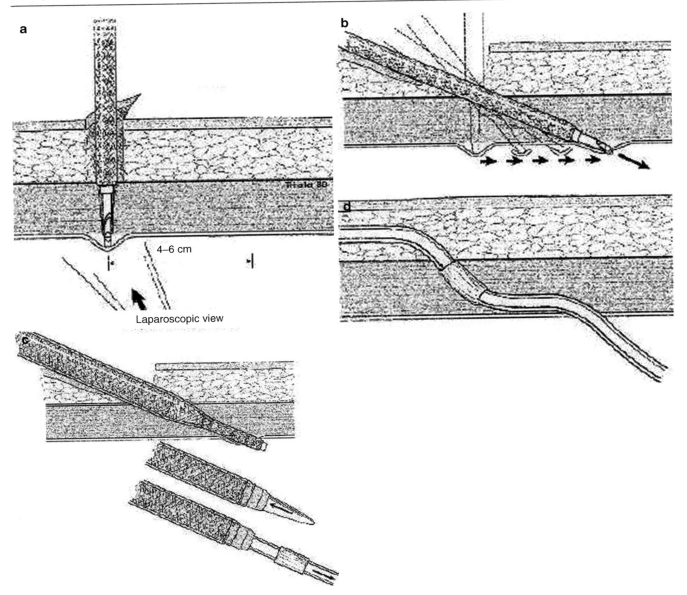

4–6 cm

Laparoscopic view

Fig. 32.10 Method of creating a long tunnel within rectus and pre-peritoneal fat to create a fixed downward direction of the PD catheter towards the pelvis (Courtesy Dr. John Crabtree). (**a**) Veress needle-expandable sleeve assembly is inserted through skin incision and anterior rectus sheath. (**b**) The needle-sleeve assembly is angled toward the pelvis, advanced down the rectus sheath, and pushed through into the peritoneal cavity at the indicated site. (**c**) The needle is removed and the expandable sleeve serves as a conduit for insertion of the dilator-cannula. The dialysis catheter over a stylet is advanced into the peritoneal cavity until the deep cuff is visible. (**d**) The cannula and stylet are withdrawn, and the catheter is pulled back until the deep cuff is just below the anterior rectus sheath

insertion or form intraperitoneal compartments that potentially contribute to poor drainage function. When these lesions are detected laparoscopically, additional ports may be inserted to permit adhesiolysis with laparoscopic scissors, cautery, or an ultrasonic shears device (ultrasonic scalpel). However, it is neither necessary nor desirable to mobilize every adhesion. Omental adhesions to the abdominal wall above the level of the pelvis that will not interfere with drainage of dialysate from the upper abdomen may even protect from omental entrapment of the catheter. Extensive

adhesiolysis to create a dialyzable space has met with variable success [11, 12]. Damage to the parietal peritoneum may result in insufficient dialyzable surface area. Immediate use of the created space by standard volumes of dialysate is necessary to prevent obliteration of the peritoneal cavity from acute adhesions between raw surface areas. Dialysate fluid leaks through laparoscopic port sites and around the catheter may still occur despite attempts to obtain watertight closure. In addition, prolonged anesthesia time and conversion to an open laparotomy to control bleeding or repair accidental enterotomies can potentially complicate such heroic attempts to create a dialyzable space.

32.5.4 Peritoneoscopic Placement

Peritoneoscopic placement of PD catheters has become popular over the last three decades by offering a method for placing peritoneal catheters under local anesthesia but providing visualization of the peritoneal space. This technique has many advantages, besides being minimally invasive. The method has the ability to ascertain proper position of the catheter within the peritoneal cavity along with the ability to directly inspect and avoid any adhesions, bowel, or omentum while reducing the risk of injury to bowel. Placement of the catheter against the parietal peritoneum in an area free of adhesions improves the likelihood of good hydraulic function of the catheter, compared to blind or dissective techniques in which the catheter can be placed under bowel loops or omentum. The minimal dissection required by this technique, and use of a Luke™ guide to place the deep cuff within the rectus muscle, results in lower risk of leakage and infections (the Luke™ guide is a recent improvement of the Y-Tec Quill™ guide marketed previously). The placement can be done under local anesthesia and with moderate conscious sedation if needed, and general anesthesia is not required. As with any other technique, the essential requirement is the operator experience. Complications such as bowel perforation are statistically no different from surgical techniques and probably less than for blind techniques. The steps of catheter placement using a peritoneoscope and the Y-Tec™ system (Medigroup, Oswego, IL) are shown in Fig. 32.11. The appearance of various adhesions as seen through the 2.2-mm Y-Tec scope is shown in Fig. 32.12.

A significant amount of experience has accumulated with the use of the peritoneoscopic technique. An initial study suggested good success of this approach [23, 37]. The technique was also compared with surgical placement of PD catheter in observational and randomized trials. A randomized controlled study of outcomes of PD catheter placed by peritoneoscopic method ($n = 76$) versus those placed by surgical method ($n = 72$) found not only a less frequent occurrence of leak or infection in early postoperative period but also a superior survival of catheter when placed peritoneoscopically (Fig. 32.13) [24]. The survival of peritoneoscopically placed catheters was superior (77.5 % at 12 months, 63 % at 24 months, and 51.3 % at 36 months) to those placed surgically (62.5 % at 12 months, 41.5 % at 24 months, and 36 % at 36 months) with $P < 0.02$, 0.01, and 0.04, respectively. Similar success was reported in another study comparing peritoneoscopic to surgical placement [25]. A recent paper described a 95 % success rate at 2 years, for PD catheters placed peritoneoscopically in the left iliac fossa [26].

Bowel injuries during PD catheter placement are rare with the peritoneoscopic technique (less than 1 in 500 cases) but use of Veress insufflation needle has made bowel perforation even more unlikely during the initial access to the peritoneal cavity [27]. The peritoneoscopic approach remains popular, especially among nephrologists though special equipment and training is required. The technique is of particular value in patients with prior surgery, to demonstrate presence and extent of adhesions.

32.5.5 Fluoroscopic Placement

Interventional nephrologists are familiar with the use of micropuncture and Seldinger techniques and have preexisting facilities for the use of fluoroscopy in a sterile environment. Fluoroscopic placement of the PD catheter has evolved in the interventional suite over the last decade. Although the technique does not allow direct visualization of the peritoneal cavity, correct position of the first entry needle within the peritoneum is easily confirmed by instillation of radiocontrast medium as shown in Fig. 32.14. Insertion of a long guidewire into the abdomen and advancing it until it forms a curve in the lower abdomen brings the wire against the parietal peritoneal surface as shown in Fig. 32.15. Inserting a dilator and split sheath then allows the catheter to follow this same course. The deep cuff is then inserted into the rectus muscle using hemostats. The success of this technique is high with a low incidence of complications [28].

The results of fluoroscopic placement of PD catheter have been studied by many authors and demonstrate a high initial technical success rate [29]. Due to the selection bias of these studies towards low-risk patients, a direct comparison of the results to results of surgical placement is unlikely to be fair. The long-term outcomes of these catheters from a study describing 10-year experience demonstrate a 14 % loss of catheters due to peritonitis, 7 % loss from pericatheter leak, 8 % from exit infection, and 2 % due to outflow failure.

The fluoroscopic method of PD catheter placement is continually being refined and improved. A recent case series reported modified fluoroscopic placement of PD catheter using ultrasound guidance to enter the peritoneal cavity under direct ultrasonic visualization to avoid injury to the bowels [30]. Additionally, the location of the epigastric vessels can also be defined using Doppler ultrasound, thus minimizing bleeding complications. The incidence of early complications was low in this series, with 3 % incidence of bowel perforation, 3 % of unsuccessful attempts, and 3 % outflow failure.

Advantages of the fluoroscopic technique include minimal invasiveness, no need of special equipment and training required for the use of peritoneoscopy, and less likelihood of

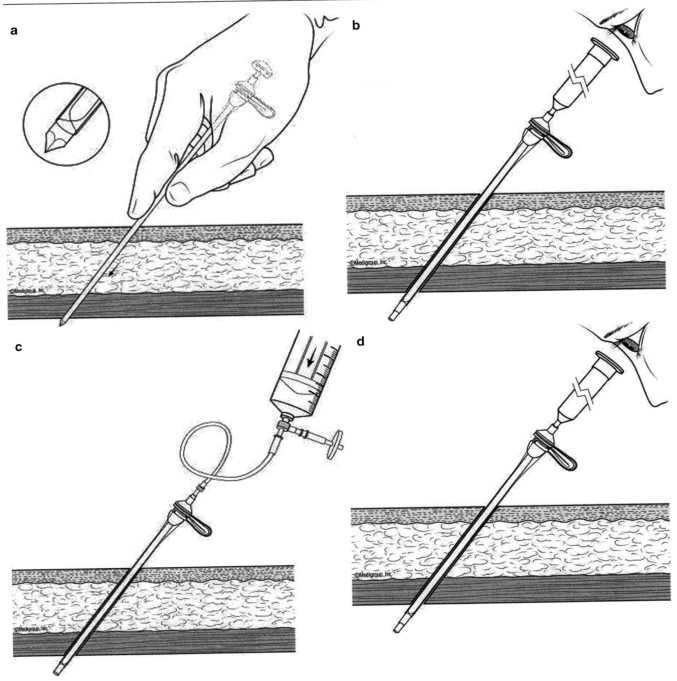

Fig. 32.11 Steps of placement of a PD catheter by peritoneoscopy using the Y-Tec™ system (Figures courtesy of Merit, Inc., now marketing Medigroup products in peritoneal dialysis). (**a**) Placement of trocar with surrounding cannula and Luke™ catheter guide, after dissection to the external rectus sheath and local anesthesia. (**b**) Inspection of the visceral peritoneal surface to determine movement with inspiration. (**c**) Infusion of air into the peritoneum with patient in Trendelenburg position. (**d**) Inspection of air space and advancement of cannula into peritoneum, into a clear space next to the parietal peritoneum and free of adhesions. (**e**) Dilation of Luke™ guide by 4- and 6-mm-diameter dilators. (**f**) Advancement of PD catheter with internal stylet, retracting stylet intermittently until deep cuff rests on outside of rectus sheath. (**g**) Advancement of cuff into rectus muscle using Cuff Implantor™. (**h**) Removal of Luke™ guide while holding the cuff in place with Cuff Implantor™. (**i**) Marking exit site and making stab incision after local anesthesia. (**j**) Pulling catheter through tunnel with Tunnelor™ tool. Tract is dilated by hemostats that are pulled into the tunnel after being lightly attached to the catheter

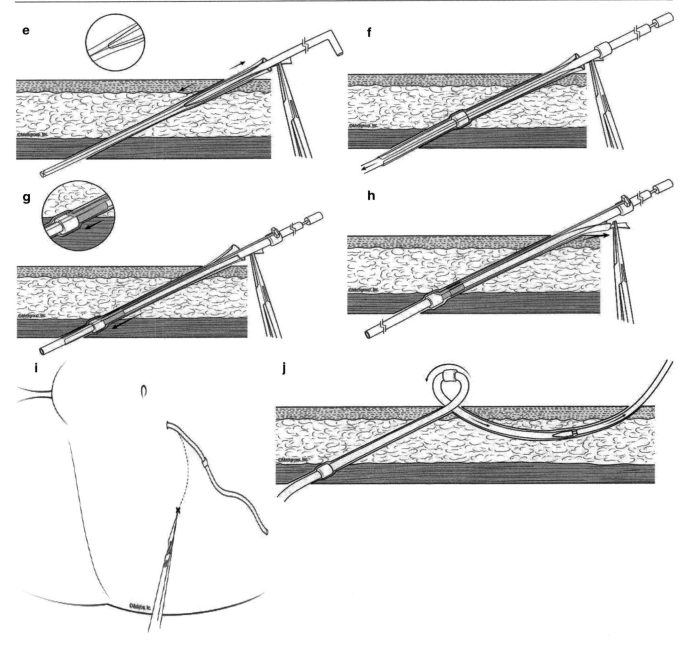

Fig. 32.11 (continued)

leakage and infection. The procedure, similar to other percutaneous techniques, can be performed under local anesthesia
and moderate conscious sedation without the need of general anesthesia. The drawbacks of the technique include the
need of fluoroscopic equipment, exposure to radiation, need
to use radiocontrast medium, relatively "blind" access of
peritoneal cavity and advancement of the catheter, and theoretical likelihood of bowel perforation. Also, a careful selection of patients is necessary to avoid placement of the
catheter against adhesions or omentum leading to poor function of the catheter.

32.5.6 Blind (Seldinger) Technique

Percutaneous placement of PD catheter with the blind
Seldinger technique was used just after split sheath catheters
became available for placement of internal jugular catheters
for dialysis in the early 1990s [31]. The technique involves
use of a needle and a guidewire, with no direct visualization
of the peritoneal cavity. A dilator and split sheath are placed
over the guidewire, allowing the catheter to follow the same
course as the guidewire into the peritoneum. The blind technique is not commonly practiced in the USA, though the

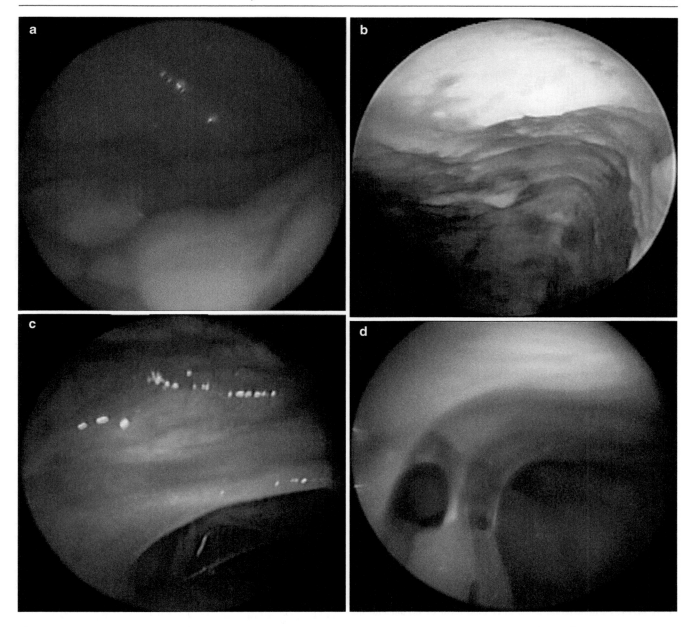

Fig. 32.12 Views of the parietal peritoneum and intraperitoneal adhesions taken through the Y-Tec™ peritoneoscope during placement of PD catheters. (**a**) Normal peritoneum, view of left lower quadrant through Y-Tec™ scope, with parietal peritoneum above and visceral peritoneum below. (**b**) Broad midline adhesion from prior midline incision. (**c**) Broad omental adhesion to anterior parietal peritoneum after fungal peritonitis. (**d**) Wispy adhesions sometimes seen in patients without prior abdominal surgery

same basic components are used in fluoroscopic placement techniques in many practices. The advantages of the blind technique include no need for expensive imaging equipment and using only local anesthesia and moderate sedation. The disadvantages are primarily from the inability to place the catheter under direct visualization of the peritoneal cavity and a risk of bowel perforation by the initial needle entry. As with the peritoneoscopic and fluoroscopic methods of placement, certain types of catheters cannot be placed using this technique (Missouri and TWH). Although the risk of

complications is intuitively high, one study found no difference in complications between catheter placed at the bedside and those placed surgically [32].

32.5.7 Relative Success of Placement Techniques

The percutaneous techniques include blind (Seldinger) technique, peritoneoscopic placement, or fluoroscopic placement.

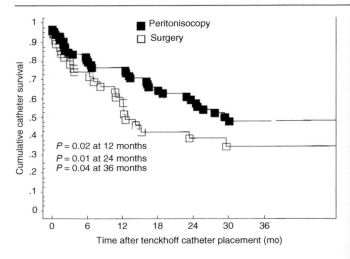

Fig. 32.13 Kaplan-Meier plot of Tenckhoff catheter survival according to the technique of placement, peritoneoscopy versus surgery (From Eklund [8])

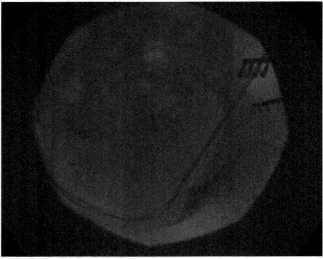

Fig. 32.15 Course of guidewire after insertion and curving into the anterior peritoneal space

operator is at least as important in PD catheter success as the exact technique chosen.

Various percutaneous and surgical techniques have been shown to be effective but appear to have differing frequencies of complications. When complications are defined as infections, outflow failure, and subcutaneous leaks, and following catheters throughout many months of function, the peritoneoscopic technique appears to have the lowest incidence of all complications at 7, 4, and 2 %, respectively. Blind technique is the next lowest with complications at 23, 16, and 11 %, respectively, and dissective or surgical placement has the highest complication rate at 45, 13, and 9 %, respectively. A note of caution is necessary however, since the comparison among the techniques may be biased by patient selection and demographics [33]. Laparoscopic techniques, when combined with omentopexy and long rectus tunnel of the catheter, provide excellent long-term and short-term catheter outcomes [5, 13, 14] but usually require a well-equipped operating room and general anesthesia.

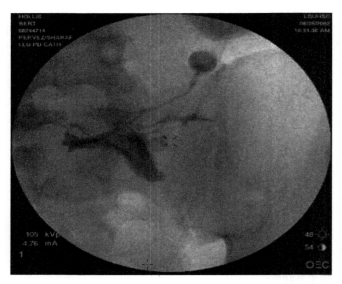

Fig. 32.14 Peritoneogram taken after placement of needle into the peritoneum during fluoroscopic PD catheter placement (Courtesy Dr. Ken Abreo)

The percutaneous techniques are at least as effective and safe as surgical placement. Moreover, there is evidence that these techniques offer lesser risk of complications and better catheter function and survival. The percutaneous techniques are tolerated better with quicker recovery than the surgical placement. Use of imaging techniques during percutaneous placement offers further enhancement of safety and represents an advance in better control of the positioning of the PD catheter. On the other hand, for all techniques there is a learning curve. One publication has demonstrated that optimal success in peritoneoscopic catheter placement by a physician occurs with about 20 procedures done [26]. The skill of the

32.6 Embedding PD Catheters and Exteriorizing

Traditional implantation of Tenckhoff catheters involves immediate exteriorization of the external segment through the skin, so that the catheter can be used for supportive PD or for intermittent infusions during the "break-in" period. In order to prevent blockage and to confirm function, the catheter is flushed at least weekly with saline or dialysate. The catheter must also be bandaged, and the skin exit site must be kept clean in the weeks after placement, to avoid bacterial contamination of the exit site. The patient must therefore be trained in some techniques of catheter care. It has always been difficult to decide when to place a PD catheter in a patient with chronic renal insufficiency. If the catheter is placed too early, the patient may spend weeks to months caring for a catheter, which is not used for dialysis. If the catheter is placed after the patient becomes uremic, then it is used for PD therapy without a "break-in" period or hemodialysis is used to provide time for ingrowth of fibrous tissue to the cuffs.

Moncrief and Popovich devised a placement technique in which the entire peritoneal catheter can be embedded or "buried" under the skin some weeks to months before it is used [34]. The catheter burying technique was first described for placement of a modified Tenckhoff catheter with a 2.5-cm-long superficial cuff, but the technique has been adopted for standard dual-cuff Tenckhoff catheters [35–37]. In the original technique, the external portion of the catheter was brought through a 2–3-cm skin exit site (much larger than the usual 0.5-cm incision). The catheter was then tied off with silk suture then coiled and placed into a "pouch" created under the skin. The skin exit site was then closed. Weeks to months later, the original skin exit site was opened, and the free end of the catheter was brought through the original skin large exit site.

Burying the entire external limb of the catheter under the skin in a subcutaneous tunnel eliminates an exit wound. Healing and tissue ingrowth into the cuffs occurs while the catheter is buried in this sterile environment. At a later date, 3–5 weeks after insertion, a small incision is made 2–4 cm distal to the subcutaneous cuff, and the external limb of the catheter is brought out through the skin. The catheter may be left in place under the skin for many months. During this time, the patient is not faced with exit-site maintenance issues or risk of infection. Full volume PD may be initiated immediately following exteriorization without concerns of pericatheter leak. The goal of burying the PD catheter was to allow ingrowth of tissue into the cuffs of the catheter without chance of bacterial colonization, and to allow the exit site to be created after tissue had fully grown into the deep and subcutaneous cuffs. Burying the catheter effectively eliminated early pericatheter leaks and decreased the incidence of peritonitis rate. In 66 months of follow-up, patients with the buried Tenckhoff catheter had peritonitis infection rates of 0.017–0.37 infections per year versus 1.3–1.9 infections per year in control patients [34]. In a study of 26 buried Tenckhoff catheters, the incidence of infection complications during PD was 0.8 infections per year, and catheter-related peritonitis was only 0.036 per patient-year [35]. A retrospective study confirmed a significantly lower catheter infection and peritonitis rate in patients having had buried catheters and a significantly longer catheter life [38], although the procedure was not effective when used for single-cuff catheters [39].

Exit-site infections were not decreased in catheters that were buried, but this is understandable, since a large exit site was created when the catheter was buried and a similarly large site was recreated when the catheter was exteriorized. Creating the "pouch" under the skin requires a considerable amount of dissection and trauma near the exit site. The size of the pocket limits the length of catheter that can be coiled and buried under the skin, limiting the external length of the catheter after exteriorization. The exit site must be opened widely to remove the catheter, because the coil rests in a position distant from the skin exit site. Subcutaneous adhesions to the silk suture around the catheter further restrict removal. Increased trauma near the exit site during placement and removal of the catheter has caused an increased incidence of early exit infection with this technique. Despite initial reports by the authors of reduction in the rate of peritonitis and colonization of bacterial biofilms in the catheter segments between the two cuffs, a controlled randomized study has failed to confirm these claims [40, 41]. A possible reason for the failure to reduce the incidence of infectious complications may be the inability of the body to provide an effective "seal" around the external cuff while the catheter is buried, partly due to the fact that the external cuff and coiled external tubing are buried in a "pocket" under the skin, according to the initially described procedure. Therefore, upon exteriorization of the catheter, the process of healing starts all over again. Prischl et al. have also reported a high incidence of seromas, subcutaneous hematomas, and fibrin thrombi postoperatively with the technique [41]. Other methods of placement such as tunneling the catheter straight towards the skin and then making a bend in the catheter and then tunneling towards a temporary exit site under the umbilicus may diminish general trauma near the external cuff, allow better bonding of the cuff to surrounding subcutaneous tissues, and diminish the size of exit site created in exteriorizing the catheter, all leading to a decreased incidence of early exit-site infection after exteriorization. To bury the external segment in a straight line, a 1-cm exit-site incision is made, and the catheter is brought through this incision in the usual manner. The catheter is filled with heparinized saline, and using a tunneling tool, the catheter is then reinserted through the exit site and tunneled for 15 cm or more in a linear direction. A linear tunneling procedure can also be done through one exit-site incision, without a need for a second incision, using the same components used during peritoneoscopic placement. We reassemble the Luke™ guide around the trocar and cannula and insert the assembly through the exit site, next to the exiting catheter. The catheter is filled with heparinized saline and plugged, and the plugged end is then advanced through the Quill guide into the tunnel. The Quill is then removed, and the exit site is closed with a subcutaneous Vicryl™ suture.

For best results, the catheter is allowed to reside in the subcutaneous tissues for a period of at least 3–5 weeks. This allows for adequate tissue ingrowth into the catheter cuffs. Secondary exteriorization of the external catheter limb can be performed under local anesthesia, by carefully incising the original 1-cm exit incision. Studies of catheters buried after surgical placement have still shown some early loss of catheters due to outflow failure, but the rates are not higher than in immediately exteriorized catheters [42].

In planning for hemodialysis of patients with ESRD, it is common practice to place a fistula or graft several months before the need for initiation of dialysis, so that they can "mature" before use. PD catheters also "mature" after placement, with fibrous tissue ingrowth into the cuffs and development of a fibrous tunnel. The fully ingrown catheter is more resistant to infection of cuffs and the surface of the catheter. The technique of burying PD catheters after placement allows this maturation to occur before use of the catheter, much as with fistulas and grafts. Burying of the external limb of the catheter can be performed as a component of any of the implantation techniques.

32.7 Catheter Repositioning

The incidence of outflow failure of peritoneal catheters is from 4 to 16 % over a mean follow-up time of 18 months. When outflow failure is accompanied by x-ray evidence of catheter migration to the upper abdomen, then omental attachment or entrapment in adhesions is highly likely. A number of options exist for resolving the problem of outflow failure and omental obstruction:

(a) Laparoscopy, freeing and repositioning the catheter, lysing adhesions, and performing an omentectomy or omentopexy if needed
(b) Guidewire repositioning of the catheter into the anterior peritoneal space with fluoroscopy
(c) Repositioning by other techniques including metal stylets, Fogarty balloons, and massage of the abdomen
(d) Placement of a new PD catheter and removal of the old catheter, which if done by peritoneoscopic technique also allows confirmation of the omental obstruction of the failed PD catheter

Most of the repositioning techniques are successful in restoring hydraulic function of the PD catheter in the short term, but long-term function of the catheters is about 50 % of those treated. Even though this success is disappointingly low, for those patients with catheters that resume hydraulic function, the reposition procedure is beneficial.

Regarding laparoscopic repositioning, Brandt and Ricanati reported on 26 procedures performed in 22 patients in the 1990s for malfunction occurring an average of 3.9 months following catheter insertion (range 0.5–18 months). Omental wrapping was present in all but three cases. Lysis of adhesions was required in 19 of 26 cases and

only repositioning in seven. Repeat laparoscopy was needed after four reocclusions. The overall success rate (defined as catheter function 30 days or more after laparoscopy) was 21/22 (96 %) [42]. Yilmazlar reported 40 consecutive patients with who underwent 46 laparoscopic correction procedures for the treatment of PD catheter malfunction between 1994 and 2004. There were 28 tip migrations (defined by the catheter being outside the pelvis) in 40 patients; 16 were without adhesions and 10 were associated with omental adhesions. Reposition and adhesiolysis were the most frequent procedures performed. Malfunction recurred in 12 patients, and 5 of them underwent 6 secondary laparoscopic procedures. Estimated primary and secondary mean catheter survival was 19.9 ± 3.32 months. The authors concluded that laparoscopic repositioning and adhesiolysis are successful in prolonging PD catheter use [43]. Crabtree reported in 2006 that omental entrapment can be relieved by laparoscopy, freeing omentum from the catheter. An omentopexy is performed to prevent recurrent obstruction, in which the greater omentum is lifted to the upper abdomen and sewn to the anterior parietal peritoneum. Crabtree stated that omentopexy can be performed much faster than omentectomy and has equal or better results [44]. Other authors have shown that similar advantages in PD catheter function can be obtained if the omentum is folded towards the upper abdomen and sewn to itself.

The most popular method of repositioning PD catheters is by fluoroscopy, using a long guidewire to bring the catheter into the anterior peritoneal space. When a long, flexible guidewire is advanced into the coiled or straight Tenckhoff catheter, the guidewire eventually forms a loop that can only fit in the anterior peritoneal space. The catheter tip is thus brought into this space, and when the guidewire is removed, the catheter will usually remain next to the parietal peritoneum. The catheter will usually be freed from omental attachment by this reposition technique. Lee reported a novel technique in which advancing one guidewire into the catheter forced it towards the pelvis and a second guidewire held the catheter in this position while the first was removed. The immediate success of the procedure was 86 % and long-term success was 59 % [45]. Jwo reported that guidewire repositioning was effective in 5 of 11 patients with outflow failure, failing in those with "severe adhesions," improper angle of insertion, or extraperitoneal location of the catheter [46]. Overall, results with stiff guidewire reposition have improved somewhat since the 1990 publication by Moss and Schwab [47]. In their study 33 patients developed catheter malfunction attributed to malposition. Forty-eight stiff-wire manipulations were performed on these patients. Thirty-eight (78 %) of the manipulations were described as successful at the time of transfer from radiology. However, only 25 (51 %) and 12 (25 %) resulted in functioning catheters at 1 week and 1 month, respectively. Only 11 of 33 patients who underwent manipulation had functional prolongation of catheter life beyond 1 month. The PD catheter was replaced by a column-disc PD catheter without additional catheter dysfunction in six patients, and the authors recommended that "catheters that repetitively malposition should be replaced with a catheter that is resistant to malpositioning." One problem with guidewire reposition is that there really is not any open space in the anterior peritoneum for the guidewire to open into, even if the abdomen is prefilled with a liter of saline or dialysate. A combination of peritoneoscopy with pneumoperitoneum and guidewire reposition might be more successful than the purely fluoroscopic techniques, for those skilled in both techniques.

Among other techniques for repositioning, the use of a stiff stylet has been the most popular: Dobrashian in 1999 reported on repositioning of PD catheters using stainless wires of 1–2-mm diameter that are bent into a "u" shape and then rotated within the PD catheter to reposition it [48]. In repositioning 18 straight PD catheters, there was technical success in 84 % but only 45 % clinical success, meaning a working PD access 6 months later. Jones reported a similar technique in 1998, and the overall success rate of catheter function was about 60 % at 1 month after the procedure [49]. Tu reported that using the hands in compression of the abdomen that many PD catheters can be freed of adhesions and restored from outflow failure. Of 30 cases of PD catheter migration, repositioning was successful on the first attempt in 9 cases, on the third attempt in 10 cases, on the seventh attempt in 7 cases, and failed in 4 cases. The overall success rate was 87 % [50]. Gadallah reported that placing a Fogarty balloon through the PD catheter and "tugging movements until proper placement of the PD catheter into the pelvis was suspected" resulted in 96 % success in restoring early and late function of these catheters [51].

A simple alternative to restore peritoneal access in a patient with outflow failure is to place a new peritoneal catheter and then remove the failed catheter. The goal is to place the new catheter through a different peritoneal entry site and in a different direction than the failed catheter, potentially minimizing the risk of outflow failure. A different type of PD catheter can also be chosen, such as a Swan Neck catheter, a catheter of differing ID or stiffness, or different tip design (straight Tenckhoff versus coiled). The new catheter can be placed at the same setting as the removal of the old catheter, but the new catheter should be placed first and then the failed catheter removed to maintain the best sterility of the operative field. After ultrasound of the rectus muscle and parietal and visceral peritoneum, a site is chosen for the deep cuff of a new peritoneal catheter (usually on the opposite side of the peritoneal cavity) from the failed catheter. If the new placement is performed by peritoneoscopy, this is the site of insertion of the cannula and Y-Tec scope. After creating a pneumoperitoneum

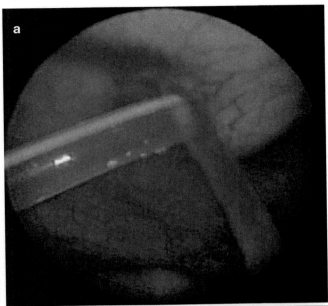
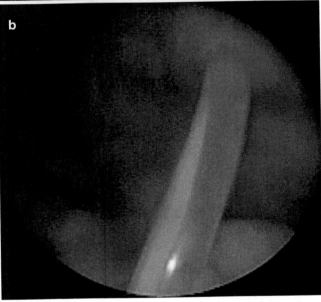

Fig. 32.16 Appearance of the deep cuff of properly inserted peritoneal catheters through the Y-Tec scope. (**a**) The catheter has a thin omental adhesion to the site of the deep cuff (**b**) normal deep cuff appearance

and viewing through the scope, the peritoneal entry site of the catheter is first located. Inspection confirms that the cuff of the failed catheter is extraperitoneal and whether there are adhesions to the site of entry, as shown in Fig. 32.16. The body of the catheter is then inspected to determine whether the tip of the catheter is lying in the anterior peritoneal space. For catheters with outflow failure and migration, usually the catheter dives into the mass of omentum and bowels, and the tip is not visible as shown in Fig. 32.17, left photograph. The tip of the Y-Tec scope can be advanced under the catheter body and the scope rotated

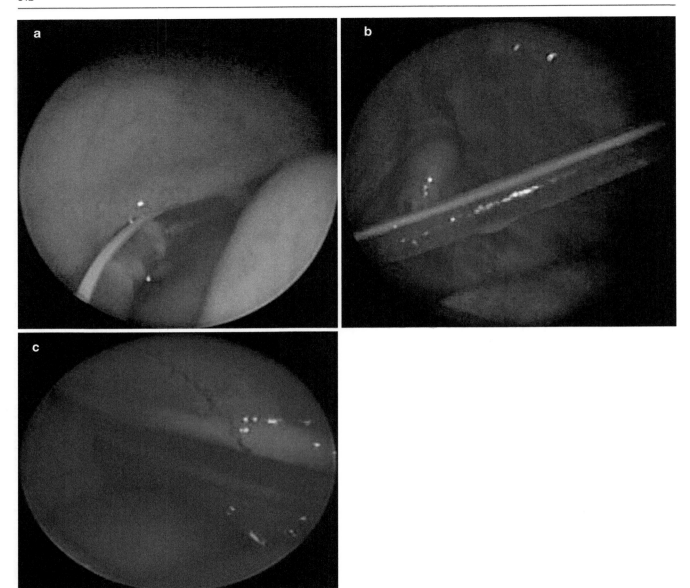

Fig. 32.17 Appearance of catheters with outflow failure and migration through the Y-Tec scope. The most common finding is that the catheter dives down into the omentum and it is immovable by mild pressure of the tip of the scope (**a**). Sometimes the catheter is covered by a thin layer of omentum, making the side holes invisible (**b**). Sometimes the catheter is held against the parietal peritoneum by a thin layer of omentum (**c**)

to put traction on the catheter. If the catheter is immovable, then it almost certainly has omental attachment. In some failed catheters, there is a thin layer of omentum over the body of the catheter as shown in Fig. 32.17, middle photograph. In others, the catheter is "plastered" against the parietal peritoneum by a thin layer of omentum, as shown in Fig. 32.17c. If gentle pressure on the catheter fails to dislodge it or bring it to the anterior peritoneal space, then a new catheter is placed through the site of the Y-Tec cannula, making sure to advance the deep cuff into the musculature. The failed catheter is then removed. The patient can

begin nighttime PD exchanges 36 h after placement of the new PD catheter. Occasionally the peritoneoscopic evaluation of a failed PD catheter indicates no omental attachment and proper position of the catheter in the anterior peritoneal space. In this case, the outflow failure is entirely "functional," and greater effort is directed to correcting constipation and assuring proper techniques of PD. If the new PD catheter is placed laparoscopically, then performing an omentopexy, lysing adhesions, and directing the new catheter through a long rectus tunnel are indicated, as described by Dr. Crabtree.

32.8 Repair of Pericatheter Leaks and Hernias

Pericatheter leaks are generally due to either outward movement of the deep cuff from the rectus muscle, a pericatheter hernia, or infection of the deep cuff. The leak may be grossly obvious when it causes a wet exit site and wet bandages, but sometimes the leak merely creates edema in the area of the deep cuff of the catheter and results in apparent outflow failure. The subcutaneous edema is best detected by grasping the subcutaneous tissue on the right and left flanks, to determine the skinfold thickness. If the skinfold thickness is greater on the catheter side of the abdomen, and if the fingers slowly move together on this side, then asymmetric edema is present. This is a sign of pericatheter dialysate leak, though sometimes it can be caused by heart failure or general fluid excess when the patient happens to sleep with the catheter side of the abdomen dependent. Ultrasound is very helpful in defining a pericatheter leak and pericatheter hernia, as described below.

If there are no signs of peritonitis or tunnel or cuff infection (such as warmth or tenderness over the tunnel and cuffs) and catheter function is excellent, then it is reasonable to repair the pericatheter leak. This can be done by the following steps:

- Anesthetize the original primary incision.
- Create a new incision through the primary incision scar, using scalpel.
- Bluntly dissect through the subcutaneous tissue to define the catheter tunnel and hernia (if present) and separate adhesions from the subcutaneous tissue to the tunnel or hernia.
- Open the tunnel or hernia and inspect the cuff. If it is covered by fibrous tissue and adhered to the tunnel or hernia surrounding it, then it is probably free of infection and the repair is possible. (If the deep cuff has no fibrous adhesion to the tunnel or hernia and is covered with exudate, then the cuff is probably infected and the repair will not be successful).
- Free the cuff from the surrounding tunnel or hernia.
- Advance the cuff into the rectus muscle using hemostats. Assure that in this position, there is no significant traction from the superficial cuff (if there is tension on the deep cuff, it will not heal in position within the rectus and the superficial cuff needs to be freed and moved closer to the deep cuff).
- While lifting the catheter upward, place a 2–0 Vicryl suture as a purse string in the external rectus sheath around the deep cuff location and tunnel or hernia. Tighten the suture, and tie and cut excess suture. Place a second purse-string suture, tighten, and tie.
- Close the primary incision with subdermal Vicryl sutures and nylon skin sutures or Steri-Strips.

This method of correction of pericatheter leak is generally successful as long as there is no infection of the deep cuff. The fibrous tissue of the tunnel in the rectus quickly bonds to the outer fibrous tissue of the cuff, in most cases. It is best to wait 3 weeks before starting PD, but if necessary the patient can perform manual exchanges or cycler therapy when inactive and mostly supine, such as from evening to morning hours, 36 h after the repair.

32.9 Catheter Removal

The physician who placed the PD catheter will be the first to be consulted if there are problems with the catheter. Interventional nephrologists and radiologists and surgeons who place PD catheters should all have the capability to remove these catheters when they fail or when the patient has unresolving or recurrent peritonitis. Electrocautery and a suction system both are of benefit in the procedure. The procedure for removal of PD catheters under local anesthesia is as follows:

- Anesthetize the original primary incision.
- Create a new incision through the primary incision scar, using a scalpel.
- Dissect through the subcutaneous tissue to define the catheter tunnel, and bluntly dissect adhesions of the subcutaneous space to the tunnel.
- Lift the tunnel and catheter to the skin surface, using a hemostat as a bridge to keep it in this position.
- Incise the tunnel using cautery or scalpel, exposing the catheter surface.
- Grasp the exposed catheter with a small hemostat. Tag the external portion with a suture, and cut the catheter between the hemostat and the suture.
- Lift the hemostat, exposing the tunnel and subcutaneous tissue around the catheter.
- Grasp the tunnel near the hemostat with toothed forceps, lift it, and cut it linearly above the catheter with scissors or cautery probe.
- Repeat cutting the tunnel until reaching the level of the deep cuff.
- If the cuff is outside the rectus muscle, incise the tunnel just below the cuff, over ½ circumference of the catheter. If the cuff is within the rectus muscle, incise fibrous tissue connections between the cuff and the muscle, then incise the peritoneal reflection over ½ circumference of the catheter. At this time retained peritoneal fluid may exit around the catheter, so a suction device is helpful.
- While lifting the catheter upward, place a 2–0 Vicryl suture in a purse-string configuration through the external rectus sheath, around the catheter entry point. Do not tighten.
- Incise the remaining tunnel or peritoneal reflection around the catheter, then remove the intraperitoneal portion of the

catheter. Pull the Vicryl suture tight and place a second purse-string suture around the first, through the external rectus sheath.

- Cut the catheter at the skin exit site.
- Retract the catheter and superficial cuff towards the primary incision.
- Grasp the tunnel near the hemostat with toothed forceps, lift it, and cut it linearly above the catheter with scissors or cautery probe.
- Repeat cutting the tunnel until reaching the level of the deep cuff.
- Incise the subcutaneous tissue connections to the subcutaneous cuff, then incise the reflection of skin attached to the cuff.
- Remove the external portion of the catheter.
- Close the primary incision with subdermal Vicryl sutures and nylon skin sutures or Steri-Strips.

32.10 Ultrasound Examination of Existing PD Catheters

There are reliable physical signs of most problems relating to PD catheters, especially those in the subcutaneous tunnel and cuffs. However, as in other areas of medicine, ultrasound imaging offers considerably more detailed information. Much can be learned using the simplest of 2D ultrasound imaging devices, such as those which are used for IJ dialysis catheter placements.

Figure 32.18 includes a number of images of various portions of normal and abnormal PD catheters. Figure 32.18a shows the normal appearance of the PD catheter within the subcutaneous tunnel. There is no shadowing from the catheter and four lines indicating inner and outer surfaces of the silicone tubing. Figure 32.18b shows

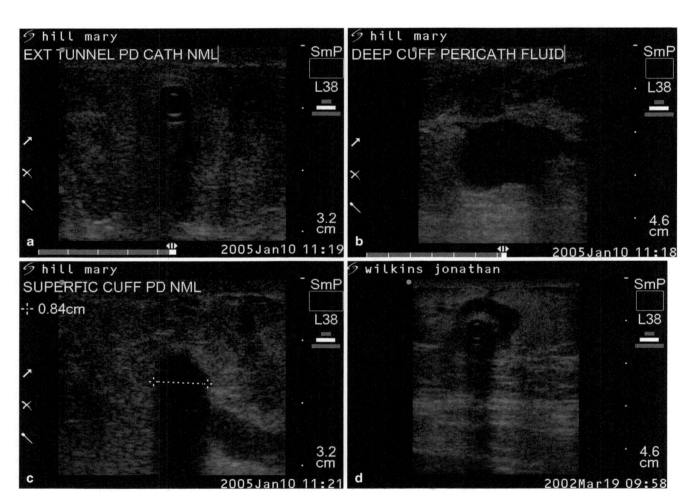

Fig. 32.18 Ultrasound appearance of various components of PD catheters. (**a**) Normal appearance of catheter in the subcutaneous tunnel. Note lack of shadowing and four lines indicating inner and outer surfaces of the silicone catheter. (**b**) Appearance of subcutaneous tunnel with fluid around the catheter. Note that the catheter surfaces are no longer visible within the fluid. (**c**) Normal appearance of the superficial cuff of a PD catheter. Note shadowing of the cuff and tissues below and no visibility of the cuff material. (**d**) Appearance of a cuff with fluid around it, with visibility of cuff material creating the "signet ring" sign. (**e**) Normal subcutaneous tunnel and catheter, in longitudinal view. (**f**) A subcutaneous tunnel and catheter which seem to disappear. Catheter is kinked progresses downward towards rectus at this point. (**g**) Deep cuff within rectus muscle. (**h**) Deep cuff within rectus muscle with fluid around the cuff

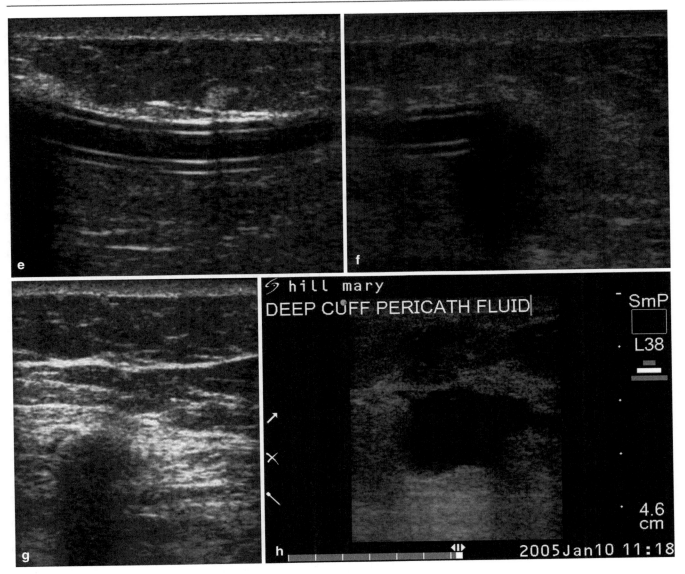

Fig.32.18 (continued)

the appearance of the PD catheter subcutaneous tunnel when there is fluid around the catheter. Note that the catheter surfaces are no longer visible within the fluid. Fluid around the catheter or around cuffs may occur with pericatheter leak, tunnel infection, or tunnel irritation. Figure 32.18c shows the normal appearance of the superficial cuff of a PD catheter. Due to the density of normal fibrous ingrowth to the cuff, ultrasound waves do not penetrate the cuff. The result is shadowing or a loss of imaging on the opposite side of the cuff, and there is no visibility of the cuff material. Figure 32.18d shows the ultrasonic image appearance of a cuff with fluid around it. The fluid around the cuff provides visibility of the cuff material, creating the "signet ring" sign. This fluid results from pericatheter fluid leak or infection or inflammation of the cuff. Figure 32.18e

shows the ultrasonic image of a normal subcutaneous tunnel and catheter, seen in longitudinal view. Figure 32.18f shows a subcutaneous tunnel tract of a PD catheter which seems to disappear. On closer inspection on several angles, the catheter was seen to be kinked and to progress downward towards the rectus muscle and deep cuff at just this point. Figure 32.18g demonstrates the normal picture of the deep cuff within rectus muscle. Note that there is shadowing underneath the cuff, indicating dense fibrous tissue ingrowth to the cuff. Figure 32.18h shows the ultrasonic image appearance of a deep cuff within the rectus muscle with fluid around the cuff. As with fluid around the catheter in the tunnel or the superficial cuff, this indicates pericatheter fluid leak, infection, or inflammation of the deep cuff.

Ultrasonic imaging is also helpful in the evaluation of hernias. With a simple ultrasound machine, the physician can determine the size of the hernia, whether there are bowel loops included, and the size and shape of the opening to the peritoneum. Repeat evaluations and printed images help to indicate whether the hernia is enlarging. All of these factors relate to the decision about whether the hernia must be repaired for the patient to remain on peritoneal dialysis. A small hernia that is stable with a small opening to the peritoneum and no bowel loops inside may be left for a while. A larger or growing hernia with bowel loops inside should be repaired as soon as possible, and this means that PD therapy must be discontinued for several weeks to allow healing of the wound.

References

1. Gokal R, Alexander S, Ash S, Chen TW, Danielson A, Holmes C, Joffe P, Moncrief J, Nichols K, Piraino B, Prowant B, Slingeneyer A, Stegmayr B, Twardowski Z, Vas S. Peritoneal catheters and exit site practice: toward optimum peritoneal access: 1998 update. Perit Dial Int. 1998;18(1):11–33.
2. Crabtree JH. Clinical biodurability of aliphatic polyether based polyurethanes as PD catheters. ASAIO J. 2003;49(3):290–4.
3. Crabtree JH. Fragmentation of polyurethane PD catheter during explantation. Perit Dial Int. 2004;24(6):601–2.
4. Twardowski ZJ, Nichols WK, Nolph KD, Khanna R. Swan neck presternal ("bath tub") catheter for PD. Adv Perit Dial. 1992;8:316–24.
5. Crabtree JH, Fishman A. Laparoscopic implantation of swan neck presternal PD catheters. J Laparoendosc Adv Surg Tech A. 2003;13:131–7.
6. Twardowski ZJ, Prowant BF, Nichols WK, Nolph KD, Khanna R. Six-year experience with Swan neck presternal pd catheter. Perit Dial Int. 1998;18:598–602.
7. Di Paolo N, Capotondo L, Sansoni E, Romolini V, Simola M, Gaggiotti E, Bercia R, Buoncristiani U, Cantù P, Concetti M, De Vecchi A, Fatuzzo P, Giannattasio M, La Rosa R, Lopez T, Lo Piccolo G, Melandr M, Vezzoli G, Orazi E, Pacitti A, Ramello A, Russo F, Napoli M, Tessarin MC. The self-locating catheter: clinical experience and follow-up. Perit Dial Int. 2004;24:359–64.
8. Eklund BH. Surgical implantation of CAPD catheters: presentation of midline incision-lateral placement method and review of 100 procedures. Nephrol Dial Transplant. 1995;10:386–90.
9. Ash SR, Daugirdas JT. Peritoneal access devices. In: Daugirdas JJ, Ing TS, editors. Handbook of dialysis. Boston: Little, Brown and Co; 1994. p. 275–300.
10. Ash SR, Nichols WK. Placement, repair, and removal of chronic peritoneal catheters. In: Gokal R, Nolph KD, editors. Textbook of PD. Dordrecht: Kluwer Academic; 1994. p. 315–33.
11. Kimmelstiel FM, Miller RE, Molinelli BM, Lorch JA. Laparoscopic management of PD catheters. Surg Gynecol Obstet. 1993;176:565–70.
12. Brandt CP, Franceschi D. Laparoscopic placement of PD catheters in patients who have undergone prior abdominal operations. J Am Coll Surg. 1994;178:515–6.
13. Crabtree JH, Fishman A. A laparoscopic approach under local anesthesia for PD access. Perit Dial Int. 2000;20:757–65.
14. Crabtree JH, Fishman A, Huen IT. Videolaparoscopic PD catheter implant and rescue procedures under local anesthesia with nitrous oxide pneumoperitoneum. Adv Perit Dial. 1998;14:83–6.
15. Draganic B, James A, Booth M, et al. Comparative experience of a simple technique for laparoscopic chronic ambulatory PD catheter placement. Aust N Z J Surg. 1998;68:735–9.
16. Gerhart CD. Needleoscopic placement of Tenckhoff catheters. JSLS. 1999;3:155–8.
17. Poole GH, Tervit P. Laparoscopic Tenckhoff catheter insertion: a prospective study of a new technique. Aust N Z J Surg. 2000;70:371–3.
18. Crabtree JH, Fishman A. Selective performance of prophylactic omentopexy during laparoscopic implantation of PD catheters. Surg Laparosc Endosc Percutan Tech. 2003;13:180–4.
19. Ogunc G. Videolaparoscopy with omentopexy: a new technique to allow placement of a catheter for continuous ambulatory PD. Surg Today. 2001;31:942–4.
20. Stone MM, Fonkalsrud EW, Salusky IB, et al. Surgical management of PD catheters in children: five-year experience with 1,800 patient-month follow-up. J Pediatr Surg. 1986;21:1177–81.
21. Rinaldi S, Sera F, Verrina E, et al. The Italian registry of pediatric chronic PD: a ten-year experience with chronic PD catheters. Perit Dial Int. 1998;18:71–4.
22. Reissman P, Lyass S, Shiloni E, et al. Placement of a PD catheter with routine omentectomy—does it prevent obstruction of the catheter? Eur J Surg. 1998;164:703–7.
23. Handt AE, Ash SR. Longevity of Tenckhoff catheters placed by the VITEC peritoneoscopic technique. Perspect Perit Dial. 1984;2:30–3.
24. Gadallah MF, Pervez A, El-Shahawy MA, Sorrells D, Zibari G, McDonald J, Work J. Peritoneoscopic versus surgical placement of PD catheters: a prospective randomized study on outcome. Am J Kidney Dis. 1999;33:118–22.
25. Pastan S, Gassensmith C, Manatunga AK, Copley JB, Smith EJ, Hamburger RJ. Prospective comparison of peritoneoscopic and surgical implantation of CAPD catheters. ASAIO Trans. 1991;37:M154–6.
26. Goh BL, Ganeshadeva Yudisthra M, Lim TO. Establishing learning curve for Tenckhoff catheter insertion by interventional nephrologist using CUSUM analysis: how many procedures and in which situation? Semin Dial. 2009;22(2):199–203.
27. Asif A, Tawakol J, Khan T, Vieira CF, Byers P, Gadalean F, Hogan R, Merrill D, Roth D. Modification of the peritoneoscopic technique of PD catheter insertion: experience of an interventional nephrology program. Semin Dial. 2004;17:171–3.
28. Zaman F, Pervez A, Atray NK, Murphy S, Work J, Abreo KD. Fluoroscopy-assisted placement of PD catheters by nephrologists. Semin Dial. 2005;18:247–51.
29. Vaux EC, Torrie PH, Barker LC, Naik RB, Gibson MR. Percutaneous fluoroscopically guided placement of PD catheters- a 10-year experience. Semin Dial. 2008;21:459–65.
30. Maya ID. Ultrasound/fluoroscopy-assisted placement of PD catheters. Semin Dial. 2007;20:611–5.
31. Zappacosta AR, Perras ST, Closkey GM. Seldinger technique for Tenckhoff catheter placement. ASAIO Trans. 1991;37:13–5.
32. Ozener C, Bihorac A, Akoglu E. Technical survival of CAPD catheters: comparison between percutaneous and conventional surgical placement techniques. Nephrol Dial Transplant. 2001;16:1893–9.
33. Asif A. PD access-related procedures by nephrologists. Semin Dial. 2004;17:398–406.
34. Moncrief JW, Popovich RP, Simmons EE, et al. The Moncrief-Popovich catheter: a new peritoneal access technique for patients on PD. ASAIO Trans. 1994;39(1):62–5.
35. Moncrief JW, Popovich RP, Simmons EE, et al. Peritoneal access technology. Perit Dial Int. 1993;13(2):S112–23.

36. Moncrief JW, Popovich RP, Oreopoulos DG, et al. Continuous ambulatory PD. In: Gokal R, Nolph KD, editors. Textbook of PD. 1st ed. Dordrecht: Kluwer Academic Publishers; 1994. p. 357–98.

37. Moncrief JW, Popovich RP, Seare W, et al. PD access technology: the Austin Diagnostic Clinic experience. Perit Dial Int. 1996;16: S327–2956.

38. Caruso DM, Gray DL, Kohr JM, Rodgers LL, Weiland DE, VanderWerf BA. Reduction of infectious complications and costs using temporary subcutaneous implantation of PD catheters. Adv Perit Dial. 1997;13:183–9.

39. Stegmayr BG, Wikdahl AM, Arnerlov C, Petersen E. A modified lateral technique for the insertion of PD catheters enabling immediate start of dialysis. Perit Dial Int. 1998;18(3):329–3158.

40. Danielsson A, Blohme L, Tranaeus A, Hylander B. A prospective randomized study of the effect of a subcutaneously "buried" PD catheter technique versus standard technique on the incidence of peritonitis and exit-site infection. Perit Dial Int. 2002;22:211–9.

41. Prischl FC, Wallner M, Kalchmair H, Povacz F, Kramar R. Initial subcutaneous embedding of the PD catheter-a critical appraisal of this new implantation technique. Nephrol Dial Transplant. 1997;12:1661–7.

42. Brandt CP, Ricanati ES. Use of laparoscopy in the management of malfunctioning PD catheters. Adv Perit Dial. 1996;12:223–6.

43. Yilmazlar T, Kirdak T, Bilgin S, Yavuz M, Yurtkuran M. Laparoscopic findings of **PD** catheter malfunction and management outcomes. Perit Dial Int. 2006;26(3):374–9.

44. Crabtree JH. Rescue and salvage procedures for mechanical and infectious complications of PD. Int J Artif Organs. 2006;29(1): 67–84.

45. Lee C-M, Ko S-F, Chen H-S, Leung T-K. Double guidewire method: a novel technique for correction of migrated Tenckhoff PD catheter. Perit Dial Int. 2003;23:587–90.

46. Jwo SC, Chen KS, Lee CM, Huang CY. Correction of migrated PD catheters using lunderquist guidewire: a preliminary report. Perit Dial Int. 2001;21(6):619–21.

47. Moss JS, Minda SA, Newman GE, Dunnick NR, Vernon WB, Schwab SJ. Malpositioned PD catheters: a critical reappraisal of correction by stiff-wire manipulation. Am J Kidney Dis. 1990;15(4):305–8.

48. Dobrashian RD, Conway B, Hutchison A, Gokal R, Taylor PM. The repositioning of migrated Tenckhoff continuous ambulatory PD catheters under fluoroscopic control. Br J Radiol. 1999;72(857): 452–6.

49. Jones B, McLaughlin K, Mactier RA, Porteous C. Tenckhoff catheter salvage by closed stiff-wire manipulation without fluoroscopic control. Perit Dial Int. 1998;18:415–8.

50. Tu W-T, Su Z, Shan Y-S. An original non-traumatic maneuver for repositioning migrated PD catheters. Perit Dial Int. 2009;29: 325–9.

51. Gadallah MF, Arora N, Arumugam R, Moles K. Role of Fogarty catheter manipulation in management of migrated, nonfunctional PD catheters. Am J Kidney Dis. 2000;35(2):301–5.

Approach to a Patient with Visceral Perforation

33

Arif Asif

Bowel perforation continues to be an important complication of peritoneal dialysis (PD) catheter insertion and is the single most important factor keeping nephrologists from performing this procedure. Although the risk of bowel perforation following a PD catheter is minimal, nephrologists and surgeons performing this procedure should be well versed in diagnosing this complication promptly and managing the patient effectively. The true incidence of bowel perforation with the peritoneoscopic technique is unknown. A recent study evaluating 750 PD catheter insertions performed by nephrologists utilizing the peritoneoscopic technique found the incidence of this complication to be 0.8 % [1]. Successful conservative management of bowel perforation using bowel rest and intravenous antibiotics has also been reported [1]. Out of 750 catheters inserted utilizing the peritoneoscopic technique, six patients suffered bowel perforation. All six cases were diagnosed and managed by the nephrologists. The diagnosis was established by direct peritoneoscopic visualization of bowel mucosa, bowel contents or hard stool, return of fecal material, or emanation of foul-smelling gas through the cannula in a majority of the cases. Upon diagnosis, all patients were maintained nothing by mouth and given intravenous triple-antibiotic therapy. Four patients recovered with conservative treatment; two eventually needed surgical interventions. Of the two patients, one was a lung transplant recipient and heavily immunosuppressed. In the second patient, the bowel rest and the antibiotics were not initiated until the next day.

Introduction of a trocar (diameter 2.2 mm) into the abdominal cavity is likely responsible for bowel injury when a PD catheter is inserted using the peritoneoscopic technique [1]. Bowel injuries due to the introduction of insufflation needles, trocars, rigid catheters, and colonoscopic examinations have been reported [2–5]. A majority of these perforations are usually small and seal spontaneously [6, 7]. These "mini-perforations" close within 24–48 h, most likely secondary to omental adherence [6–8]. Simkin and Wright [8] provided direct evidence of the self-sealing nature of bowel perforations sustained during PD catheter insertion. During surgical exploration, they observed sealed bowel perforations that were sustained during PD catheter insertion 12–16 h earlier.

To further minimize/avoid the risk of perforation, we have modified the peritoneoscopic technique. A Veress needle instead of a trocar is utilized to gain access to the abdominal cavity [9]. In contrast to the sharp tip of the trocar, the Veress needle has a blunt, self-retracting end. In addition, the Veress needle is only 14 gauge as opposed to the 2.2 mm diameter of the trocar. After the same skin incision and blunt dissection as used in the standard peritoneoscopic technique, the anterior rectus sheath is identified and local anesthesia infiltrated. At this point, a Veress insufflation needle (Ethicon Endo-Surgery Inc., Cincinnati, OH) is introduced into the abdominal cavity at the site chosen for trocar insertion. Two distinct "pops" are discerned similar to the cannula and trocar of the peritoneoscopic technique. Four to five hundred cubic centimeters of air are infused into the abdominal cavity through the needle using the insufflation device provided by the Y-Tech kit (Medigroup, Naperville, IL) to create an air-filled space between the peritoneal surface of the anterior abdominal wall and the bowel loops. The Veress needle is then removed. At this point, the trocar and cannula are introduced into this space in the abdominal cavity. The remainder of the steps are similar to the peritoneoscopic insertion technique. Veress needle insertion adds 2–3 min to the procedure time. Using Veress needle, we did not encounter a single perforation in 82 consecutive PD catheter insertions [9].

In summary, the peritoneoscopic technique of PD catheter insertion allows for the diagnosis of bowel perforation to be made immediately and implement therapeutic measures promptly. A majority of these patients can be successfully managed conservatively with close monitoring of vital signs,

A. Asif, MD, FASN, FNKF
Division of Nephrology and Hypertension,
Albany Medical College, 25 Hackett Blvd, MC 69,
Albany, NY 12206, USA
e-mail: asifa@mail.amc.edu, aasif@med.miami.edu

A.S. Yevzlin et al. (eds.), *Interventional Nephrology*,
DOI 10.1007/978-1-4614-8803-3_33, © Springer Science+Business Media New York 2014

serial abdominal examination, bowel rest, and broad-spectrum intravenous antibiotics [1]. With this approach, patients who do not need surgical intervention can be identified and unnecessary laparotomy is avoided. Clinical deterioration and signs of peritoneal irritation should prompt a surgical consult.

References

1. Asif A, Byers P, Vieira CF, Merrill D, Gadalean F, Bourgoignie JJ, Leclercq B, Roth D, Gadallah MF. Bowel perforation peritoneoscopic placement of peritoneal dialysis catheter and bowel perforation: experience of an interventional nephrology program. Am J Kidney Dis. 2003;42:1270–4.
2. Asif A, Byers P, Gadalean F, Roth D. Peritoneal dialysis underutilization: the impact of an interventional nephrology peritoneal dialysis access program. Semin Dial. 2003;16:266–71.
3. Reich H. Laparoscopic bowel injury. Surg Laparosc Endosc. 1992; 2:74–8.
4. Birns MT. Inadvertent instrumental perforation of the colon during laparoscopy: nonsurgical repair. Gastrointest Endosc. 1989;35: 54–6.
5. Nomura T, Shirai Y, Okamoto H, Hatakeyama K. Bowel perforation caused by silicone drains: a report of two cases. Surg Today. 1998;28:940–2.
6. Christie JP, Marrazzo 3rd J. "Mini-perforation" of the colon–not all postpolypectomy perforations require laparotomy. Dis Colon Rectum. 1991;34:132–5.
7. Damore II LJ, Rantis PC, Vernava III AM, Longo WE. Colonoscopic perforations. Etiology, diagnosis, and management. Dis Colon Rectum. 1996;39:1308–14.
8. Simkin EP, Wright FK. Perforating injuries of the bowel complicating peritoneal catheter insertion. Lancet. 1968;1:64–6.
9. Asif A, Tawakol J, Khan T, Vieira CF, Byers P, Gadalean F, Hogan R, Merrill D, Roth D. Modification of the peritoneoscopic technique of peritoneal dialysis catheter insertion: experience of an interventional nephrology program. Semin Dial. 2004;17:171–3.

Index

A.S. Yevzlin et al. (eds.), *Interventional Nephrology*,
DOI 10.1007/978-1-4614-8803-3, © Springer Science+Business Media New York 2014

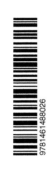